Laryngopharyngeal and Gastroesophageal Reflux

Craig H. Zalvan
Editor

Laryngopharyngeal and Gastroesophageal Reflux

A Comprehensive Guide to Diagnosis, Treatment, and Diet-Based Approaches

Springer

Editor
Craig H. Zalvan
ENT and Allergy Associates
LLP; Voice and Swallow Division
Tarrytown, NY
USA

The Institute for Voice and Swallowing Disorders
Phelps Hospital, Northwell Health
Sleepy Hollow
NY, USA

Professor of Otolaryngology
Donald and Barbara Zucker School of Medicine at
Hofstra/Northwell Health, Phelps Hospital Campus
Sleepy Hollow
NY, USA

Speech and Communication Department at Mercy College
Dobbs Ferry
NY, USA

ISBN 978-3-030-48889-5 ISBN 978-3-030-48890-1 (eBook)
https://doi.org/10.1007/978-3-030-48890-1

This Springer imprint is published by the registered company Springer Nature Switzerland AG
The registered company address is: Gewerbestrasse 11, 6330 Cham, Switzerland

Foreword

Reflux is a normal physiologic process experienced by all of us. The stomach needs to vent gas. Symptoms of reflux are ubiquitous and affect nearly a quarter of our population. Complications of excessive reflux can be considerable and range from mild swallowing difficulty to esophageal cancer and death. An incomplete understanding of the anatomy and physiology of the aerodigestive tract as it relates to reflux in health and disease has led to confusion, missed diagnoses, and inappropriate and unnecessary treatments. ***Laryngopharyngeal and Gastroesophageal Reflux*** unites some of the brightest and most innovative minds in the field to thoroughly elucidate the comprehensive diagnosis and management of this enigmatic physiologic process and its disorders. Congratulation Dr. Zalvan on a job well done!

Peter C. Belafsky, MD, MPH, PhD
pbelafsky@gmail.com
http://ucdvoice.org
Department of Otolaryngology/Head and Neck Surgery
Center for Voice and Swallowing, Davis School of Medicine
Sacramento, CA, USA

University of California, Davis School of Medicine
Sacramento, CA, USA

University of California, Davis School of Veterinary Medicine
Sacramento, CA, USA

Foreword

Gastroesophageal reflux disease (GERD) became a recognized clinical entity in the mid-1930s following two basic discoveries. The first was in 1929 when Chevalier Jackson reported the first description of pre-moribund esophagitis using a rigid endoscope outfitted with a recently introduced electric light [1]. The second was in 1935 when Asher Winkelstein used a newly lighted esophagoscope to describe diffuse inflammation of the esophagus without ulceration in 5 patients who complained of heartburn and regurgitation [2]. Today GERD is the most prevalent upper gastrointestinal disorder in clinical practice.

In 1934, a year before Asher Winkelstein's publication, G.W. Bray published an article suggesting a link between upper gastrointestinal symptoms and airway disease [3]. Stimulated by this hypothesis, subsequent studies sought to confirm aspiration as a contributing factor to the poorly understood laryngeal and respiratory conditions. It was not until 1979 that the link between airway symptoms and the reflux of gastric contents was first documented and treatment of the reflux disease was shown to eliminate the airway symptoms [4]. Today, this association is thought to account for 10% of patients presenting to an ear, nose, and throat (ENT) specialist [5]. It is estimated that up to 75% of patients with refractory ear, nose, and throat complaints, the retrograde flow of gastric contents into the esophagus and pharynx is likely the cause [6]. These symptoms are collectively referred to as extra-esophageal manifestations of GERD or the symptoms of laryngo-pharyngeal reflux (LPR). Their management requires an understanding of what is known about the pathogenesis of the symptoms and the difficulties in determining the cause of the symptoms and an appreciation for how effective medical or surgical therapy is in relieving the symptoms. Hence the importance of the book you are about to read.

The general premise of the book is a compilation of the most current approaches to the diagnosis and treatment of LPR/GERD in one comprehensive medical text. An interesting additional component is the treatment of LPR/GERD with a diet-based approach and how this can be incorporated into the treatment paradigm for all that is GERD. Enjoy.

Tom R. DeMeester, MD
Department of Surgery
Keck School of Medicine, University
of Southern California
Los Angeles, CA, USA

References

1. Jackson C. Peptic ulcer of the esophagus. JAMA. 1929;92:369–72.
2. Winkelstein A. Gastro-intestinal tract. 1st ed. Oxford University Press; 1942.
3. Bray GW. Recent advances in the treatment of asthma and hay fever. Practitioner. 1934;34:368–71.
4. Pellegrini CA, DeMeester TR, Johnson LF, Skinner DB. Gastroesophageal reflux and pulmonary aspiration: incidence, functional abnormality, and results of surgical therapy. Surgery. 1979;86:110–19.
5. Drug VL, Cobzeanu D, Papaghuic C, et al. Gastrooesophageal reflux involvement in ENT disorders. Rev Med Chir Soc Med Nat Iasi. 2005;109:220–2.
6. Poelmans J, Feenstra L, Tack J. Determinants of long-term outcome of patients with reflux related ear, nose, and throat symptoms. Dig Dis Sci. 2006;51:282–8.

Foreword

A Must Read

I write this support letter because yet another illness, acid reflux (heartburn, indigestion, gastroesophageal reflux disease—GERD and throat clearing, water-brash, hoarseness, cough, Laryngopharyngeal Reflux (LPR)), is added to a growing list of "Western' diseases that can be controlled by a whole food plant-based (WFPB) diet. By "control," I refer both to prevention of future disease and treatment of existing disease using variations of the same dietary protocol. This illness is profoundly distressing, both because it affects as many as 40–50% of individuals in the USA; because it associates with a broad spectrum of illnesses like cardiovascular disease, asthma, chronic cough, sinusitis, and irritable bowel syndrome; and because treatment of its symptoms with drugs is only transient. Symptoms are often experienced as chest discomfort resulting from excess acid regurgitated from the stomach into the proximal end of the esophagus as well as acid reflux affecting the throat with cough, voice changes, and swallowing issues. As a result, the most common pharmaceutical protocols are designed to reduce the formation of gastric acid by proton pump inhibitors (PPIs). However, they exhibit only limited reduction in discomfort that is likely to be transient.

I do not find it surprising that this disease with its multiple associations with other diseases should respond to a WFPB diet. We now know that the nutritional expression of this diet comprises countless, biologically plausible factors operating in synchrony to promote and restore health throughout the body. They include several systems involved in hormonal, enzymatic, immunologic, neurologic, digestive, and circulatory function.

This is a much-needed book that should be useful both by medical professionals and the public alike. On the basis of my information at this time, I am confident that we will come to realize that a long-term dietary strategy for disease control like that described in this book will supersede the pharmacologic and surgical procedures now being used.

T. Colin Campbell, PhD
Emeritus of Nutritional Biochemistry
Cornell University
Ithaca, NY, USA

Preface

Reflux, a common malady in modern society, evokes many thoughts of symptoms, physical findings, and disease states. Images of someone holding their chest from burning are the hallmark of gastroesophageal reflux disease (GERD) and has been in the forefront of medicine for centuries. GERD represents the classic constellation of symptoms including heartburn, indigestion, chest discomfort, back pain, early satiety, and abdominal discomfort. Laryngopharyngeal reflux (LPR), popularized in the 1990s [1], refers to symptoms of throat clearing, coughing, voice changes, throat pain, waterbrash or "sour" throat, and dysphagia. Both types of reflux disease have become a multi-billion-dollar industry fueled from diagnostic testing to pharmacological treatment.

LPR is thought to occur more in the daytime and while upright, while GERD tends to occur more at night and while supine, though both have significant overlap in timing and severity. Recent data suggest a high degree of overlap, with over 70% of LPR patients demonstrating GERD on pH impedance testing. Non-acid and mixed acid exposures, especially with reflux episodes of aerosolized gastric contents, occur more frequently in LPR patients, with most demonstrating concurrent GERD episodes. Both disease states are thus more appropriately thought of as a spectrum of one reflux syndrome with protean manifestations [2].

LPR has garnered many names over the century. Reflux laryngitis, silent reflux, laryngeal reflux, gastro-pharyngeal reflux, pharyngoesophageal reflux, supra-esophageal reflux, extraesophageal reflux, and atypical reflux are used throughout the GI and ENT literature. Given the varied nomenclature, it is not hard to realize that LPR adoption, as a medical entity, has taken time in the medical community. In addition, LPR symptoms have considerable overlap with other common diseases such as allergy, sinusitis, asthma, and upper respiratory infections. Thus, there has been a delay in adoption which has led to a delay in diagnosis and treatment of this entity. Even within the otolaryngology community, significant differences in awareness and understanding of LPR exist between the general otolaryngologist and the laryngologist specializing in throat-related conditions which includes LPR [3]. Patient adoption of LPR as a cause of their symptoms has also been difficult. Most patients when told they have "reflux" will argue that they do not have classic heartburn, which they associate with a reflux diagnosis. Only through careful explanation and review of the patient history and exam and an explanation of LPR as a distinct disease presentation will a patient adopt this diagnosis.

GERD is very prevalent in modern societies. In the USA, 18–27% of individuals have reflux in some form or another [4]. Primary care has seen a steady and continued increase in patients with reflux symptoms, with over 20% of office visits being reflux symptom related [5]. Most have had reflux at some point, either transiently or on a more long-term basis. This disease process is costly with nearly $150 billion US dollars spent per year [6]. Some suggest that LPR is far more expensive to diagnose and treat than GERD with LPR costs up to 5.6 times higher than GERD making reflux overall one of the most expensive medical conditions. More than half of these costs are due to medication alone [7]. From the viewpoint of morbidity and mortality, upper aerodigestive tract cancers have been increasing over the last half century with esophageal adenocarcinoma incidence increasing at an alarming rate [8]. With over 18,000 new cases yearly in the USA, with a 5-yr survival rate of only 20%, the emotional and financial costs are enormous [9]. Cancers of the pharynx, larynx, tonsils, and sinuses have been associated with GERD (technically LPR) suggesting reflux is possibly a cause and at least a co-factor in the development and propagation of these malignancies [10].

Over the last few decades, we have seen an evolution of the thought process behind these reflux disorders. Initially patient diagnosis and treatment of reflux resided in the gastroenterology domain. More recently, otolaryngologists, laryngologists in particular, have taken on the domain of extra-esophageal reflux disease and are now the primary caregivers for patients with LPR. Additionally, treatment of pulmonary manifestations is often now in the domain of the laryngologist. However, it is very important to mention that this disease is truly a spectrum of shared pathophysiology, presentation, treatment, and outcome that is best managed by a multispecialty team approach. The "Reflux Center" approach combines laryngologists, gastroenterologists, and thoracic surgeons together to manage patients presenting with the entire spectrum of reflux disease. This collaboration ensures a more accurate diagnosis, focuses on a more diet-based approach initially while offering more conservative interventions when required. Ultimately, failure to improve results in the patient's full access to the spectrum of interventions, including surgical [11].

This text is a culmination of a change in thought process bringing together what is known and current in gastroesophageal reflux (GERD) together with a comprehensive explanation and description of the known laryngopharyngeal reflux (LPR) literature. With chapters written by experts from around the world, this text aims to deliver what is current in reflux recognition, diagnosis, reflux-related complications, and the various treatment modalities. This is the first textbook to combine the most up-to-date knowledge of both LPR and GERD meant for both specialties and the general medicine population. Completely unique to the reflux literature is a section detailing the substantial benefits of a mostly plant-based, Mediterranean style diet in the treatment of reflux disease. The overall health benefits of a plant-based diet will be discussed and include guidance on how to transition the diets of both the reader as well as the patient.

After an introduction to the pertinent anatomy and physiology of the laryngopharynx, esophagus and stomach, and history of reflux disease, the book will be divided into two disease parts: LPR and GERD. The LPR part will delve into a detailed analysis of the disease presentation. Symptoms and physical findings will be reviewed in the context of the literature and experience, all leading toward the diagnostic workup and evaluation. Current standard of care for diagnosis, or lack thereof, will be discussed in detail as will the decision making in this process. Review of various types of pH testing, modified barium swallow in the differential diagnosis, the utility of pepsin testing and manometry in the workup, and eventual diagnosis of LPR will be presented. Additionally, the role of LPR with other diseases of the head and neck, such as sinusitis and pulmonary disease, will also be discussed as part of a unified upper aerodigestive tract.

The second disease part will focus on GERD presentation and diagnosis. Mirroring the first part, the history and physical examination will be reviewed in detail. GERD presentation, the topic of non-erosive esophagitis, and functional dyspepsia will give the reader an understanding of the multifaceted presentation that exists with this disease. Long-term exposure to reflux can result in esophagitis, Barrett's esophagus, with the potential for esophageal adenocarcinoma. Next, current standard diagnostic testing will be reviewed including pH testing, manometry, and esophagoscopy. The gold standards of diagnostic testing will be explained giving the reader an understanding of the most commonly used criteria for diagnosis of reflux.

Treatment of both LPR and GERD will be considered together in the third part. Over-the-counter remedies, herbal and alternative approaches, and the spectrum of pharmacological interventions will be discussed in detail. The current controversy over proton pump inhibitor use will be outlined and explained. More conservative endoscopic interventions within the esophagus will be defined and reviewed as less invasive approaches for those failing dietary, behavioral, and pharmacological interventions. Finally, the gamut of surgical management will be evaluated.

The fourth part of this text is an evolution of thought regarding treatment of reflux. Historical analysis of treatment evolution culminates in a broad coverage of modern treatment options. Dietary and behavioral modifications will be identified and stressed as the single most important treatment approach. Medications, both over-the-counter and prescribed, will be covered in detail, together with a broad understanding of their efficacy in LPR and GERD. Next, interventional approaches will be discussed from the least to most invasive. Current treatment outcomes, bolstered by the current literature, for these approaches will be evaluated, providing the reader with a comprehensive assessment of treatment options to help formulate an acceptable plan for the individual patient.

Getting back to diet is the basis for the fifth and final section of this part. Diet and behavioral modifications, in general, have been poorly studied in the LPR and GERD literature. Yet despite the lack of randomized controlled studies of these measures, they are often recommended. Modern medicine's focus tends to be on prescriptions and interventions and often fails to encourage and promote diet as a primary treatment modality. Most patients expect a prescription for their malady and look for a pill to alleviate their problem. Few manage to initiate and most certainly maintain the dietary and behavioral modifications leading to overall failure to improve and in most cases progression of the disease state. This section will review the results of LPR treatment using a plant-based, Mediterranean style diet and alkaline water regimen giving outcomes as well as, if not better than, PPI therapy [12]. The concept of using diet to treat LPR is based on the wealth of information demonstrating the overall health benefits of plant-based diets in improving most of the chronic diseases plaguing modern society. These health benefits will be reviewed with references intended to encourage the reader to explore the literature and develop their own understanding of this concept. Encouraging patients to read and learn about diet and health is likely the most important step in improving their disease. The text will provide direction to the caregiver on how to transition to a mostly plant-based diet. Review of myths, effects of diet in the setting of other disease states, and dietary consequences will be explained. Guidelines on how to transition diet, dining out while maintaining a plant-based diet, and how to wean off medication, such as PPI, will be provided.

Overall, our aim is to provide the medical community with a resource to understand, teach, and provide the latest in LPR and GERD information to the caregiver and subsequently the patient. Focusing on dietary transition is meant to improve reflux without the use or need for medication and surgery with the intended consequences of improved overall health for the individual and society.

Sleepy Hollow, NY, USA Craig H. Zalvan, MD, FACS

References

1. Koufman JA. The otolaryngologic manifestations of gastroesophageal reflux disease. Laryngoscope. 1991;101(Supplement 53):1–78.
2. Lechien JR, Bobin F, Muls V, Eisendrath P, Horoi M, Thill MP, Dequanter D, Durdurez J, Rodriguez A, Saussez S. Gastroesophageal reflux in laryngopharyngeal reflux patients: Clinical features and therapeutic response. Laryngoscope. 2019. https://doi.org/10.1002/lary.28482.
3. Lechien JR, Allen J, Mouawad F, Ayad T, Barillari MR, Huet K, Crevier-Buchman L, Hans S, Karkos PD, Eun YG, Bobin F, Saussez S, Akst LM. Do laryngologists and general otolaryngologists manage laryngopharyngeal reflux differently? Laryngoscope. 2020. https://doi.org/10.1002/lary.28484.
4. El-Serag 2014 - El-Serag HB, Sweet S, Winchester CC, Dent J. Update on the epidemiology of gastro-oesophageal reflux disease: a systematic review. Gut. 2014;63(6):871–80.
5. Altman KW, Stephens RM, Lyttle CS, Weiss KB. Changing impact of gastroesophageal reflux in medical and otolaryngology practice. Laryngoscope. 2005;115(7):1145–53.
6. Peery AF, Dellon ES, Lund J, et al. Burden of gastrointestinal disease in the United States: 2012 update. Gastroenterology. 2012;143(5):1179–87.
7. Francis DO, Rymer JA, Slaughter JC, Choksi Y, Jiramongkolchai P, Ogbeide E, Tran C, Goutte M, Garrett CG, Hagaman D, Vaezi MF. High economic burden of caring for patients

with suspected extraesophageal reflux. Am J Gastroenterol. 2013;108(6):905–11. https://doi.org/10.1038/ajg.2013.69. Epub 2013 Apr 2.

8. Lepage C, Drouillard A, Jouve JL, Faivre J. Epidemiology and risk factors for oesophageal adenocarcinoma. Dig Liver Dis. 2013;45:625–629.
9. Siegel R, Naishadham D, Jemal A. Cancer statistics, 2012. CA Cancer J Clin 2012;62:10–29.
10. Riley CA, Wu EL, Hsieh MC, Marino MJ, Wu XC, McCoul ED. Association of gastroesophageal reflux with malignancy of the upper aerodigestive tract in elderly patients. JAMA Otolaryngol Head Neck Surg. 2018;144(2):140–8. https://doi.org/10.1001/jamaoto.2017.2561.
11. https://phelps.northwell.edu/gastroenterology/reflux-center-of-westchester.
12. Zalvan CH, Hu S, Greenberg B, Geliebter J. Comparison of alkaline water and mediterranean diet vs proton pump inhibition for treatment of laryngopharyngeal reflux. JAMA Otolaryngol Head Neck Surg. 2017;143(10):1023–29. https://doi.org/10.1001/jamaoto.2017.1454.

Acknowledgment

Writing a book and including authors from around the country and world is not a simple task. This process takes time, organization, and cooperation from all involved. I am eternally grateful for the contributions from all of the authors in this text. Their attention, commitment, and excellent synthesis of the information for their topic has made this text an important contribution to the education of medical personnel, students, and public seeking information on the topics of laryngopharyngeal (LPR) and gastroesophageal reflux (GERD) as well as a diet-based approach to treatment.

This textbook represents the first comprehensive approach to the topics of reflux and diet and could not have been created without acknowledging those who have molded my thinking throughout my career. Springer Nature saw the importance of combining both LPR and GERD given the disease is a continuum and not distinct entities. More importantly is the identification of diet playing a larger role in chronic disease, of which reflux is included.

My special thanks to a host of mentors that have helped mold my thinking in the field of laryngology (voice and swallowing disorders) and a diet-based approach to treatment of reflux. Dr. Andrew Blitzer, my fellowship director, mentor, and friend, changed the direction of my professional life and opened my eyes and thinking to laryngology. Drs. Jonathan Aviv and Jaime Koufman introduced and solidified the concepts of pepsin, acidic diets, and dietary approaches to treating reflux. A heartfelt thanks to Drs. Brian Benson, Daniel Novakovik, Jan Geliebter, and Omar Gonzalez for their advice, discourse, and friendship through this process.

Introducing the concept of diet and chronic disease treatment, Dr. T. Colin Campbell deserves a notable mention as the father of this field of medicine. His early insight and steadfast movement toward a plant-based diet as the means to prevent and reverse much of our chronic disease has been the basis to my approach to treating reflux with diet.

Dr. Peter Stein who edited much of the gastroenterological contributions has been supportive throughout the process. His conversations, ideas, editing, and friendship have helped me push through the process.

I want to thank Eva Cerrato for her tireless work to keep my practice running perfectly during the time of my writing, as she always does.

Most importantly, I want to acknowledge my family. Coren, Hana, and Max have endured countless hours of typing, reading, editing, and conversation, all of which kept me away for short periods of time from them. Their endless love, support, encouragement, and welcome distractions made this possible. Sorry Louie for the missed dog walks. Special thanks to Hana for her image of the larynx entitled "Laryngeal Abd-straction."

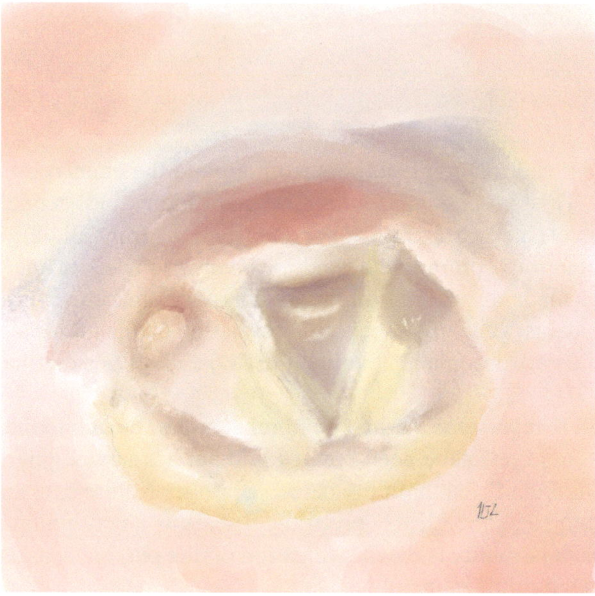

Craig H. Zalvan, MD, FACS

Contents

Editor Biography

Craig H. Zalvan, MD, FACS is the Medical Director at the Institute for Voice and Swallowing Disorders and Chief of Otolaryngology at Phelps Hospital, Northwell Health, Sleepy Hollow, New York, USA.

He is a Professor of Otolaryngology at the Donald and Barbara Zucker School of Medicine at Hofstra/Northwell and a partner at ENT and Allergy Associates, LLP in New York. He maintains an Adjunct Clinical Professorship of Otolaryngology at New York Medical College, Valhalla, New York, and an Adjunct Professor in the Department of Communications, Speech Department, at Mercy College, Dobbs Ferry, New York.

Dr. Zalvan completed his residency training in Otolaryngology/Head & Neck Surgery at the Manhattan Eye, Ear & Throat Hospital and at the New York Presbyterian Hospital. In addition, he has been trained at Memorial Sloan Kettering Cancer Center, New York Hospital-Cornell Medical Center, and Lenox Hill Hospital. He went on to complete his Fellowship in Laryngology with Dr. Andrew Blitzer: Voice and Swallowing Disorders at Roosevelt Hospital/St. Luke's Medical Center. Dr. Zalvan's specialties include adult and pediatric voice and swallowing disorders, professional voice disorders, vocal fold paralysis, spasmodic dysphonia, neurolaryngology, laryngopharyngeal reflux, the aging voice, Zenker's diverticulum, laryngeal cancer, and chronic cough.

Dr. Zalvan has introduced numerous laryngological techniques to the Hudson Valley NY region including injection laryngoplasty, medialization thyroplasty, transnasal esophagoscopy, office-based laryngeal and pharyngeal KTP laser procedures, as well as the entire spectrum of operative laryngology.

Dr. Zalvan lectures nationally and internationally with numerous presentations, publications, and research projects on topics such as: chronic cough, laryngopharyngeal reflux treatment with plant-based diet, laryngeal EMG, dysphagia, laryngeal sensory testing, and many other IRB-approved studies.

Dr. Zalvan has a special focus on treating reflux disease with a mostly plant-based, Mediterranean style diet with publications in *JAMA* and *The Laryngoscope* highlighting the improvement in results over medications with additional health benefits of preventing and reversing many chronic diseases.

Contributors

Jacqui E. Allen University of Auckland, Auckland, New Zealand

Kenneth W. Altman Geisinger Health System, Geisinger Commonwealth School of Medicine, Department of Otolaryngology – Head & Neck Surgery, Danville, PA, USA

Linda Arpino Life Focus Nutrition, LLC, Stamford, CT, USA

Jonathan E. Aviv Department of Otolaryngology, Icahn School of Medicine, Mount Sinai, New York, NY, USA

Voice and Swallowing Center, ENT and Allergy Associates, LLP, New York, NY, USA

Brian Benson Department of Otolaryngology-Head & Neck Surgery, Hackensack Meridian School of Medicine at Seton Hall University, Nutley, NJ, USA

Craig Berzofsky Center for Voice and Swallowing, White Plains Hospital, White Plains, NY, USA

John W. Blackett Division of Digestive and Liver Diseases, Columbia University Medical Center, New York, NY, USA

Jonathan M. Bock Department of Otolaryngology & Communication Sciences, Division of Laryngology & Professional Voice, Medical College of Wisconsin, Milwaukee, WI, USA

Andrea Bracciante-Ely, MS Sp, CCC-SLP Speech and Hearing Center,Institute for Voice and Swallowing Disorders, Phelps Hospital, Northwell Health, Sleepy Hollow, NY, USA

Thomas L. Carroll Department of Otolaryngology-Head and Neck Surgery, Harvard Medical School, Boston, MA, USA

Division of Otolaryngology, Department of Surgery, Brigham and Women's Hospital, Boston, MA, USA

John O. Clarke Esophageal Program, Division of Gastroenterology & Hepatology, Stanford University, Redwood City, CA, USA

Sina Dadafarin Department of Microbiology and Immunology, Department of Otolaryngology, New York Medical College, Valhalla, NY, USA

Corina Din-Lovinescu Department of Otolaryngology-Head and Neck Surgery, Rutgers New Jersey Medical School, Newark, NJ, USA

Paula Dinu, MS, CCC-SLP-BRSS Speech and Hearing Center, Institute for Voice and Swallowing Disorders, Phelps Hospital, Northwell Health, Sleepy Hollow, NY, USA

Lorella Fanti Vita-Salute San Raffaele University - IRCCS San Raffaele Scientific Institute, Division of Gastroenterology and Gastrointestinal Endoscopy, Milan, Italy

Muhammad Farooq Hackensack Meridian School of Medicine at Seton Hall University, Nutley, NJ, USA

Camille Finck Research Committee, Laryngopharyngeal Reflux Study Group of Young-Otolaryngologists of the International Federations of Oto-rhino-laryngological Societies (YO-IFOS), Paris, France

Department of Otolaryngology-Head & Neck Surgery, CHU de Liege, Liege, Belgium

Hans F. Fuchs Department of General, Visceral, Cancer and Transplant Surgery, University of Cologne, Cologne, Germany

Jan Geliebter Department of Microbiology and Immunology, Department of Otolaryngology, New York Medical College, Valhalla, NY, USA

David M. Gutman Zucker School of Medicine at Hofstra/Northwell Health, Hempstead, NY, USA

Shirley Hu Department of Otolaryngolgy, New York Eye and Ear Infirmary of Mt. Sinai, New York, NY, USA

Caroline Hudson Baylor College of Medicine, Department of Otolaryngology – Head & Neck Surgery, Houston, TX, USA

Ralph A. Iannuzzi Department of Otolaryngology, Plastic Surgery and Cosmetic Services, and Allergy, Atrius Health, Boston, MA, USA

Aaron J. Jaworek, MD Drexel University College of Medicine, Department of Otolaryngology – Head and Neck Surgery, Philadelphia, PA, USA

Temple University Lewis Katz School of Medicine, Department of Otolaryngology – Head and Neck Surgery, Philadelphia, PA, USA

Daniela Jodorkovsky Division of Digestive and Liver Diseases, Columbia University Medical Center, New York, NY, USA

Nikki Johnston Department of Otolaryngology and Communication Sciences, Division of Laryngology and Professional Voice and Pediatric Otolaryngology, Department of Microbiology and Immunology, Milwaukee, WI, USA

Division of Research, Medical College of Wisconsin, Milwaukee, WI, USA

Deya Jourdy Rhinology, Endoscopic Sinus & Skull Base Surgery, Otolaryngology & Neurosurgery, New York Medical College, Phelps Hospital, Northwell Health, Sleepy Hollow, NY, USA

ENT and Allergy Associates, LLP, Sleepy Hollow, NY, USA

Ameet Kamat Sinus and Skull Base Surgery, White Plains Hospital Physician Associates, Department of Otolaryngology, NY Medical College, Valhalla, NY, USA

Sarah Kidwai Department of Otolaryngology—Icahn School of Medicine at Mount Sinai, New York, NY, USA

Jerome R. Lechien Research Committee, Laryngopharyngeal Reflux Study Group of Young-Otolaryngologists of the International Federations of Oto-rhino-laryngological Societies (YO-IFOS), Paris, France

Department of Otolaryngology-Head & Neck Surgery, Foch Hospital, Paris, France

Laboratory of Human Anatomy and Experimental Oncology, Faculty of Medicine, UMONS Research Institute for Health Sciences and Technology, University of Mons (UMons), Mons, Belgium

Michel de Lorgeril Laboratoire Coeur et Nutrition, School of Medicine, Grenoble Alps University, Grenoble, France

Giorgia Mazzoleni Ospedale "Treviglio-Caravaggio" di Treviglio ASST Bergamo Ovest, Treviglio (Bg), Italy

Dolores T. Mueller Department for General, Visceral, Cancer and Transplant Surgery, University Hospital Cologne, Cologne, Deutschland

Claude Nganzeu Medical College of Wisconsin, Milwaukee, Milwaukee, WI, USA

Daniel Novakovic University of Sydney, Dr Liang Voice Program, Central Clinical School, Faculty of Medicine and Health, Sydney, Australia

Lena C. O'Flynn Department of Otolaryngology – Head and Neck Surgery, Massachusetts Eye and Ear, Boston, MA, USA

Department of Neurology, Massachusetts General Hospital, Boston, MA, USA

Jing-Yin Pang Khoo Teck Puat Hospital, Yishun Central, Singapore, Singapore

University of Sydney, Dr Liang Voice Program. Central Clinical School, Faculty of Medicine and Health, Sydney, Australia

Darren Rohan Northwell Health, Donald and Barbara Zucker School of Medicine at Hofstra/Northwell, Hempstead, NY, USA

Maria Carolina Rojido, MD, MHA Plant-based Nutrition Certificate, Freelance Medical Writer, Ségoufielle, France

Patricia Salen Laboratoire Coeur et Nutrition, School of Medicine, Grenoble Alps University, Grenoble, France

Henya Sandhaus Otolaryngology - Head and Neck Surgery, Southern Illinois University, Springfield, IL, USA

Kristina Simonyan Department of Otolaryngology – Head and Neck Surgery, Massachusetts Eye and Ear, Boston, MA, USA

Department of Neurology, Massachusetts General Hospital, Boston, MA, USA

Department of Otolaryngology – Head and Neck Surgery, Harvard Medical School, Boston, MA, USA

Peter H. Stein Division of Gastroenterology, Phelps Hospital Northwell Health, Sleepy Hollow, NY, USA

Pier Alberto Testoni Vita-Salute San Raffaele University - IRCCS San Raffaele Scientific Institute, Division of Gastroenterology and Gastrointestinal Endoscopy, Milan, Italy

Sabrina Gloria Giulia Testoni Vita-Salute San Raffaele University - IRCCS San Raffaele Scientific Institute, Division of Pancreatico-Biliary Endoscopy, Milan, Italy

Steven A. Thau Board Certified in Pulmonary, Critical Care, Sleep Medicine and Hospice and Palliative Care, Phelps Hospital/Northwell Health, Sleepy Hollow, NY, USA

Raj K. Tiwari Department of Microbiology and Immunology, Department of Otolaryngology, New York Medical College, Valhalla, NY, USA

George Triadafilopoulos Stanford University School of Medicine, Stanford, CA, USA

Nimish Vakil University of Wisconsin School of Medicine and Public Health, Madison, WI, USA

Diana M. Winston Comartin Division of Gastroenterology, Phelps Hospital Northwell Health, Sleepy Hollow, NY, USA

Alexis Worthley Department of Otolaryngology – Head and Neck Surgery, Massachusetts Eye and Ear, Boston, MA, USA

Department of Neurology, Massachusetts General Hospital, Boston, MA, USA

Erick Yuen Department of Otolaryngology—New York Medical College, School of Medicine, Valhalla, NY, USA

Craig H. Zalvan ENT and Allergy Associates, LLP; Voice and Swallow Division, Tarrytown, NY, USA

The Institute for Voice and Swallowing Disorders, Phelps Hospital, Northwell Health, Sleepy Hollow, NY, USA

Professor of Otolaryngology at the Donald and Barbara Zucker School of Medicine at Hofstra/Northwell, Phelps Hospital Campus, Sleepy Hollow, NY, USA

Adjunct Professor, Speech and Communication Department at Mercy College, Dobbs Ferry, NY, USA

Part I
Laryngopharyngeal and Upper Gastroenterological Anatomy and Physiology

Chapter 1
Relevant Anatomy of the Head and Neck

Sina Dadafarin, Jan Geliebter, Raj K. Tiwari, and Craig H. Zalvan

Oral Cavity

The oral cavity is the opening to the digestive and respiratory tracts. It extends from the oral fissure to the palatine tonsils posteriorly and is bounded superiorly by the palate and inferiorly by the tongue and floor of the mouth. The roof of the mouth is made of the hard palate anteriorly and soft palate posteriorly (Fig. 1.1). There are small perforations throughout the palate that allows secretions of the palatine glands, located just deep to the palatine mucosa, to enter and lubricate the oral cavity. While the hard palate is composed of bone covered by a thin mucosa, the soft palate is composed of skeletal muscle that can be tensed and elevated to simultaneously block the opening to the nasal cavity while allowing a bolus of food to pass through during swallowing. The tongue is a large, mobile muscular tissue that covers most of the mouth floor. It is composed of layers of muscle that are oriented in a

S. Dadafarin · J. Geliebter (✉) · R. K. Tiwari
Department of Microbiology and Immunology, Department of Otolaryngology,
New York Medical College, Valhalla, NY, USA
e-mail: sina_dadafarin@student.nymc.edu; jan_geliebter@nymc.edu; raj_tiwari@nymc.edu

C. H. Zalvan
The Institute for Voice and Swallowing Disorders, Phelps Hospital, Northwell Health,
Sleepy Hollow, NY, USA

Otolaryngology, New York Medical College, Valhalla, NY, USA

ENT and Allergy Associates, LLP, Tarrytown, NY, USA

Communication at Mercy College, Dobbs Ferry, NY, USA
e-mail: czalvan1@northwell.edu

C. H. Zalvan (ed.), *Laryngopharyngeal and Gastroesophageal Reflux*,
https://doi.org/10.1007/978-3-030-48890-1_1

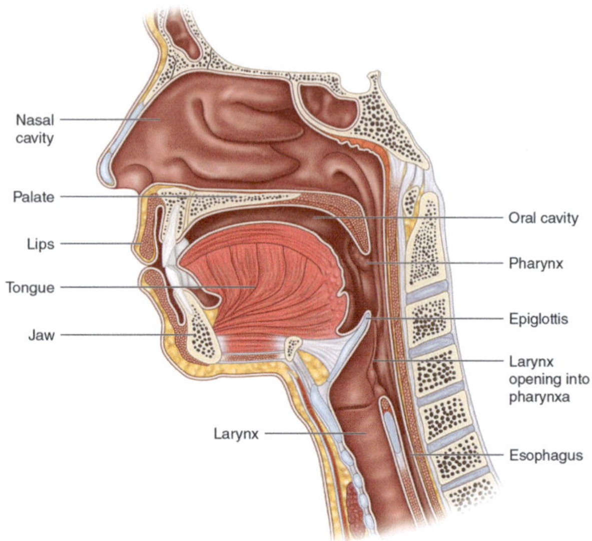

Fig. 1.1 Cross-sectional anatomy of the head and neck ("Head and Neck Overview" from http://training.seer.cancer.gov/head-neck/anatomy/overview.html). (Images were obtained from Wikimedia Commons (https://commons.wikimedia.org) and are in the public domain in their country of origin and the United States)

variety of directions to allow a wide range of motion. Furthermore, the mucosa contains many papillae that hold tactile sensory afferents, taste buds, and secretory ducts of serous glands of the tongue. The tongue has a unique pattern of sensory innervation owing to the types of sensory information (tactile and taste) as well as the distinct embryologic origins of the anterior and posterior tongue. Innervation for taste and sensation to the posterior third of the tongue is provided by the glossopharyngeal nerve, while the anterior two-thirds receive taste sensation from the chorda tympani branch of the facial nerve and tactile sensation from the mandibular branch of the trigeminal nerve.

The remaining floor of the mouth is composed of a variety of muscles, including the genioglossus, mylohyoid, and anterior bellies of the digastric. The posterior belly of the digastric is a separate muscle that attaches to the mastoid process and is tethered to the anterior belly by a common tendon that is anchored to the hyoid bone (Fig. 1.2). Together, the digastric muscles act to elevate the hyoid bone during swallowing. The mucosa overlying this region receives sensory innervation by the mandibular division of the trigeminal nerve.

Inferior and lateral to the tongue lies the paired sublingual glands. These predominately mucous glands are just deep to the mucosa of the floor of the mouth and border the mandible laterally. There are numerous openings to the sublingual glands that lie underneath the anterior tip of the tongue. The second major pair of glands of the mouth are the submandibular glands predominately located inferior to the mylohyoid, but portions of the gland can be superior to the muscle (Fig. 1.3). The submandibular duct runs anteriorly and superiorly and opens just lateral to the frenulum of the tongue bilaterally. This region is often called the sublingual caruncle. There

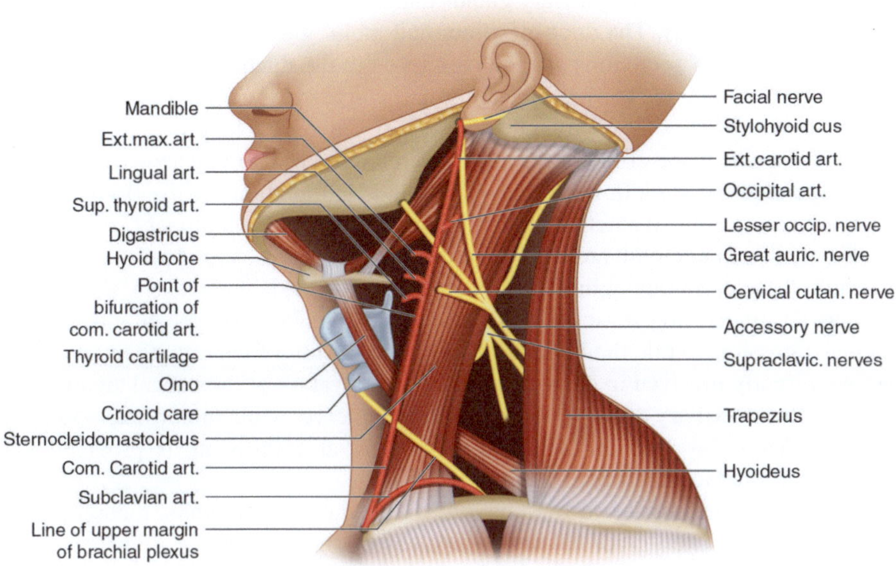

Fig. 1.2 Nervous distribution of the neck and relationship of the digastric muscles with the hyoid bone ("Plate 1210" of Henry Gray's *Anatomy of the Human Body*). (Images were obtained from Wikimedia Commons (https://commons.wikimedia.org) and are in the public domain in their country of origin and the United States)

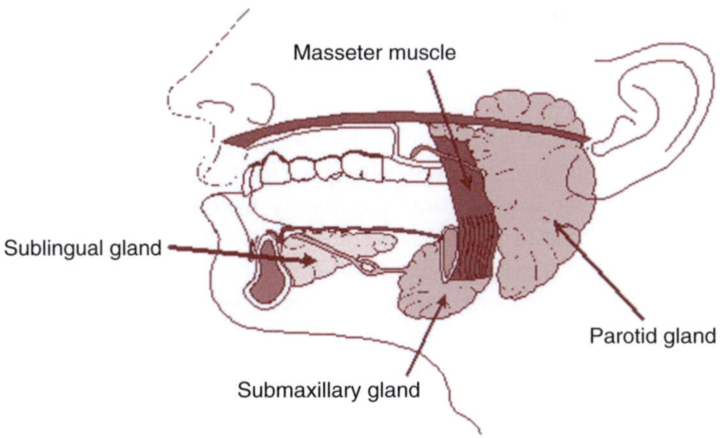

Fig. 1.3 Location and relationships of major salivary glands ("Salivary Glands" from https://training.seer.cancer.gov/head-neck/anatomy/salivary.html). (Images were obtained from Wikimedia Commons (https://commons.wikimedia.org) and are in the public domain in their country of origin and the United States)

are also hundreds of minor salivary glands that contribute to lubrication and protection of the oral cavity. The ducts of minor and major glands play a role in altering the composition of secretions as they pass through the ducts. These secretions are composed of protective enzymes, mucins, and electrolytes which prevent bacterial establishment in the oral cavity, raise the pH of saliva, and help break down food [1]. Bicarbonate is the critical acid buffer secreted by the salivary acini in response to neuroendocrine stimuli, including sympathetic stimulation via the B-adrenergic receptors and parasympathetic stimulation via M1 and M3 receptors [2].

The walls of the mouth are composed of muscles, nerves, and glands covered by a stratified squamous epithelium. The buccinators line the lateral walls of the mouth, and, as the underlying muscles of the cheek, are involved in speech and making facial expression. While the buccinators assist in pushing food onto the teeth, they are not directly involved in chewing. Sensory innervation of the buccal area is provided by the maxillary division of the mandibular nerve, while motor innervation to the buccinators, as well as other muscles of facial expression, is provided via branches of the facial nerve.

There are four muscles of mastication: the masseter, temporalis, medial pterygoid, and lateral pterygoid. All are innervated by the mandibular division of the trigeminal nerve. The parotid gland, a large serous gland that sits anterior to the ear, is superficial to the masseter on each side of the face. Key vessels and nerves penetrate and course through the parotid, including the facial nerve and external carotid artery. The parotid duct passes anteriorly and horizontally from the gland and punctures the buccinator muscle near the anterior border of the masseter (Fig. 1.3). When examining the mouth, the opening to the parotid duct can be seen lateral to the second maxillary molar teeth.

Nasal Cavity

The nasal cavity is bound anteriorly by the limen nasi, posteriorly at the choana, superiorly by the skull base, and inferiorly by the hard palate. The lateral wall of the nasal cavity has three bony protrusions covered by mucosa that extend medially and inferiorly called turbinates or concha. The space underlying each turbinate is a meatus where the openings to the paranasal sinuses reside (Fig. 1.4). The sphenoethmoidal recess, as well as the opening of the sphenoid sinus, is located at the posterior end of the superior meatus. Along the middle meatus lies the semilunar hiatus, a crescent-shaped fissure that extends alongside the uncinate process. The opening to the frontonasal sinus is located at the anterior aspect of the semilunar hiatus while the maxillary sinus opens near the medial or posterior end of the hiatus.

The superior nasal concha and the roof of the nose are considered the olfactory region. The sensation of smell is provided by olfactory nerves directly entering this region from the olfactory bulb of the brain via perforation of the cribriform plate. In the posterio-lateral wall of the nasopharynx at the level of the inferior turbinate is the opening of the Eustachian tube. The tube acts as a passage for air between the

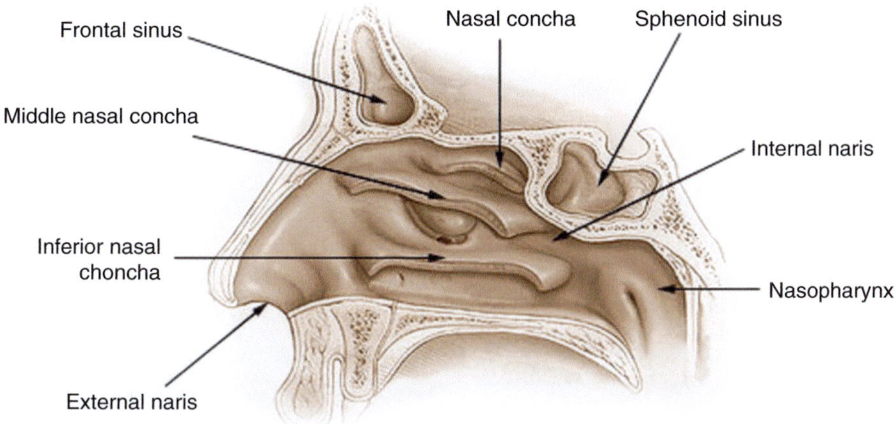

Fig. 1.4 Nasal cavity and sinuses ("Nose and Nasal Cavity" from http://training.seer.cancer.gov/images/anatomy/respiratory/nose_nasal_cavities.jpg). (Images were obtained from Wikimedia Commons (https://commons.wikimedia.org) and are in the public domain in their country of origin and the United States)

nasopharynx and the middle ear. While the Eustachian tube is collapsed at rest, contraction of the muscles of the soft palate during swallowing opens it and allows pressure equalization for the middle ear.

Pharynx

The pharynx is anatomically divided into three regions: the nasopharynx, oropharynx, and laryngopharynx (Fig. 1.5). The nasopharynx begins posterior to the choana, the opening to the nasal cavity, and ends at the nasal surface of the soft palate. The nasopharyngeal tonsil, commonly referred to as the adenoid, is located along the wall of the nasopharynx posterior to the middle and lower turbinates. The adenoids are unencapsulated lymphoid tissue, and, together with the palatine, lingual, and tubal tonsils, they create a ring of tonsillar tissue known as Waldeyer's ring that acts as a first line of defense against potential pathogens entering the oral and nasal cavities. The oropharynx is bounded superiorly at the level of the hard palate and inferiorly by the hyoid bone. The base of the tongue, soft palate, palatine tonsils, as well as the tonsillar pillars are located within this region.

The superior pharyngeal constrictor begins at the pharyngeal tubercle on the base of the skull and attaches anteriorly to the pterygoid hamulus and pterygomandibular raphe (Fig. 1.6). The middle constrictor originates from the posterior median raphe and attaches to the hyoid bone as well as the stylohyoid ligament (Fig. 1.6). The inferior constrictor is divided into a superior portion, the thyropharyngeus, and inferior portion, the cricopharyngeus. In conjunction with the cervical

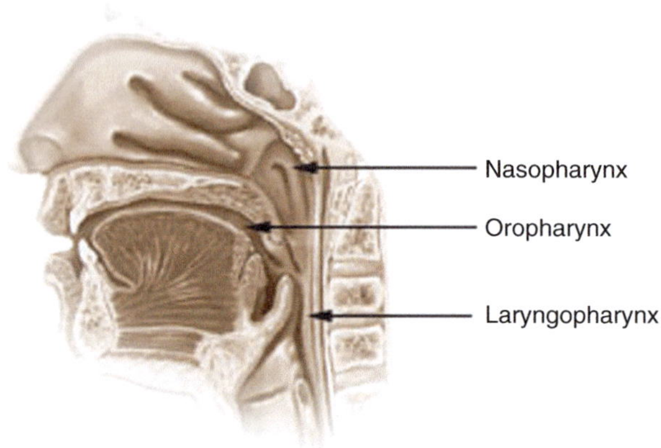

Fig. 1.5 Location of the nasopharynx, oropharynx, and laryngopharynx ("Pharynx" from http://training.seer.cancer.gov/module_anatomy/images/illu_pharynx.jpg). (Images were obtained from Wikimedia Commons (https://commons.wikimedia.org) and are in the public domain in their country of origin and the United States)

esophagus, these muscles create the upper esophageal sphincter. This sphincter is constitutively contracted to act as a barrier between the pharynx and esophagus and intermittently relaxes to allow passage of food. The cricopharyngeus is histologically unique compared to other skeletal muscles in the pharynx as its fibers do not all run in parallel but rather as a mesh of fibers running in a variety of directions. The cricopharyngeus is innervated by a plexus generated by branches of the pharyngeal vagus nerve, including the superior laryngeal nerve and recurrent laryngeal nerve, as well as the glossopharyngeal nerve and sympathetics from the superior cervical ganglion. The triangular area created by the two bands of the cricopharyngeus and their junction with the thyropharyngeus is called Killian's triangle. This is a weak area of the hypopharynx that is prone to pulsion diverticulum called Zenker's diverticulum [3].

All the pharyngeal constrictors are innervated by branches of the vagus nerve via the pharyngeal plexus. The pharyngeal wall is composed predominately of squamous epithelium covering the entirety of the pharyngeal constrictors. Sensory innervation of the pharyngeal mucosa is provided by the glossopharyngeal nerve. The epithelium on the posterior wall of the pharynx acts as the anterior bound of the retropharyngeal space.

The esophagus begins inferior to the cricopharyngeal muscle. It is attached to the posterior aspect of the trachea by a fibroelastic membrane and creates a complete cylindrical passage for food to travel en route to the stomach. The upper third of the esophagus is predominately skeletal muscle and contracts voluntarily, while the lower two-thirds are composed of smooth muscles and contract via involuntary peristalsis. The mucosa, similar to the pharynx, is composed of stratified squamous epithelium overlying the musculature. Sympathetic and parasympathetic innervation is provided by the sympathetic trunk and vagus nerve, respectively.

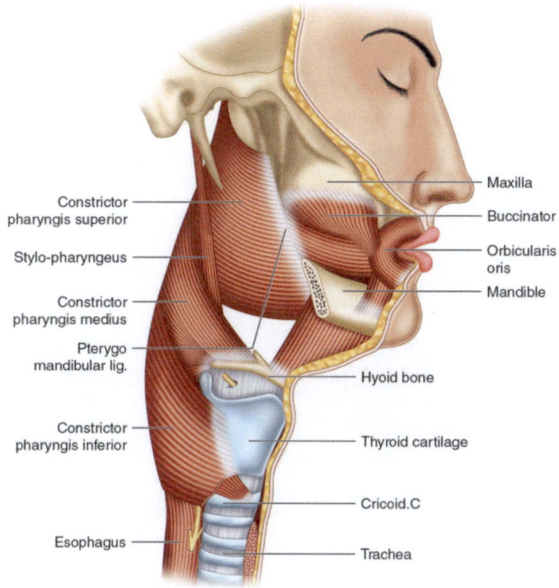

Fig. 1.6 Pharyngeal constrictors ("Plate 380" of Henry Gray's *Anatomy of the Human Body*). (Images were obtained from Wikimedia Commons (https://commons.wikimedia.org) and are in the public domain in their country of origin and the United States)

Larynx

The larynx is a complex apparatus of cartilages, muscles, ligaments, and membranes that acts as the passageway between the oropharynx and trachea. While most commonly considered as the organ responsible for phonation, the primary function of the larynx is to protect the airway. Key structural components are formed by nine cartilages. The epiglottis, thyroid, and cricoid cartilages are the largest and can be viewed by directly observing the inside of the mouth or the neck (Fig. 1.7). The arytenoid, cuneiform, and corniculate are present in pairs bilaterally and are located within the interior of the larynx.

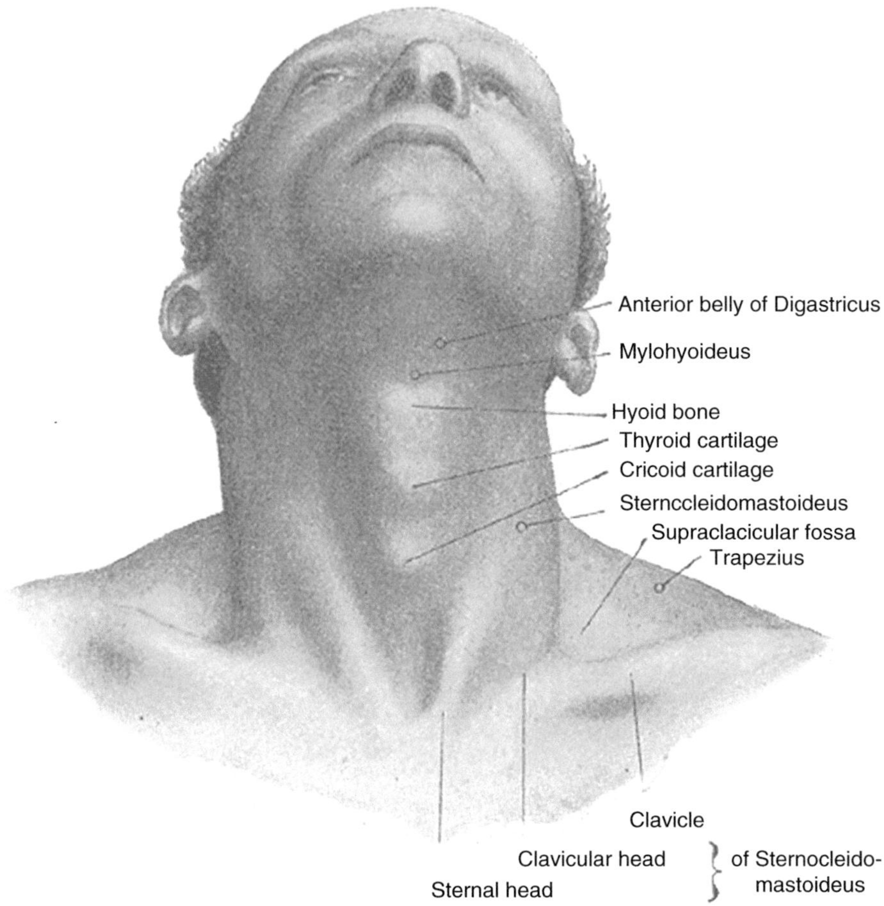

Fig. 1.7 View of the anterior neck and cartilaginous protrusions ("Plate 1195" of Henry Gray's *Anatomy of the Human Body*). (Images were obtained from Wikimedia Commons (https://commons.wikimedia.org) and are in the public domain in their country of origin and the United States)

The epiglottis is an elastic cartilaginous flap that originates posterior to the root of the tongue and projects superiorly behind the tongue and hyoid bone. Between the epiglottis and the back of the tongue is a recess called the vallecula which can trap food or foreign bodies. During swallowing, the hyoid bone, along with the rest of the laryngeal apparatus, deflects the epiglottis downward and prevents the bolus of food from entering the laryngeal inlet, an opening formed by the aryepiglottic folds and the posterior surface of the epiglottis. The aryepiglottic folds extend from the lateral edges of the epiglottis to the cuneiform and corniculate cartilages and come together to form the interarytenoid notch. A pear-shaped recess called the piriform sinus is formed by the lateral surface of the aryepiglottic folds and the mucosa covering the inner surface of the thyroid cartilage. This recess can trap food entering the larynx, and deep to its mucous membrane lies the internal laryngeal nerve, a branch of the superior laryngeal nerve.

The thyroid cartilage is a large, V-shaped shield formed by two plates that join anteriorly at the center of the neck between the levels of the C4 and C5 vertebrae. The cartilage surrounds the larynx anteriorly, and the angle at the center forms a protrusion called the laryngeal prominence or Adam's apple. During puberty, the size of this prominence increases in males relative to females. The thyroid cartilage is attached to the hyoid bone via the thyrohyoid ligament and the cricoid inferiorly by the cricothyroid joint. The cricoid forms the inferior bound of the larynx. Its name comes from the Greek word for ring as it is the only completely circumferential cartilage in the airway.

The interior larynx is divided into three spaces: the supraglottis, glottis, and epiglottis. These regions are determined by the location of the vocal folds, where the supraglottis is above, the subglottis below, and the glottis at the level of the folds. Within the supraglottis are two thick folds of mucous membrane called the vestibular folds, or the false vocal folds, that cover the underlying true vocal folds (Fig. 1.8). The space between the vestibular folds is the vestibule, while the airway compartments that extend laterally and superiorly underneath the vestibular folds are the ventricles. The glottis is composed of the true vocal folds and the rima glottidis, the orifice created between the vocal folds when they are abducted.

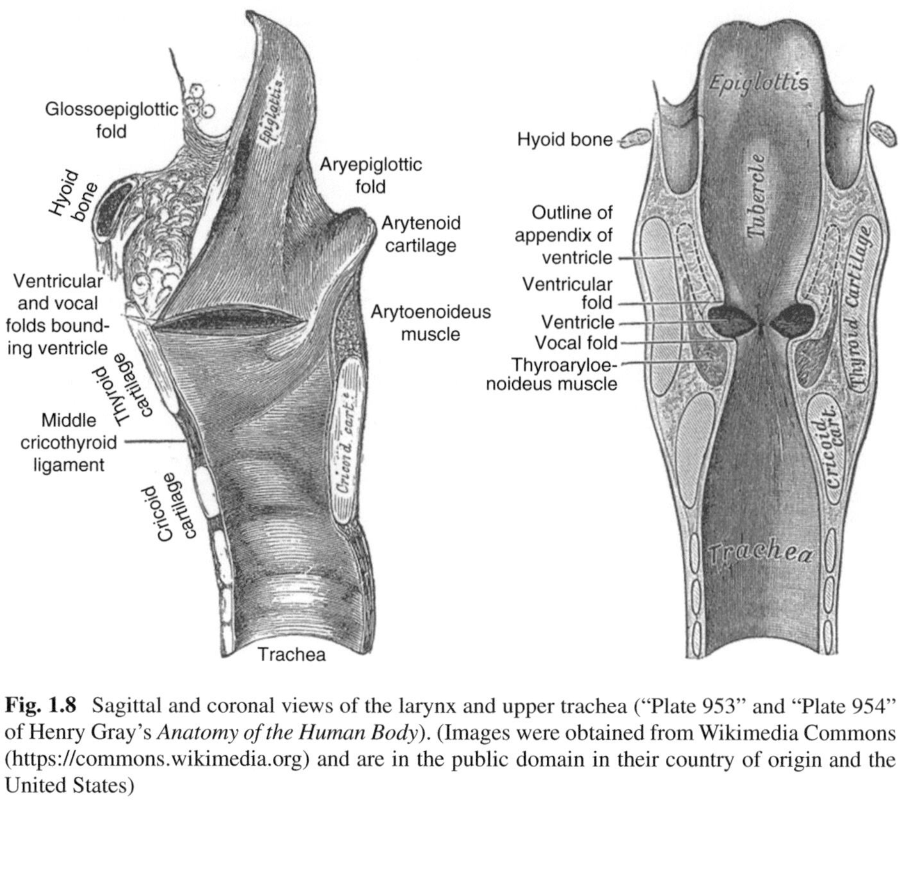

Fig. 1.8 Sagittal and coronal views of the larynx and upper trachea ("Plate 953" and "Plate 954" of Henry Gray's *Anatomy of the Human Body*). (Images were obtained from Wikimedia Commons (https://commons.wikimedia.org) and are in the public domain in their country of origin and the United States)

Two triangular-shaped cartilages called the arytenoids sit atop the posterior aspect of the cricoid and are attached to the true vocal folds by their medial processes (often called the vocal process) (Fig. 1.8). The arytenoids have a wide range of movements allowing subsequent movement of the vocal folds. There are many intrinsic muscles of the larynx that manipulate the arytenoids to tense, loosen, adduct, or abduct the vocal folds. The posterior cricoarytenoideus attaches the posterior cricoid cartilage to the arytenoids and acts as the sole abductor of the vocal folds. In contrast, the lateral cricoarytenoids, internal thyroarytenoids, external thyroarytenoids, and interarytenoids contract to adduct the vocal. The thyroarytenoids can also contract to bring the arytenoids forward to reduce the tension of the vocal cords, leading to a deeper pitch. The vocalis muscles that attach directly to parts of the vocal folds and conus elasticus increase tension and produce higher pitch. The cricothyroid is located outside of the larynx, and contraction results in tipping of the thyroid cartilage forward, resulting in tensing of the vocal folds to, like the vocalis muscles, increase the pitch.

The recurrent laryngeal nerve provides motor input for all internal muscles of the larynx excluding the cricothyroid. Injury to the recurrent nerve, which may be a complication from thyroid surgery, results in impairment of ipsilateral vocal fold movement and hoarseness. Bilateral injury prevents closure of the vocal folds during swallowing and poses a serious risk of aspiration. The superior laryngeal nerve branches into internal and external divisions. The internal division provides sensory innervation to the upper portion of the laryngeal apparatus from the epiglottic regions to the vocal folds. The external division provides motor innervation to the pharyngeal constrictors as well as the cricothyroid.

References

1. Melvin JE, Yule D, Shuttleworth T, Begenisich T. Regulation of fluid and electrolyte secretion in salivary gland acinar cells. Annu Rev Physiol. 2005;67(1):445–69. https://doi.org/10.1146/annurev.physiol.67.041703.084745.
2. Lee MG, Ohana E, Park HW, Yang D, Muallem S. Molecular mechanism of pancreatic and salivary gland fluid and HCO3 secretion. Physiol Rev. 2012;92(1):39–74. https://doi.org/10.1152/physrev.00011.2011.
3. Ferreira LEVVC, Simmons DT, Baron TH. Zenker's diverticula: pathophysiology, clinical presentation, and flexible endoscopic management. Dis Esophagus. 2008;21(1):1–8. https://doi.org/10.1111/j.1442-2050.2007.00795.x.

Chapter 2
Esophagus Anatomy: Cricopharyngeus and Lower Esophagus as Sphincters

Peter H. Stein

The esophagus is composed of three distinct anatomic components, comprising the cervical, thoracic, and abdominal segments. The cervical esophagus begins below the vocal cords, behind the trachea. The thoracic esophagus comprises the majority of what one typically considers when describing esophageal anatomy and function, sitting posterior to the trachea and left atrium of the heart and anterior to the thoracic spine. A small segment of the esophagus enters below the diaphragm into the stomach and creates a small indentation on the underside of the liver [1] (Fig. 2.1).

The upper quarter of the esophagus is primarily striated muscle, meaning that each individual has control over the contractions of this segment of the esophagus [2]. A transition zone begins approximately a quarter of the way down the esophagus, where both striated and smooth muscles are present. This transition further continues to all smooth muscle roughly halfway down the esophagus.

The esophagus acts primarily as a conduit for food contents exiting the mouth and entering the stomach. Two distinct sphincters control the passage of food along this tract, not only allowing the passage of food distally from the mouth through the esophagus into the stomach but in addition preventing the reflux of stomach contents retrograde back into the esophagus and mouth.

The first of these sphincters is marked by the transition from the pharynx to the esophagus, where the cricopharyngeus muscle lies [2]. This marks the transition from the pharynx to the esophagus. Thus, when food passes beyond the cricopharyngeus, the pharyngeal phase of swallowing ends, and the esophageal phase begins. At this anatomic location, a narrow band of muscle fibers exists just below the cricoid cartilage which functions as a sphincter for the upper esophagus. Muscle tone of the esophageal lumen is greatest at this level. Although this is not a true "sphincter" in the strictest sense of the word, it functions as such, preventing esophageal

P. H. Stein (✉)
Division of Gastroenterology, Phelps Hospital Northwell Health, Sleepy Hollow, NY, USA
e-mail: pstein2@northwell.edu

C. H. Zalvan (ed.), *Laryngopharyngeal and Gastroesophageal Reflux*,
https://doi.org/10.1007/978-3-030-48890-1_2

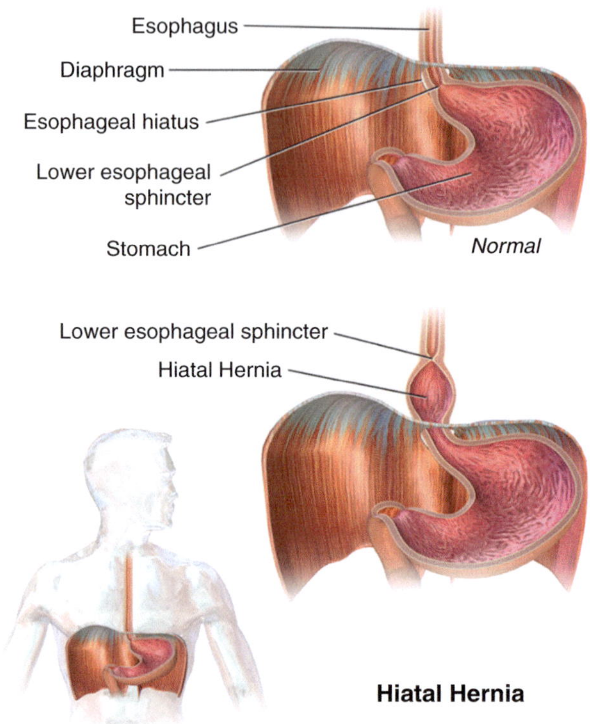

Fig. 2.1 Illustration of the esophageal segments. (Courtesy of IntechOpen.com)

contents from refluxing into the trachea. The controlled act of swallowing (as this area is still comprised of striated muscle) acts to relax this muscle [2].

As we travel further distally into the esophagus, we come to the distal aspect where the esophagus enters the crus of the diaphragm. Here lies the lower esophageal sphincter (LES) – again, not a true "sphincter," but rather a complex anatomic structure acting as such, preventing stomach contents from refluxing into the esophagus {picture}. This complex structure sits at the gastroesophageal (GE) junction and makes up roughly the bottom 3–4 cm of the esophagus. The proximal portion normally sits 1–2 cm above the squamocolumnar junction (where the mucosa changes from esophageal to gastric tissue) within the thoracic cavity. The distal segment is approximately 2 cm below the squamocolumnar junction, residing in the abdominal cavity below the diaphragm. At rest, this "sphincter" is tonically contracted, preventing retrograde flow of gastric contents into the esophagus. As one swallows, peristaltic contractions allow the LES to relax, allowing food contents to pass integrate from the esophagus into the stomach.

What makes up the LES? This complex anatomic structure is comprised of at least six distinct components, each providing their own unique function. Muscle fibers from the right crus of the diaphragm wrap tightly around the distal esophagus, creating a band or angle at the GE junction. The diaphragm contributes to the LES most during inspiration, when the crura contract and compress the esophagus, preventing passage of a food bolus. Extrinsic "squeezing" of the esophagus occurs during inspiration, as the lungs expand and press nearly circumferentially on the esophagus. Measured pressures in the esophagus tend to be highest during times of increased abdominal pressure, such as coughing, sneezing, bending, and straining of the abdominal muscles.

A thickening of the circular and longitudinal muscles of the esophagus exists at the LES. The thickest components sit 1–2 cm above the GE junction. This allows for tonic contractions of this area of the esophagus, again preventing reflux of stomach contents.

The small intra-abdominal component of the esophagus plays a role as well. The intrathoracic esophagus as mentioned above is significantly affected by inspiration. During inspiration, the diaphragm contracts and pulls the lungs inferiorly, creating negative pressure in the intrathoracic esophagus, which is countered by positive pressure in the intrabdominal esophagus. As the LES lies just below the diaphragm in the upper abdomen, this pressure difference aids in keeping this distal most portion of the esophagus tonically contracted. When a hiatal hernia is present (meaning the LES sits within the thorax), this pressure difference is negated removing a vital component of the LES function (Fig. 2.2).

Gastric cardia muscles are contiguous with the inner circular muscle layers of the esophagus. As these gastric muscles meet the distal esophagus at the location of the LES, they wrap around the esophagus, acting as a "sling" or muscular collar. This "sling" formation of these muscle fibers exerts pressure on the distal most aspect of the esophagus, contributing to the sphincter-like anatomy.

Lastly, a sharp angle is created by the entry of the esophagus into and through the diaphragm, termed the "angle of His." As the esophagus enters the stomach, it makes an oblique bend, creating a sharp angle that acts as a "flap-valve."

The resting LES pressure is controlled by hormonal, muscular, and neuronal mechanisms. Variations in the basal LES pressure are based on time of day, in addition to various circulating peptides, hormones, foods, and drugs – many of which go well beyond the scope of this text. The highest LES pressure exists at night, preventing reflux of food contents as we are sleeping. The lowest LES pressure is after meals.

As one can see, the LES is a complex structure with multiple subtle yet important components. If any of these components develops a defect, or malfunctions, the function of the LES can become compromised leading to GERD-related symptoms. Initially the esophagus was thought of as a simple tubular conduit for food contents from the mouth into the stomach. In reality, it is quite complex. Small abnormalities in esophageal anatomy can have great effects on function, leading to symptoms or GERD-related complications.

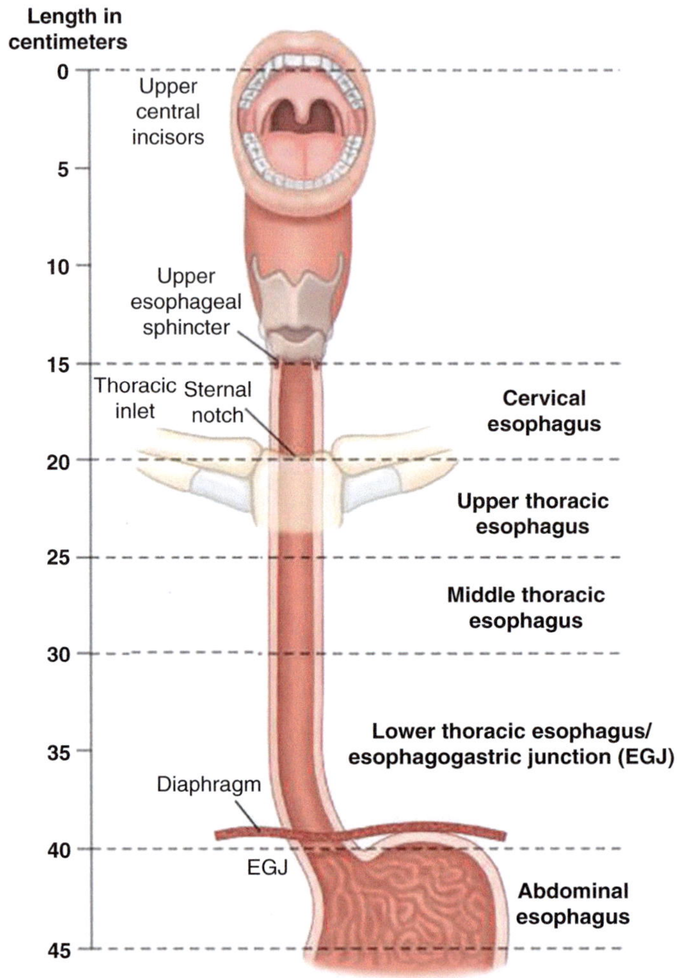

Fig. 2.2 Illustration of a hiatal hernia. (Courtesy of wikimediacommons.org)

References

1. Gray H, Bannister LH, Berry MM, Williams PL, editors. Gray's anatomy: the anatomical basis of medicine and surgery. New York: Churchill Livingstone; 1995.
2. Floch MH, Kowdley KV, et al. Netter's gastroenterology. Philadelphia: Saunders Elsevier; 2010. p. 1–83.

Chapter 3
Relevant Stomach and Intestine Anatomy

Peter H. Stein

In order to understand GERD and its associated complications, it is important to understand gastric and duodenal anatomy, as these organs are intricately tied to the process of GERD. The gastrointestinal tract from the mouth to the anus is one long tubular series of connected structures, all working dynamically in a complex manner. It would be impossible to separate out the function of one portion of the gastrointestinal tract without considering the function of the immediately adjacent portions. This clearly applies to the disease process of GERD, where the esophagus is the primary affected portion. Although our focus traditionally rests on esophageal disease, the contributions of the stomach, duodenum, and additional associated anatomy cannot be ignored.

The stomach acts as a reservoir to hold food contents after passage through the esophagus. It sits just below the diaphragm and passes slightly leftward, with the abdominal wall and a portion of the left lung anterior and the pancreas and spleen posterior [1, 2] (Fig. 3.1). After food is swallowed, it passes through the esophagus into the stomach where it is held to begin digestion. Digestion truly begins in the mouth with chewing and exposure to saliva with a small number of digestive enzymes; however, we commonly think of the stomach as the first site of extensive digestive enzyme exposure. In the stomach, food contents are soaked in acidic stomach secretions that include hydrochloric acid, pepsin, gastric lipase, and intrinsic factor [3]. The stomach acts as a stopgap, slowing the passage of food to allow for adequate breakdown of food contents. Slowly, these digesting gastric contents are churned into smaller particles that are then released through the pylorus into the first portion of the small intestine (the duodenum) in a carefully controlled fashion. This process is controlled through neurologic and hormonal pathways that are beyond the scope of this text.

P. H. Stein (✉)
Division of Gastroenterology, Phelps Hospital Northwell Health, Sleepy Hollow, NY, USA
e-mail: pstein2@northwell.edu

C. H. Zalvan (ed.), *Laryngopharyngeal and Gastroesophageal Reflux*,
https://doi.org/10.1007/978-3-030-48890-1_3

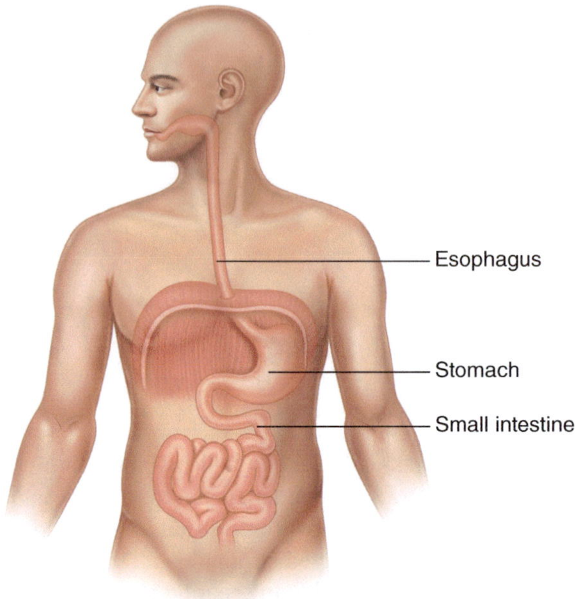

Fig. 3.1 Illustration of normal upper gastrointestinal tract anatomy

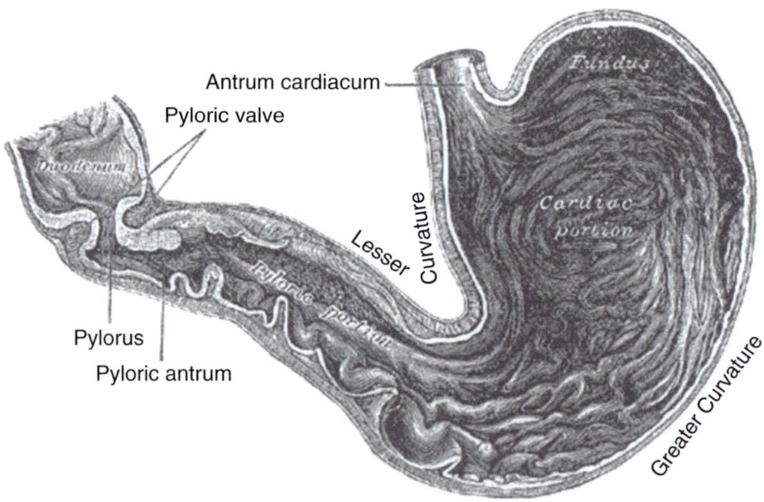

Fig. 3.2 Illustration of gastric anatomy (wikimediacommons.org)

The first portion of the stomach is termed the cardia, which is the point where the esophagus enters the stomach (Figs. 3.2 and 3.3). The cardia constitutes the first few centimeters of the stomach and quickly transitions into the gastric body and fundus. The fundus sits on the left side of the stomach and is the portion that relaxes and expands during eating to accommodate a large meal [2]. Without this accommoda-tion, one would not be able to take in a large meal, resulting in food contents either

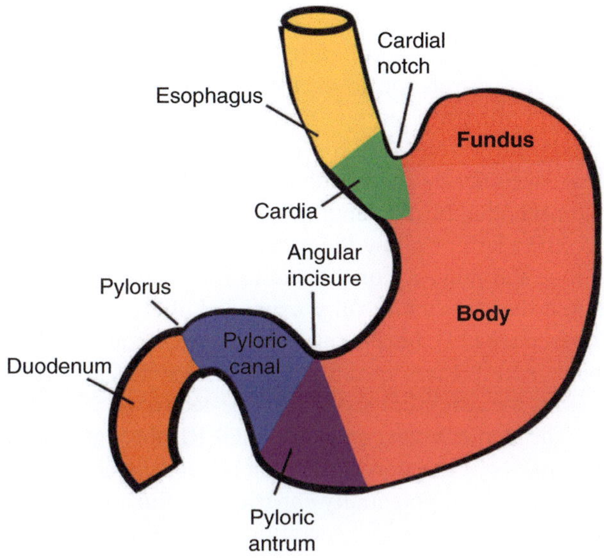

Fig. 3.3 Illustration of gastric anatomy (wikimediacommons.org)

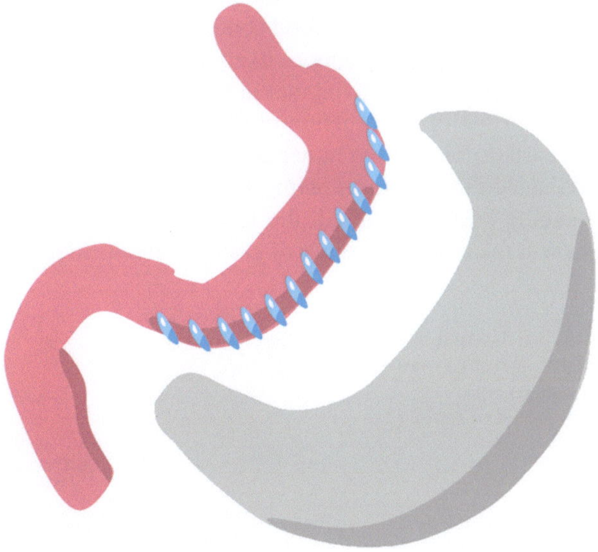

Fig. 3.4 Illustration of gastric sleeve anatomy (wikimediacommons.org)

refluxing back into the esophagus or being forced distally into the intestines. This exact process occurs in patients who have had their stomachs surgically altered in the setting of bariatric surgeries, such as a gastric sleeve. The gastric sleeve procedure surgically removes or endoscopically restricts the gastric fundus (Fig. 3.4). Gastric accommodation drastically decreases resulting in the inability to take in large volumes of solid food. Unfortunately, a common side effect of this procedure is reflux of acidic gastric contents into the distal esophagus, resulting in GERD-related symptoms [4].

The main portion of the stomach is termed the body of the stomach. The left side is the greater curvature, while the right side is the lesser curvature – names reflecting their size in relation to each other. The body of the stomach transitions into the antrum, the distal portion that is thickly muscular. This portion grinds and churns food prior to releasing contents through the pylorus into the proximal small intestine, specifically the duodenal bulb. The pylorus, which is the opening from the stomach into the duodenum, is controlled by a sphincter which contracts and relaxes to either halt or allow the passage of food contents into the duodenum (Fig. 3.5). Along the majority of the stomach lining exist folds termed rugae, which flatten when the stomach is fully expanded after a large meal. These folds increase the surface area [2]. Each area of the stomach contains mucosa that serves specific purposes and releases specific digestive enzymes and hormones, in conjunction allowing for the careful digestion of ingested food.

The stomach can contribute to GERD through a number of means. As mentioned previously, if the stomach cannot adequately accommodate ingested food contents, the patient will potentially experience reflux of acidic gastric contents. The stomach produces highly acidic secretions, which are the main culprit in GERD. Patients experience GERD-related symptoms not because of ingested acidic or other caustic food types, but rather from refluxing acidic gastric contents. If the stomach produces an excess of acidic food contents, or does not allow timely passage of gastric acid, the patient will be more likely to pass these acidic contents into their esophagus resulting in GERD symptoms. Lastly, proximal gastric anatomy makes up a large portion of the function of the complex lower esophageal sphincter, which is not a true sphincter but rather an interplay between a series of small muscle groups and anatomic structures acting in a sphincter-like fashion. If the proximal gastric anatomy becomes altered, the lower esophageal sphincter may lose its ability to prevent the abnormal reflux of gastric contents into the distal esophagus [5, 6].

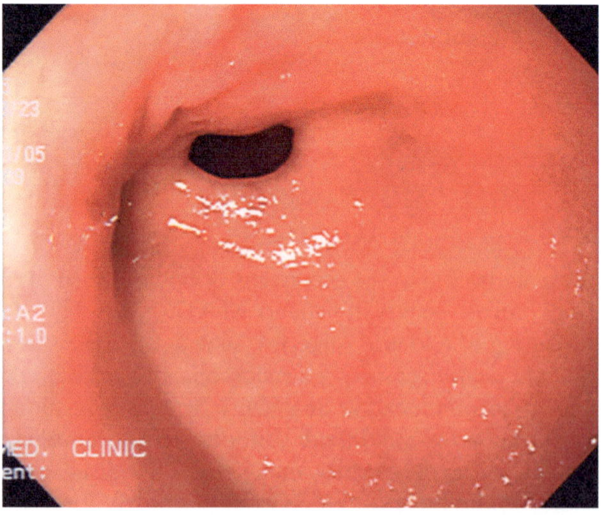

Fig. 3.5 Normal appearing gastric pylorus (wikimedia-commons.org)

Partially digested stomach contents are released into the small intestine. The small intestine is at least 20 feet in length and is divided into three parts: duodenum, jejunum, and ileum (Fig. 3.6). The duodenum is the most proximal section, which is further subdivided into four parts (first, second, third, and fourth portions of the duodenum). The entirety of the duodenum is approximately 30 cm in length and forms a C-shape around the head of the pancreas [2].

The small bowel normally plays a small role in the pathophysiology of GERD. Typically, the first part of the duodenum, termed the "duodenal bulb," accepts partially digested food readily from the stomach through the pylorus, which is the junction between the antrum of the stomach and the duodenum. This is carefully controlled by a sphincter at this location, releasing gastric food contents into the duodenum when appropriate. Food then travels past the duodenal bulb into the second portion, where the major papilla allows for drainage of pancreatic and biliary secretions into the duodenum, furthering the digestive process.

An improperly functioning pylorus can indirectly lead to reflux. If the pylorus is incompetent, meaning that the sphincter in this area does not contract properly, food can rapidly pass into the intestines. Passage of contents would be free to pass in a retrograde fashion, leading to the potential reflux of bile acids. Their interaction with pepsin and gastric acid can potentially lead to injury of the esophagus [7]. Few adequate treatments exist for this form of reflux, although the coating agent, carafate, has been used with some efficacy in this scenario.

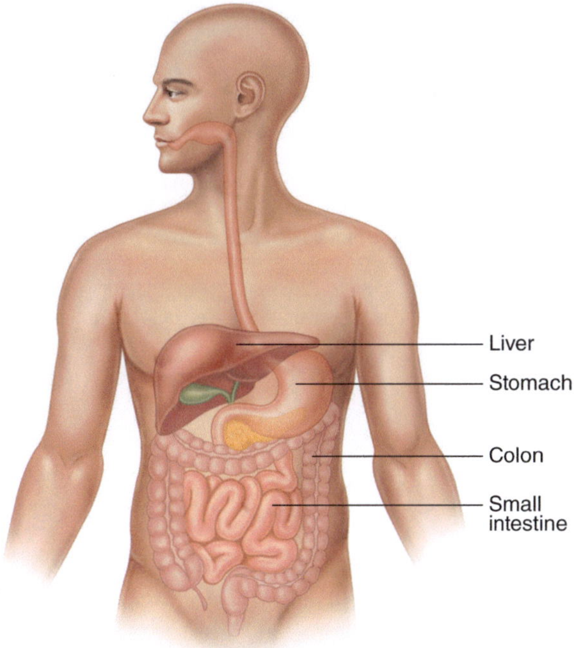

Fig. 3.6 Illustration of normal gastrointestinal tract anatomy showing the small intestine and colon in relation to additional abdominal anatomy

The corollary of an incompetent pylorus – a stenotic or poorly relaxing pylorus – can lead to significant reflux as well. If the stomach cannot adequately pass partially digested food contents into the duodenum, the ability of the proximal stomach to accommodate large food volumes will be challenged, leading to reflux of food contents into the esophagus. A "raft" of gastric acid can accumulate along the proximal margin of this large volume of gastric food contents, floating below or into the lower esophagus. This process is the same as that of gastroparesis, where the stomach fails to pass food contents in a timely fashion into the small intestine [8]. One can view these two processes as equivalent in terms of GERD-related symptoms, as both inadequate gastric motility and an inadequately relaxing pylorus will ultimately have the same effect proximally: the backup of gastric contents into the distal esophagus. As we have seen, the stomach and, to a lesser degree, the duodenum play vital roles in the etiology of GERD. One cannot view the function of the esophagus without considering the function of the stomach and duodenum.

References

1. Gray H, Bannister LH, Berry MM, Williams PL, editors. Gray's anatomy: the anatomical basis of medicine and surgery. New York: Churchill Livingstone; 1995.
2. Floch MH, Kowdley KV, et al. Netter's gastroenterology. Philadelphia: Saunders, Elsevier; 2010. p. 87–155.
3. Schubert ML, Peura DA. Control of gastric acid secretion in health and disease. Gastroenterology. 2008;134:1842.
4. Viscido G, Gorodner V, Signorini F, et al. Laparoscopic sleeve gastrectomy: endoscopic findings and gastroesophageal reflux symptoms at 18-month follow-up. J Laparoendosc Adv Surg Tech A. 2018;28:71.
5. Jones MP, Sloan SS, Rabine JC, et al. Hiatal hernia size is the dominant determinant of esophagitis presence and severity in gastroesophageal reflux disease. Am J Gastroenterol. 2001;96:1711.
6. Boeckxstaens G, El-Serag HB, Smout AJ, Kahrilas PJ. Symptomatic reflux disease: the present, the past, and the future. Gut. 2014;63:1185.
7. Souza RF. The role of acid and bile reflux in esophagitis and Barrett's metaplasia. Biochem Soc Trans. 2010;38:348.
8. Vijayvargiya P, Jameie Oskooei S, Camilleri M, et al. Association between delayed gastric emptying an upper gastrointestinal symptoms: a systematic review and meta-analysis. Gut. 2019;68:804.

Chapter 4
Gastric Acid and Pepsin Roles in Reflux Disease

Claude Nganzeu, Jonathan M. Bock, and Nikki Johnston

Gastric Acid

Secretion of Gastric Acid

Gastric acid is produced by highly differentiated epithelial cells in the fundic glands of the gastric mucosa called parietal cells. Parietal cells contain an extensive secretory network, called canaliculi, from which gastric acid is secreted into the lumen of the stomach. Gastric acid is approximately pH 2 in the lumen of the stomach, the acidity being maintained by H^+/K^+ ATPase proton pumps. The resulting highly acidic environment in the stomach lumen causes proteins from food to denature, thus exposing the protein's peptide bonds. Additionally, the acidic environment of the stomach inhibits growth of many microorganisms; the gut's bacterial load is controlled, and this helps prevent infection.

C. Nganzeu
Medical College of Wisconsin, Milwaukee, WI, USA
e-mail: cnganzeu@mcw.edu

J. M. Bock
Department of Otolaryngology & Communication Sciences, Division of Laryngology & Professional Voice, Medical College of Wisconsin, Milwaukee, WI, USA
e-mail: jbock@mcw.edu

N. Johnston (✉)
Department of Otolaryngology and Communication Sciences, Division of Laryngology and Professional Voice and Pediatric Otolaryngology, Department of Microbiology and Immunology, Milwaukee, WI, USA
e-mail: njohnston@mcw.edu

C. H. Zalvan (ed.), *Laryngopharyngeal and Gastroesophageal Reflux*,
https://doi.org/10.1007/978-3-030-48890-1_4

Gastric acid secretion happens in several steps. Chloride and hydrogen ions are secreted separately from the cytoplasm of parietal cells and mixed in the canaliculi ultimately forming hydrochloric acid (HCl). This acid is then secreted into the lumen of the oxyntic gland and gradually reaches the stomach lumen. Chloride and sodium ions are secreted actively from the cytoplasm of the parietal cell into the lumen of the canaliculus. This creates a negative potential of −40 mV to −70 mV across the parietal cell membrane that causes potassium and sodium ions to diffuse from the cytoplasm into the parietal cell canaliculi. The enzyme carbonic anhydrase catalyzes the reaction between carbon dioxide and water to form carbonic acid. This acid immediately dissociates into hydrogen and bicarbonate ions. The hydrogen ions leave the cell through H^+/K^+ ATPase antiporter pumps. At the same time, sodium ions are actively reabsorbed. The majority of secreted potassium and sodium ions therefore return to the cytoplasm. The highest concentration of gastric acid that reaches the stomach is 160 mM in the canaliculi. This is about three million times that of arterial blood but is isotonic with other bodily fluids. The lowest pH of the secreted acid is 0.8, but as the acid is diluted in the stomach lumen with other secretions, the intragastric pH will range between 1 and 3.

Nerves and hormones are responsible for gastric acid secretion. Stomach glands receive stimuli from the brain, stomach, and small intestine to modulate gastric acid secretion. These stimulations are done in three phases called the cephalic, gastric, and intestinal phases [1, 2]. The cephalic phase, also called the reflex phase, occurs prior to food entering the stomach. This phase is relatively brief and occurs when the brain receives sensory input after the sight, smell, taste, or even the thought of food. The brain then relays the signal to the gastric mucosa to increase gastric juice production for digestion. The gastric phase is the longest of all three phases, lasting around 3–4 hours [3]. This occurs when food enters the lumen of the stomach and causes it to distend. Distention then activates stretch receptors, and the stretch receptors stimulate the vagus nerve, mediated by gastrin-releasing peptide (GRP) and neurocrine bombesin, through the parasympathetic pathway, and cause the secretion of acetylcholine. Acetylcholine increases production of gastric juice. As proteins are digested in the stomach, this increases pH in the stomach lumen. The rise in the pH induces the secretion of gastrin from G cells located in the pyloric antrum of the stomach. Gastrin binds to cholecystokinin B receptors and causes the release of histamine from enterochromaffin-like (ECL) cells. Histamine binds to H_2 receptors of the parietal cells causing H^+/K^+ ATPase pumps to insert in the parietal cells' canaliculi and transport H^+ into the stomach lumen to create gastric acid [1–3]. The intestinal phase is a relatively brief phase that occurs in the duodenum. When chyme enters the duodenum, the small intestine's mucosa cells secrete intestinal gastrin, which increases gastric juice secretion. Gastric juice secretion is inhibited by enterogastric reflex that is activated when chyme, filling the duodenum, causes distention. The enterogastric reflex is important for the closure pyloric sphincter to prevent further entry of chyme in the small intestine [1–3].

Regulation of Secretion

Gastric acid production is regulated by both the autonomic nervous system and several hormones. The parasympathetic nervous system, via the vagus nerve, and the hormone gastrin stimulate the parietal cell to produce gastric acid, both directly acting on parietal cells and indirectly by stimulating secretion of the hormone histamine from ECL cells. Vasoactive intestinal peptide, cholecystokinin, and secretin all inhibit production. The production of gastric acid in the stomach is tightly regulated by positive regulators and negative feedback mechanisms. Four types of cells are involved in this process: parietal cells, G cells, D cells, and ECL cells. In addition, the endings of the vagus nerve (CN X) and the intramural nervous plexus in the digestive tract also significantly influence secretion. Nerve endings in the stomach secrete two stimulatory neurotransmitters: acetylcholine and GRP. Their action is both direct on parietal cells and mediated through the secretion of gastrin from G cells and histamine from ECL cells. Gastrin acts on parietal cells directly and indirectly too, by stimulating the release of histamine. The release of histamine is the most important positive regulatory mechanism of the secretion of gastric acid in the stomach. Its release is stimulated by gastrin and acetylcholine and inhibited by somatostatin.

Neutralization of Gastric Acid

In the duodenum, gastric acid is neutralized by sodium bicarbonate secreted from the pancreas, the liver, and Brunner's glands of the duodenum. This also blocks gastric enzymes that have their pH optima in the acid range. The secretion of sodium bicarbonate from the pancreas is stimulated by secretin. This polypeptide gets activated and secreted from S cells in the mucosa of the duodenum and jejunum when the pH in the duodenum falls below 4.5–5. This neutralization is described by the equation:

$$HCL + NaHCO_3 \leftrightarrow NaCl + H_2CO_3$$

This carbonic acid instantly decomposes into carbon dioxide and water and is eliminated through the kidneys in urine.

Role of Gastric Acid in Disease

In hypochlorhydria and achlorhydria, there is low or no gastric acid in the stomach, potentially leading to problems as the disinfectant properties of the gastric lumen are decreased. In such conditions, there is greater risk of infections of the digestive tract (such as infection with *Helicobacter* bacteria). In Zollinger-Ellison syndrome and hypercalcemia, there are increased gastrin levels, leading to excess gastric acid production, which can cause gastric ulcers. Reflux of gastric acid into the esophagus (gastroesophageal reflux, GER) and more proximally into the laryngopharynx (laryngopharyngeal reflux, LPR) and other extra-esophageal sites (extra-esophageal reflux, EER) also causes significant injury and disease.

Pharmacology

Acid secretion is mediated principally by acetylcholine and gastrin inducing increased cytosolic calcium and histamine activating adenylate cyclase and producing cAMP. All these hormones regulate the activity of the H^+/K^+ ATPase pumps on the parietal cells to control gastric acid production. Extensive research on the mechanism of the production of gastric acid and the discovery of specific receptor subtypes allowed the creation of potent drugs that efficiently inhibit gastric acid secretion. The receptors targeted by competitive inhibitors are muscarinic M1-3-receptors and histamine H_2 receptors, and the receptors targeted by non-competitive inhibitors are H^+/K^+ ATPase enzymes [4].

H_2-Receptor Antagonists

H_2 inhibitors such as cimetidine, famotidine, ranitidine, and nizatidine are used as first-line therapy in peptic ulcer disease and also used for situational relief of reflux symptoms induced by certain activities, for example, in patients who experience heartburn during running. It is recommended that H_2_receptor antagonists are taken 1 hour prior to the activity that causes reflux symptoms. While they are effective in up to 80% of GERD patients [5], they are only effective in approximately 50% of LPR patients [6]. This is because H_2-receptor antagonists merely reduce acid production by blocking stimulation of the parietal cell. The laryngeal epithelium is more sensitive to injury from gastric acid compared to the esophagus, and thus more complete acid suppression is required [7, 8].

M1-Receptor Antagonists

M1-receptor antagonists such as pirenzepine and telenzepine are used to treat peptic ulcer disease and reflux esophagitis. They suppress acid production by inhibiting the release of stimulatory neurotransmitters. Other antimuscarinic antagonists such as atropine, methylscopolamine, and propantheline are potent antagonists of gastric acid secretion; however, they are not often used in treatment of GER or LPR due to side effects such as photophobia, mydriasis, tachycardia, ileus, blurred vision, and urinary retention [9].

Proton Pump Inhibitors

Proton pump inhibitors (PPIs) such as omeprazole, lansoprazole, esomeprazole, pantoprazole, rabeprazole, and dexlansoprazole irreversibly inhibit H^+/K^+ATPase enzyme. By targeting the terminal step in production, they prevent secretion of HCl and thus are potent gastric acid-suppressing agents, which are effective for the treatment of GERD. Although PPIs remain the mainstay for treatment of GERD, there is poor evidence for their efficacy in the treatment of airway reflux-mediated disease including LPR [10]. It is widely believed that the upper airway is more sensitive to reflux than the esophagus and hence that higher-dose PPIs are necessary for the control of LPR-related symptoms [11–13]. At this time, placebo-controlled studies have by and large not shown a significant therapeutic benefit to PPI used in LPR [14–19]. Although some studies have noted evidence of symptomatic improvement with PPI therapy [20, 21], upon review of these two studies, it has been argued that the affected patients only had significant improvement of gastroesophageal reflux symptoms, rather than improvement of upper airway symptoms [18]. Arguments can be made that these studies were done prior to the era of combined hypopharyngeal-esophageal impedance with dual pH probe testing and that the diagnosis of non-acid reflux was incomplete. In light of the poor data for the efficacy of acid suppression in treatment of EER, the American Gastroenterological Association has specifically recommended against the empiric use of PPIs for suspected LPR unless there are concomitant symptoms of GERD [22]. Likely as a result of the paucity of alternative effective therapies, however, PPIs continue to be used for LPR [18, 23], and indeed the American Academy of Otolaryngology–Head and Neck Surgery has recommended empiric use of high-dose PPI therapy for suspected LPR, with laparoscopic fundoplication proposed as an alternative to medical management [12]. A survey from the American Bronchoesophagological Association reported that the twice-daily PPIs remain a popular first-line therapy for LPR [24].

Prokinetic Agents

Prokinetic agents such as metoclopramide and cisapride are used in reflux patients who have dyspeptic symptoms such as nausea, vomiting, and abdominal bloating. These drugs increase lower esophageal sphincter pressure and accelerate esophageal acid clearance and gastric emptying. Their use has fallen out of favor in recent [25]. Problems with cardiac arrhythmias and drug-associated deaths led to removal of cisapride from the US market in 2000 [26]. Their results as single-agent therapy for GER or LPR have been disappointing. Some patients are intolerant of the medicines' side-effect profiles including diarrhea or cramping, and treatment success with acid suppression has been variable and limited.

Sucralfate

Sucralfate is used in the treatment of GER and stress ulcers and may be useful in the treatment of LPR. Sucralfate is a locally acting substance that reacts with HCl to form a cross-linking viscous material that acts as an acid buffer for up to 8 hours. It attaches to proteins on the surface of ulcers, such as albumin and fibrinogen, to form stable and insoluble complexes, creating a barrier against gastric refluxate. In addition, it prevents back diffusion of hydrogen ions and absorbs both pepsin and bile acids further preventing damage by reflux.

Alginate

Alginate anti-reflux preparations are widely used for the treatment of GER. They react with stomach acid to form a gel raft which floats on top of the stomach, helping to keep gastric contents in the stomach and preventing GER. Several studies have shown the efficacy of Gaviscon Advance (Reckitt Benckiser, Kingston-upon-Thames, UK) in the treatment of LPR. This alginate preparation is licensed in the UK for the treatment of LPR but is not currently available in the USA. Treatment with Gaviscon Advance, either alone or in conjunction with a PPI, was found to be significantly beneficial in improving symptoms, laryngeal findings, and patient quality of life compared to control [27].

Surgical Management of Reflux

Laparoscopic fundoplication and magnetic ring procedures are well-established, reliable options for the surgical management of GERD. In contrast to the predictable improvement seen in the treatment of GERD, research on the efficacy of anti-reflux surgery in the treatment of LPR is mixed, with various studies showing resolution of symptoms ranging from 63% up to 85% of patients [28–30]. Hypotheses for this variance range from differences in surgical technique to differences in patient selection criteria. In particular, it has been observed that patients with more severe stereotypical GERD symptoms are more likely to benefit from anti-reflux surgery [28, 31], and in particular patients with preoperative heartburn and pH < 4 for over 12% of a 24-hour period have been found to have a 90% probability of symptomatic improvement [31].

Pepsin

History

Pepsin is the principal proteolytic enzyme in the stomach. It is found in all vertebrates studied like mammals and fishes. Pepsin was the first enzyme to be discovered. It was discovered in 1836 by German physiologist Theodor Schwann named pepsin from the Greek word pepsis, meaning "digestion." In 1930, pig pepsin, after urease, became the second enzyme to be crystallized by American biochemist John H. Northrop using dialysis, filtration, and cooling. The crystallization of these enzymes was important in demonstrating that enzymes were proteins with a defined structure [32].

Structure

Pepsin's primary structure is composed of 326 amino acid residues and has a molecular weight of around 35,000 daltons. Its secondary structure is a single-chain peptide consisting mainly of beta sheets (Fig. 4.1). Pepsin is composed of two homologous domains (N-terminal and C-terminal domains) that fold to create a tertiary structure made of two nearly identical and symmetrical lobes. Each lobe is made of two beta-sheets and two short alpha-helices. A six-stranded, antiparallel beta-sheet connects the two lobes and allows the formation of the catalytic site in a deep cleft. The catalytic site is made of two aspartate residues (Asp32 and Asp 215) and activated when one aspartate is protonated and the other is deprotonated [32]. Pepsin is created in the chief cells of the stomach mucosa. It has multiple isoenzymes with the most common isoenzymes named isoenzymes 1–6. Isoenzyme 3 makes the largest proportion of total pepsin at 80%, with isoenzymes 3B making 70% of total enzyme activity. Isoenzymes 1 and 2 makes less than 6% proportion of total pepsin; pepsin 4 is not active; pepsin 5 makes 6–7% of enzyme activity; and

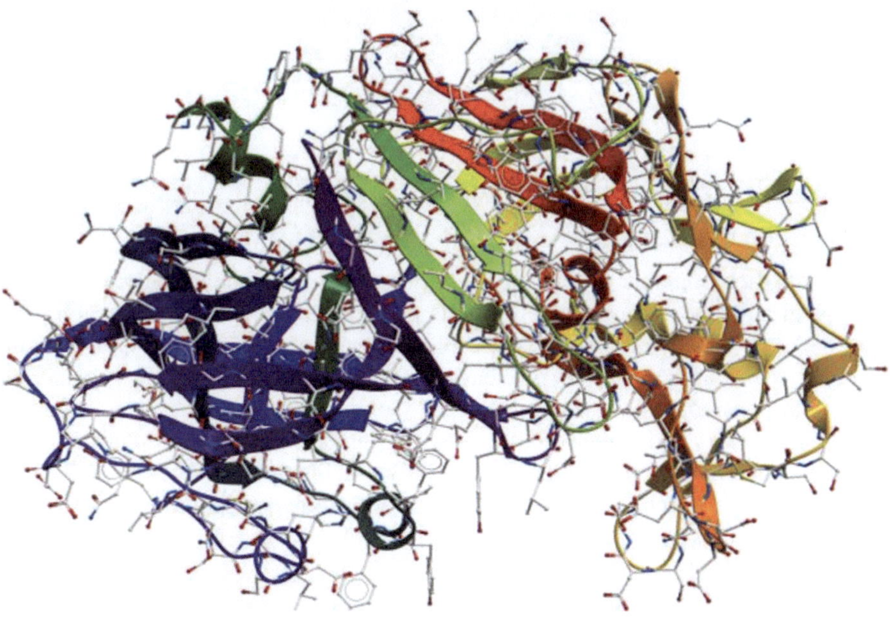

Fig. 4.1 Secondary structure of pepsin (https://sciencestruck.com/pepsin-enzyme-structure-function-important-facts)

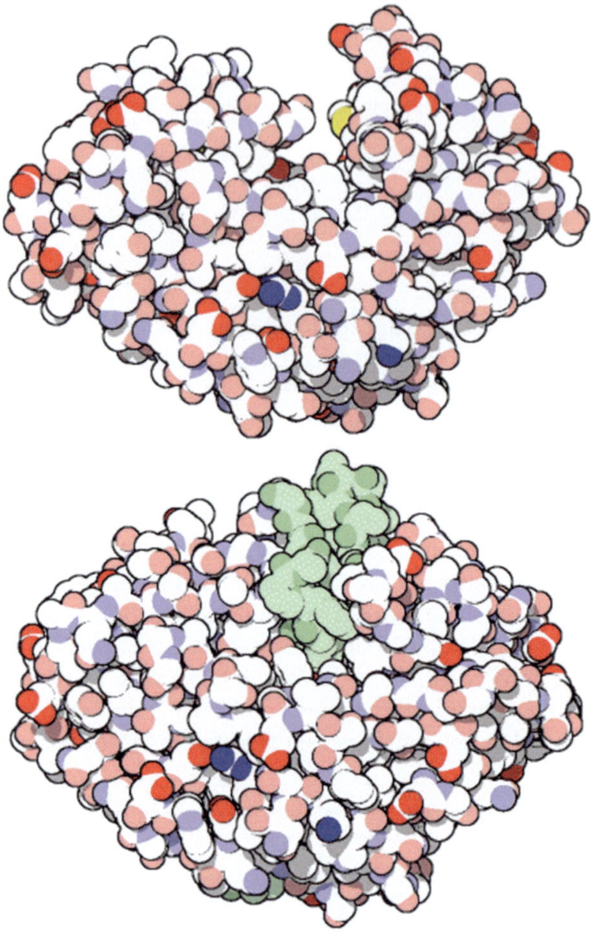

Fig. 4.2 Tertiary structure of pepsin (top) and pepsinogen (bottom). (Image from the RCSB PDB December 2000 Molecule of the Month feature by David Goodsell)

pepsin 6 is the remainder of the zymogen [33]. Pepsin is made initially as an inactive pre-proenzyme. The pre-proenzyme is made of signal protein, activation peptide, and active enzyme. As the molecule is inserted in the rough endoplasmic reticulum, the signal peptide is cleaved, creating the proenzyme, pepsinogen (Fig. 4.2). Pepsinogen is transported to the Golgi apparatus, where it is stored in secretory granules and released in the stomach lumen by exocytosis. Pepsinogen's primary structure has an additional of 44 amino acids that occlude the active site groove. In the stomach lumen, the chief cells secrete pepsinogen, which is hydrolyzed by HCl, creating its active protein, pepsin (Fig. 4.2).

Pepsin Physiology and Role in Digestion

Pepsin is the main digestive enzyme in the stomach. Its principal role is digesting protein in the stomach. It is released from chief cells as pepsinogen, its inactive form, to prevent digestion of protective proteins in the gastric mucosa. Pepsin release is activated by the same neural and hormonal modulators that stimulate gastric acid release. Gastrin, acetylcholine, and histamine stimulate parietal cells to secrete chloride and hydrogen ions via the H^+/K^+ ATPase pump to form HCl. Similarly, in chief cells, gastrin and acetylcholine from vagus nerve activation induces the release of pepsinogen. The presence of HCl in the lumen creates the acidic environment that allows pepsinogen to unfold and cleave itself in an autocatalytic fashion, thereby generating pepsin (Fig. 4.3). Pepsin then cleaves the 44 amino acids from pepsinogen creating more pepsin. Pepsin will digest up to 20% of ingested protein's amide bonds by cleaving preferentially after the N-terminal of amino acids (Fig. 4.4), especially aromatic amino acids such as phenylalanine, tryptophan, and tyrosine. Pepsin exhibits preferential cleavage for hydrophobic, preferably aromatic, residues in P1 and P1' positions. Increased susceptibility to hydrolysis occurs if there is a sulfur-containing amino acid close to the peptide bond, which has an aromatic amino acid. For example, pepsin cleaves Phe-Val, Gln-His, Glu-Ala, Ala-Leu, Leu-Tyr, Tyr-Leu, Gly-Phe, Phe-Phe, and Phe-Tyr bonds in the B chain of insulin. Peptides may be further digested by other proteases in the duodenum and eventually absorbed in the intestine. Pepsin is stored as pepsinogen so it will only be released when needed and does not digest the body's own proteins in the stomach's lining.

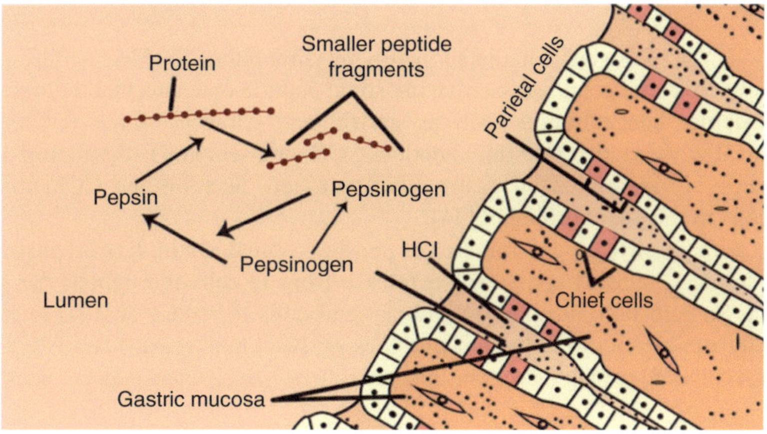

Fig. 4.3 Process involved in the cleavage of pepsinogen to pepsin (https://sciecestruck.com/pepsin-enzyme-function-important-facts)

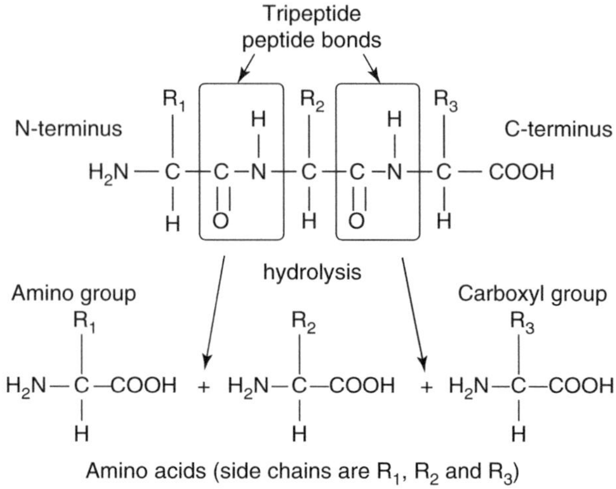

Fig. 4.4 Reaction involved in the cleavage of peptide bonds in amino (https://sciencestruck.com/pepsin-enzyme-structure-function-important-facts)

Pepsin is maximally active at pH 1.5–2.5 but has activity up to pH 6.5. While inactive at pH 6.5 and above, it remains stable to pH 8. The enzyme is not irreversibly inactivated (denatured) until pH 8. While the stomach is designed to resist damage by pepsin, reflux of pepsin into the esophagus and laryngopharynx causes damage even above pH 4. Pepsin is considered an important etiological factor in reflux disease of the aero-digestive tract and a biomarker for reflux, whose levels and acidity can be related to the severity of damage.

Physiologic Agonists and Antagonists

Secretion of pepsinogen is mediated mainly by stimulators of cAMP synthesis such as secretin, histamine, and vasoactive intestinal peptide or agents that increase cytosolic calcium concentration such as gastrin and cholecystokinin (CCK) [34]. Additionally, vasoactive intestinal peptide, CCK, and secretin's stimulation of pepsin release is independent of gastric acid secretion. Secretin and CCK stimulate chief cells to release pepsinogen [34].

The primary physiologic inhibitor of pepsin is somatostatin. Excess gastric acid in the stomach induces somatostatin release from D cells throughout the gastric mucosa. Somatostatin directly inhibits parietal cells to reduce acid secretion and indirectly inhibits acid production by blocking histamine release from ECL cells and mast cells and gastrin secretion, as a consequence, decreasing pepsin release [35].

Plant-Based Versus Animal-Based Digestion

Proteins are hydrolyzed to smaller peptide units by pepsin in the gastric lumen before complete degradation to individual amino acids in the small intestines. All proteins are not degraded equally. Some proteins are harder to digest than others and can survive fully intact or partially degraded to the large intestines. The level of digestion depends on the source (plant-based vs animal-based proteins) and the processing conditions of the proteins altering proteins' digestive susceptibility. Animal-based proteins are more easily digestible (>90%) than plant-based proteins (70–90%) [36]. This difference in digestibility may be due to some antinutritional factors present in some plant proteins. Legumes, cereals, potatoes, and tomatoes have proteins that inhibit proteolysis by pepsin and other gastrointestinal proteases. Tannins (polyphenols) found in vegetables, grains, and fruits decrease activity of gut enzymes by binding to proteases and dietary proteins and inhibiting hydrolysis through allosteric inhibition of proteases or destabilization of the enzymes' structures [36, 37]. Phytic acid, also found in plants and grains, is shown to inhibit digestibility. Many plants contain complex carbohydrates that surround their proteins and prevent enzymes from protein degradation by digestive enzymes [36, 38]. There is lack of data on the effect of plant protein on gastrin secretion; however, in 1988, Mcarthur et al. performed a study comparing the effect of soy proteins versus beef proteins on gastrin release in ten normal subjects. The results showed that there was about 30–40% less acid secretion and 65–75% less gastrin secretion when individuals consumed soy proteins versus beef proteins [39]. Less gastric acid and gastrin stimulation may also decrease the secretion of pepsin and, thus, be beneficial for relief of reflux symptoms in patients with LPR and GERD. In essence, the presence of protein inhibitors in plant-based proteins may be important in the use of Mediterranean diet style as therapy for GER or LPR. Martinucci et al., in a clinical study, measured the multichannel intraluminal impedance and pH (MII-pH) in 165 patients with heartburn after a 1-day consumption of Mediterranean diet and animal protein divided into 2 separate meals [40]. The results revealed that consumption of animal proteins raised acid about three times higher compared to vegetable proteins (acid exposure time (AET) −1 h, 3.3 +/− 2.7% vs 0.9+/− 1.4%); furthermore, patients who consumed animal proteins experienced higher reflux events to those who consumed plant proteins (total reflux events: 12.4+/− 9 vs 6.3+/− 3.9) [40]. Similarly, Zalvan et al. compared the efficacy of alkaline water and Mediterranean diet versus PPI therapy in the treatment of LPR through a retrospective study from 2010 to 2015 [41]. Utilizing a six-point reduction or improvement in Reflux Symptom Index (RSI) score, the study results showed no statistically significant difference in the number of six-point reduction in RSI score in patients on PPI therapy to those on the Mediterranean style diet; 54% and 62.6%, respectively, attained a six-point reduction in RSI score. Notably, patients on Mediterranean style had a statistically higher mean percent reduction in RSI compared to patients on PPI therapy, 39.8% and 27.2%, respectively [41]. In conclusion, the study demonstrated that there is no statistically significant difference in the efficacy of PPIs versus Mediterranean diet style in the treatment of LPR; moreover, other studies clearly show the advantage of vegetal proteins in the treatment of GERD and LPR symptoms.

Mediator of Cell Damage and Role in Disease

In vitro studies have shown that via receptor-mediated endocytosis, non-acid pepsin can enter the epithelium of the hypopharynx and larynx [42, 43]. Following endocytosis, receptors and ligands are sorted within weakly acidic late endosomes and the trans-reticular Golgi (TRG) raising the possibility of pepsin transport via these pathways. Immuno-electron microscopic findings have supported this notion, having identified co-localization of pepsin with the late endosome marker Rab-9 and the TRG marker TRG-46 [44]. The TRG has a weakly acidic pH (pH 5), at which pepsin has roughly 40% of its maximal activity [42, 45]; as such, inactive pepsin might potentially be taken up by laryngeal epithelial cells and be activated within intracellular compartments of low pH, setting the stage for intracellular damage. Exposure of hypopharyngeal cells to pepsin at pH 7 has been shown to induce the expression of several pro-inflammatory cytokines and receptors, including IL-1α, the neutrophil chemoattractant IL-8, and the eosinophil colony-stimulating factor IL-5 [43]. Conversely, exposure of laryngeal epithelium to pepsin has been shown to deplete protective proteins such as Sep70 and carbonic anhydrase-III, implying multiple pathways by which pepsin-mediated cell damage might contribute to ongoing inflammation and the endoscopic findings of LPR disease [42]. Moreover, the aforementioned pro-inflammatory cytokine profile, induced in hypopharyngeal tissues independent of acidic refluxate, is similar to that expressed in reflux esophagitis and which is known to contribute to ongoing inflammation in the pathophysiology of GERD [43].

The above research identifies a novel mechanism by which pepsin might induce cellular injury and inflammation irrespective of the acidity of the extracellular environment, potentially proffering an explanation for the persistence of chronic mucosal inflammation, symptoms, and endoscopic findings in many patients with reflux-attributed laryngeal pathology in spite of therapy with high-dose acid suppression. While pepsin has long been known to play an etiologic role in GERD due to its proteolytic activity in the low-pH environment induced by GER episodes, the finding of potentially active intracellular pepsin and induction of a pro-inflammatory response suggests a role for pepsin in reflux-mediated disease of the airway where pH may be less clinically relevant. The receptor-mediated uptake of nonacid pepsin, as can occur following LPR, and any inflammatory or neoplastic changes which may occur as a result [46–48], cannot be prevented by PPIs, which only address acid production in gastric mucosa. As the role of pepsin in LPR-mediated mucosal damage seems to involve its activation within more acidic intracellular compartments or through dysregulation or activation of cell signaling cascades [44], the amelioration of the acidic environment of gastric refluxate with PPI or H_2-receptor antagonists may not adequately address pepsin-mediated inflammatory changes.

Therapeutic Target

As discussed above, PPIs continue to be commonly used in clinical practice for the treatment of airway reflux disease including LPR in spite of poor evidence for their efficacy [14–19], with approximately $26 billion spent yearly for this indication [49]. In light of the inefficacy of PPI therapy for LPR and its associated costs and potential risks, there is substantial interest in an alternative modality for the treatment of LPR [33, 50, 51]. Pepsin represents an exciting potential novel target for future therapies, particularly for patients who experience symptoms refractory to PPI therapy in light of its role in nonacid LPR [33, 44]. Two mechanisms by which pepsin might be targeted have been identified: irreversible inactivation and via receptor antagonism [33, 44]. While the first of these would prevent pepsin's reactivation within the acidic environment of intracellular compartments, the latter would prevent its endocytosis. Although pepstatin A is a potent inhibitor of pepsin activity and is currently commercially available, its poor pharmacokinetics and water-soluble characteristics make it a poor candidate for the purpose of treating LPR. As such, novel agents targeting pepsin are currently in development and represent an exciting potential avenue for the treatment of reflux-mediated disease including LPR.

References

1. William Sircus WTK. Human digestive system. Encyclopedia Britannica. 2018: Encyclopedia Britannica, inc; 2018.
2. Kim E, Barrett P. Gastric secretion. Gastrointestinal physiology. 2nd ed. New York: McGraw-Hill; 2014.
3. The Digestive System. In: Campus B, editor. Anatomy and physiology opentextbc.ca: Open Book Publishing.
4. Shamburek RD, Schubert ML. Pharmacology of gastric acid inhibition. Baillieres Clin Gastroenterol. 1993;7(1):23–54. Epub 1993/03/01.
5. Sontag S, Robinson M, McCallum RW, Barwick KW, Nardi R. Ranitidine therapy for gastroesophageal reflux disease. Results of a large double-blind trial. Arch Intern Med. 1987;147(8):1485–91. Epub 1987/08/01.
6. Scott M, Gelhot AR. Gastroesophageal reflux disease: diagnosis and management. Am Fam Physician. 1999;59(5):1161–9, 99. Epub 1999/03/24.
7. Koufman JA. The otolaryngologic manifestations of gastroesophageal reflux disease (GERD): a clinical investigation of 225 patients using ambulatory 24-hour pH monitoring and an experimental investigation of the role of acid and pepsin in the development of laryngeal injury. Laryngoscope. 1991;101(4 Pt 2 Suppl 53):1–78. Epub 1991/04/01.
8. Little JPMB, Glock MS, et al. Extraesophageal pediatric reflux: 24-hour double-probe pH monitoring of 222 children. Ann Otol Rhinol Laryngol Suppl. 1997;169:1–16.
9. Aihara T, Nakamura E, Amagase K, Tomita K, Fujishita T, Furutani K, Okabe S. Pharmacological control of gastric acid secretion for the treatment of acid-related peptic disease: past, present, and future. Pharmacol Ther. 2003;98(1):109–27. Epub 2003/04/02.

10. Martinucci I, Guidi G, Savarino EV, Frazzoni M, Tolone S, Frazzoni L, Fuccio L, Bertani L, Bodini G, Ceccarelli L, Savarino V, Marchi S, de Bortoli N. Vegetal and animal food proteins have a different impact in the first postprandial hour of impedance-pH analysis in patients with heartburn. Gastroenterol Res Pract. 2018;2018:7. https://doi.org/10.1155/2018/7572430.
11. Ford CN. Evaluation and management of laryngopharyngeal reflux. JAMA. 2005;294(12):1534–40. https://doi.org/10.1001/jama.294.12.1534. Epub 2005/09/29.
12. Koufman JA. Laryngopharyngeal reflux is different from classic gastroesophageal reflux disease. Ear Nose Throat J. 2002;81(9 Suppl 2):7–9. Epub 2002/10/02.
13. Park W, Hicks DM, Khandwala F, Richter JE, Abelson TI, Milstein C, Vaezi MF. Laryngopharyngeal reflux: prospective cohort study evaluating optimal dose of proton-pump inhibitor therapy and pretherapy predictors of response. Laryngoscope. 2005;115(7):1230–8. https://doi.org/10.1097/01.MLG.0000163746.81766.45. Epub 2005/07/05.
14. Eherer AJ, Habermann W, Hammer HF, Kiesler K, Friedrich G, Krejs GJ. Effect of pantoprazole on the course of reflux-associated laryngitis: a placebo-controlled double-blind crossover study. Scand J Gastroenterol. 2003;38(5):462–7. Epub 2003/06/11.
15. El-Serag HB, Lee P, Buchner A, Inadomi JM, Gavin M, McCarthy DM. Lansoprazole treatment of patients with chronic idiopathic laryngitis: a placebo-controlled trial. Am J Gastroenterol. 2001;96(4):979–83. https://doi.org/10.1111/j.1572-0241.2001.03681.x. Epub 2001/04/24.
16. Noordzij JP, Khidr A, Evans BA, Desper E, Mittal RK, Reibel JF, Levine PA. Evaluation of omeprazole in the treatment of reflux laryngitis: a prospective, placebo-controlled, randomized, double-blind study. Laryngoscope. 2001;111(12):2147–51. https://doi.org/10.1097/00005537-200112000-00013. Epub 2002/01/22.
17. Steward DL, Wilson KM, Kelly DH, Patil MS, Schwartzbauer HR, Long JD, Welge JA. Proton pump inhibitor therapy for chronic laryngo-pharyngitis: a randomized placebo-control trial. Otolaryngol Head Neck Surg. 2004;131(4):342–50. https://doi.org/10.1016/j.otohns.2004.03.037. Epub 2004/10/07.
18. Vaezi MF. Benefit of acid-suppressive therapy in chronic laryngitis: the devil is in the details. Clin Gastroenterol Hepatol. 2010;8(9):741–2. https://doi.org/10.1016/j.cgh.2010.05.024. Epub 2010/07/14.
19. Wo JM, Koopman J, Harrell SP, Parker K, Winstead W, Lentsch E. Double-blind, placebo-controlled trial with single-dose pantoprazole for laryngopharyngeal reflux. Am J Gastroenterol 2006;101(9):1972–1978; quiz 2169. https://doi.org/10.1111/j.1572-0241.2006.00693.x . Epub 2006/09/14.
20. Lam PK, Ng ML, Cheung TK, Wong BY, Tan VP, Fong DY, Wei WI, Wong BC. Rabeprazole is effective in treating laryngopharyngeal reflux in a randomized placebo-controlled trial. Clin Gastroenterol Hepatol. 2010;8(9):770–6. https://doi.org/10.1016/j.cgh.2010.03.009. Epub 2010/03/23.
21. Reichel O, Dressel H, Wiederanders K, Issing WJ. Double-blind, placebo-controlled trial with esomeprazole for symptoms and signs associated with laryngopharyngeal reflux. Otolaryngol Head Neck Surg. 2008;139(3):414–20. https://doi.org/10.1016/j.otohns.2008.06.003. Epub 2008/08/30.
22. Kahrilas PJ, Shaheen NJ, Vaezi MF, Hiltz SW, Black E, Modlin IM, Johnson SP, Allen J, Brill JV, American Gastroenterological A. American Gastroenterological Association Medical Position Statement on the management of gastroesophageal reflux disease. Gastroenterology. 2008;135(4):1383–91, 91 e1–5. Epub 2008/09/16. doi: https://doi.org/10.1053/j.gastro.2008.08.045.
23. Barry DW, Vaezi MF. Laryngopharyngeal reflux: more questions than answers. Cleve Clin J Med. 2010;77(5):327–34. https://doi.org/10.3949/ccjm.77a.09121. Epub 2010/05/05.
24. Gooi Z, Ishman SL, Bock JM, Blumin JH, Akst LM. Changing patterns in reflux care: 10-year comparison of ABEA members. Ann Otol Rhinol Laryngol. 2015;124(12):940–6. https://doi.org/10.1177/0003489415592407. Epub 2015/06/21.
25. De Caestecker J. Prokinetics and reflux: a promise unfulfilled. Eur J Gastroenterol Hepatol. 2002;14(1):5–7.

26. Wysowski DK, Corken A, Gallo-Torres H, Talarico L, Rodriguez EM. Postmarketing reports of QT prolongation and ventricular arrhythmia in association with cisapride and Food and Drug Administration regulatory actions. Am J Gastroenterol. 2001;96(6):1698–703. https://doi.org/10.1111/j.1572-0241.2001.03927.x. Epub 2001/06/23.
27. McGlashan JA, Johnstone LM, Sykes J, Strugala V, Dettmar PW. The value of a liquid alginate suspension (Gaviscon Advance) in the management of laryngopharyngeal reflux. Eur Arch Otorhinolaryngol. 2009;266(2):243–51. https://doi.org/10.1007/s00405-008-0708-7. Epub 2008/05/29.
28. Lugaresi M, Aramini B, Daddi N, Baldi F, Mattioli S. Effectiveness of antireflux surgery for the cure of chronic cough associated with gastroesophageal reflux disease. World J Surg. 2015;39(1):208–15. https://doi.org/10.1007/s00268-014-2769-7. Epub 2014/09/06.
29. Faruqi S, Sedman P, Jackson W, Molyneux I, Morice AH. Fundoplication in chronic intractable cough. Cough. 2012;8(1):3. https://doi.org/10.1186/1745-9974-8-3. Epub 2012/07/21. PubMed PMID: 22812601; PMCID: PMC3499264.
30. Hoppo T, Komatsu Y, Jobe BA. Antireflux surgery in patients with chronic cough and abnormal proximal exposure as measured by hypopharyngeal multichannel intraluminal impedance. JAMA Surg. 2013;148(7):608–15. https://doi.org/10.1001/jamasurg.2013.1376. Epub 2013/05/24.
31. Francis DO, Goutte M, Slaughter JC, Garrett CG, Hagaman D, Holzman MD, Vaezi MF. Traditional reflux parameters and not impedance monitoring predict outcome after fundoplication in extraesophageal reflux. Laryngoscope. 2011;121(9):1902–9. https://doi.org/10.1002/lary.21897. Epub 2011/10/26.
32. Reginald H, Garrett CMG. Mechanisms of enzyme action. In: Lockwood L, editor. Biochemistry. 4th ed. Boston: Mary Finch; 2010. p. 419–48.
33. Bardhan KD, Strugala V, Dettmar PW. Reflux revisited: advancing the role of pepsin. Int J Otolaryngol. 2012;2012:646901. https://doi.org/10.1155/2012/646901. Epub 2012/01/14. PubMed PMID: 22242022; PMCID: PMC3216344.
34. Raufman JP. Gastric chief cells: receptors and signal-transduction mechanisms. Gastroenterology. 1992;102(2):699–710. Epub 1992/02/01.
35. Vijay Kumar Bansal SKG, Goswami DS, Singla S, Rahar S, Kumar S. Herbal approach to peptic ulcer disease-review. J Biosci Tec. 2009;1:52–8.
36. Dallas DC, Sanctuary MR, Qu Y, Khajavi SH, Van Zandt AE, Dyandra M, Frese SA, Barile D, German JB. Personalizing protein nourishment. Crit Rev Food Sci Nutr. 2017;57(15):3313–31. https://doi.org/10.1080/10408398.2015.1117412. Epub 2015/12/30. PubMed PMID: 26713355; PMCID: PMC4927412.
37. Tanja D, Velickovic C, Stanic-Vucinic DJ. The role of dietary phenolic compounds in protein digestion and processing technologies to improve their antinutritive properties. Comp Rev Food Sci Food Safety. 2018;17(1):82.
38. Santos-Hernandez M, Miralles B, Amigo L, Recio I. Intestinal signaling of proteins and digestion-derived products relevant to satiety. J Agric Food Chem. 2018;66(39):10123–31. https://doi.org/10.1021/acs.jafc.8b02355. Epub 2018/07/31.
39. McArthur KE, Walsh JH, Richardson CT. Soy protein meals stimulate less gastric acid secretion and gastrin release than beef meals. Gastroenterology. 1988;95(4):920–6. Epub 1988/10/01.
40. Martinucci I, Guidi G, Savarino EV, Frazzoni M, Tolone S, Frazzoni L, Fuccio L, Bertani L, Bodini G, Ceccarelli L, Savarino V, Marchi S, de Bortoli N. Vegetal and animal food proteins have a different impact in the first postprandial hour of impedance-ph analysis in patients with heartburn. Gastroenterol Res Pract. 2018;2018:7572430. https://doi.org/10.1155/2018/7572430. Epub 2018/06/01. PubMed PMID: 29849599; PMCID: PMC5933063.
41. Zalvan CH, Hu S, Greenberg B, Geliebter J. A comparison of alkaline water and mediterranean diet vs proton pump inhibition for treatment of laryngopharyngeal reflux. JAMA Otolaryngol

Head Neck Surg. 2017;143(10):1023–9. https://doi.org/10.1001/jamaoto.2017.1454. Epub 2017/09/08. PubMed PMID: 28880991; PMCID: PMC5710251.

42. Johnston N, Dettmar PW, Bishwokarma B, Lively MO, Koufman JA. Activity/stability of human pepsin: implications for reflux attributed laryngeal disease. Laryngoscope. 2007;117(6):1036–9. https://doi.org/10.1097/MLG.0b013e31804154c3. Epub 2007/04/10.
43. Johnston N, Wells CW, Samuels TL, Blumin JH. Pepsin in nonacidic refluxate can damage hypopharyngeal epithelial cells. Ann Otol Rhinol Laryngol. 2009;118(9):677–85. https://doi.org/10.1177/000348940911800913. Epub 2009/10/09.
44. Johnston N, Wells CW, Samuels TL, Blumin JH. Rationale for targeting pepsin in the treatment of reflux disease. Ann Otol Rhinol Laryngol. 2010;119(8):547–58. https://doi.org/10.1177/000348941011900808. Epub 2010/09/24.
45. Piper DW, Fenton BH. pH stability and activity curves of pepsin with special reference to their clinical importance. Gut. 1965;6(5):506–8. https://doi.org/10.1136/gut.6.5.506. Epub 1965/10/01. PubMed PMID: 4158734; PMCID: PMC1552331.
46. Johnston N, Yan JC, Hoekzema CR, Samuels TL, Stoner GD, Blumin JH, Bock JM. Pepsin promotes proliferation of laryngeal and pharyngeal epithelial cells. Laryngoscope. 2012;122(6):1317–25. https://doi.org/10.1002/lary.23307. Epub 2012/05/10. PubMed PMID: 22570308; PMCID: PMC3816638.
47. Kelly EA, Samuels TL, Johnston N. Chronic pepsin exposure promotes anchorage-independent growth and migration of a hypopharyngeal squamous cell line. Otolaryngol Head Neck Surg. 2014;150(4):618–24. https://doi.org/10.1177/0194599813517862.. Epub 2014/01/01. PubMed PMID: 24376122; PMCID: PMC4423599.
48. Pearson JP, Parikh S, Orlando RC, Johnston N, Allen J, Tinling SP, Johnston N, Belafsky P, Arevalo LF, Sharma N, Castell DO, Fox M, Harding SM, Morice AH, Watson MG, Shields MD, Bateman N, McCallion WA, van Wijk MP, Wenzl TG, Karkos PD, Belafsky PC. Review article: reflux and its consequences–the laryngeal, pulmonary and oesophageal manifestations. Conference held in conjunction with the 9th International Symposium on Human Pepsin (ISHP) Kingston-upon-Hull, UK, 21–23 April 2010. Aliment Pharmacol Ther. 2011;33 Suppl 1:1–71. Epub 2011/03/05. https://doi.org/10.1111/j.1365-2036.2011.04581.x.
49. Francis DO, Rymer JA, Slaughter JC, Choksi Y, Jiramongkolchai P, Ogbeide E, Tran C, Goutte M, Garrett CG, Hagaman D, Vaezi MF. High economic burden of caring for patients with suspected extraesophageal reflux. Gastroenterol. 2013;108(6):905–11. https://doi.org/10.1038/ajg.2013.69. Epub 2013 Apr 2.
50. Belafsky PC. PRO: empiric treatment with PPIs is not appropriate without testing. Am J Gastroenterol. 2006;101(1):6–8.. Epub 2006/01/13. https://doi.org/10.1111/j.1572-0241.2006.00448_2.x.
51. Carroll TL, Werner A, Nahikian K, Dezube A, Roth DF. Rethinking the laryngopharyngeal reflux treatment algorithm: evaluating an alternate empiric dosing regimen and considering up-front, pH-impedance, and manometry testing to minimize cost in treating suspect laryngopharyngeal reflux disease. Laryngoscope. 2017;127(Suppl 6):S1–S13. https://doi.org/10.1002/lary.26806. Epub 2017/08/27

Chapter 5
Neural Control of the Laryngopharynx

Lena C. O'Flynn, Alexis Worthley, and Kristina Simonyan

The Laryngopharynx and the Vagus Nerve

The laryngopharynx, including the hypopharynx, is a cavity that is part of the pharynx. It acts as a point of division between the larynx and esophagus and is a crucial structural component that allows swallowing of food and water as well as the production of speech. Its main structures include the posterior pharyngeal wall, pyriform sinuses, and post-cricoid area [1].

The laryngopharynx is innervated by the vagus nerve (also referred to as cranial nerve X or the vagal nerve) [2]. The vagus nerve is a significant physiological component of the parasympathetic nervous system [3]. It is the tenth of 12 pairs of cranial nerves that originate in the brain and pass through apertures in the skull to supply sense organs and muscles of the head, neck, and viscera [4, 5]. The vagus nerve contains both afferent and efferent fibers. The efferent fibers originate from motor neurons of the vagus nerve, which have their cell bodies in the medullary

---

Authors "Lena C. O'Flynn and Alexis Worthley" were contributed equally to this chapter.

L. C. O'Flynn · A. Worthley
Department of Otolaryngology – Head and Neck Surgery, Massachusetts Eye and Ear, Boston, MA, USA

Department of Neurology, Massachusetts General Hospital, Boston, MA, USA
e-mail: LenaCarolyn_Oflynn@MEEI.HARVARD.EDU; Alexis_Worthley@MEEI.Harvard.edu

K. Simonyan (✉)
Department of Otolaryngology – Head and Neck Surgery, Massachusetts Eye and Ear, Boston, MA, USA

Department of Neurology, Massachusetts General Hospital, Boston, MA, USA

Department of Otolaryngology – Head and Neck Surgery, Harvard Medical School, Boston, MA, USA
e-mail: Kristina_Simonyan@MEEI.Harvard.edu

C. H. Zalvan (ed.), *Laryngopharyngeal and Gastroesophageal Reflux*,
https://doi.org/10.1007/978-3-030-48890-1_5

nuclei and carry neural impulses from the central nervous system to different muscles in the human body for movement production. Afferent fibers of the vagus nerve originate from sensory neurons, which have their cell bodies in the vagus nerve ganglia, and carry neural impulses from sensory organs to the central nervous system. These signals travel to the thalamus, which further projects to the cortex.

The vagus nerve is the longest and most widely distributed of the cranial nerves and is unique in its asymmetrical structure. It is comprised of several branches that spread extensively throughout the face, thorax, and abdomen to supply the laryngopharynx, larynx, ear, epiglottis, tongue, trachea, bronchi, heart, and gastrointestinal tract [5]. In this chapter, we will focus on the branches of the vagus nerve innervating the neck that are important for the function of the laryngopharynx. These branches include the superior laryngeal nerve, recurrent laryngeal nerve, and pharyngeal nerve [6, 7]. These nerve fibers originate in different nuclei within the medulla and can be motor, sensory, and secretomotor [8]. We will first provide an overview of the structure and function of pertinent nuclei in the medulla. Then, we will examine the neural pathways of the three vagus nerve branches present, from their origins in the medulla to their presence in the vagus ganglia.

Vagus Nerve Nuclei

The fibers that comprise the vagus nerve have endings in different nuclei within the medulla. These nuclei include the dorsal motor nucleus, nucleus solitarius, nucleus ambiguus, and the spinal trigeminal nucleus. Each of these nuclei is a paired, bilateral, and symmetrical structure located in the vagal complex of the medulla oblongata [9].

Dorsal Motor Nucleus

The dorsal motor nucleus is located in the dorsomedial caudal part of the medulla which is a general visceral, motor, and sensory mixed center [9, 10]. It sends parasympathetic signals to the viscera, heart, bronchi, and alimentary tract via general visceral efferent fibers and receives sensory signals from the larynx, lungs, pharynx, heart, and alimentary tract. The dorsal motor nucleus also receives input from the brainstem and higher brain regions, including reticular formation, nucleus solitarius, hypothalamus, and olfactory system.

Solitary Tract Nucleus (Nucleus of the Tractus Solitarius)

The solitary tract nucleus is a vertical agglomeration of sensory nuclei embedded in the dorsomedial medulla. It serves as a primary sensory recipient of sensorimotor, viscerosensory, autonomic, and gustatory inputs. The nucleus is intersected by the solitary tract, which expands longitudinally through the medulla and is composed of fibers from the glossopharyngeal, facial, and vagus nerves [11]. The solitary tract nucleus receives sensory information from mechano- and chemoreceptors in the peripheral nervous system and is responsible for the gastrointestinal, cardiovascular, and respiratory functions [12]. After these reflexes have been initiated, signals are sent to other medullary nuclei to coordinate the action of emesis.

Additionally, the solitary tract nucleus receives information from other peripheral nerves, brainstem structures, spinal cord, and cerebellar structures. The solitary tract nucleus projects to the central nucleus of the amygdala, hippocampus, thalamus, nucleus accumbens, and the bed nucleus of stria terminalis [13]. These connections provide the solitary tract nucleus with direct influence over higher autonomic systems, the amygdala-hippocampus-entorhinal cortex pathway of the limbic system, and extrapyramidal motor systems [14, 15].

Nucleus Ambiguus

The nucleus ambiguus is located in the medullary reticular formation and contributes to the efferent portion of the vagus and glossopharyngeal nerves. The nucleus ambiguus provides motor innervation to the pharynx, palate, and larynx for phonation and swallowing [16, 17].

Spinal Trigeminal Nucleus

The spinal trigeminal nucleus is located in the dorsal pons and receives sensory information regarding deep touch, temperature, and pain from the ear, the posterior cranial fossa, and the mucosa of the larynx [16]. It is a minor contributor to the vagus nerve and receives information from the trigeminal, facial, and glossopharyngeal nerves. The spinal trigeminal nucleus projects to the medial thalamus [18].

Cranial Nerve Fibers

There are seven types of cranial nerve fibers that project from nuclei within the medulla. These fibers include general visceral efferents and afferents, special visceral efferents and afferents, and somatic efferents and afferents [19]. Of these seven types of nerve fibers, four are constituents of the vagus nerve: general somatic afferents, general visceral afferents and efferents, and special visceral efferents [18].

The general somatic afferent fibers of the vagus nerve receive sensory information from the pharynx, larynx, trachea, esophagus, external auditory meatus, and auricle [18, 20, 21]. The fibers have their cell bodies in the superior ganglion. Signals travel up through the jugular foramen to the spinal trigeminal nucleus [16, 21].

General visceral afferent fibers relay pain or reflex sensations. They also transmit sensory information from the pharynx, larynx, trachea, esophagus, heart, lungs, stomach, and thoracoabdominal viscera down to the splenic flexure, aortic arch baroreceptors, and aortic body. Information in the vagus transmitted by way of general visceral afferent fibers relays to the solitary tract nucleus through the nodose ganglion [16, 20–22].

General visceral efferent fibers originate in the dorsal motor vagal nucleus and are relevant to visceral autonomic innervation [16]. These fibers send parasympathetic signals to the lungs and heart and innervate gastrointestinal smooth muscles and glands [10]. They also deliver secretomotor innervation to pharyngeal and laryngeal mucosa, the ganglia in the walls of thoracic organs, and esophageal, hepatic, celiac, gastric, and celiac plexus [8, 20].

Special visceral efferent fibers, also called branchiomotor fibers, provide motor innervation for phonation and swallowing. They originate in the nucleus ambiguus, specifically supplying striated musculature of the soft palate, pharynx, larynx, and branchial arches via the vagus nerve [16, 20].

The Vagus Nerve Ganglia

The different nerve fibers emerge from each vagal nucleus at the postero-lateral sulcus and unite to form a single trunk at the lateral aspect of the medulla. This trunk leaves the skull through the jugular foramen [8]. The nerve forms two consecutive ganglia that are exclusively sensory and contain somatic, general visceral, and special visceral afferent neurons [18]. They are separated by the jugular foramen. These ganglia are bilateral structures that create the right and left vagus nerve and are considered part of the peripheral nervous system.

Superior (Jugular) Ganglion

The superior ganglion provides sensory innervation to the auricular and meningeal branches of the vagus nerve [10]. In doing so, the structure communicates with the glossopharyngeal nerve, accessory nerve, the sympathetic trunk, and the superior cervical sympathetic ganglion [18].

Inferior (Nodose) Ganglion

The inferior ganglion is larger than the superior ganglion and is located below the superior ganglion. It contains most of the visceral afferent cell bodies and provides innervation to the visceral branches. This structure communicates with the hypoglossal nerve, the superior sympathetic ganglion, and the loop between the first and second cervical nerves [10, 18].

Neck Branches of the Vagus Nerve

Recurrent Laryngeal Nerve

The recurrent laryngeal nerve contains sensory, motor, and autonomic fibers [23]. Specifically, the recurrent laryngeal nerve is comprised of special visceral efferents and general visceral afferents, and thus it receives innervation from the nucleus ambiguus and sends information from sensory stimuli to the nucleus solitarius. Special visceral afferent fibers innervate laryngeal muscles, while general visceral afferent fibers supply the subglottic mucosa [20, 24].

Superior Laryngeal Nerve

The superior laryngeal nerve is divided up into an internal and external branch. It is comprised of special visceral efferent and general visceral afferent fibers, meaning it receives innervation from the nucleus ambiguus and sends information from sensory stimuli to the nucleus solitarius, respectively. Special visceral efferent fibers comprise the external branch of the superior laryngeal nerve and innervate the cricothyroid muscle. General visceral afferent fibers comprise the internal branch and supply the supraglottic mucosa [20, 24].

Pharyngeal Branches

The pharyngeal branches of the vagus nerve supply the pharynx. They contain both sensory and motor fibers. These branches are made of special visceral efferent fibers and general visceral afferent fibers. Therefore, they receive innervation from the nucleus ambiguus and supply sensory information to the spinal trigeminal nucleus, respectively [18, 20, 25].

Superior Cardiac Nerve

The superior cardiac nerve supplies the heart. It is comprised of general visceral afferent fibers. Therefore, it sends information from sensory stimuli to the nucleus solitarius [18, 20].

Conflict of Interest No authors have any pertinent disclosures or conflicts of interest.

References

1. Emura F, Baron TH, Gralnek IM. The pharynx: examination of an area too often ignored during upper endoscopy. Gastrointest Endosc. 2013;78(1):143–9.
2. Mu L, Sanders I. Sensory nerve supply of the human Oro- and laryngopharynx: a preliminary study. Anat Rec. 2000;258(4):14.
3. Breit S, et al. Vagus nerve as modulator of the brain-gut Axis in psychiatric and inflammatory disorders. Front Psych. 2018;9:44.
4. Chavez-Barba O, et al. Imaging anatomy of the cranial nerves using 3.0 Tesla MRI: a practical review for clinicians. Gaceta Medica De Mexico. 2011;147(6):11.
5. Morani A, Ramani N, Wesolowski J. Skull Base, orbits, temporal bone, and cranial nerves: anatomy on MR imaging. Magn Reson Imaging Clin N Am. 2011;19(3):17.
6. Stephens RE, Wendel KH, Addington WR. Anatomy of the internal branch of the superior laryngeal nerve. Clin Anat. 1999;12(2):79–83.
7. De Gama BZ, et al. The sympathetic and parasympathetic contributions to the cardiac plexus: a fetal study. Int J Morphol. 2012;30(4):7.
8. Ellis H, Feldman S, Harrop-Griffiths W. Anatomy for anaesthetists. 8th ed. Malden: Blackwell Science; 2004.
9. Mussa BM, Verberne AJ. The dorsal motor nucleus of the vagus and regulation of pancreatic secretory function. Exp Physiol. 2013;98(1):25–37.
10. Berthoud HR, Neuhuber WL. Functional and chemical anatomy of the afferent vagal system. Auton Neurosci. 2000;85(1–3):1–17.
11. Hayakawa T, et al. Subnuclear distribution of afferents from the oral, pharyngeal and laryngeal regions in the nucleus tractus solitarii of the rat: a study using transganglionic transport of cholera toxin. Neurosci Res. 2001;39(2):221–32.
12. Cutsforth-Gregory JK, Benarroch EE. Nucleus of the solitary tract, medullary reflexes, and clinical implications. Neurology. 2017;88(12):1187–96.
13. Dietrich S, et al. A novel transcutaneous vagus nerve stimulation leads to brainstem and cerebral activations measured by functional MRI. Biomed Tech (Berl). 2008;53(3):104–11.
14. Kraus T, et al. BOLD fMRI deactivation of limbic and temporal brain structures and mood enhancing effect by transcutaneous vagus nerve stimulation. J Neural Transm (Vienna). 2007;114(11):1485–93.
15. Groves DA, Bowman EM, Brown VJ. Recordings from the rat locus coeruleus during acute vagal nerve stimulation in the anaesthetised rat. Neurosci Lett. 2005;379(3):174–9.
16. Hirsch WL, et al. Anatomy of the brainstem: correlation of in vitro MR images with histologic sections. AJNR Am J Neuroradiol. 1989;10(5):923–8.
17. Simonyan K, Horwitz B. Laryngeal motor cortex and control of speech in humans. Neuroscientist. 2011;17(2):197–208.
18. Standring S, Borley NR, Gray H. Gray's anatomy: the anatomical basis of clinical practice. 40th ed., anniversary edition. Edinburgh: Churchill Livingstone/Elsevier; 2008.
19. Sonne J, Lopez-Ojeda W. Neuroanatomy, cranial nerve, in StatPearls. 2019. Treasure Island (FL).
20. Binder D, Sonne D, Fischbein N. Cranial nerves: anatomy, pathology, imaging. New York: Thieme; 2010.
21. Naidich T, et al. Duvernoy's atlas of the human brain stem and cerebellum: high-field MRI: surface anatomy, internal structure, vascularization and 3D sectional anatomy. Vienna: Springer Vienna; 2009.
22. Li BY, et al. Unmyelinated visceral afferents exhibit frequency dependent action potential broadening while myelinated visceral afferents do not. Neurosci Lett. 2007;421(1):62–6.
23. Dilworth TF. The nerves of the human larynx. J Anat. 1921;56(1):4.
24. Monkhouse S. Cranial nerves: functional anatomy. Cambridge, UK, New York: Cambridge University Press; 2006.
25. Yoshida Y, et al. Sensory innervation of the pharynx and larynx. Am J Med. 2000;108(Suppl 4a):51S–61S.

Chapter 6
Peripheral Neural Regulation of the Laryngopharynx

Caroline Hudson and Kenneth W. Altman

Peripheral Neural Regulation of the Laryngopharynx

Peripheral Course of the Vagus Nerve

Peripherally, the vagus nerve exits the skull through the posterolateral portion of the jugular foramen called the pars vascularis and then runs with the internal carotid artery within the carotid sheath, with the artery lying anteromedial to the nerve and the jugular vein lying laterally. In the upper mediastinum, the right and left vagus nerves take different courses. The right vagus nerve crosses the right subclavian artery anteriorly and then travels into the adipose tissue behind the innominate vessels. It then courses medially and posteriorly toward the right side of the trachea. Then, the nerve travels superiorly, posterior to the hilum of the right lung and then medially toward the esophagus. Here, it forms the esophageal plexus with the left vagus nerve. The left vagus nerve descends anterior to the left subclavian artery, entering the thorax between subclavian and left common carotid arteries. It descends on the left side of the aortic arch and travels posterior to the phrenic nerve. It then travels superiorly posterior to the hilum of the left lung and traverses inferomedially to reach the esophagus and join the right vagus nerve to form the esophageal plexus [1].

The vagus nerve has several branches, and in this section, we will focus on the branches of the vagus nerve located in the neck and highlight their anatomic

C. Hudson
Baylor College of Medicine, Department of Otolaryngology – Head & Neck Surgery, Houston, TX, USA
e-mail: caroline.hudson@bcm.edu

K. W. Altman (✉)
Geisinger Health System, Geisinger Commonwealth School of Medicine, Department of Otolaryngology – Head & Neck Surgery, Danville, PA, USA
e-mail: kaltman@geisinger.edu

C. H. Zalvan (ed.), *Laryngopharyngeal and Gastroesophageal Reflux*,
https://doi.org/10.1007/978-3-030-48890-1_6

pathways. These branches are the recurrent laryngeal nerve, superior laryngeal nerve, pharyngeal branches, and superior cardiac nerve [2].

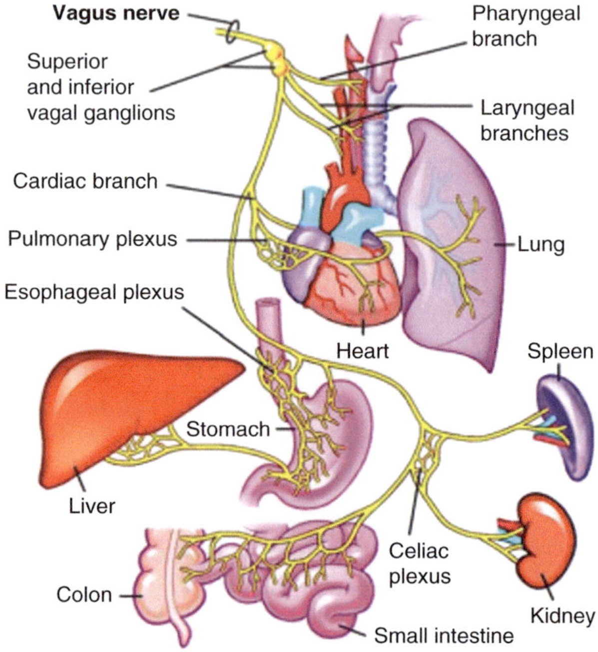

Illustration of the VN anatomy. (Retrieved October 7, 2019 from http://medical-dictionary.thefreedictionary.com/vagus+nerve)

Recurrent Laryngeal Nerve

All intrinsic laryngeal muscles apart from the cricothyroid muscle are innervated by the recurrent laryngeal nerve, also known as the inferior laryngeal nerve. The right recurrent laryngeal nerve branches from the vagus nerve just distal to the right subclavian artery. It travels superiorly in the tracheoesophageal groove to enter the larynx between the esophagus and the cricopharyngeus muscle. The left recurrent laryngeal nerve has a similar course as the right but remains anterior to the subclavian artery and loops around the arch of the aorta on the left side, distal to the ligamentum arteriosum at the level of the aorto-pulmonary window. From this point, it ascends along the left tracheoesophageal groove toward the larynx. Both the left and right recurrent laryngeal nerves enter the larynx through the inferior constrictor muscles at the level of the cricothyroid joint. The nerve passes under the ligament of Berry before entering the larynx [3].

Superior Laryngeal Nerve

The superior laryngeal nerve branches from the vagus nerve near the inferior half of the nodose ganglion, roughly 40 mm above the carotid bifurcation and 36 mm below the jugular foramen. It then travels inferiorly, dividing into the internal and external branches. The internal branch pierces the thyrohyoid membrane and provides sensory innervation to the supraglottis, whereas the external branch travels to and innervates the cricothyroid muscle. There is some variation in the course of the superior laryngeal nerve, specifically relating to the superior constrictor as well as the superior thyroid vessels. At the tip of the hyoid, the superior laryngeal nerve divides into internal and external branches. The internal branch, which supplies sensory innervation to the majority of the supraglottic mucosa, has three divisions: first, middle, and inferior. The external branch travels with the superior thyroid vessels inferiorly to the inferior pharyngeal constrictor, supplying the cricothyroid muscle. The ramus communicans, also known as the nerve of Galen, connects the superior and the recurrent laryngeal nerves. It provides motor innervation to the tracheoesophageal mucosa and smooth muscle [4].

Superior Cardiac Nerve

The superior cardiac nerve has two to three branches. These branches communicate with the sympathetic fibers.

Pharyngeal Branches

The pharyngeal branches, containing both sensory and motor fibers, arise from the inferior ganglion. The motor branches cross between the external and internal carotid artery and travel to the middle constrictor muscle and then reach the pharyngeal plexus, which is formed by the glossopharyngeal nerve and the sympathetic chain. Branches from the pharyngeal plexus supply the pharyngeal mucous membranes and muscles excluding the tensor palatini. Vagal fibers from the pharyngeal plexus also form the intercarotid plexus, located at the carotid bifurcation. These fibers mediate impulses sent from carotid body chemoreceptors [5, 6].

Laryngopharyngeal Sensitivity Receptors

Sensory receptors are the starting point for neural activity [7, 8]. The receptors outlined in this section include the following:

- *TRPV1*: transient receptor/ion channel potential vanilloid 1, stimulated by acids, protons and capsaicin
- *TRPA1*: transient receptor potential ankyrin, stimulated by cigarette smoke and toluene diisocyanate
- *Cough receptors*: myelinated nerves with a conduction velocity of 5 m/s
- *RAR*: rapidly adapting receptors, a type of mechanoreceptor
- *SAR*: slowly adapting receptors, sense stretch
- *C-fiber afferent nerves*: small diameter, slow-conducting nerve (velocity of <1–2 m/s)

C-Fibers

The majority of bronchopulmonary vagal afferent nerves are unmyelinated C-fibers. In addition to their conduction velocity (<1 m/s), airway vagal afferent C-fibers are distinguished from lung stretch receptors in a number of ways. C-fibers are relatively insensitive to mechanical stimulation and lung inflation. C-fibers also are sensitive to capsaicin and bradykinin and activate ion channels, including TRPV1 (e.g., capsaicin, protons) and TRPA1 (e.g., ozone, allyl isothiocyanate).

Other inflammatory mediators and environmental irritants that selectively activate C-fibers include prostaglandin E2, ozone, nicotine, adenosine, and serotonin. Bronchopulmonary afferent C-fiber subtypes have been described in several species, with subtypes being differentiated by their ganglionic origin (nodose vs. jugular), sites of termination in the airway/lungs, chemical sensitivity, neurochemistry, and reflexes initiated by their activation. It is unknown whether similar physiologic distinctions between bronchial and pulmonary afferent C-fibers can be defined in humans. Neurokinins, such as substance P, are uniquely expressed by airway C-fibers in animals.

Mechanoreceptor: Widdicombe Cough Receptors

More than 50 years ago, John Widdicombe described a type of myelinated vagal afferent nerves innervating the airway that play an essential role in cough reflexes of anesthetized cats. He called these afferent nerves "cough receptors," a flawed term, but one that has persisted in the literature since. Widdicombe's claims have been substantiated in multiple studies since, and it is now well-established that, in addition to C-fibers, a subset of myelinated vagal afferent mechanoreceptors plays an essential role in laryngeal sensitivity. Cough receptors differ from C-fibers and lung stretch receptors by their axon conduction speed. Cough receptor axon conduction velocity is 5 m/s, which is faster than C-fibers (<2 m/s) but slower than lung stretch receptors (15 m/s). These mechanoreceptors also differentiate themselves with their insensitivity to capsaicin, as they do not normally express the ion channels TRPV1 or TRPA1. Cough receptors are, however, activated by protons, possibly through expression of acid-sensing ion channels.

Widdicombe, at various times since his seminal work, referred to cough receptors by other terms, including irritant receptors and rapidly adapting receptors (RARs). Although cough receptors are myelinated and adapt rapidly to a tactile rather than stretch-like mechanical stimulation, cough receptors are simply RARs that innervate the extrapulmonary airways. RARs primarily innervate the intrapulmonary airways, whereas cough receptor terminations are found exclusively in the extrapulmonary airways (larynx, trachea, mainstem bronchi). Furthermore, unlike RARs, cough receptors are unresponsive to a wide variety of spasmogens, irritants, and autacoids that induce airway smooth muscle contraction and decrease lung compliance (e.g., histamine, ATP, methacholine, substance P, leukotriene C4, neurokinin A, 5-hydroxytryptamine, and adenosine). All of these stimuli have been shown to activate RARs.

RAR/SAR

Rapidly adapting receptors (RARs) and slowly adapting receptors (SARs) are lung stretch receptors characterized by their responses to sustained lung inflation and deflation. RARs and SARs are both activated by sustained lung inflation, but RARs are active predominately during the dynamic phase of lung inflation, whereas SARs continue firing throughout lung distension.

Receptor	Stimuli	Myelinated?	Conduction velocity (m/s)
TRPV1	Acids, protons, and capsaicin	N/A	N/A
TRPA1	Cigarette smoke, toluene diisocyanate	N/A	N/A
Cough receptors	Protons	Yes	5
RAR	Wide variety of spasmogens, irritants, and autacoids. Lung inflation	Yes	4–18
SAR	Lung inflation	Yes	15
C-fibers	Capsaicin and bradykinin, protons, nicotine, and the TRPA1 agonists cinnamaldehyde and AITC	Mostly no	<1

The precise anatomy of RAR terminations in the airway wall is not well understood. Studies suggest that RARs terminate in or beneath the epithelium in the intrapulmonary airways. This location might explain RAR sensitivity patterns to lung collapse and deflation. However, RAR responsiveness to alterations in dynamic lung compliance also suggests a likely association with airway smooth muscle. RARs may, thus, be better thought of as dynamic airway mechanoreceptors. SARs are highly sensitive to the mechanical forces imposed upon the lung during breathing. SAR activity sharply increases during inspiration and peaks just before the initiation of expiration. SARs are therefore thought to be the primary afferent fibers involved in the Hering-Breuer inflation reflex, which terminates inspiration when the lungs are adequately inflated and initiates expiration. Anatomically, SAR terminal structures have been identified in the intrapulmonary airways and lungs of rabbits. These terminals assume a complex and varying position within the airway wall but are found primarily in the peripheral airways (associated with alveoli or bronchioles).

Proposed Mechanisms of Hypersensitivity

Laryngeal sensitivity can be related to a type of sensory neuropathy. The apparent paradox of hypersensitivity is that sensory neuropathy is generally thought of as a reduction of nerve sensitivity, yet the clinical presentation is that of a hyperexcitable condition. Neurogenic cough, a type of hypersensitivity, often presents after a viral infection, so it is helpful to consider the evidence and mechanisms of virally induced nerve injury in the larynx and elsewhere [9, 10]. In otolaryngology, strong anecdotal evidence supports a viral causality for sudden sensorineural hearing loss, vestibular neuronitis, facial palsy, and idiopathic vocal paralysis. Association with herpes simplex virus, varicella zoster, Epstein-Barr virus, cytomegalovirus, and human immunodeficiency virus (HIV) have all been documented. The mechanism of injury causing a neuropathy in these and other conditions has been investigated, and the thought is damage may occur indirectly to the nerve through its blood supply, as is the case with varicella zoster viral-induced optic neuropathy and its association with temporal artery vasculitis and hepatitis B virus-induced Guillain-Barre syndrome and its link to mononeuritis multiplex. Viral infection may also have a direct effect on the nervous system, as with cases of HIV peripheral neuropathy where viral RNA has been seen in the spinal cord, as well as in hepatitis C virus infection found in diffuse tissues throughout the body.

Multiple factors can act concurrently to induce airway hypersensitivity, including topical airway infectious agents, viscosity of the airway mucus, inflammatory cytokines, gene regulation producing pathologically altered mucus, and the temperature and pH of the airway surface [11, 12].

Activity within the submucosa, including vascular dilation and smooth muscle constriction, can affect sensory receptor excitability. Neurokinin and substance P have been shown to affect C-fiber and cough receptor excitability in guinea pigs, though this has not yet been documented in humans [13].

Laryngopharyngeal Sensitivity: Etiologies Beyond Reflux

Functional laryngeal disorder may be considered a diagnosis of exclusion in patients who do not have objective findings of reflux on pH testing and in whom other etiologies of laryngeal dysfunction – such as Parkinson disease, multiple sclerosis, amyotrophic lateral sclerosis, essential tremor, and dystonia – have been ruled out. Laryngeal hypersensitivity can be a common feature of neuropathic laryngeal pathologies with overlapping symptoms such as paradoxical vocal fold movement, globus pharyngeus, chronic cough, and muscle tension dysphonia [14, 15]. Certain events have been proposed as possibly pre-disposing people to develop laryngeal sensitization, such as an aspiration event, history of intubation, upper respiratory tract infection, asthma, and chronic rhinosinusitis.

Quantitative testing such as hypertonic saline challenge, capsaicin cough reflex sensitivity, acoustic voice testing, timed swallow test, cough frequency monitor, and the voice stress test have been shown to be significantly impaired in patients with functional laryngeal disorder. Below is a brief description of these quantitative voice measures.

The *hypertonic saline challenge test* acts as a physical stimulus to the walls of the airway, aimed at causing bronchoconstriction to assess airway hyperresponsiveness in patients with normal spirometry.

The *capsaicin cough reflex test* uses solutions of capsaicin in varying concentrations delivered in a nebulized fashion aimed at triggering an airway response to assess airway dynamics.

The *timed swallow test* measures the swallowing speed in ml/s and is highly sensitive and moderately specific for neurogenic etiologies of dysphagia.

The *acoustic voice test* consists of recording a speaking or singing voice and measuring acoustic parameters including pitch, loudness, and range with computer software. Cough frequency monitors are objective tools to measure the frequency and quality of cough using microphones. *Voice stress testing* aims to assess the frequency of the voice when certain questions are posed to the patient in order to make predictions on that person's thoughts and behaviors.

Multiple studies have tried to evaluate the role of laryngeal hypersensitivity with tests using a combination of patient-reported outcome measures and direct testing using laryngoscopy or laryngeal electromyography [16]; however, use of these tests in the clinical setting is limited by variable sensitivity and specificity, as well as lack of access to equipment. Therefore, diagnosis of laryngeal sensitivity is often made clinically after exclusion of other etiologies.

The symptoms of laryngopharyngeal reflux can be sensory alone, a combination of sensory and true reflux exacerbation, or reflux alone. These sensory changes are the main reason the gold standard remains elusive. Testing focused on reflux alone will not capture the alterations in sensory receptors, and addressing these sensory changes can be critical for controlling symptom severity.

There is also evidence to suggest that viral infection may indirectly upregulate the cough reflex via the sensitizing effects of cytokines and inflammatory cells induced by the infecting virus [17]. Viral infection of bronchial cells has been demonstrated to induce upregulation of acid (ASIC) receptors, TRPV1 and TRPA1 channels potentially increasing sensitivity [18]. In addition, a direct sensitizing effect on afferent nerves of the airway needs to be considered also. Sensory nerves themselves have been shown to express the viral receptor ICAM-1, in addition to toll-like receptors (TLRs), which have an integral role in host immunologic defense during microbial infection. Reducing triggers, such as nasal drainage and reflux, can improve cough severity by decreasing stimulation of a hypersensitive laryngopharynx [19]. More research is needed to elucidate precisely how viruses may exert a direct effect on human airway sensory nerves and consequently laryngeal hypersensitivity.

Conflict of Interest Neither author has any pertinent disclosures or conflicts of interest.

References

1. Dankbaar JW, Pameijer FA. Vocal cord paralysis: anatomy, imaging and pathology. Insights Imaging. 2014;5(6):743–51. https://doi.org/10.1007/s13244-014-0364-y.
2. Doty RW. Influence of stimulus pattern on reflex deglutition. Am J Physiol Legacy Content. 1951;166(1):142–58.
3. Steele CM, Miller AJ. Sensory input pathways and mechanisms in swallowing: a review. Dysphagia. 2010;25(4):323–33. https://doi.org/10.1007/s00455-010-9301-5.
4. Orestes MI, Chhetri DK. Superior laryngeal nerve injury: effects, clinical findings, prognosis, and management options. Curr Opin Otolaryngol Head Neck Surg. 2014;22(6):439–43. https://doi.org/10.1097/MOO.0000000000000097.
5. Yuan H, Silberstein SD. Vagus nerve and vagus nerve stimulation, a comprehensive review: part I. Headache. 2015;56(1):71–8. https://doi.org/10.1111/head.12647.
6. Hejal R, Strohl KP, Erokwu B, Cherniack NS, Haxhiu MA. Pathways and mechanisms involved in neural control of laryngeal submucosal gland secretion. J Appl Physiol. 1993;75(6):2347–52. https://doi.org/10.1152/jappl.1993.75.6.2347.
7. Canning BJ, Chang AB, Bolser DC, et al. Anatomy and neurophysiology of cough: CHEST guideline and expert panel report. Chest. 2014;146(6):1633–48. https://doi.org/10.1378/chest.14-1481.
8. Du Q, Liao Q, Chen C, Yang X, Xie R, Xu J. The role of transient receptor potential vanilloid 1 in common diseases of the digestive tract and the cardiovascular and respiratory system. Front Physiol. 2019;10:1064.
9. Altman KW, Noordzij JP, Rosen CA, Cohen S, Sulica L. Neurogenic cough. Laryngoscope. 2015;125(7):1675–81. https://doi.org/10.1002/lary.25186.
10. Chung KF, McGarvey L, Mazzone SB. Chronic cough as a neuropathic disorder. Lancet Respir Med. 2013;1(5):414–22. https://doi.org/10.1016/s2213-2600(13)70043-2.
11. Javorkova N, Varechova S, Pecova R, Tatar M, Balaz D, Demeter M, Hyrdel R, Kollarik M. Acidification of the oesophagus acutely increases the cough sensitivity in patients with gastro-oesophageal reflux and chronic cough. Neurogastroenterol Motility. 2018;20:119–24. https://doi.org/10.1111/j.1365-2982.2007.01020.x.
12. Johnston N, Yan JC, Hoekzema CR, et al. Pepsin promotes proliferation of laryngeal and pharyngeal epithelial cells. Laryngoscope. 2012;122(6):1317–25. https://doi.org/10.1002/lary.23307.
13. Canning BJ. Afferent nerves regulating the cough reflex: mechanisms and mediators of cough in disease. Otolaryngol Clin N Am. 2010;43(1):15–vii. https://doi.org/10.1016/j.otc.2009.11.012.
14. Patel DA, Blanco M, Vaezi MF. Laryngopharyngeal reflux and functional laryngeal disorder: perspective and common practice of the general gastroenterologist. Gastroenterol Hepatol (N Y). 2018;14(9):512–20.

15. Ryan NM, Vertigan AE, Gibson PG. Chronic cough and laryngeal dysfunction improve with specific treatment of cough and paradoxical vocal fold movement. Cough. 2009;5:4. https://doi.org/10.1186/1745-9974-5-4. Published 2009 Mar 17.
16. Zalvan CH, Yuen E, Thomas AM, Benson BE. Laryngeal electromyographic findings in a cohort of recalcitrant chronic neurogenic cough patients. J Voice. 2020:S0892-1997(19)30633-2. doi: 10.1016/j.jvoice.2020.01.024. Online ahead of print. J Voice. 2020. PMID: 32146037.
17. Undem BJ, Zaccone E, McGarvey L, Mazzone SB. Neural dysfunction following respiratory viral infection as a cause of chronic cough hypersensitivity. Pulm Pharmacol Ther. 2015;33:52–6. https://doi.org/10.1016/j.pupt.2015.06.006.
18. Omar S, Clarke R, Abdullah H, et al. Respiratory virus infection up-regulates TRPV1, TRPA1 and ASICS3 receptors on airway cells. PLoS One. 2017;12(2):e0171681. https://doi.org/10.1371/journal.pone.0171681. eCollection 2017
19. Zalvan CH, Berzofsky C, Tiwari R, Geliebter J. Trigger reduction prior to systemic drugs for neurogenic chronic cough. Laryngoscope. 2019;129(1):198–202.

Chapter 7
Peripheral and Central Hypersensitivity

Craig H. Zalvan

The etiology of LPR is likely multifactorial, representing a series of events and factors that culminate in the onset and propagation of the disease state. The diagnosis of LPR rests in the constellation of presenting symptoms. Symptoms represent sensory information conveyed by peripheral stimulation and central processing that result in the "sensation" of a stimuli. During this peripheral and central stimulation, neuromodulation can take place leading to peripheral and central hypersensitivity leading to a heightened perception of sensory symptoms potentially triggering exaggerated motor responses. The upper aerodigestive tract contains a large array of peripheral receptors with cross communication between neuronal endings through ion channels. Local hypersensitivity can be stimulated by inflammation through viral upper respiratory infection, reflux, extreme temperature exposure, chemical exposure, repetitive trauma, allergens, and other infectious sources. Specifically, transient receptor potential (TRP) ion channels TRPV1 and TRPA1 mediate sensory responses to inflammation, thermal change, and chemical exposure [1]. Viral infection of respiratory cells has been shown to demonstrate upregulation of these various TRP ion channels and more consequential to reflux disease, the acid sensing ion channel, ASIC3 receptors, postulated to result in a hypersensitive state from both upregulation of receptor expression and potentiation of peripheral stimulation through adjacent neuronal signaling [2]. These ASIC3 receptors are transmembrane ion channels located throughout the peripheral and central nervous system and are activated by a decrease in the extracellular pH. Increased tissue inflammation,

C. H. Zalvan (✉)
The Institute for Voice and Swallowing Disorders, Phelps Hospital, Northwell Health, Sleepy Hollow, NY, USA

Professor of Otolaryngology at the Donald and Barbara Zucker School of Medicine at Hofstra/Northwell, Phelps Hospital Campus, Sleepy Hollow, NY, USA

Communication, Speech Department at Mercy College, Dobbs Ferry, NY, USA

ENT and Allergy Associates, LLP; Voice and Swallow Division, Tarrytown, NY, USA
e-mail: czalvan@entandallergy.com; https://www.westchestervoicedoc.com

C. H. Zalvan (ed.), *Laryngopharyngeal and Gastroesophageal Reflux*,
https://doi.org/10.1007/978-3-030-48890-1_7

localized drop in pH, and viral mediation can upregulate these ion channels within nocioreceptors, proprioceptors, thermoreceptors, and chemoreceptors leading to increased neuronal sensitivity to basal and subclinical stimulation as well as heightened response to pathological stimulation. Chronic, recurrent inflammation from LPR can also induce these peripheral changes due to repeat stimulation leading to hypersensitive mucosal tissue. Ultimately, in a state of hypersensitivity, even exposure to normal basal levels of acidic material can produce symptoms of LPR. Even stimulation from other materials, basal amounts of sinus drainage, oral secretions, food, and drinking can lead to chronic symptoms of LPR such as globus, post-nasal drip (PND), and repeat throat clearing, symptoms commonly diagnosed (or misdiagnosed) as LPR. Acidic food and beverages consumed are likely as important in LPR symptomatology as is true reflux. Acid is acid, and stimulation from either direction, either consumed or refluxed, can result in sensory receptor activation. Humans have PND with at least a liter of sinus and oral secretions "dripping" daily. In the absence of a pathological sinus state such as allergy or sinusitis, both of which would have significant other concomitant symptoms and findings, the normal basal rate of drainage can be "sensed" in those with a hypersensitive pharynx. Evidence of mechanoreceptor sensitization following inflammation supports the notion that basal stimulation can lead to an exaggerated response [3]. Chronic reflux exposure of the laryngopharyngeal tissues can theoretically induce these states of hypersensitivity leading to the chronic symptoms of throat clearing, globus, and PND sensation, even in the absence of pathological reflux exposure. Conversely, pathological reflux in the setting of hypersensitivity can provoke an exaggerated sensory stimulation.

Repeat inflammation locally results in elevated levels of inflammatory cytokines leading to increases in local neurotransmitters. This persistent peripheral inflammation can result in second-order neuronal hyperexcitability within the brainstem [4]. This central hyperexcitability can then lead to efferent discharge resulting in many of the sequelae of LPR such as laryngospasm, coughing, throat clearing, and vocal fold dysfunction. Other receptors, such as the rapidly adapting receptors (RAR) within the airways and c-fibers, when stimulated, can lead to discharge of the efferent parasympathetic reflexes resulting in cough [5]. Vagal afferents traveling through the nodose ganglia to the brainstem converge on the brainstem nucleus of the solitary tract. Various subpopulations of neurons project to other cranial nerve centers. Lacrimal glands, nasal cavity glands, and other cranial nerve-controlled functions can be reflexively activated by peripheral stimuli of the aerodigestive tract, potentially adding to the plethora of symptoms patients with LPR describe [6]. Similarly, patients with chronic neurogenic cough can exhibit a hypersensitive laryngeal state that when stimulated results in coughing spasms often associated with epiphora, rhinorrhea, sneeze, acute vocal strain from laryngospasm, and nausea with or without vomiting. These symptoms can follow the onset of a neurogenic cough suggesting concurrent brainstem efferent discharge. Electromyographic data of thyroarytenoid muscles in patients with refractory chronic cough suggests bilateral vagal neuropathy is possibly present from either a bilateral peripheral event or a more centrally mediated insult [7].

The sensory feedback of the laryngopharyngeal tissues is far more complex than vagally mediated afferents and reflexes and includes contributions from the sensory pathways of the olfactory, trigeminal, and glossopharyngeal nerves. Repeat stimulation of these neural endings, triggered by the many stimuli, such as chemical, temperature, and pressure (food and mucus) can result in chronic peripheral stimulation leading to central hypersensitization causing the symptoms of globus, burning, and throat discomfort.

Reflux hypersensitivity is not limited to the laryngopharynx. The esophagus, also innervated by the vagus nerve, can demonstrate similar hypersensitivity changes resulting in a range of symptoms that mimic those of true GERD. With prolonged acid exposure times and increased acid production in the setting of normal physical findings, NERD, or non-erosive reflux disease, can be considered. In these instances, like in the laryngopharynx, heightened sensitivity to acid can result in symptoms of GERD. In cases where there are normal acid exposure times, symptoms can also be encountered in states of hypersensitivity, referred to as functional heartburn [8]. As with the laryngopharynx, upregulation of TRPV1 channels has been demonstrated in the functional, hypersensitive esophagus. Protease-activated receptor 2, another acid sensing receptor, has similarly been shown to be upregulated [9].

Chronic pain syndromes suggest a model and mechanism similar to the hypersensitive laryngopharynx. Repeat stimulation at the peripheral level from injury or inflammation results in neuronal upregulation of receptors and neuronal hypersensitivity ultimately culminating in central modulation and a central state of heightened sensitivity with concurrent sensory, motor, and emotional response. Initial insult, exposure to inflammatory agents, and upregulation of peripheral receptors can result in central hypersensitivity through altered central processing, psychological influences with alterations of the limbic system, and alteration of autonomic output [10, 11]. Repetitive peripheral stimulation or acute inflammation-induced peripheral hypersensitivity can lead to both peripheral and central allodynia, or exaggerated pain response, thermal hypersensitivity, paresthesia, and areas of hyperalgesia throughout the laryngopharynx and esophagus.

Perhaps a more descriptive nomenclature should be applied to patients presenting with LPR symptomatology, namely, LPSS or laryngopharyngeal sensory syndrome. LPSS is the constellation of "symptoms" such as globus, throat clearing, PND sensation, tickle/trigger sensations, burning, altered taste, and mucus sensation that many patients present to the otolaryngologist. Many are diagnosed with LPR given the similarity to the typical symptoms of LPR; however, it is quite probable that many of these patients have a hypersensitive state and thus LPSS. LPR is thus likely overdiagnosed in a significant portion of these patients. These heightened sensory states may be involved in laryngospasm, vocal cord dysfunction, and chronic neurogenic cough with episodes triggered by multiple types of exposure, of which reflux is included. Even in patients with LPR, according to the model of hypersensitivity, they too likely have a state of LPSS leading to more pronounced and bothersome symptoms.

What remains to be determined is the initial cause or trigger of LPR and LPSS. Historically, patients often report the onset of LPR-like symptoms after the onset and resolution of a viral upper respiratory infection. Nasal symptoms, congestion, headache, and acute vocal changes resolve, but persistent throat clearing, globus, coughing, or burning persist for weeks, months, and even years. Thus, the concept of a "post-viral refluxopathy" must be considered. We know viruses induce many neuromotor and sensory changes. Bell's palsy, post-herpetic pain, acute vocal paralysis, and acute neurosensory hearing loss are all examples of a post-viral neuropathy. Similarly, a post-viral upper respiratory infection can affect the vagus nerve leading to these sensory and motor symptoms. Potentially, a viral gastroenteritis could theoretically affect esophageal sensory and motor function in a similar fashion. The vagus is one of the strongest stimulants of gastrin secretion and acid release. Additionally, the vagus is responsible for controlling esophageal sensation, motor and peristaltic reflexes, gastric emptying, and sensitivity of the esophagus and stomach. Therefore, exposure to upper respiratory and gastroenterological viral infection could lead to mucosal damage and inflammation resulting in neuronal hypersensitivity changes. A perfect storm is likely the pathophysiological mechanism: isolated events likely do not lead to disease states; however, viral illness, exposure to local and systemic factors, and sensory changes likely contribute to the disease states of LPR or LPSS and GERD.

In conclusion, the peripheral and central states of sensitivity should be taken into consideration when working with a patient who describes upper aerodigestive symptoms suggestive of LPR and GERD. A history of symptoms commencing after a viral respiratory event, a noxious exposure, or physical trauma should entertain the possibility of hypersensitivity of the laryngopharynx and esophagus [12]. The absence of physical findings or response to reflux treatment can indicate hypersensitivity and thus suggest altered treatment regimens, such as the use of trigger reduction paradigms and neuromodulating medications [13].

References

1. Bessac B, Jordt SE. Breathtaking TRP channels: TRPA1 and TRPV1 in airway chemosensation and reflex control. Physiology. 2008;23:360–70.
2. Omar S, Clarke R, Abdullah H, Brady C, Corry J, Winter H, Touzelet O, Power UF, Lundy F, McGarvey LP, Cosby SL. Respiratory virus infection up-regulates TRPV1, TRPA1 and ASICS3 receptors on airway cells. PLoS One. 2017;12(2):e0171681. https://doi.org/10.1371/journal.pone.0171681.
3. Carr MJ, Lee LY. Plasticity of peripheral mechanisms of cough. Respir Physiol Neurobiol. 2006;152:298–311.
4. Driessen AK, McGovern AE, Narula M, et al. Central mechanisms of airway sensation and cough hypersensitivity. Pulm Pharmacol Ther. 2017;47:9–15. https://doi.org/10.1016/j.pupt.2017.01.010. Epub 2017 Jan 27.
5. Canning BJ. Anatomy and neurophysiology of the cough reflex. Chest. 2006;129:33S–47S.
6. Mazzone SB. An overview of the sensory receptors regulating cough. Cough. 2005;1(2):1–9.
7. Drossman DA, Crazziari R, Talley NJ, Thompson WG, Whitehead WE. The Rome II multinational working teams. Rome II: the functional gastrointestinal disorders. 2nd ed. McLean: Degnon Associates, Inc.; 2000.

8. Zalvan CH, Yuen E, Thomas AM, Benson BE. Laryngeal Electromyographic Findings in a Cohort of Recalcitrant Chronic Neurogenic Cough Patients. J Voice. 2020;5:pii:S0892-1997;(19):30633–2. https://doi.org/10.1016/j.jvoice.2020.01.024.
9. Yoshida N, Kuroda M, Suzuki T, et al. Role of nociceptors/neuropeptides in the pathogenesis of visceral hypersensitivity of nonerosive reflux disease. Dig Dis Sci. 2013;58:2237–43.
10. Naliboff BD, Mayer M, Fass R, et al. The effect of life stress on symptoms of heartburn. Psychosom Med. 2004;66:426–34.
11. Miwa H, Kondo T, Oshima T, Fukui H, Tomita T, Watari J. Esophageal sensation and esophageal hypersensitivity – overview from bench to bedside. J Neurogastroenterol Motil. 2010;16:353–62.
12. Yamasaki T, Fass R. Reflux hypersensitivity: a new functional esophageal disorder. J Neurogastroenterol Motil. 2017;23(4):495–503. https://doi.org/10.5056/jnm17097.
13. Zalvan C, Berzofsky C, Tiwari R, Geliebter J. Trigger reduction prior to systemic drugs for neurogenic chronic cough. Laryngoscope. 2019;129(1):198–202. https://doi.org/10.1002/lary.27459.. Epub 2018 Aug 10

Chapter 8
A Brief History of Reflux Disease

Brian Benson, Corina Din-Lovinescu, and Muhammad Farooq

Early Understanding of Dyspepsia

For most of human history, the esophagus has been a poorly understood organ of the digestive tract. In ancient times, physicians referred to the esophagus as a "humble" organ because it was not associated with many diseases other than that occurring due to obstruction with a swallowed food bolus or foreign object. In fact, there is speculation that the Greek term, oisophagos, could be interpreted as "osier" "eater" in a reference to willow branches (osier) used to treat esophageal obstruction. The first description of inflammation of the esophagus dates back to the second century by the Greek physician, surgeon, and philosopher Galen. While the description was incomplete, Galen introduced the association of dysphagia secondary to the inflamed esophagus [1, 2].

The hallmark symptom of reflux esophagitis, a burning sensation within the central chest, remained a topic of confusion partially due to underappreciation of the esophagus as a separate organ from that of the mouth or the stomach and due to lack of clear understanding of the anatomy and physiology of the esophagus. The modern term dyspepsia, referred to as "dyspepsia" in the 1650s, was defined as "imbecility of the stomach" but was commonly used as catch-all term for all upper abdominal discomfort [1]. The term "hartburning," in reference to epigastric

B. Benson (✉)
Department of Otolaryngology-Head & Neck Surgery, Hackensack Meridian School of Medicine at Seton Hall University, Nutley, NJ, USA
e-mail: BrianE.Benson@HackensackMeridian.org

C. Din-Lovinescu
Department of Otolaryngology-Head and Neck Surgery, Rutgers New Jersey Medical School, Newark, NJ, USA

M. Farooq
Hackensack Meridian School of Medicine at Seton Hall University, Nutley, NJ, USA
e-mail: muhammad.farooq1@student.shu.edu

C. H. Zalvan (ed.), *Laryngopharyngeal and Gastroesophageal Reflux*,
https://doi.org/10.1007/978-3-030-48890-1_8

discomfort, as opposed to an embittered mental state, was used as early as 1591. Despite the lack of anatomic understanding and physiologic evidence, the idea that heartburn could be due to reflux of gastric contents gained some acceptance, as evidenced by the practices of such as by John Gerard, master surgeon of London, who stated in 1597 that "a small stonecrop (a small flowering plant that grows among stones) is good for hart-burne." The symptoms of heartburn, although associated with the consumption of poor quality food, were assumed to be cardiac in nature, partially due to the location of the discomfort but also because of the perceived dominant role of the heart in the body at that time. Hence, the terms "cardalgia" or "cardiodynia" were also used to refer to these symptoms.

Coining the Term Esophagitis

More modern descriptions of esophagitis can be found in literature of the late 1700s and 1800s by Frank, Velpeau, Knott, and many others, although the use of the term "esophagitis" in the English language is credited to the otolaryngologist Morell Mackenzie in 1884, whose extensive text described inflammatory conditions of the upper esophagus due to infectious agents and corrosive damage [3]. Mackenzie did not, however, propose that inflammation of the pharynx and larynx could be caused by reflux of gastric contents. Although the notion of gastric contents causing distal esophageal ulceration was supported by Baron Carl von Rokitansky in the late 1800s, the concept of reflux esophagitis remained controversial. The advent of improved endoscopic instrumentation in the late 1800s aided descriptions of esophageal disease. However, the otolaryngologist Chevalier Jackson reported in 1929 only 88 cases of esophagitis in 4000 consecutive esophagoscopies [4]. At the same time, the understanding of gastric ulcer disease was also transforming, and these insights would impact the modern concept of reflux disease.

Beginning in the Renaissance, anatomic studies described gastric ulcers. As the topic of gastric ulcer gained increasing recognition, controversy regarding the pathogenesis of gastric ulcers developed. In 1853, Rudolf Virchow, a German physician and a pathologist, proposed that gastric ulcers were the product of gastric mucosa vessel occlusion and infarction followed by digestion of the necrotic areas by the gastric juice [5]. In contrast, Julius Cohnheim, a German pathologist and the pioneer in experimental histology, and Franz Riegel, a German internist and gastroenterologist, argued during the late 1800s and early 1900s that gastric ulcer formation was due to damage by increased hydrochloric acid secretion [5]. Even as the hyperchlorhydria theory gained popularity, there were others, such as G. Bottcher, one of the first gastric bacteriologists, and Edward C. Rosenow, who proposed that hematogenous bacterial invasion was the most important factor in the genesis of the gastric ulcer formation [5]. By the beginning of the twentieth century, however, the hyperchlorhydria theory became the most widely accepted, especially after the creation and invention of the gastric pouch by Ivan Pavlov, a Russian physiologist, and the recognition of the role of gastric acid [5].

First Description of Gastroesophageal Reflux

Although reflux esophagitis (peptic ulcer of the esophagus) had been described in the early twentieth century by Jackson, Tileston, and others, the modern framework for the reflux entity commonly known as gastroesophageal reflux disease (GERD) is attributed to Asher Winkelstein, a gastroenterologist, who in 1934 described "diffuse esophageal inflammation without a definite ulcer" in a patient with heartburn [6]. With the development of the fully flexible endoscope in 1957, large numbers of individuals underwent esophagoscopy. Multiple grading systems have been proposed to more accurately standardize the extent of esophagitis. The Los Angeles classification system, created in 1994, is the most frequently used system [7].

Building upon the hyperchlorhydria hypothesis of gastric ulcer formation, an acid perfusion test developed by Bernstein and Baker in 1958 demonstrated the direct relationship between acidification and reflux disease symptoms [8]. Interestingly, Bernstein and Baker noted that acid perfusion only reliably reproduced heartburn symptoms in patients with a prior history of reflux symptoms and not in controls. Subsequently, Behar et al. showed that in a cohort of 77 patients with chronic heartburn and regurgitation, only 61% had endoscopically visible esophagitis [9]. The advent of ambulatory pH monitoring enabled the identification of patients with reflux disease without esophageal ulceration. DeMeester et al. found that more than half of patients with symptoms of reflux disease, but without mucosal breaks noted on endoscopy, had abnormal pH probe monitoring results [10]. Today, it is accepted that most patients with esophageal reflux symptoms have non-erosive esophagitis (NERD).

Mechanisms of GERD: Hiatal Hernias, Transient Relaxation Events, and the Acid Pocket

While it is generally accepted that symptoms of reflux disease are mediated by reflux of gastric contents, the pathophysiologic mechanisms that lead to reflux events, the epithelial changes associated with reflux, and sensory neuron alterations that may predispose to symptoms are poorly understood. During the first half of the twentieth century, the presence of a hiatus hernia (herniation of the stomach through the diaphragmatic hiatus) was the leading theory used to explain reflux esophagitis. The newly discovered technique of contrast radiography showed dramatic images of this previously neglected clinical entity, which was first described in 1580 by Ambroise Paré [11]. Surgical intervention to correct the hiatus hernia was promoted by thoracic surgeons until the mid-twentieth century, when convincing evidence for the existence of the lower esophageal sphincter and multiple reports of a high frequency of hiatal hernia in asymptomatic patients shifted attention to lower esophageal sphincter incompetence [12]. Esophageal manometry studies in the 1980s revealed that reflux events were not associated with low resting pressure of the lower esophageal sphincter but rather transient relaxation events (TLESR), during which symptomatic individuals were more likely to have acid reflux events [13, 14]. Increased distensibility of the esophagogastric junction has also been implicated in GERD, presumably by allowing greater volumes of refluxate per event [15]. In addition to TLESR, the role of the crural diaphragm in reflux prevention was also confirmed in the 1980s. Coordinated phrenic inhibition of contraction of the crural diaphragm, in conjunction of the vagal mediated inhibition of the intrinsic muscle fibers of the esophagus, results in TLESR [16]. Although the vagal innervation of the gastroesophageal junction was described in 1906, it was not until the 1990s and 2000s that it was demonstrated that the majority of the relaxation of the LES was mediated by the vagus nerve via the neurotransmitter glutamate [17, 18].

During the early twentieth century, several investigators studying peptic ulcer disease noticed that stomach contents high in the fundus remained acidic, while the remainder of the stomach contents was less acidic, due to the buffering action of the food bolus [19]. A well-known paradox of GERD is that most symptoms occur in the post-prandial period, when the pH of the stomach contents would be expected to be increased. While TLESR are associated with the post-prandial period, the acidity of the refluxate was lower than expected. In 2001, investigators re-discovered a phenomenon referred to as the "Acid Pocket" using pH electrode studies, which identified a small 2 cm region of increased acidity just below the LES [20]. This finding, in addition to the fact that the acid pocket is longer (3–6.5 cm) in patients suffering from GERD, offered an explanation for the highly acidic refluxate in post-prandial GERD. Furthermore, patients with large hiatal hernias have been shown to have a supradiaphragmatic location of the acid pocket, a known risk factor for acid reflux during TLESRs [21].

Cellular Basis of GERD

As understanding of the complex mechanical aspects of GERD accelerated over the past century, so did appreciation of the cellular and neurophysiologic mechanisms of GERD. In 1970, histologic findings of basal cell hyperplasia and elongated papillae of esophageal mucosa of individuals with reflux disease both with and without mucosal breaks were reported [22]. One decade later, transmission electron microscopy identified dilated intracellular spaces (DIS) in the esophageal mucosa of rabbits that had been exposed to acid. In 1996, these same findings were reported in humans with GERD [23]. It is postulated that DIS is a consequence of increased permeability due to exposure to acid, proteolytic enzymes, and bile acids. Furthermore, it is postulated that increased permeability of the squamous epithelium allows those same agents to stimulate sensory nerve endings in patients without mucosal breaks. In vivo techniques to measure the permeability of the esophageal epithelium using impedance monitoring and electrical tissue impedance spectroscopy have been developed recently and may be clinically useful diagnostic modality [24, 25].

The elucidation of ultrastructural cellular changes associated with GERD led investigators to postulate that stimulation of afferent nerves could lead to receptor upregulation through the release of inflammatory mediators. Multiple receptors involved in peripheral sensitization have been identified in the past 20 years. The transient receptor vanilloid-1 receptor (TRPV1) expression is increased in inflamed esophageal mucosa and may result in increased production of substance P and CGRP, thus promoting additional inflammation of the epithelial barrier [26]. Central sensitization may also play a role in esophageal hypersensitivity. Functional MRI has been used to demonstrate how acid stimulation of the esophagus results in cortical activity [27, 28].

Laryngopharyngeal Reflux

The rapid increase in the understanding of the pathophysiology of reflux disease due to improved imaging techniques, fiberoptic and digital imaging technology, pH probe testing, esophageal manometry, as well as medical and surgical treatments during the past 30 years has also been accompanied by a recognition of extra-esophageal manifestation of reflux disease. The first report in the otolaryngology literature of a laryngeal contact ulcer in 1968 preceded widespread consensus among otolaryngologists by more than 20 years [29]. In 1991, Koufman coined the term laryngopharyngeal reflux (LPR) to describe a diverse set of otolaryngic symptoms in a large case series of individuals suspected of having GERD, the majority of whom had positive pH probe studies, and a large minority of whom exhibited reflux into the pharynx [30]. A consensus statement by the American Academy of Otolaryngology/Head and Neck Surgery in 1996 supported the concept that reflux is associated with laryngopharyngeal as well as pulmonary manifestations [31]. LPR was differentiated from GERD in that it is associated with daytime and upright reflux, is associated with less heartburn symptoms, and is mediated by UES dysfunction, in addition to the well-known GERD risk factors.

The pathophysiology of LPR is incompletely understood, but significant progress has been made over the past several decades. In 2010, investigators described edema of the lamina propria, hyperplasia of the submucosal glands, and muscle atrophy in laryngeal specimens exposed to acid [32, 33]. In addition, dilated intracellular spaces of the hypopharyngeal mucosa were identified in patients with LPR symptoms by Amin and colleagues [34]. Decreased E-cadherin, an adhesion molecule required for cellular barrier function that is also thought to be a tumor suppressor in epithelial carcinoma, has been found to be decreased in patients with LPR [35]. Similarly, mucin gene expression is also decreased in patients with LPR [36].

Johnston and collaborators described pepsin and carbonic anhydrase isoenzyme III as markers for LPR in 2003 and subsequently elucidated another mechanism of laryngeal injury via receptor-mediated endocytosis of laryngopharyngeal pepsin in 2009 [37, 38].

Establishing the diagnosis of LPR using both qualitative and quantitative techniques remains challenging. While ambulatory multichannel intraluminal impedance-pH monitoring is considered the gold standard for establishing the diagnosis of LPR, there is still debate regarding testing methods as well as the definition of an abnormal study. Despite these drawbacks, a 2005 meta-analysis found statistically significant variation in upper probe measurements between normal subjects and those with LPR [39]. Unfortunately, the initially promising results of oropharyngeal pH testing have not been supported in follow-up studies [40, 41].

Since performing pH probe studies on every patient with suspected LPR is not feasible, alternative strategies to establish the diagnosis of LPR based upon reported symptoms, laryngoscopy findings, and response to empiric treatment are commonly employed. Symptoms of LPR commonly include throat clearing, coughing, hoarseness, and globus sensation. Additional symptoms including sore throat, mild dysphagia, and halitosis have been described in LPR patients, although most patients do not report classic GERD symptoms such as heartburn. Belafsky et al. developed a validated Reflux Symptom Index in 2002, although the poor specificity of laryngopharyngeal symptoms has resulted in lack of correlation with pH probe findings [39, 42].

Laryngeal examination findings including edema (especially infraglottic edema, referred to as pseudosulcus), erythema, granulomas, contact ulcers, as well as subglottic stenosis, leukoplakia, dysplasia, and laryngeal carcinoma have been associated with LPR. Belafsky et al. also developed a validated reflux finding score (RFS) based upon findings consistent with laryngeal inflammation: pseudosulcus, ventricular obliteration, erythema, vocal fold edema, diffuse laryngeal edema, posterior commissure hypertrophy, granuloma, and thick endolaryngeal mucus [42]. Despite the clinical utility of the RFS, poor inter-relater reliability and correlation with pH probe results also plague this tool as well as the RSI [39, 43].

Empiric treatment with proton pump inhibitors is a well-accepted diagnostic tool, whereby resolution of symptoms is considered a diagnostic confirmation of LPR [44]. Patients are typically treated with a 3-month course of a twice-daily proton pump inhibitor as well as diet modifications.

In 2015, Hyat et al. described salivary pepsin levels as a diagnostic test for GERD [45]. More recently, the measurement of saliva and nasal lavage pepsin levels has been shown to have a positive correlation with MII-pH results in two prospective studies [46].

Other Extra-Esophageal Manifestations of GERD

Other extra-esophageal manifestations of GERD, particularly in upper and lower airway diseases, have also recently become more widely described. As of 2006, the Montreal definition and classification of GERD recognized laryngitis, cough, asthma, and dental erosions as possible GERD syndromes [47]. Asthma is thought to be linked to GERD via damage to the bronchial tree after exposure to acid reflux or via vagal nerve stimulation from the esophagus. While it is unclear if GERD precedes asthma, or if asthma triggers GERD, we know that there is a higher prevalence of GERD symptoms in patients with asthma compared to those without asthma and that antireflux therapy reduces asthma medication use [48]. Similarly, GERD has also been shown to increase risk for chronic rhinosinusitis in both adults and children [49]. One hypothesis for this finding is that acid, pepsin and trypsin, which may reflux into the nasopharynx and sinuses, can irritate and injure the sinonasal mucosa. GERD is also one of the most common causes of chronic cough via stimulation of the esophageal-bronchial reflex through afferent nerves in the distal esophagus or via microaspiration into the airway [50]. Furthermore, chronic bronchitis, idiopathic pulmonary fibrosis, chronic obstructive pulmonary disease, and obstructive sleep apnea are additional respiratory disorders which have been associated with GERD [51]. Lastly, dental erosions, carries, and tooth hypersensitivity have also been shown to be increased in patients with GERD [52].

Modern Risk Factors

In the twenty-first century, GERD has become widely recognizable by physicians and patients alike, with an estimated 18–28% of the North American population experiencing some sort of reflux disease at least once in their life [53]. Multiple etiologies have now been linked to GERD, including lifestyle choices such as consumption of certain types of food and drinks, certain analgesic intake, smoking, and increased body mass index (BMI), in addition to non-modifiable risk factors including male sex, older age, race, and presence of *Helicobacter pylori* bacteria. As such, the cornerstone of modern-day GERD treatment has focused on lifestyle modifications in order to limit hazardous exposures.

Conclusion

While the modern-day term GERD was first described by Winkelstein in the twentieth century, the symptoms of GERD or dyspepsia have been present and documented in human history for centuries dating back to the early 1500s. The advent of endoscopic instrumentation in the late 1800s in combination with the popularization of the hyperchlorhydria theory in the early twentieth century provided the groundwork for the basis of GERD. Esophageal pH probe and contrast radiography studies, in addition to histologic and electron microscopy studies, provided an anatomical and cellular basis for GERD in the late twentieth century. More recently, extra-esophageal manifestations of GERD, including LPR, have been elucidated and recognized as important entities.

References

1. Modlin IM, Kidd M, Lye KD. Historical perspectives on the treatment of gastroesophageal reflux disease. Gastrointest Endosc Clin N Am. 2003;13(1):19–55, vii–viii
2. Malfertheiner MV, Fill S, Kidd M, Modlin IM. The elucidation of peptic esophagitis: from Hamperl to heartburn. Z Gastroenterol. 2007;45(11):1164–8. https://doi.org/10.1055/s-2007-963476.
3. Mackenzie M. Diseases of the throat and nose, vol. 2. London: Churchill; 1884.
4. Jackson C. Peptic ulcer of the esophagus. JAMA. 1929;92:369–72.
5. Zucker GM, Clayman CB. Landmark perspective: Bertram W. Sippy and ulcer disease therapy. JAMA. 1983;250(16):2198–202.
6. Winkelstein A. Peptic esophagitis: a new clinical entity. JAMA. 1935;104(11):906–9.
7. Sami SS, Ragunath K. The Los Angeles classification of gastroesophageal reflux disease, video. J Encyclop GI Endosc. 2013;1(1):103–4.
8. Berstein LM, Baker LA. A clinical test for esophagitis. Gastroenterology. 1958;34:760–81.
9. Behar J, Biancani P, Sheahan DG. Evaluation of esophageal tests in the diagnosis of reflux esophagitis. Gastroenterology. 1976;71:9–15.
10. DeMeester TR, Wang CI, Wernly JA, Pellegrini CA, Little AG, Klementschitsch P, et al. Technique, indications, and clinical use of 24 hour esophageal pH monitoring. J Thorac Cardiovasc Surg. 1980;79:656–70.
11. Pare A. Diaphragmatic hernia, [part 2]. Arch Surg. 1928;16:386–415.
12. Palmer ED. The hiatus hernia-esophagitis-esophageal stricture complex: twenty year prospective study. Am J Med. 1968;44(4):566–79.
13. Dent J, Dodds WJ, Friedman RH, Sekiguchi T, Hogan WJ, Arndorfer RC, Petrie DJ. Mechanism of gastroesophageal reflux in recumbent asymptomatic human subjects. J Clin Invest. 1980;65(2):256–67.
14. Sifrim D, Holloway R. Transient lower esophageal sphincter relaxations: how many or how harmful? Am J Gastroenterol. 2001;9:2529–31.
15. Pandolfino JE, Shi G, Trueworthy B, Kahrilas PJ. Esophagogastric junction opening during relaxation distinguishes nonhernia reflux patients, hernia patients, and normal subjects. Gastroenterology. 2003;125:1018–24. https://doi.org/10.1016/S0016-5085(03)01210-1.
16. Mittal RK, Balaban DH. The esophagogastric junction. N Engl J Med. 1997;336:924–32.
17. Tileston W. Peptic ulcer of the oesophagus. Am J Med Sci. 1906;132:240–65.
18. Zagorodnyuk V, Chen BN, Brookes SJ. Intraganglionic laminar endings are mechanotransduction sites of vagal tension receptors in the guinea pig stomach. J Physiol Lond. 2001;534:255–68.
19. Hurst AF. The sensibility of the alimentary canal. London: Oxford University Press; 1911.
20. Fletcher J, Wirz A, Young J, Vallance R, McColl KE. Unbuffered highly acidic gastric juice exists at the gastroesophageal junction after a meal. Gastroenterology. 2001;121:775–83.
21. Beaumont H, Bennink RJ, de Jong J, Boeckxstaens GE. The position of the acid pocket as a major risk factor for acidic reflux in healthy subjects and patients with GORD. Gut. 2010;59:441–51.
22. Ismail-Beigi F, Horton PF, Pope CE. Histological consequences of gastroesophageal reflux in man. Gastroenterology. 1970;58(2):163–74.
23. Tobey NA, Carson JL, Alkiek RA, et al. Dilated intercellular spaces: a morphological feature of acid reflux–damaged human esophageal epithelium. Gastroenterology. 1996;111:1200–5.
24. Farre R, Blondeau K, Clement D, et al. Evaluation of oesophageal mucosa integrity by the intraluminal impedance technique. Gut. 2011;60:885–92.
25. Wiejenborg PW, Rohof WOA, Ackermans LMA, Verheij J, Smout AJPM, Bredenoord AJ. Electrical tissue impedance spectroscopy: a novel device to measure esophageal mucosal integrity changes during endoscopy. Neurogastroenterolog Motil. 2013;25:574–E458.

26. Matthews PJ, Aziz Q, Facer P, Davis JB, Thompson DG, Anand P. Increased capsaicin receptor TRPV1 nerve fibres in the inflamed human oesophagus. Eur J Gastroenterol Hepatol. 2004;16:897–902.
27. Sarkar S, Aziz Q, Woolf CJ, et al. Contribution of central sensitisation to the development of non-cardiac chest pain. Lancet. 2000;356:1154–9.
28. Lawal A, Kern M, Sanjeevi A, Antonik S, Mepani R, Rittmann T, et al. Neurocognitive processing of esophageal central sensitization in the insula and cingulate gyrus. Am J Physiol Gastrointest Liver Physiol. 2008;294:G787–94.
29. Cherry J, Margulies SI. Contact ulcer of the larynx. Laryngoscope. 1968;78(11):1937–40.
30. Koufman JA. The otolaryngologic manifestations of gastroesophageal reflux disease (GERD): a clinical investigation of 225 patients using ambulatory 24-hour pH monitoring and an experimental investigation of the role of acid and pepsin in the development of laryngeal injury. Laryngoscope. 1991;101:1–78.
31. Koufman J, Sataloff RT, Toohill R. Laryngopharyngeal reflux: consensus conference report. J Voice. 1996;10:215–6.
32. Habesoglu TE, et al. Histological changes of rat soft palate with exposure to experimental laryngopharyngeal reflux. Auris Nasus Larynx. 2010;37:730–6.
33. Bulmer DM, et al. Laryngeal mucosa: its susceptibility to damage by acid and pepsin. Laryngoscope. 2010;120:777–82.
34. Amin SM, et al. Laryngopharyngeal reflux with sore throat: an ultrastructural study of oropharyngeal epithelium. Ann Otol Rhinol Larngol. 2009;118:362–7.
35. Reichel O, Mayr D, Durst F, Berghaus A. E-cadherin but not B-catenin expression is decreased in laryngeal biopsies from patients with laryngopharyngeal reflux. Eur Arch Otorhinolaryngol. 2008;265:937–42.
36. Samuels TL, Handler E, Syring LI, et al. Mucin gene expression in human laryngeal epithelia: effect of laryngopharyngeal reflux. Ann Otol Rhinol Laryngol. 2008;117:688–95.
37. Johnston N, Knight J, Dettma PW, Lively MO, Koufman J. Pepsin and carbonic anhydrase isoenzyme III as diagnostic markers for laryngopharyngeal reflux disease. Laryngoscope. 2004;114:2129–34.
38. Johnston N, et al. Pepsin in nonacidic refluxate can damage hypopharyngeal epithelial cells. Ann Otol Rhinol Laryngol. 2009;118:677–85.
39. Merati AL, Lim HJ, Ulualp SO, Toohill RJ. Meta-analysis of upper probe measurements in normal subjects and patients with laryngopharyngeal reflux. Ann Otol Rhinol Laryngol. 2005;114:177–82.
40. Wiener GJ, Tsukashima R, Kelly C, Wold E, Schmeltzer M, Bankert C, Fisk L, Vaezi M. Oropharyngeal pH monitoring for the detection of liquid and aerosolized supraesophageal gastric reflux. J Voice. 2009;23(4):498–504.
41. Mazzoleni G, Vailati C, Lisma DG, Testoni PA, Passarentti S. Correlation between oropharyngeal pH-monitoring and esophageal pH-impedance monitoring in patients with suspected GERD-related extra-esophageal symptoms. Neurogastroenterol Motil. 2014;26(11):1557–64.
42. Belafsky PC, Postma GN, Koufman JA. Validity and reliability of the reflux symptom index (RSI). J Voice. 2002;16:274–7.
43. Branski R, Bhattacharyya N, Shapiro J. The reliability of the assessment of endoscopic laryngopharyngeal reflux disease. Laryngoscope. 2002;112(6):1019–24.
44. Abou-Ismail A, Vaezi MF. Evaluation of patients with suspected laryngopharyngeal reflux: a practical approach. Curr Gastroenterol Rep. 2011;13:213–8.
45. Hayat JO, Gabieta-Somnez S, Yazaki E, et al. Pepsin in saliva for the diagnosis of gastroesophageal reflux disease. Gut. 2015;64:373–80.
46. Weitzendorfer M, Antoniou SA, Schredl P, et al. Pepsin and oropharyngeal pH monitoring to diagnose patients with laryngopharyngeal reflux. Laryngoscope. 2019; https://doi.org/10.1002/lary.28320.

47. Vakil N, van Zanten SV, Kahrilas P, et al. The Montreal definition and classification of gastroesophageal reflux disease: a global evidence-based consensus. Am J Gastroenterol. 2006;101:1900–20.
48. Havermann BD, Henderson CA, El-Serag HB. The association between gastro-oesophageal reflux disease and asthma: a systematic review. Gut. 2007;56:1654–64.
49. Lin YH, Chang TS, Yao YC, Li YC. Increased risk of chronic sinusitis in adults with gastroesophgeal reflux disease: a nationwide population-based cohort study. Medicine (Baltimore). 2015;94(39):e1642. https://doi.org/10.1097/MD.0000000000001642.
50. Irwin RS. Chronic cough due to gastroesophageal reflux disease: ACCP evidence-based clinical practice guidelines. Chest. 2006;129:80S–94S.
51. Gaude GS. Pulmonary manifestations of gastroesophageal reflux disease. Ann Thorac Med. 2009;4(3):115–23. https://doi.org/10.4103/1817-1737.53347.
52. Ranjitkar S, Kaidonis JA, Smales RJ. Gastroesophageal reflux disease and tooth erosion. Int J Dent. 2012;2012:479850. https://doi.org/10.1155/2012/479850.
53. Yamasaki T, Hemond C, Eisa M, Ganocy S, Fass R. The changing epidemiology of gastroesophageal reflux disease: are patients getting younger? J Neurogastroenterol Motil. 2018;24(4):559–69. https://doi.org/10.5056/jnm18140.

Part II
Laryngopharyngeal Reflux: LPR

Chapter 9
Laryngopharyngeal Reflux (LPR) Overview and Introduction

Craig H. Zalvan

One of the primary objectives of this text is to summarize and detail what is known about LPR in a comprehensive manner to provide the reader the tools to identify, diagnose, and treat. LPR is a relatively new diagnosis whose name was coined by Dr. Jamie Koufman in the 1990s to outline a constellation of symptoms and findings of the head and neck region. This section will outline the history of reflux, followed by the symptoms, differential diagnosis, and diagnostic workup of LPR based on what is current. Medicine, like philosophy, evolves as we learn. Having a strong foundation in what is accepted knowledge of LPR today will help set the stage for better understanding and thus treatment of diseases of the head and neck tomorrow.

Drs. Benson and Din-Lovinescu detail the history of reflux treatment from ancient Greek solutions borne of trial and error to modern science extracting molecular interventions from physiologic pathways elucidated from modern benchtop science. Perhaps illuminating, and one of the goals of this project, is realizing the transition from initial diet and herbal-based treatments to pharmacological intervention has now begun to trend back toward diet, the final component of this text.

LPR, to this day, remains a controversial topic. Diagnosis is strongly rooted in the presenting symptoms of the patient as well as the physical findings, yet a gold standard remains elusive. Symptoms of LPR encompass an enormous range of head and neck manifestations of disease with none being pathognomonic for reflux. The physical findings are based on a collection of findings, essentially highlighting inflammation and mucosal change. However, the overlap of LPR and many other disease presentations remains quite high and often difficult to distinguish. Drs.

C. H. Zalvan (✉)
ENT and Allergy Associates, LLP; Voice and Swallow Division, Tarrytown, NY, USA

The Institute for Voice and Swallowing Disorders at Phelps Hospital, Northwell Health, Sleepy Hollow, NY, USA

Professor of Otolaryngology at the Donald and Barbara Zucker School of Medicine at Hofstra/Northwell, Phelps Hospital Campus, Sleepy Hollow, NY, USA
e-mail: czalvan1@northwell.edu

C. H. Zalvan (ed.), *Laryngopharyngeal and Gastroesophageal Reflux*,
https://doi.org/10.1007/978-3-030-48890-1_9

Novakovic and Pang tackle the next task of outlining the current presentation and physical findings most often described in patients with LPR. They review the subjective and objective rating scales, with their deficiencies, that help one arrive at the diagnosis. As LPR is an inflammatory disease, contribution to other head and neck manifestations can occur, and many of these disease processes are reviewed. Following, Drs. Lechien, Finck, and Carroll describe the process in which reflux can result in mucosal and inflammatory changes of the vocal folds resulting in the onset and propagation of mucosal disease. A detailed description of the pathophysiology of reflux-induced changes helps with understanding the mechanism leading to improved diagnosis. As stated earlier, there are many confounding factors that cause laryngopharyngeal disease. Reflux can be causative or contributory. LPR can exacerbate underlying mucosal disease, trigger sensory responses, and worsen other pathophysiologic processes such as sinusitis and pulmonary disease, which are both reviewed in the final chapters of this section by Drs. Kamat, Jourdy, Kidwai, and Yuen examining sinus disease and Drs. Thau, Zalvan, and Stein reviewing pulmonary disease.

Diagnostic testing is possibly the most controversial topic of LPR. There is no gold standard. Without a gold standard, subjective and objective testing has no real basis of comparison and is thus flawed with decreased sensitivity and specificity. Yet despite this lack of gold standard, multiple objective tests have been created and are utilized daily. Dr. Iannuzzi will review these diagnostic tests. Response to treatment, pH testing, manometry, swallow testing, and other less utilized diagnostic modalities are reviewed in detail. More important than the test is the interpretation of the results in the setting of the clinical presentation. Drs. Nganzeu, Bock, Zalvan, and Johnston review pepsin testing as a newer modality of testing. The current understanding of true LPR suggests that pepsin is the mediator of inflammation in the setting of an acidic environment. Therefore, the presence of pepsin in saliva should suggest reflux of gastric contents is present. Once again, the interpretation of these results is the key to making the diagnosis. Pepsin and acid together have to be present in order to cause pathophysiologic changes. However, understanding sensory changes can coexist leading to states of hypersensitivity must also be taken into consideration. High subjective scores in the absence of pepsin and/or acid suggest neurosensory changes as does normal to elevated acid in the setting of no pepsin.

Given the high prevalence of reflux in modern society, which is the primary factor for esophageal adenocarcinoma, evaluation of the esophagus has become necessary for the practitioner who cares for reflux patients. LPR patients are at risk of developing cancer and should be evaluated when appropriate. Trans-nasal esophagoscopy was developed to perform evaluation of the entire upper digestive tract from the pharynx to the stomach. Dr. Allen highlights the evolution and importance of this technique, together with a detailed explanation of the indications, process, and findings.

There are many diseases of the pharynx and swallowing mechanism that can cause symptoms like that of LPR. A synopsis of related findings by the speech pathology (SLP) team helps outline their role in identifying different pathologies that either coexist with reflux, contribute to reflux, or merely mimic their symptoms. Bracciante-Ely and Dinu, SLP, highlight these findings while providing an understanding of the SLP role.

The final chapters in this section review the contribution of LPR to the development of sinus and pulmonary disease, as mentioned above.

Chapter 10
Laryngopharyngeal Reflux: Symptoms, Physical Findings, Differential Diagnosis, and Manifestations

Jing-Yin Pang, Daniel Novakovic, and Craig H. Zalvan

Introduction

Laryngopharyngeal reflux (LPR) is an important and common condition seen in otolaryngology practice. It refers to a constellation of symptoms involving the laryngopharynx and upper airways caused by the backward passage of gastric contents beyond the upper esophageal sphincter. The term LPR has been used interchangeably with extraesophageal reflux, gastroesophageal reflux, reflux laryngitis and supraesophageal reflux. Out of all these terms, LPR is the term accepted by the American Academy of Otolaryngology: Head and Neck Surgery [1].

With increasing recognition of this condition and an estimated prevalence of up to 10% of outpatients visiting ear, nose, and throat (ENT) departments, this translates to significant healthcare costs [2, 3].

J.-Y. Pang
Khoo Teck Puat Hospital, Yishun Central, Singapore, Singapore

University of Sydney, Dr Liang Voice Program. Central Clinical School, Faculty of Medicine and Health, Sydney, Australia
e-mail: pang.jing.yin@ktph.com.sg

D. Novakovic (✉)
University of Sydney, Dr Liang Voice Program. Central Clinical School, Faculty of Medicine and Health, Sydney, Australia

C. H. Zalvan
ENT and Allergy Associates, LLP; Voice and Swallow Division, Tarrytown, NY, USA

The Institute for Voice and Swallowing Disorders, Phelps Hospital, Northwell Health, Sleepy Hollow, NY, USA

Professor of Otolaryngology at the Donald and Barbara Zucker School of Medicine at Hofstra/Northwell, Phelps Hospital Campus, Sleepy Hollow, NY, USA

Speech and Communication Department at Mercy College, Dobbs Ferry, NY, USA
e-mail: czalvan1@northwell.edu

C. H. Zalvan (ed.), *Laryngopharyngeal and Gastroesophageal Reflux*,
https://doi.org/10.1007/978-3-030-48890-1_10

The etiology of LPR is not well understood. Gastroenterologists may consider LPR to be a manifestation of gastroesophageal reflux disease (GERD), but with the support of otolaryngologists, LPR is now recognized as a distinct and separate entity [1]. Patients with LPR often do not have heartburn which is the most common (classic) symptom of GERD. As such, mucosal injury may manifest as esophagitis on esophagoscopy in patients with GERD. Patients with LPR, however, usually have a negative or normal esophagoscopy which does not necessarily rule out LPR [4]. Histological features of the larynx and pharynx vary between the end organs specific to each condition. In contrast to the esophagus which is lined by tough, stratified squamous epithelium, the larynx and pharynx are devoid of this acid clearance mechanism, rendering them more susceptible to chemical trauma from pepsin and acid [5, 6]. Additionally, carbonic anhydrase is thought to play a vital protective mechanism in the larynx and there is some evidence that this may be disrupted in patients with LPR [7, 8]. Esophageal motility differences may underpin the reason why LPR patients are more likely to have a reflux event in an upright position compared with GERD patients [9].

Symptoms

The most common presenting symptoms of a patient with LPR include a sensation of a lump or ball in the throat (globus pharyngeus), chronic cough or throat clearing, dysphagia, dysphonia, postnasal drip, excessive mucus in the throat, and altered taste sensation in the mouth or water brash [1, 2, 10]. These symptoms are often intermittent, or chronic intermittent, corresponding to the occurrence of refluxate in the larynx but often persisting beyond a single reflux event. Dysphonia, when exacerbated by LPR, is often described as morning hoarseness with a deeper, gravelly type voice. Vocal issues often improve upon throat clearing of thick mucus and as the morning progresses. Mucus is often thicker in patients with LPR, reflecting the mucosal inflammation reducing bicarbonate secretion, more viscous mucin, and other physiological changes that are not well understood. This thicker mucus alone can elicit symptoms of throat clearing, PND sensation, and globus by direct contact with mucosa as well as by stimulation of the hypersensitive laryngopharyngeal sensory neurons.

Belafsky and colleagues designed the Reflux Symptom Index (RSI) to help raise the clinical suspicion of LPR in patients presenting to the ENT clinic [11, 12]. The RSI (Table 1) is a self-administered questionnaire comprising nine questions. Based on normative pH data, an RSI of more than 10 is associated with a high likelihood of LPR based on dual-probe pH study. There are however limitations to the RSI.

LPR symptoms are usually nonspecific and can be found in patients without reflux or in association with other conditions affecting the larynx. The RSI also does not take into consideration other important LPR symptoms such as sore throat, odynophagia, ear fullness/pressure, and halitosis [13, 14]. The RSI has not been reproduced on a larger scale to provide greater sensitivity and specificity. Lastly, the RSI does not take into consideration the frequency of symptoms. Symptom evaluation is based on a 5-point Likert scale score which can vary across cultural backgrounds.

Interestingly, one of the measures (#9) includes GERD symptoms of heartburn, indigestion, and acid regurgitation. Nearly a third of people with GERD have LPR symptoms, while 20–50% of people with LPR complain of typical GERD symptoms. Given the overlap anatomically, there is likely a greater overlap of symptoms from both diseases which can lead to a falsely elevated score. Despite the shortcomings, the RSI is used in nearly every study evaluating LPR and provides an excellent framework and language to follow a patient's response to treatment and provide a degree of severity of symptoms. However, given there is no gold standard diagnostic test, the use of the RSI has also led to a significant overdiagnosis and treatment of this disease. Hoarseness, for example, is rarely caused by LPR alone, though it can be exacerbated in the presence of acid and pepsin. Other causes of hoarseness should be sought after such as sulcus or scar, vocal paresis, or other mucosal issues. In addition, other symptoms in the RSI can be caused by a myriad of other diseases. Postnasal drip can certainly be a symptom of sinonasal inflammation and allergy. The sensation of drainage can also be reported because of pharyngeal hypersensitivity to the normal basal level of drainage from the sinuses. Humans normally have at least a liter of drainage from the nasal cavities into the throat daily. Some patients are hypersensitive and report feeling this normal basal level of drainage. Additional potential symptoms of LPR missing from the RSI include respiratory symptoms of stridor and laryngospasm, Eustachian tube dysfunction-related symptoms, halitosis, eructation, and tonsil stones. Many symptoms included in the RSI can arise from neurosensory changes and can lead to a falsely elevated score.

Given the overlap of symptoms and potential involvement of the entire upper aerodigestive tract with reflux disease, overlap of symptoms is common and expected. Under the direction of Lechien et al., the LPR study group of the Young Otolaryngologists of the International Federation of Oto-Rhino-Laryngological Societies (YO-IFOS) created the Reflux Symptom Score (RSS) [15], a patient-reported outcome questionnaire, to further enhance an LPR diagnosis by taking into account ENT, digestive, and respiratory symptoms and disease impact on quality of life. It has also been validated for use in the assessment of therapeutic responses in suspected and confirmed LPR patients.

The Reflux Symptom Index (Belafsky et al., 2002)

Within the past month, how did the following problems affect you?	0 = No problem 5 = Severe problem					
Hoarseness or a problem with your voice	0	1	2	3	4	5
Clearing your throat						
Excess throat mucus or postnasal drip						
Difficulty swallowing food, liquids, or pills						
Coughing after you ate or after lying down						
Breathing difficulties or choking episodes						
Troublesome or annoying cough						
Sensations of something sticking in your throat or a lump in your throat						
Heartburn, chest pain, indigestion, or stomach acid coming up						

Clinical Manifestations

The clinical manifestations of LPR range from benign throat disturbances to neoplastic lesions although a clear cause-and-effect relationship is difficult to prove.

Laryngeal manifestations of LPR include:

- Granuloma formation
- Subglottic stenosis
- Laryngospasm
- Paradoxical vocal cord motion
- Laryngeal cancer

Extra-laryngeal manifestations include:

- Sinusitis
- Otitis media
- Pulmonary fibrosis
- Asthma

Laryngeal Granuloma

Laryngeal arytenoid granulomas arise from (physical or chemical) trauma to the posterior glottis. When discovered, these granulomas should raise the clinical suspicion of LPR. However, other proposed etiologies include vocal trauma from repeated throat clearing and shouting, vocal misuse, and trauma associated with endotracheal intubation [16]. Additionally, neuropathic changes to the recurrent laryngeal or vagus nerve, either from a viral mechanism or post-intubation, can result in continued asymmetric posterior glottic forces resulting in localized trauma. In the setting of trauma and acid, granulation forms and persists. The continued imbalance can result in continued granulation or recurrent lesions post-removal.

Support for reflux as a cause of laryngeal granuloma was demonstrated in a study by Delahunty and Cherry [17]. The investigators successfully induced the formation of vocal process granulomas through atraumatic application of gastric secretions on the vocal fold mucosa in dogs. In a more recent study, Ogawa et al. demonstrated that only GERD is an independent etiological factor retarding the resolution of laryngeal granulomas in patients on pharmacological therapy [18].

Management of laryngeal granulomas requires aggressive anti-reflux therapy, lifestyle modifications, and adjuvant speech therapy. These were successful in achieving resolution of most of the granulomas and preventing recurrence [19, 20]. Surgery is generally reserved for cases requiring histological diagnosis or when the granuloma causes airway compromise. Novel techniques include chemodenervation with botulinum toxin injections [21, 22] and augmentation injection laryngoplasty to overcome underlying glottal insufficiency that may be causing compensatory adductor hyperfunction [23] (Fig. 10.1).

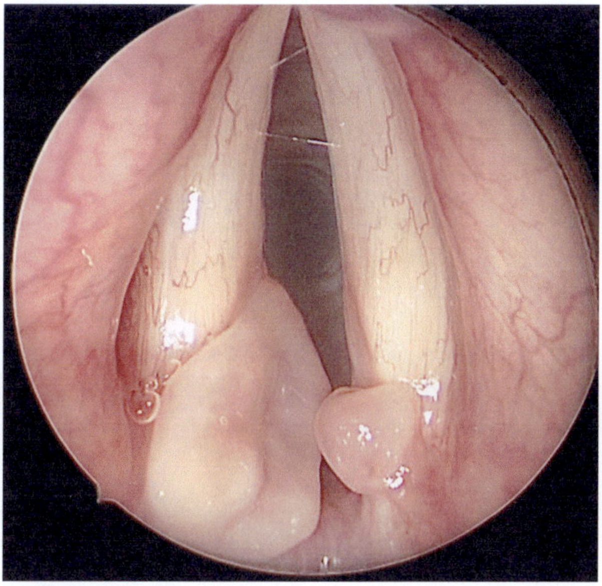

Fig. 10.1 Image of the larynx with a large lobular granuloma of the left posterior vocal process; smaller granuloma opposite on the right posterior vocal process

Subglottic Stenosis

There are some studies which have demonstrated an association between LPR and subglottic stenosis [5, 24]. The hypothesis is that reflux of gastric contents into the upper airway elicits an abnormal response of epithelial cells to injury, resulting in inflammation, fibrosis, and subsequent scar formation in the airway [25, 26].

Blumin and Johnston detected the presence of pepsin in up to 59% of larynges in patients with idiopathic subglottic stenosis, implicating the contributory role of LPR in its development [24]. But a few years later, they went on to demonstrate that in vitro acute exposure of pepsin to subglottic mucosa of patients with iSGS does not provide evidence of a direct causal role for development of fibrosis in epithelial cell cultures [27]. Though the exact cause of subglottic stenosis is not known and varies from idiopathic to iatrogenic, added inflammation from reflux is thought to interfere with healing and promote granulation and is associated with recurrence.

Hence, the relationship between reflux and subglottic stenosis is not well understood. Combining anti-reflux therapy with surgical management would be a reasonable approach (Fig. 10.2).

Laryngeal Malignancies

The association between tobacco, alcohol, and laryngeal malignancies is well known. The strength of association between gastroduodenal contents and extraesophageal cancer is weak. Some studies did not show GERD as an independent risk

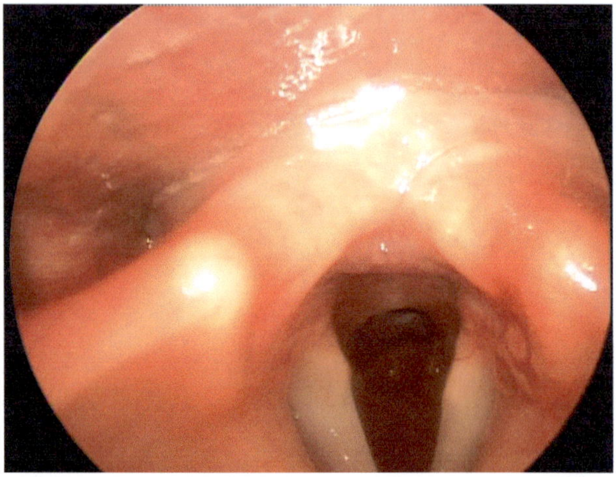

Fig. 10.2 Laryngeal image of 1.4 cm subglottic stenosis at the junction of the proximal trachea

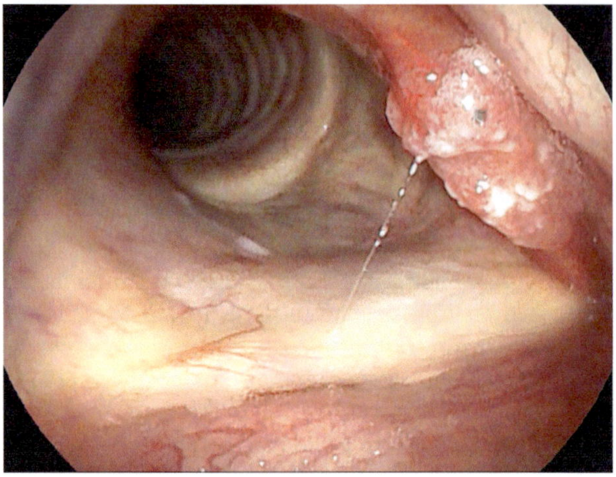

Fig. 10.3 Laryngoscopic image of a left exophytic, bulky vocal fold carcinoma

factor for cancer in multivariate analysis when tobacco and alcohol consumption are considered [28]. Other studies, including a meta-analysis, do show GERD as an independent risk factor especially in nonsmokers [29–32] (Fig. 10.3).

Inducible Laryngeal Obstruction/Paradoxical Vocal Fold Motion

Inducible laryngeal obstruction (ILO), also known as paradoxical vocal fold motion (PVFM) or vocal cord dysfunction (VCD), is characterized by inappropriate vocal cord adduction of more than 50% during the respiratory cycle (especially inspiration) leading to intermittent episodes of acute functional airway obstruction [33]. Its symptoms closely mimic wheezing or stridor, and the condition is frequently misdiagnosed as asthma or upper airway obstruction.

Maschka et al. proposed that PVFM might represent a spectrum of underlying diseases that manifest as a single clinical entity [34]. His group described cases of PVFM due to medical conditions such as brainstem compression and airway irritants. This was further supported by Perkner et al. who identified common irritants as ammonia, cleaning chemicals, organic solvents, flux flames, or smoke. These agents trigger off an alteration in vagally mediated laryngeal tone, lowering the threshold for irritant stimuli producing inspiratory adduction [35].

Because of the consistently observed high prevalence of reflux disease in patients with PVFM, an association between LPR and PVFM has been drawn. The proposed mechanism is accentuation of the glottic closure reflex secondary to acid damage of the laryngeal mucosa [36].

Management of PVFM requires identification and management of the underlying triggers (e.g., chemical, thermal, exercise) and psychological factors. If there is an association with LPR or GERD, appropriate medical therapy may be required. Speech therapy techniques are aimed at expiration and abdominal breathing in a relaxed throat breathing pattern. Psychological interventions include psychotherapy, behavioral therapy, and relaxation techniques to combat anxiety [37]. Combining a trigger reduction approach using respiratory retraining therapy, psychotherapy, nasal irrigation with saline and nasal steroid with antihistamine spray, and a 90% plant-based, Mediterranean style diet led to resolution and improvement in a study by Zalvan et al. [38].

There is still a great need for more research into elucidating the underlying pathogenesis and optimum management of PVFM. While many theories and treatments have been suggested, the underlying pathophysiology remains only partially described.

Asthma

Asthma is a heterogeneous clinical syndrome characterized by nonspecific airway hyperresponsiveness and inflammation [39]. Triggers of asthma include viruses, allergens, occupational exposures, exercise, and smoking. Related comorbidities include GERD and obesity [40].

The relationship between GERD, LPR, and asthma is complex, but the potential link between them can be explained by the following mechanisms:

1. Acid exposure to the distal esophagus can stimulate vagal nerve afferent fibers, resulting in bronchoconstriction and increased respiratory resistance [41].
2. Direct exposure of the trachea, bronchi, and lungs via microaspiration may induce bronchoconstriction and asthma.
3. Attenuation of the pharyngo-cricopharyngeal reflex may result in the inability of the upper esophageal sphincter to contract appropriately in the face of reflux events, exposing the unprotected laryngeal mucosa to refluxate [42].

While there is a strong link between GERD and asthma, the role of LPR, which is considered to be a separate entity from GERD, is underexplored. The diagnosis of LPR should be considered in patients with difficult-to-treat asthma as treatment may provide an improvement in LPR and asthma symptoms [43].

Chronic Cough

Chronic and recurrent cough is a costly and frustrating medical condition prompting over 10% of office visits yearly. Acute cough is frequently, and appropriately, attributed to viral infections of the upper respiratory tract, allergy and sinus inflammation, though typically presenting with other signs and symptoms of those disease states [44]. When cough recurs and persists beyond the acute state, it is considered chronic. Chronic cough is often diagnosed as asthma. Asthma should be considered in the setting of typical expiratory wheeze, sputum eosinophilia, methacholine challenge testing revealing reversible airway disease and most importantly a good response to the plethora of inhaled medication. However, patients often do not have these typical parameters, and upon further detailed questioning, the "wheeze" is actually occurring during inhalation at the level of the vocal folds and is thus "stridor." Hypersensitivity of the laryngopharynx, often from a post-viral vagal neuropathy, can result in coughing from multiple triggers such as cold air, talking, eating, or drinking and odors [45]. This type of neurogenic cough is often resistant to typical treatment for asthma, sinusitis, or allergy. Trigger reduction, focusing on decreasing the basal nasal drainage and decreasing reflux, can improve this type of cough in over 70% of patients with at least a 50% reduction in their cough [46]. Thus, reflux can play a significant role in triggering cough in states of hypersensitivity. This is likely due to the upregulation of acid sensing receptors in neurons of the laryngopharynx in the post-neuropathic state. LPR alone can trigger coughing. Direct reflux of acidic contents can stimulate ongoing cough, either with irritation of the laryngopharyngeal mucosa or direct penetration with or without aspiration of gastric contents. Cough due to LPR typically, though not always, is more of a wet cough, often with mucus production. Patients often awaken at night coughing and note increased coughing in the morning that tends to resolve when the mucus is clear. pH testing often reveals long periods of nocturnal acidity, even mildly, with coughing in the morning. The voice of these patients can also be slightly lower in pitch and more gravelly due to laryngeal edema.

Idiopathic Pulmonary Fibrosis

Idiopathic pulmonary fibrosis (IPF) is a chronic fibrotic lung disease with a median survival ranging from 2 to 3 years from the time of diagnosis [47]. The mechanisms leading to IPF remain unknown. To date, no cure is available and treatment strategies show little effect [48]. GERD has been previously associated with a number of interstitial lung diseases (ILDs) [49]. The etiology is long-term, repeated tracheobronchial aspiration of small amounts of gastric contents over time [50] and recent investigations demonstrating disease stabilization or delayed disease progression following medical or surgical treatment of GERD [51, 52].

Chronic Rhinosinusitis

Chronic rhinosinusitis (CRS) refers to inflammation of the nose and paranasal sinuses of more than 12 weeks' duration. It is a heterogeneous condition with varying etiologies including bacteria, fungi, viruses, biofilms, allergy, genetic conditions, and anatomic/innate factors. LPR has also been implicated as a factor contributing to the pathogenesis of CRS. It has been postulated that the direct exposure of gastric contents to the nasopharynx and nasal cavity results in mucosal injury, edema, and impaired mucociliary transport [53]. Several studies have shown a higher incidence of reflux events in patients with CRS, especially those refractory to medical and/or surgical therapy [54] with a corresponding reduction in subjective and objective assessment measures following medical therapy [55, 56].

Otitis Media Effusion

Otitis media with effusion (OME) in adults is less prevalent than in the pediatric population but still causes considerable morbidity. Etiologies and risk factors for adult OME are local malignancy, sinonasal disease, Eustachian tube dysfunction, allergies, and smoking. It has been suggested that LPR may have a role in the etiology of adult OME with some studies reporting a higher prevalence of OME in patients with LPR [57].

Special Consideration of Reflux in the Pediatric Age Group

There has been an increasing awareness of extraesophageal reflux in the pathogenesis and management of a variety of conditions involving the pediatric airway. The former has been implicated in conditions such as sinusitis, otitis media, laryngomalacia, recurrent croup, and other respiratory conditions including asthma, recurrent pneumonia, chronic cough, and even sleep apnea [58].

As with adult conditions, the link between reflux and the above conditions is unclear. One reason for the paucity of evidence is the inability to have conclusive, objective testing for LPR in the pediatric age group and the lack of robust evidence linking GERD as the cause of respiratory or ENT disorders.

Differential Diagnoses of LPR

Laryngopharyngeal reflux is a chronic condition that results from repeated extraesophageal exposure to gastric refluxate. As such, other conditions that cause chronic laryngitis should be considered in the differential diagnosis.

If the patient presents with an acute time course with fever, malaise, and sore throat, an infectious origin should be considered. Common bacterial pathogens include group A streptococcus and *Haemophilus influenzae*. Typical viral pathogens include parainfluenza, influenza, rhinovirus, adenovirus, and herpes simplex.

Acute laryngeal edema without infective symptoms could be suggestive of an anaphylactic or allergic reaction, especially if there is associated lip or tongue swelling.

In more chronic forms of laryngitis, infectious granulomatous diseases such as tuberculosis (*Mycobacterium tuberculosis*), leprosy (*Mycobacterium leprae*), actinomycosis (*Actinomyces bovis* or *israelii*), and syphilis (*Treponema pallidum*) should be considered. Granulomatous fungal infections can also affect the larynx, including candidiasis (*Candida albicans*), blastomycosis (*Blastomyces dermatitidis*), histoplasmosis (*Histoplasma capsulatum*), and aspergillosis (*Aspergillus fumigatus*). Noninfectious granulomatous diseases of the larynx include sarcoidosis and Wegener's granulomatosis. Autoimmune diseases such as rheumatoid arthritis, systemic lupus erythematosus, pemphigoid, relapsing polychondritis, and amyloidosis often have coexistent systemic symptoms [59, 60].

Other conditions can present with similar symptoms of LPR in the absence of frank laryngeal inflammation. Laryngeal sensory dysfunction is thought to play an important role in conditions including chronic refractory cough, ILO/PVFM, and muscle tension dysphonia. These conditions alone can mimic the symptoms of LPR even when it is absent. Furthermore, variable laryngeal hypersensitivity may help explain why some people are more likely to manifest the symptoms of LPR even in the presence of physiological reflux, whereas others remain minimally or relatively asymptomatic.

Physical Examination

Common LPR findings are posterior commissure hypertrophy, laryngeal/arytenoid inflammation, and thick endolaryngeal mucus. These changes occur as a result of mucosal irritation by refluxate from the stomach and inflammatory changes to the upper aerodigestive tract mucosa.

The majority of clinical research that have studied LPR signs use the Reflux Finding Score (RFS) to judge whether pathophysiologic reflux is present or not. The RFS is an eight-item scale that attempts to document the clinical severity of LPR using discrete scoring of possible inflammation at various points in the larynx. These findings include varying degrees of edema of the vocal folds and below the vocal folds (subglottic edema), ventricular obliteration or lateral vocal fold edema, erythema and/or hyperemia of the arytenoids and interarytenoid region, diffuse laryngeal edema involving the other structures of the larynx, posterior commissure hypertrophy or pachydermia of the glottis, granuloma or granulation formation, and the presence of thick endolaryngeal mucus. A score of >11 is thought to be suggestive of LPR [61] (Figs. 10.4, 10.5, and 10.6).

However, there are problems with the RFS. It does not take into account the myriad of other clinical signs that characterize LPR, such as laryngeal keratosis, posterior pharyngeal wall edema, and erythema with post-cricoid mucosal crowding, cobblestoning of the pharynx, "strawberry" nasopharynx (pockmarked nasopharyngeal tissues resembling a strawberry surface), lingual tonsil

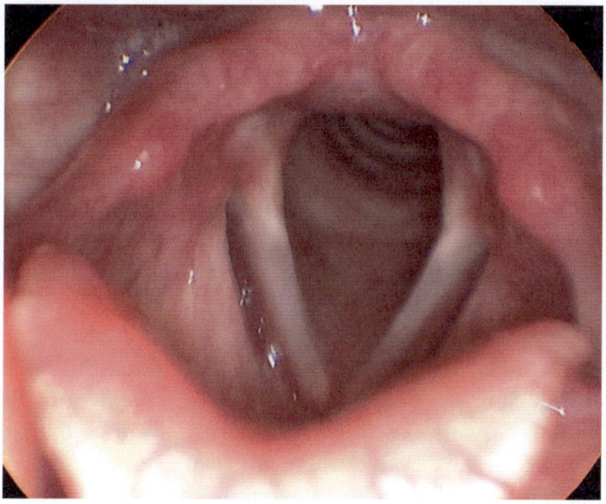

Fig. 10.4 Laryngoscopic image of normal vocal folds

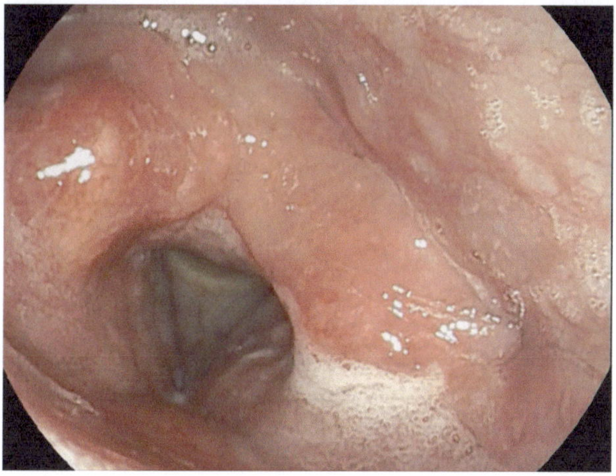

Fig. 10.5 Image of diffuse edema of the interarytenoid region, arytenoids, sub vocal fold region, and vocal folds; diffuse mucosal thickening, thick endolaryngeal mucus, and erythema

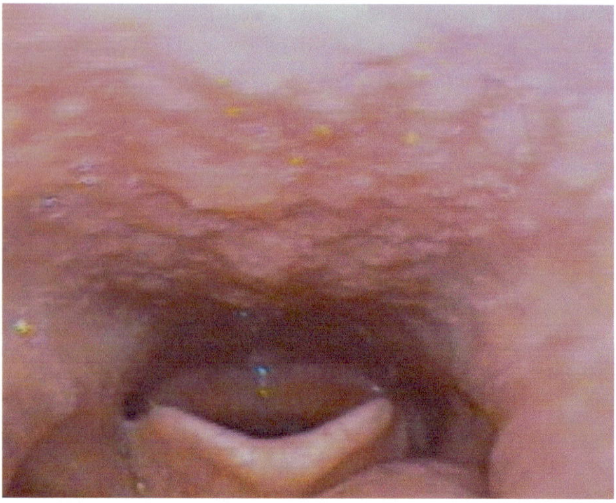

Fig. 10.6 Image of the posterior pharyngeal wall with raised mucosal glandular cobblestoning

hypertrophy, anterior tongue mucosal hypertrophy, and erythema of the anterior pillar [3, 62, 63]. RFS in clinical practice has also been shown to have poor inter-rater and intra-rater reliability [38] and may not correlate with pharyngeal pH probe studies or response to therapy [6]. In addition, some signs such as true vocal cord edema, interarytenoid hyperplasia, and arytenoid erythema that are utilized in the RFS have been found in non-reflux controls as well as other conditions [64]. Additionally, there is poor correlation between the RSI and the RFS, likely because there is no gold standard diagnostic test and both are subjective scoring systems. The RFS is subject to timing and presentation by the patient as well as subjective interpretation of the findings of the laryngopharynx by the observer. As a result of these issues, the laryngoscopic exam is not currently thought to be an accurate means of LPR diagnosis. However, the RFS score does provide a framework for identifying findings that could potentially signify the presence, or absence, of LPR. Additionally, these descriptive terms provide a lexicon for communicating findings to other healthcare workers and patients and can be helpful in describing the severity of findings (Fig. 10.7).

To address the deficiencies in the RFS, Lechien et al. have created a validated scoring system, the Reflux Sign Assessment (RSA). Like the RFS, a point system is assigned to various subcomponents of the laryngopharyngeal anatomy. In addition the RSA includes oropharyngeal findings. A score > 14 suggests the presence of LPR. High rates of intra- and inter-related concordance were present suggesting reliability. Treatment of LPR resulted in a demonstrable change in the RSA [65].

Some investigators have used computer color analysis of documented videolaryngoscopic examinations to provide quantitative data on the degree of erythema in the posterior commissure and have found it useful as a quantitative means of diagnosis and documentation of treatment outcomes for reflux laryngitis [66].

Fig. 10.7 Image of the nasopharynx with stippling of the nasopharyngeal mucosa

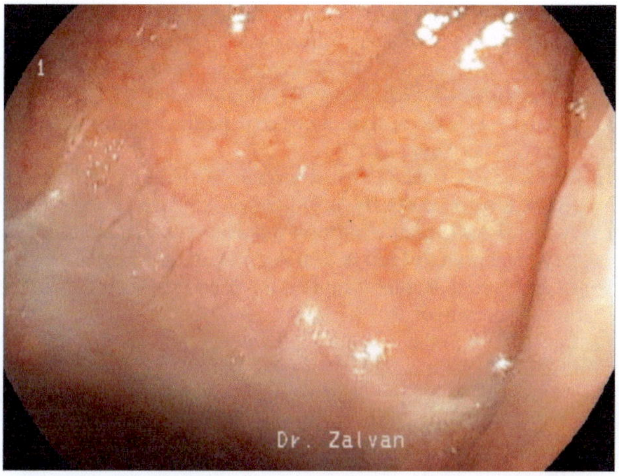

Summary

Although LPR is a common condition presenting in the ENT clinic, its evaluation is complex. Unfortunately, there is no gold standard for diagnosis of LPR, and clinical judgment is relied heavily upon when making a diagnosis. A considerable amount of research is needed to understand the pathophysiology of LPR and its association with other otolaryngological conditions.

References

1. Koufman JA, et al. Laryngopharyngeal reflux: position statement of the committee on speech, voice, and swallowing disorders of the American Academy of Otolaryngology-Head and Neck Surgery. Otolaryngol Head Neck Surg. 2002;127(1):32–5.
2. Koufman JA. The otolaryngologic manifestations of gastroesophageal reflux disease (GERD): a clinical investigation of 225 patients using ambulatory 24-hour pH monitoring and an experimental investigation of the role of acid and pepsin in the development of laryngeal injury. Laryngoscope. 1991;101(4 Pt 2 Suppl 53):1–78.
3. Lee YS, et al. Prospective, observational study using rabeprazole in 455 patients with laryngopharyngeal reflux disease. Eur Arch Otorhinolaryngol. 2011;268(6):863–9.
4. Koufman JA, et al. Prevalence of esophagitis in patients with pH-documented laryngopharyngeal reflux. Laryngoscope. 2002;112(9):1606–9.
5. Little FB, et al. Effect of gastric acid on the pathogenesis of subglottic stenosis. Ann Otol Rhinol Laryngol. 1985;94(5 Pt 1):516–9.
6. Johnson PE, et al. Ambulatory 24-hour double-probe pH monitoring: the importance of manometry. Laryngoscope. 2001;111(11 Pt 1):1970–5.
7. Johnston N, et al. Cell biology of laryngeal epithelial defenses in health and disease: further studies. Ann Otol Rhinol Laryngol. 2003;112(6):481–91.
8. Gill GA, et al. Laryngeal epithelial defenses against laryngopharyngeal reflux: investigations of E-cadherin, carbonic anhydrase isoenzyme III, and pepsin. Ann Otol Rhinol Laryngol. 2005;114(12):913–21.

9. Postma GN, et al. Esophageal motor function in laryngopharyngeal reflux is superior to that in classic gastroesophageal reflux disease. Ann Otol Rhinol Laryngol. 2001;110(12):1114–6.
10. Wiener GJ, et al. Chronic hoarseness secondary to gastroesophageal reflux disease: documentation with 24-h ambulatory pH monitoring. Am J Gastroenterol. 1989;84(12):1503–8.
11. Belafsky PC, et al. Symptoms and findings of laryngopharyngeal reflux. Ear Nose Throat J. 2002;81(9 Suppl 2):10–3.
12. Belafsky PC, Postma GN, Kourman JA. Validity and reliability of the reflux symptom index (RSI). J Voice. 2002;16(2):274–7.
13. Avincsal MO, et al. Halitosis associated volatile sulphur compound levels in patients with laryngopharyngeal reflux. Eur Arch Otorhinolaryngol. 2016;273(6):1515–20.
14. Chen M, et al. Reflux symptom index and reflux finding score in 91 asymptomatic volunteers. Acta Otolaryngol. 2018;138(7):659–63.
15. Lechien JR, et al. Validity and reliability of the reflux symptom score. Laryngoscope. 2020;130:E94.
16. Feder RJ, Michell MJ. Hyperfunctional, hyperacidic, and intubation granulomas. Arch Otolaryngol. 1984;110(9):582–4.
17. Delahunty JE, Cherry J. Experimentally produced vocal cord granulomas. Laryngoscope. 1968;78(11):1941–7.
18. Ogawa M, et al. The results of Kaplan-Meier and multivariate analyses of etiological factors related to the outcome of combined pharmacological therapy against laryngeal granuloma. Acta Otolaryngol. 2016;136(11):1141–6.
19. Tsunoda K, et al. An effective management regimen for laryngeal granuloma caused by gastroesophageal reflux: combination therapy with suggestions for lifestyle modifications. Acta Otolaryngol. 2007;127(1):88–92.
20. Havas TE, Priestley J, Lowinger DS. A management strategy for vocal process granulomas. Laryngoscope. 1999;109(2 Pt 1):301–6.
21. Fink DS, et al. Interarytenoid botulinum toxin injection for recalcitrant vocal process granuloma. Laryngoscope. 2013;123(12):3084–7.
22. Pham Q, et al. Botulinum toxin injections into the lateral cricoarytenoid muscles for vocal process granuloma. J Voice. 2018;32(3):363–6.
23. Hu HC, et al. Office-based autologous fat injection laryngoplasty for vocal process granuloma. J Voice. 2016;30(6):758.e7–758.e11.
24. Blumin JH, Johnston N. Evidence of extraesophageal reflux in idiopathic subglottic stenosis. Laryngoscope. 2011;121(6):1266–73.
25. Namba DR, et al. Rapamycin inhibits human laryngotracheal stenosis-derived fibroblast proliferation, metabolism, and function in vitro. Otolaryngol Head Neck Surg. 2015;152(5): 881–8.
26. Mark EJ, et al. Idiopathic tracheal stenosis: a clinicopathologic study of 63 cases and comparison of the pathology with chondromalacia. Am J Surg Pathol. 2008;32(8):1138–43.
27. McCann AJ, et al. The role of pepsin in epithelia-mesenchymal transition in idiopathic subglottic stenosis. Laryngoscope. 2019;130:154.
28. Francis DO, et al. Reevaluation of gastroesophageal reflux disease as a risk factor for laryngeal cancer. Laryngoscope. 2011;121(1):102–5.
29. Vaezi MF, et al. Laryngeal cancer and gastroesophageal reflux disease: a case-control study. Am J Med. 2006;119(9):768–76.
30. Qadeer MA, Colabianchi N, Vaezi MF. Is GERD a risk factor for laryngeal cancer? Laryngoscope. 2005;115(3):486–91.
31. Langevin SM, et al. Gastric reflux is an independent risk factor for laryngopharyngeal carcinoma. Cancer Epidemiol Biomark Prev. 2013;22(6):1061–8.
32. Bacciu A, et al. Effects of gastroesophageal reflux disease in laryngeal carcinoma. Clin Otolaryngol Allied Sci. 2004;29(5):545–8.
33. Christopher KL, et al. Vocal-cord dysfunction presenting as asthma. N Engl J Med. 1983;308(26):1566–70.

34. Maschka DA, et al. A classification scheme for paradoxical vocal cord motion. Laryngoscope. 1997;107(11 Pt 1):1429–35.
35. Perkner JJ, et al. Irritant-associated vocal cord dysfunction. J Occup Environ Med. 1998;40(2):136–43.
36. Balkissoon R, Kenn K. Asthma: vocal cord dysfunction (VCD) and other dysfunctional breathing disorders. Semin Respir Crit Care Med. 2012;33(6):595–605.
37. Murry T, et al. Respiratory retraining therapy and management of laryngopharyngeal reflux in the treatment of patients with cough and paradoxical vocal fold movement disorder. Ann Otol Rhinol Laryngol. 2006;115(10):754–8.
38. Paul BC, et al. Diagnostic accuracy of history, laryngoscopy, and stroboscopy. Laryngoscope. 2013;123(1):215–9.
39. Busse WW. Biological treatments for severe asthma: a major advance in asthma care. Allergol Int. 2019;68(2):158–66.
40. Dougherty RH, Fahy JV. Acute exacerbations of asthma: epidemiology, biology and the exacerbation-prone phenotype. Clin Exp Allergy. 2009;39(2):193–202.
41. Kollarik M, Ru F, Undem BJ. Acid-sensitive vagal sensory pathways and cough. Pulm Pharmacol Ther. 2007;20(4):402–11.
42. In AJ, Ngu MC, Breslin AB. Pathogenesis of chronic persistent cough associated with gastroesophageal reflux. Am J Respir Crit Care Med. 1994;149(1):160–7.
43. Eryuksel E, et al. Treatment of laryngopharyngeal reflux improves asthma symptoms in asthmatics. J Asthma. 2006;43(7):539–42.
44. Irwin RS, Boulet LP, Cloutier MM. Managing cough as a defense mechanism and as a symptom. A consensus panel report of the American College of Chest Physicians. Chest. 1998;114(2 Suppl Managing):133S–81S.
45. Altman KW, Noordzij JP, Rosen CA, et al. Neurogenic cough. Laryngoscope. 2015;125(7):1675–81. https://doi.org/10.1002/lary.25186. Epub 2015 Feb 3.
46. Zalvan C, Berzofsky C, Tiwari R, Geliebter J. Trigger reduction prior to systemic drugs for neurogenic chronic cough. Laryngoscope. 2019;129(1):198–202.
47. Nathan SD, et al. Long-term course and prognosis of idiopathic pulmonary fibrosis in the new millennium. Chest. 2011;140(1):221–9.
48. Noble PW, et al. Pirfenidone in patients with idiopathic pulmonary fibrosis (CAPACITY): two randomised trials. Lancet. 2011;377(9779):1760–9.
49. Hoppo T, Komatsu Y, Jobe BA. Gastroesophageal reflux disease and patterns of reflux in patients with idiopathic pulmonary fibrosis using hypopharyngeal multichannel intraluminal impedance. Dis Esophagus. 2014;27(6):530–7.
50. Savarino E, et al. Gastro-oesophageal reflux and gastric aspiration in idiopathic pulmonary fibrosis patients. Eur Respir J. 2013;42(5):1322–31.
51. Raghu G, et al. Sole treatment of acid gastroesophageal reflux in idiopathic pulmonary fibrosis: a case series. Chest. 2006;129(3):794–800.
52. Lee JS, et al. Gastroesophageal reflux therapy is associated with longer survival in patients with idiopathic pulmonary fibrosis. Am J Respir Crit Care Med. 2011;184(12):1390–4.
53. Ren JJ, et al. PepsinA as a marker of laryngopharyngeal reflux detected in chronic rhinosinusitis patients. Otolaryngol Head Neck Surg. 2017;156(5):893–900.
54. Lupa M, DelGaudio JM. Evidence-based practice: reflux in sinusitis. Otolaryngol Clin N Am. 2012;45(5):983–92.
55. Habermann W, et al. Short-term therapeutic trial of proton pump inhibitors in suspected extraesophageal reflux. J Voice. 2002;16(3):425–32.
56. El-Serag HB, et al. Lansoprazole treatment of patients with chronic idiopathic laryngitis: a placebo-controlled trial. Am J Gastroenterol. 2001;96(4):979–83.
57. Karyanta M, Satrowiyoto S, Wulandari DP. Prevalence ratio of otitis media with effusion in laryngopharyngeal reflux. Int J Otolaryngol. 2019;2019:7460891.
58. Karkos PD, et al. Laryngeal manifestations and pediatric laryngopharyngeal reflux. Am J Otolaryngol. 2006;27(3):200–3.

59. Ohki M, Kikuchi S. Nasal, oral, and pharyngolaryngeal manifestations of pemphigus vulgaris: endoscopic ororhinolaryngologic examination. Ear Nose Throat J. 2017;96(3):120–7.
60. Hamdan AL, Sarieddine D. Laryngeal manifestations of rheumatoid arthritis. Autoimmune Dis. 2013;2013:103081.
61. Belafsky PC, Postma GN, Koufman JA. The validity and reliability of the reflux finding score (RFS). Laryngoscope. 2001;111(8):1313–7.
62. Habermann W, et al. Reflux symptom index and reflux finding score in otolaryngologic practice. J Voice. 2012;26(3):e123–7.
63. Chappity P, et al. Proton pump inhibitors versus solitary lifestyle modification in management of laryngopharyngeal reflux and evaluating who is at risk: scenario in a developing country. Clin Med Insights Ear Nose Throat. 2014;7:1–5.
64. Hicks DM, et al. The prevalence of hypopharynx findings associated with gastroesophageal reflux in normal volunteers. J Voice. 2002;16(4):564–79.
65. Lechien JR, Rodriguez A, Dequanter D, et al. Validity and reliability of the reflux sign assessment (RSA). Ann Otol Rhinol Laryngol. 2019; https://doi.org/10.1177/0003489419888947.
66. Hanson DG, Jiang J, Chi W. Quantitative color analysis of laryngeal erythema in chronic posterior laryngitis. J Voice. 1998;12(1):78–83.

Chapter 11
Association Between Laryngopharyngeal Reflux and Benign Lesions of the Vocal Folds

Jerome R. Lechien, Camille Finck, and Thomas L. Carroll

Background and Epidemiology

Laryngopharyngeal reflux (LPR) symptoms are found in approximately 10–30% of outpatients visiting Otolaryngology – Head and Neck Surgery Departments in Western countries [1] and up to 50% of patients in voice centers [2]. In that respect, LPR has long been suspected to play a key role in the development of hoarseness [3, 4], and benign lesions of the vocal folds (BLVF), especially nodules, polyps, and hemorrhages, and Reinke's edema [5–8]. Nowadays, the mechanisms underlying the association between LPR and BLVF are still unknown [9]. However, the issue

J. R. Lechien (✉)
Research Committee, Laryngopharyngeal Reflux Study Group of Young-Otolaryngologists of the International Federations of Oto-rhino-laryngological Societies (YO-IFOS), Paris, France

Department of Otolaryngology-Head & Neck Surgery, Foch Hospital, Paris, France

Laboratory of Human Anatomy and Experimental Oncology, Faculty of Medicine, UMONS Research Institute for Health Sciences and Technology, University of Mons (UMons), Mons, Belgium
e-mail: Jerome.Lechien@umons.ac.be

C. Finck
Research Committee, Laryngopharyngeal Reflux Study Group of Young-Otolaryngologists of the International Federations of Oto-rhino-laryngological Societies (YO-IFOS), Paris, France

Department of Otolaryngology-Head & Neck Surgery, CHU de Liege, Liege, Belgium

T. L. Carroll
Department of Otolaryngology-Head and Neck Surgery, Harvard Medical School, Boston, MA, USA

Division of Otolaryngology, Department of Surgery, Brigham and Women's Hospital, Boston, MA, USA
e-mail: tcarroll@bwh.harvard.edu

C. H. Zalvan (ed.), *Laryngopharyngeal and Gastroesophageal Reflux*,
https://doi.org/10.1007/978-3-030-48890-1_11

remains important regarding the direct and indirect costs of BLVF in the USA. BLVF is one of the three most prevalent conditions associated with dysphonia, with treatment costs ranging from US $577.18 to US $953.21 per patient, per year [10, 11]. Pharmacy claims accounted for 20.1–33.3%, procedure claims 50.4–69.9%, and medical encounter claims 16.3–8.6% of overall direct costs, while anti-reflux drugs accounted for 10% of annual direct costs [10]. A better understanding of the mechanisms associating LPR and the development of BLVF appears important from a public health perspective.

In this chapter, we aim to evaluate the different clinical and basic science studies linking LPR to the development of BLVF, including nodules, polyps, hemorrhagic lesions, cysts, Reinke's edema, and sulcus vocalis.

Reflux and Voice Disorder

Experimental Studies

To understand the potential mechanisms associating reflux and BLVF, one must have a knowledge of the mechanisms underlying the macro- and micromodifications of the histology of the mucosa of the vocal folds (VFs) and their related impact on the vibratory process. Twenty experimental studies have been conducted over the past two decades that demonstrate the impact of reflux on the vocal folds. Two-thirds of these studies are focused on human VF samples and the other third on animal models (especially on pigs and dogs because of their physiologic and immunologic similarities) [12]. The findings of these studies may be grouped according to two areas: the inflammatory process of the VF mucosa related to reflux and the impact of reflux on the defense mechanisms of the laryngeal mucosa.

Inflammatory Reaction Related to Pepsin

The inflammatory reaction appears to be due to pepsin deposition in the upper aerodigestive tract mucosa. Pepsin is a proteolytic enzyme active to some degree at any pH between 1.5 and 6.0. A longer exposure time may be necessary at pH 5 to produce lesions [13–15]. Pepsin is well known in gastroenterology due to its important involvement in the development of esophagitis in patients with gastroesophageal reflux disease (GERD) [16]. The mechanisms, however, of the toxicity of pepsin in the upper aerodigestive tract mucosa remain unclear. Pepsin has extracellular and intracellular toxicities partially because inactivated pepsin molecules have good stability over time in the laryngeal epithelium and remain as potential irritants longer than the duration of a single reflux episode. In practice, the reactivation of pepsin is mediated by the next acidic reflux episode, an acid dietary intake (extracellular pepsin) [15, 17], or through the lower pH environment in the mitochondrial Golgi apparatus leading to activation of endocytosed pepsin. Regardless of how pepsin is activated by a lower pH environment, intracellular injuries and the development of an inflammatory reaction ensue [13, 17]. Pepsin endocytosis results in mitochondrial damage [13] and promotes the expression of many genes involved in the recruitment of inflammatory cells, migration, differentiation, growth, and angiogenesis [14, 18, 19]. The changes in the transcript levels of many pro-inflammatory genes can then occur in the epithelial cells of the VFs [20, 21]. Laryngeal epithelium is highly vulnerable to pepsin and these mechanisms. Pepsin would also ensure a chronic inflammatory reaction through additional alterations of the expression of growth factors involved in wound repair and angiogenesis [22, 23].

Pepsin is the most studied molecule in the development of the LPR inflammatory reaction in upper aerodigestive tract mucosa, but it does not act alone. One study has investigated the occurrence of bile acids in saliva, and these authors found that the level of bile acids was significantly higher in patients with LPR than in the controls [24]. Based on a recent study that did not find significant correlation either between the extracellular pepsin concentration and the proximal reflux episodes or the number and duration of reflux episodes and the clinical outcomes, it was suggested that reflux episodes may lead to the deposit of a mosaic of toxic gastrointestinal enzymes in the laryngopharyngeal mucosa, i.e., pepsin, lipase, bile salts, and trypsin. More complex mechanisms than those currently understood are likely [25].

Defense Mechanisms of the Vocal Folds

Experimental studies demonstrate that pepsin impairs the defense mechanism of the mucosa of the VFs, thus favoring inflammation, epithelial injuries, and the development of BLVF [9, 17]. Three main defense mechanisms impaired by pepsin have been identified: carbonic anhydrase (CA) activity, heat shock protein integrity, and the composition of mucin.

CA is the main pH-regulating enzyme located in the laryngeal mucosa [26]. It has been shown in a porcine model that acid and pepsin stress may acutely increase bicarbonate production by laryngeal epithelial cells, thus decreasing cell membrane transepithelial resistance [27, 28]. This adaptive and reversible response to mucosal injury, mediated by the intracellular CA isoform III [29], plays a key role in the neutralization of refluxed gastric acid, thus reducing pepsin's activity. Several studies report that chronic acidic and pepsin exposure reduce the expression of CA III in VF mucosa in both human [29–31] and animal [15] laryngeal samples at pH levels of 1.5 and 3.0 [15]. Thus, there is a positive correlation between the presence of pepsin and the lack of CAIII expression in VFs [31, 32].

The production of mucin is the second defense mechanism that is impaired in reflux patients. Hydrated mucin is one element of the mucus physical barrier between the extracellular environment and epithelial cells and contributes to the hydration and lubrication of the VF surfaces [33, 34]. The hydration of mucins is important for the determination of the volume of the mucus gel that contributes to the rheological properties of the VF and mediates binding and sequestration of a range of host defense factors. Some experimental studies demonstrated that reflux is associated with a cellular upregulation of mucin and other genes involved in inflammatory reactions (including vascular endothelial growth factor, fibroblast growth factor 2, matrix metalloproteinase 1, CA III, and Sep70). It has been demonstrated that MUC4 and MUC5AC gene expressions are decreased in laryngeal biopsies of VFs from LPR patient [29]. The depletion of MUC genes related to chronic LPR compromises epithelial restoration after chronic injury, leaving the epithelium more vulnerable [17].

The third noxious impact of LPR on VF defense mechanisms is the depletion of squamous epithelial heat shock protein which is involved in cellular protection from stress. Three studies reported a depletion of squamous epithelial heat shock protein 70 (Sep70) by acidic pepsin, suggesting an increased risk of VF trauma [15, 30, 35].

Morphological Changes of the Vocal Folds

The VF epithelium is composed of stratified squamous cells (eight layers) connected by apical junctional complexes that form a resistant barrier to mechanical and chemical stress [36]. The inflammatory reaction related to LPR causes dilatation of the intracellular spaces of the VF epithelium [15]. Specifically, intracellular epithelial pepsin decreases the expression of some cell adhesion molecules such as E-cadherin, supporting a defect in the integrity of the laryngeal epithelial barrier [29, 32, 37]. It is not clear whether the reduction in E-cadherin expression is related to the downstream inflammatory reaction from, or the direct effect of, acidic pepsin [32]. A canine model of LPR showed that the chronic exposure of VFs to gastroduodenal content (pepsin, bile salts, etc.) leads to substantial laryngeal mucosal changes including intraepithelial inflammation, VF squamous mucosal thickening and metaplasia, ulcers, erosions, stromal and peri-glandular infiltrations, and fibrosis [21, 38]. Other studies confirmed thickening of the mucosa of VFs exposed to reflux [38, 39]. Thus, the increase of intercellular spaces of the VF epithelium, as shown in human and animal models, favors the development of microtrauma, an important step in the development of BLVF [40, 41].

Clinical Studies

The observations of the experimental studies may help explain the findings of clinical studies. Most clinical studies, investigating hoarseness associated with reflux, found evidence of alterations in the vibratory process of the VFs through acoustic and aerodynamic measurements. Overall, aerodynamic (i.e., maximum phonation time) and acoustic (i.e., jitter and shimmer) measurements are better in healthy individuals than in patients with suspected or confirmed LPR.

Most clinical studies report an improvement in the inflammatory laryngostroboscopic findings (i.e., sticky mucus, posterior commissure hypertrophy, VF ulcerations, redness, edema, and granulation) after treatment [42]. These results, however, are biased due to the investigative physicians not assessing the laryngeal signs in a blinded manner to the patients' symptoms [43]. Studies investigating the changes of aerodynamic findings reported mixed results [44, 45], with only a few studies considering important objective physiologic evaluations such as transglottic airflow, subglottic pressure, and/or phonatory quotient [45–48]. Acoustic measurements offer indirect information about the vibrational characteristics of the VFs and are historically considered more able to detect subtle voice changes as compared to perceptual analysis alone [49]. Clinical studies tend to report significant pre- to posttreatment improvement of both jitter and shimmer, acoustic cues assessing perturbations of the frequency, and the intensity of voice, respectively [44, 47, 50–53].

In summary, regarding both experimental and clinical studies, LPR is likely associated with micro- and macroscopic changes of the mucosa of the VFs, leading to voice impairments, and related compensation mechanism (laryngeal hyperfunction, etc.) [17, 45]. In that respect, a recent multifactorial model of etiology and pathophysiology of hoarseness related to reflux has been proposed which includes the aforementioned mechanisms (Fig. 11.1).

Reflux and Benign Lesion of the Vocal Folds

Definition and Classification of Benign Lesions of the Vocal Folds

Thanks to the original work of Hirano [54], it is known that the human VFs have a very specialized and unique laminar histologic architecture. The vibratory tissue of the VFs, the lamina propria (LP), is organized in three layers differing in their composition of extracellular matrix (ECM) which is filled with a variety of macromolecules (fibrous proteins collagen and elastin, interstitial molecules mainly represented by glycosaminoglycans, proteoglycans, and glycoproteins) [55].

The superficial layer of the LP (SLLP), also called Reinke's space, plays a major role in the natural oscillatory function of the VFs. The SLLP is a very thin layer (0.3–0.5 mm) with a loose fibrous scaffolding and high concentration of hyaluronic acid. SLLP is also the only layer of the LP containing decorin, a small proteoglycan able to attach to collagen type I and II, modifying their assembly and reducing the fiber size. Molecular composition and fiber arrangement inside the SLLP allows a low viscosity, flexibility of the tissue, and also resistance to excessive deformation [56, 57]. Together with the epithelium, the SLLP forms the "mucosal cover" responsible for the mucosal wave, propagating on a more rigid "body" made up of the deep LP, vocal ligament, and thyroarytenoid muscle [57]. The VF epithelium is securely attached to the underlying SLLP by the epithelial basal lamina and anchoring fibers forming together the basement membrane (BM) zone [58].

In disease states, vibratory and nonvibratory trauma (including LPR) leads to benign vocal fold lesions by altering the structure and biomechanical properties of the Reinke's space. The SLLP is the more fragile layer, and vocal fold lesions

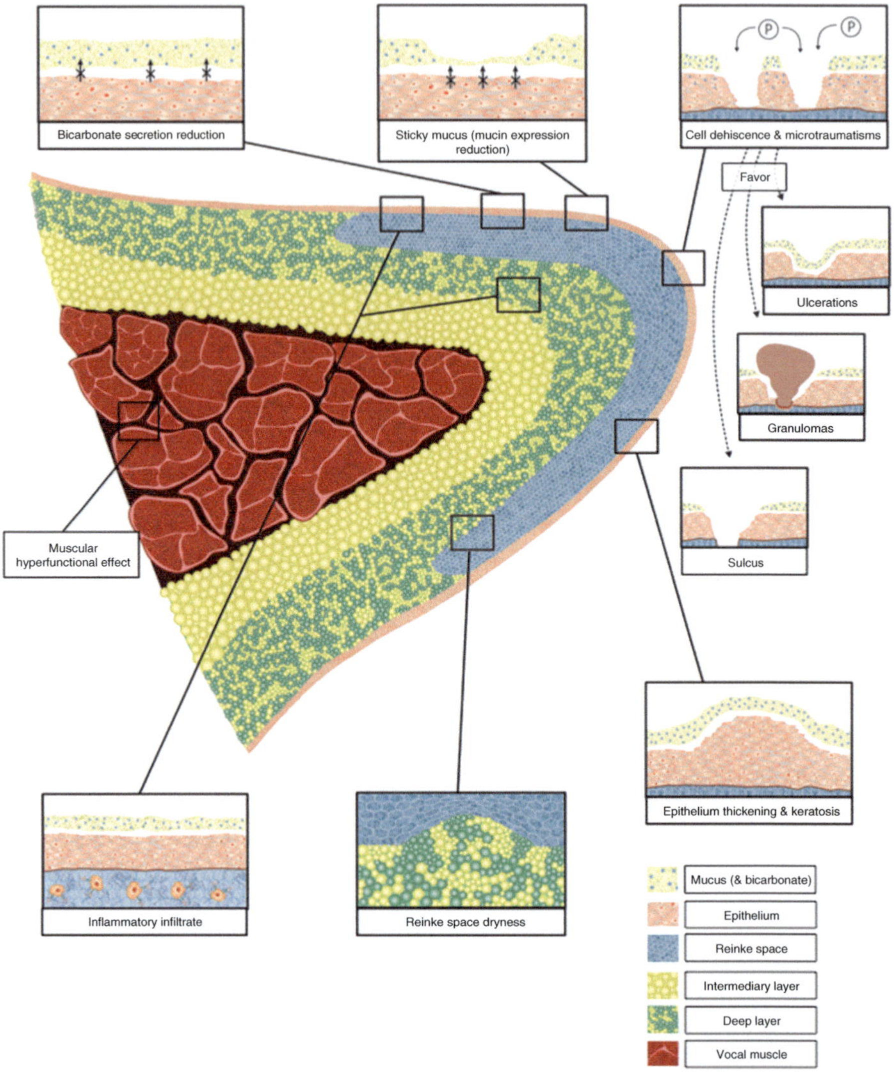

Fig. 11.1 The pathophysiological mechanisms of the development of hoarseness related to reflux. Reflux leads to several mechanisms, i.e., the reduction of bicarbonate secretion, the presence of sticky mucus (related to the reduction of the mucin expression), cell dehiscence and microtraumas in the vibrating epithelium (which favors the occurrence of ulcerations, granulomas, and sulcus), epithelium thickening and keratosis, Reinke's space dryness, inflammation infiltrate, and muscular hyperfunctional effect (compensatory behavior). The ulcerations and granulomas could be associated with VF scare, but that needs future studies to be demonstrated. The blue layer in this figure may correspond to superficial lamina propria. (This figure is from Lechien et al., J Voice (2016) [17]). Abbreviation: P pepsin

usually occur in this layer. They are the consequence of both tissue destruction and tissue response to trauma [59].

Classification of BLVFs is difficult because clinical, etiopathogenic, or histological criteria can be used to name them. Unfortunately, phoniatricians and phonomicrosurgeons do not reach consensus on the macroscopic appearance, the videostroboscopic features, and the pathogenic mechanisms of BLVFs. Pathogenic mechanisms remain mostly unknown, with the exception of a few (such as nodules).

What appears to be functionally important in the formation of BLVFs is how the SLLP is altered: thickness, pliability, and deformation of Reinke's space are the main features permitting a proposed, original classification system of BLVFs.

Four lesion types are proposed:

- Occupying lesions (epidermoid and mucous intracordal cysts, hemorrhagic lesions)
- Destructive lesions (sulci, vergetures, scars, mucosal bridges)
- Occupying and destructive lesions (nodules and subepithelial fibrosis)
- Deforming lesions (all types of edema, pseudocysts, some polyps)

Occupying Lesions (Mucous and Epidermoid Cysts, Posthemorrhagic Masses)

Mucous cysts are unilateral lesions thought to form from obstruction of a mucous gland naturally located on the inferior aspect of the VF. They are not considered by all to be related to excessive voice use [60].

Epidermoid cysts contain keratin debris and are more common than mucous cysts. For a long time considered to be congenital [61], previous papers lead to another physiopathological possibility: effortful phonation and excessive vocal demands induce a lesion of the SLLP, followed by a pathological healing process trapping epithelial cells inside the SLLP [60]. This mechanism could explain the high prevalence of such lesions (frequently bilateral) in singers, teachers, coaches, etc.

Posthemorrhagic lesions including vocal fold hemorrhages and hemorrhagic polyps are more frequently unilateral than bilateral. They often appear following an intense and temporary vocal effort, a Valsalva maneuver, coughing efforts [60], and voice use in a noisy environment [62]. They would be more likely to occur in patients on aspirin, those with laryngeal inflammation and irritation, and premenopausal women due to the hormonal changes associated with the menstrual cycle.

Destructive Lesions (Sulci, Vergetures, Mucosal Bridges, and Scars)

Destructive lesions are characterized by loss of the SLLP [63]. The lesions may be congenital [61] or acquired (i.e., sequel of traumatic lesion of the SLLP: excessive vocal charge [60], post-iatrogenic lesion [64] [i.e., post-microsurgical scars], or toxic or inflammatory trauma).

Occupying and Destructive Lesions (Nodules and Subepithelial Fibrosis)

Nodules appear as a slight convexity of the free edge of the bilateral VFs and cause decreased pliability during vibration. BM zone changes have been demonstrated in VF nodules including abnormal thickening of the BM as well as dislocation and fragmentation of the basal lamina. Authors have also reported abnormal deposition of fibronectin and collagen in the subepithelial region [65, 66]. Physiopathological mechanisms underlying the development of nodules could include excessive voice use leading to localized destruction of the BM and the progressive invasion of the SLLP by fragments of BM and other factors involved in an abnormal healing process.

Subepithelial fibrosis is rarely described but has the same characteristics as nodules with the exception of deformation of the free edge of the VFs. Both lesions represent a localized destruction and occupation of SLLP, starting at the level of the epithelial BM.

Deforming Lesions (Edema, Pseudocysts, and Polyps)

Deforming lesions are characterized by an excessive amount of ECM of the SLLP leading to deformation of the free edge of the VFs. Pliability is variable and sometimes greatly reduced. Unilateral or bilateral edema may be a consequence of excessive voice use or due to toxic or inflammatory lesions of the vocal cover as is seen in particular patients who smoke tobacco [67]. Pseudocysts are unilateral lesions, more frequently observed in women, that appear as a translucent and very superficial blister; its etiology remains unknown, but it is theorized that a unilateral VF paresis has been suspected [68]. Polyps are deforming lesions that are thought to result after hemorrhage.

To date, 35 papers have explored, directly or indirectly, the relationship between LPR and BLVF [9].

Reflux and Nodules

The association between LPR and nodules has been evaluated in more than ten studies [9]. Some suggest the coexistence of both conditions in patients with suspected LPR [69–72] as well as in voice professionals in other papers [7, 71, 73–75]. In all of these studies, however, the LPR diagnosis has not been made through objective reflux testing. There are only five studies that investigated the relationship between nodules and reflux where reflux was diagnosed through objective methods [5, 75–79]. Twenty years ago, the initial studies of Kuhn et al. and Ulualp et al. reported a significantly higher prevalence of pharyngeal acid reflux events in patients with nodules in comparison with healthy subjects [5, 79]. Ulualp et al. identified LPR in 78% of patients with nodules, while 64% of nodule patients in Kuhn et al. revealed coexisting LPR [5, 79]. In these two studies, LPR was present in only 18% and 21% of healthy individuals who composed the control groups. Along the same vein, Beltis et al. identified 60% of patients with nodules that also had LPR [76]. In contrast, Chung et al. did not identify a significantly higher prevalence of LPR, a pathological reflux finding score, or an elevated reflux symptom index score in patients with nodules compared to subjects who complained of LPR symptoms without BLVF [77]. None of these authors used impedance-pH monitoring to determine if nonacid and/or mixed LPR was present in their patients.

Using a Western blot approach, Tasli et al. did not find pepsin molecules in vocal fold nodule specimens of patients who underwent phonosurgery [80]. These authors only analyzed the nodule tissue and did not evaluate the mucosa of the vocal folds (the area where pepsin was identified in previous studies) [81].

In summary, and based on the few studies that used objective testing for the LPR diagnosis, LPR appears more prevalent in patients with nodules than in healthy controls.

Reflux and Reinke's Edema

In 2009, Chung et al. identified an LPR-related symptom prevalence of 90% in patients with Reinke's edema, which was significantly higher than in patients who did not have Reinke's edema [77]. Similarly, Beltis et al. identified an LPR prevalence of 67% in patients with Reinke's edema after diagnosing LPR by pH monitoring [76]. The association between LPR, laryngitis, and Reinke's edema was supported in a large cohort of patients who had gastrointestinal (GI) endoscopy [82]. Another study reported that nonsmoker LPR patients with Reinke's edema had more inflammatory histopathological findings in the laryngeal mucosa than those without reflux [83]. Kantas et al. observed that the persistence of LPR after surgery negatively influenced the re-epithelialization of vocal folds in patients who underwent phonosurgery for polyps and Reinke's edema [78].

Reflux, Hemorrhage, and Polyps

As was seen with the research on nodules and Reinke's edema, only a few studies used an objective approach to identify reflux in patients with hemorrhages or polyps of the vocal folds; the majority of studies report low levels of evidence in the demonstration of an association between LPR and polyps [7, 70, 84–86]. Among the two studies that used pH monitoring for the LPR diagnosis, significant reflux events were identified in 75% of patients with polyps, while only 37% of healthy controls had positive pH monitoring [76, 77]. Similarly to nodules, LPR may negatively influence voice outcomes of patients after surgery for polyps. Those patients without LPR had better perceptual voice quality outcomes after surgery than those with LPR [84].

Reflux and Cysts

The relationship between LPR and vocal fold cysts is still poorly studied. Nacci et al. exhibited a higher prevalence of cysts in singing students who had higher clinical scores of reflux (Reflux Symptom Index and Reflux Finding Score) in comparison with non-singing students [73]. In the same way, Perez Fernandez et al. observed a higher prevalence of cysts and LPR in teachers [74]. Wang et al. suggested that patients who underwent phonosurgery for vocal fold retention cysts had better post-operative perceptual voice quality improvements if they did not have LPR symptoms [84]. In the majority of these studies, there was no histopathological information about the type of cysts (mucous versus epidermoid).

Reflux and Sulcus Vocalis

Similar to what was seen in cysts and LPR, Nacci et al. found a higher prevalence of sulcus vocalis in singing students who also have higher reflux symptom score [73]. Myint et al. showed that opera students with suspected LPR had a higher prevalence of sulcus vocalis than students without LPR symptoms [87]. Again, authors did not use an objective approach for the diagnosis of LPR in these studies, thus limiting the establishment of clear conclusions.

Perspectives

According to experimental and clinical studies, caustic mucosal exposure from reflux would increase the susceptibility of the vocal fold mucosa to injury and subsequent nodules, polyps, and Reinke's edema formation. In practice, the pathophysiological model would be more complex than what is offered here, as many other risk factors of mucosal injury must be considered (tobacco, laryngopharyngeal allergy, pollution, etc.). In practice, objective methods of diagnosing LPR remain unavailable to most, and in the literature on this subject no author employs pH-impedance testing to consider the acidity or lack thereof of the refluxate nor has a true gold standard diagnostic test been validated for LPR. In studies that do employ pH testing, oropharyngeal pH monitoring and dual pH probe testing have also afforded a wide range of results given the lack of a gold standard true diagnostic test of LPR. While all manners of pH measurement are sensitive to detect the pH level of the involved structures, pH alone is clearly not the only criteria required for an LPR diagnosis. The heterogeneity between studies regarding inclusion, exclusion, and diagnostic criteria, as well as clinical outcomes for the diagnosis, explains the variability of results between experimental studies and clinical observation. As new research is considered and studies are designed, it seems important to consider LPR as a potential risk factor in the development of BLVF in high-risk, high-voice-use professionals. Future studies using the best current diagnostic tools (pH monitoring, pepsin, and trypsin detection) and tissue analysis to detect the presence of histologic evidence suggestive of LPR should be considered. A better understanding of the relationship between reflux and vocal fold pathology could lead to reductions in both the cost and effort that are associated with the treatment of BLVF for both clinicians and patients.

References

1. Lechien JR, Akst LM, Hamdan AL, Schindler A, Karkos PD, Barillari MR, Calvo-Henriquez C, Crevier-Buchman L, Finck C, Eun YG, Saussez S, Vaezi MF. Evaluation and management of laryngopharyngeal reflux disease: state of the art review. Otolaryngol Head Neck Surg. 2019;160(5):762–82.
2. Koufman JA, Aviv JE, Casiano RR, Shaw GY. Laryngopharyngeal reflux: position statement of the committee on speech, voice, and swallowing disorders of the American Academy of Otolaryngology-Head and Neck Surgery. Otolaryngol Head Neck Surg. 2002;127(1):32–5.
3. Sataloff RT. Professional singers: the science and art of clinical care. Am J Otolaryngol. 1981;2(3):251–66.
4. Deveney CW, Benner K, Cohen J. Gastroesophageal reflux and laryngeal disease. Arch Surg. 1993;128(9):1021–5; discussion 1026–7
5. Kuhn J, Toohill RJ, Ulualp SO, et al. Pharyngeal acid reflux events in patients with vocal cord nodules. Laryngoscope. 1998;108(8 Pt 1):1146–9.
6. Sandokji AM, Al-Karawi MA, Sanai FM. Transnasal upper gastrointestinal endoscopy in detection of gastroesophageal reflux disease induced vocal cord polyp. Saudi Med J. 2000;21(8):780–1.
7. Pereira ER, Tavares EL, Martins RH. Voice disorders in teachers: clinical, videolaryngoscopical, and vocal aspects. J Voice. 2015;29(5):564–71.
8. Preciado J, Pérez C, Calzada M, Preciado P. Prevalence and incidence studies of voice disorders among teaching staff of La Rioja, Spain. Clinical study: questionnaire, function vocal examination, acoustic analysis and videolaryngostroboscopy. Acta Otorrinolaringol Esp. 2005;56(5):202–10.
9. Lechien JR, Saussez S, Nacci A, Barillari MR, Rodriguez A, Le Bon SD, Crevier-Buchman L, Harmegnies B, Finck C, Akst LM. Association between laryngopharyngeal reflux and benign vocal folds lesions: a systematic review. Laryngoscope. 2019; https://doi.org/10.1002/lary.27932.
10. Cohen SM, Kim J, Roy N, et al. Direct health care costs of laryngeal diseases and disorders. Laryngoscope. 2012;122:1582–8.
11. Stachler RJ, Francis DO, Schwartz SR, et al. Clinical practice guideline: hoarseness (dysphonia) (update). Otolaryngol Head Neck Surg. 2018;158(1_suppl):S1–S42.
12. Birchall MA, Bailey M, Barker EV, Rothkötter HJ, Otto K, Macchiarini P. Model for experimental revascularized laryngeal allotransplantation. Br J Surg. 2002;89(11):1470–5.
13. Johnston N, Wells CW, Samuels TL, Blumin JH. Pepsin in nonacidic refluxate can damage hypopharyngeal epithelial cells. Ann Otol Rhinol Laryngol. 2009;118(9):677–85.
14. Ylitalo R, Thibeault SL. Relationship between time of exposure of laryngopharyngeal reflux and gene expression in laryngeal fibroblasts. Ann Otol Rhinol Laryngol. 2006;115(10):775–83.
15. Johnston N, Dettmar PW, Bishwokarma B, Lively MO, Koufman JA. Activity/stability of human pepsin: implications for reflux attributed laryngeal disease. Laryngoscope. 2007;117(6):1036–9.

16. Roberts NB. Review article: human pepsins - their multiplicity, function and role in reflux disease. Aliment Pharmacol Ther. 2006;24(Suppl 2):2–9.
17. Lechien JR, Saussez S, Harmegnies B, Finck C, Burns JA. Laryngopharyngeal reflux and voice disorders: a multifactorial model of etiology and pathophysiology. J Voice. 2017;31(6):733–52.
18. Johnston N, Wells CW, Blumin JH, Toohill RJ, Merati AL. Receptor-mediated uptake of pepsin by laryngeal epithelial cells. Ann Otol Rhinol Laryngol. 2007;116(12):934–8.
19. Johnston N, Wells CW, Samuels TL, Blumin JH. Rationale for targeting pepsin in the treatment of reflux disease. Ann Otol Rhinol Laryngol. 2010;119(8):547–58.
20. Bulmer DM, Ali MS, Brownlee IA, Dettmar PW, Pearson JP. Laryngeal mucosa: its susceptibility to damage by acid and pepsin. Laryngoscope. 2010;120(4):777–82.
21. Cohen SM, Huang S, Garrett CG, Courey MS. Acute histologic effects of extraesophageal reflux on vocal fold healing. Ann Otol Rhinol Laryngol. 2005;114(4):296–303.
22. Hom DB. Growth factors and wound healing in otolaryngology. Otolaryngol Head Neck Surg. 1994;110(6):560–4.
23. Lord RV, Park JM, Wickramasinghe K, et al. Vascular endothelial growth factor and basic fibroblast growth factor expression in esophageal adenocarcinoma and Barrett esophagus. J Thorac Cardiovasc Surg. 2003;125(2):246–53.
24. Sereg-Bahar M, Jerin A, Jansa R, Stabuc B, Hocevar-Boltezar I. Pepsin and bile acids in saliva in patients with laryngopharyngeal reflux – a prospective comparative study. Clin Otolaryngol. 2015;40(3):234–9.
25. Bobin F, Journe F, Lechien JR. Saliva pepsin level of laryngopharyngeal reflux patients is not correlated with reflux episodes. Laryngoscope. 2019; https://doi.org/10.1002/lary.28260.
26. Axford SE, Sharp N, Ross PE, et al. Cell biology of laryngeal epithelial defenses in health and disease: preliminary studies. Ann Otol Rhinol Laryngol. 2001;110(12):1099–108.
27. Erickson E, Sivasankar M. Simulated reflux decreases vocal fold epithelial barrier resistance. Laryngoscope. 2010;120(8):1569–75.
28. Erickson-Levendoski E, Sivasankar MP. Role for ion transport in porcine vocal fold epithelial defense to acid challenge. Otolaryngol Head Neck Surg. 2012;146(2):272–8.
29. Johnston N, Bulmer D, Gill GA, et al. Cell biology of laryngeal epithelial defenses in health and disease: further studies. Ann Otol Rhinol Laryngol. 2003;112(6):481–91.
30. Min HJ, Hong SC, Yang HS, Mun SK, Lee SY. Expression of CAIII and Hsp70 is increased the mucous membrane of the posterior commissure in laryngopharyngeal reflux disease. Yonsei Med J. 2016;57(2):469–74.
31. Johnston N, Knight J, Dettmar PW, Lively MO, Koufman J. Pepsin and carbonic anhydrase isoenzyme III as diagnostic markers for laryngopharyngeal reflux disease. Laryngoscope. 2004;114(12):2129–34.
32. Gill GA, Johnston N, Buda A, et al. Laryngeal epithelial defenses against laryngopharyngeal reflux: investigations of E-cadherin, carbonic anhydrase isoenzyme III, and pepsin. Ann Otol Rhinol Laryngol. 2005;114(12):913–21.
33. Ali MS, Pearson JP. Upper airway mucin gene expression: a review. Laryngoscope. 2007;117(5):932–8.
34. Sivasankar M, Erickson E, Schneider S, Hawes A. Phonatory effects of airway dehydration: preliminary evidence for impaired compensation to oral breathing in individuals with a history of vocal fatigue. J Speech Lang Hear Res. 2008;51(6):1494–506.
35. Hoppo T, Zaidi AH, Matsui D, Martin SA, Komatsu Y, Lloyd EJ, Kosovec JE, Civitarese AA, Boyd NH, Shetty A, Omstead AN, Smith E, Jobe BA. Sep70/Pepsin expression in hypopharynx combined with hypopharyngeal multichannel intraluminal impedance increases diagnostic sensitivity of laryngopharyngeal reflux. Surg Endosc. 2018;32(5):2434–41.
36. Hirano M. Morphological structure of the vocal cord as a vibrator and its variations. Folia Phoniatr (Basel). 1974;26(2):89–94.
37. Reichel O, Mayr D, Durst F, Berghaus A. E-cadherin but not beta-catenin expression is decreased in laryngeal biopsies from patients with laryngopharyngeal reflux. Eur Arch Otorhinolaryngol. 2008;265(8):937–42.

38. Adhami T, Goldblum JR, Richter JE, Vaezi MF. The role of gastric and duodenal agents in laryngeal injury: an experimental canine model. Am J Gastroenterol. 2004;99(11):2098–106.
39. Shimazu R, Kusano K, Kuratomi Y, Inokuchi A. Histological changes of the pharynx and larynx in rats with chronic acid reflux esophagitis. Acta Otolaryngol. 2009;129(8):886–92.
40. Rees LE, Pazmany L, Gutowska-Owsiak D, et al. The mucosal immune response to laryngopharyngeal reflux. Am J Respir Crit Care Med. 2008;177(11):1187–93.
41. Hu Y, Xu X, Xu L, Lai C, Zhang T. Dilated intercellular space in the larynx and esophagus of a rabbit reflux model. Auris Nasus Larynx. 2013;40(4):379–82.
42. Lechien JR, Saussez S, Schindler A, Karkos PD, Hamdan AL, Harmegnies B, De Marrez LG, Finck C, Journe F, Paesmans M, Vaezi MF. Clinical outcomes of laryngopharyngeal reflux treatment: a systematic review and meta-analysis. Laryngoscope. 2019;129(5):1174–87.
43. Chang BA, MacNeil SD, Morrison MD, Lee PK. The reliability of the reflux finding score among general otolaryngologists. J Voice. 2015;29(5):572–7.
44. Lechien JR, Finck C, Khalife M, Huet K, Delvaux V, Picalugga M, Harmegnies B, Saussez S. Change of signs, symptoms and voice quality evaluations throughout a 3- to 6-month empirical treatment for laryngopharyngeal reflux disease. Clin Otolaryngol. 2018;43(5):1273–82.
45. Lechien JR, Finck C, Costa de Araujo P, Huet K, Delvaux V, Piccaluga M, Harmegnies B, Saussez S. Voice outcomes of laryngopharyngeal reflux treatment: a systematic review of 1483 patients. Eur Arch Otorhinolaryngol. 2017;274(1):1–23.
46. Hamdan AL, Sharara AI, Younes A, Fuleihan N. Effect of aggressive therapy on laryngeal symptoms and voice characteristics in patients with gastroesophageal reflux. Acta Otolaryngol. 2001;121(7):868–72.
47. Wan Y, Yan Y, Ma F, et al. LPR: how different diagnostic tools shape the outcomes of treatment. J Voice. 2014;28(3):362–8.
48. Sahin M, Kirazli T, Ogut MF, Akyildiz NS, Bor S. The effect of antireflux surgery on laryngeal symptoms, findings and voice parameters. Eur Arch Otorhinolaryngol. 2015;272(11):3375–83.
49. Lechien JR, Huet K, Khalife M, et al. Impact of laryngopharyngeal reflux on subjective and objective voice assessments: a prospective study. J Otolaryngol Head Neck Surg. 2016;45(1):59.
50. Jin BJ, Lee YS, Jeong SW, Jeong JH, Lee SH, Tae K. Change of acoustic parameters before and after treatment in laryngopharyngeal reflux patients. Laryngoscope. 2008;118(5):938–41.
51. Ogut F, Ersin S, Engin EZ, et al. The effect of laparoscopic Nissen fundoplication on laryngeal findings and voice quality. Surg Endosc. 2007;21(4):549–54.
52. Shaw GY, Searl JP. Laryngeal manifestations of gastroesophageal reflux before and after treatment with omeprazole. South Med J. 1997;90(11):1115–22.
53. Park JO, Shim MR, Hwang YS, et al. Combination of voice therapy and antireflux therapy rapidly recovers voice-related symptoms in laryngopharyngeal reflux patients. Otolaryngol Head Neck Surg. 2012;146(1):92–7.
54. Hirano M, Kurita S, Nakashima T. The structure of the vocal folds. In: Stevens KN, Hirano M, editors. Vocal fold physiology. Tokyo: University of Tokyo press; 1981.
55. Alberts B, Johnson A, Walter P, Lewis J, Raff M, Roberts K. Cell junction, cell adhesion and the extra- cellular matrix. In: McDonald Institute for Archaeological research, editor. Molecular biology of the cell. New York, London: Garland Science; 2008.
56. Gray SD, Titze IR, Chan R, Hammond TH. Vocal fold proteoglycans and their influence on biomechanics. Laryngoscope. 1999;109:845–54.
57. Finck C, Lejeune L. Structure and oscillatory function of the vocal folds. In: Brudzynski SM, editor. Handbook of mammalian vocalization. San Diego: Elsevier Academic Press; 2010.
58. Tateya T, Tateya I, Bless DM. Immuno-scanning electron microscopy of collagen types I and III in human vocal fold lamina propria. Ann Otol Rhinol Laryngol. 2007;116:156–9.
59. Finck C, Lefebvre P. Implantation of esterified hyaluronic acid in micro-dissected Reinke's space after vocal fold microsurgery: first clinical experiences. Laryngoscope. 2005;115:1841–7.

60. Bastian RW. Benign vocal fold mucosal disorders. In: Cummings CW, Frederckson JM, Harker LA, Krause CJ, Schuller DE, Richardson MA, editors. Otolaryngology & head neck surgery, vol. 5. 3rd ed. St Louis: Mosby; 1998.
61. Garcia Martins RH, et al. Sulcus vocalis: probable genetic etiology. Rev Bras Otorrinolaringol. 2007;73(4):573.
62. Rontal E, Rontal M, Jacob HJ, Rolnick MI. Vocal cord dysfunction- an industrial health hazard. Ann Otol Rhinol Laryngol. 1979;88:818–21.
63. Ford CN. Advances and refinements in Phonosurgery. Laryngoscope. 1999;109:1891–900.
64. Benninger MS, Alessi D, Archer S, Bastian R, Ford C, Koufman J, Sataloff RT, Spiegel JR, Woo P. Vocal fold scarring: current concepts and management. Otolaryngol-Head Neck Surg. 1996;115:474–82.
65. Gray SD, Hammond E, Hanson DF. Benign pathologic responses of the larynx. Ann Otol Rhinol Laryngol. 1995;104:13–8.
66. Gray SD. Basement membrane zone injury in vocal nodules. In: Gauffin J, Hammarberg B, editors. Vocal fold physiology: acoustic, perceptual, and physiological aspects of voice mechanisms. San Diego: Whurr Publishers, Singular publishing group; 1991.
67. Zeitels SM, Hillman RE, Bunting GW, Vaughn T. Reinke's edema: phonatory mechanisms and management strategies. Ann Otol Rhinol Laryngol. 1997;106(7 Pt 1):533–43.
68. Koufman JA, Belafsky PC. Unilateral or localized Reinke's edema (pseudocyst) as a manifestation of vocal fold paresis: the paresis podule. Laryngoscope. 2001;111:576–80.
69. de Bortoli N, Nacci A, Savarino E, et al. How many cases of laryngopharyngeal reflux suspected by laryngoscopy are gastroesophageal reflux disease-related? World J Gastroenterol. 2012;18(32):4363–70.
70. Arruda Henry MA, Martins RH, Lerco MM, Carvalho LR, Lamônica-Garcia VC. Gastroesophageal reflux disease and vocal disturbances. Arq Gastroenterol. 2011;48(2):98–103.
71. Van Houtte E, Van Lierde K, D'Haeseleer E, Claeys S. The prevalence of laryngeal pathology in a treatment-seeking population with dysphonia. Laryngoscope. 2010;120(2):306–12.
72. Catalano F, Terminella C, Grillo C, Biondi S, Zappalà M, Bentivegna C. Prevalence of oesophagitis in patients with persistent upper respiratory symptoms. J Laryngol Otol. 2004;118(11):857–61.
73. Nacci A, Baracca G, Romeo SO, et al. Endoscopic and phoniatric evaluation in singing students. J Voice. 2017. pii: S0892-1997(17)30305-3.
74. Pérez Fernández CA, Preciado LJ. Vocal fold nodules. Risk factors in teachers. A case control study design. Acta Otorrinolaringol Esp. 2003;54(4):253–60.
75. Lundy DS, Casiano RR, Sullivan PA, Roy S, Xue JW, Evans J. Incidence of abnormal laryngeal findings in asymptomatic singing students. Otolaryngol Head Neck Surg. 1999;121(1):69–77.
76. Beltsis A, Katsinelos P, Kountouras J, et al. Double probe pH-monitoring findings in patients with benign lesions of the true vocal folds: comparison with typical GERD and the effect of smoking. Eur Arch Otorhinolaryngol. 2011;268(8):1169–74.
77. Chung JH, Tae K, Lee YS, et al. The significance of laryngopharyngeal reflux in benign vocal mucosal lesions. Otolaryngol Head Neck Surg. 2009;141(3):369–73.
78. Kantas I, Balatsouras DG, Kamargianis N, Katotomichelakis M, Riga M, Danielidis V. The influence of laryngopharyngeal reflux in the healing of laryngeal trauma. Eur Arch Otorhinolaryngol. 2009;266(2):253–9.
79. Ulualp SO, Toohill RJ, Shaker R. Pharyngeal acid reflux in patients with single and multiple otolaryngologic disorders. Otolaryngol Head Neck Surg. 1999;121(6):725–30.
80. Tasli H, Eser B, Asik MB, Birkent H. Does pepsin play a role in etiology of laryngeal nodules? J Voice. 2018. pii: S0892-1997(18)30041-9.
81. Lechien JR, Saussez S, Harmegnies B, Finck C. Laryngopharyngeal reflux as causative factor of vocal fold nodules. J Voice. 2018. pii: S0892-1997(18)30223-6.

82. Katsinelos P, Kountouras J, Chatzimavroudis G, et al. Should inspection of the laryngopharyngeal area be part of routine upper gastrointestinal endoscopy? A prospective study. Dig Liver Dis. 2009;41(4):283–8.
83. Kamargiannis N, Gouveris H, Katsinelos P, et al. Chronic pharyngitis is associated with severe acidic laryngopharyngeal reflux in patients with Reinke's edema. Ann Otol Rhinol Laryngol. 2011;120(11):722–6.
84. Wang CT, Lai MS, Hsiao TY. Comprehensive outcome researches of intralesional steroid injection on benign vocal fold lesions. J Voice. 2015;29(5):578–87.
85. Akdogan MV, Erinanc H, Topal O, Erbek SS. Expression of a disintegrin and metalloproteinase-33 protein in vocal fold polyp(s). J Laryngol Otol. 2015;129(7):688–92.
86. Siupsinskiene N, Jurgutaviciute V, Katutiene I, Janciauskas D, Vaitkus S, Adamonis K. Helicobacter pylori infection in laryngeal diseases. Eur Arch Otorhinolaryngol. 2013;270(8):2283–8.
87. Myint C, Moore JE, Hu A, Jaworek AJ, Sataloff RT. A comparison of initial and subsequent follow-up strobovideolaryngoscopic examinations in singers. J Voice. 2016;30(4):472–7.

Chapter 12
Diagnostic Approach to Laryngopharyngeal Reflux

Ralph A. Iannuzzi

Introduction

The diagnosis of laryngopharyngeal reflux (LPR) presents significant challenges despite its first being recognized as a distinct clinical entity decades ago. There remains considerable controversy over what the most reliable diagnostic criteria are and what diagnostic modality is preferred. There is no gold standard [1]. Currently, a combination of clinical history, physical findings on laryngoscopy, and a variety of somewhat nonspecific tests are employed by practitioners to evaluate patients with suspected LPR. In this chapter, we will detail a variety of available diagnostic options for LPR, presenting the advantages and the disadvantages of each.

Barium Esophagram

The barium esophagram, or barium swallow, is one of the oldest diagnostic tests for evaluation of upper gastrointestinal disorders predating modern endoscopy. It remains a useful screen for luminal disorders including stricture, tumors, and hiatal hernia. It may demonstrate backflow but has a significant false-negative rate, thus limiting its benefit in patients with suspected LPR. Kimura et al. demonstrated barium esophagram as a useful predictor of response to empiric treatment [2], but it offers no practical advantages over therapeutic trial.

R. A. Iannuzzi (✉)
Department of Otolaryngology, Plastic Surgery and Cosmetic Services, and Allergy, Atrius Health, Boston, MA, USA
e-mail: Ralph_iannuzzi@atriushealth.org

C. H. Zalvan (ed.), *Laryngopharyngeal and Gastroesophageal Reflux*,
https://doi.org/10.1007/978-3-030-48890-1_12

Therapeutic Trial

Empiric therapeutic trial of antisecretory therapy with acid-reducing agents, in particular, twice daily proton pump inhibitors, has long been felt by many to be the most optimum approach in patients with suspected LPR. In fact, in 2009 the American Academy of Otolaryngology published guidelines on hoarseness wherein patients were evaluated with a reflux symptom index and reflux finding score [3]. If greater than 13 or 7, respectively, Ford recommended empiric treatment with twice daily PPI therapy for 3–6 months and pH monitoring for patients who failed to show improvement after the initial 3 months [4]. Despite the accepted safety of PPI therapy, it is suggested that there are significant rates of adverse events including, but not limited to, osteoporosis, an increased rate of pneumonia [5], increased potential for rates of cardiovascular disease [6], nephrotoxicity [7], hepatotoxicity [8], and greater risk for cancer of the esophagus and stomach [9]. In addition, much has been written about the association of PPI use and cognitive impairment; however, Goldstein et al. [10] and other authors had confirmed this concern that continuous PPI use does not cause cognitive decline [11, 12]. These studies suggest a potential correlation in large-scale data analysis that long-term PPI use might confer an increase in risk to these various diseases and certainly to at-risk populations. However, interpretation of retrospective data and large cohort studies must be weighed against potential benefits. The primary goal should be to limit the use of long-term pharmacotherapy. Most authors recommend 8–12 weeks of empiric twice daily PPI therapy in combination with lifestyle modifications for patients with suspected LPR [13].

Therapeutic trial is a reasonable initial approach in patients with suspected laryngopharyngeal reflux disease; however, the subjective nature of symptom reporting, as well as the inter- and intra-observer variability, calls this approach into question. In addition, controlled studies have demonstrated symptom improvement in placebo groups. Given the aforementioned concerns in regard to long-term PPI use, diet and lifestyle modifications should be an additional consideration. Zalvan et al. demonstrated that alkaline water, a Mediterranean-style, plant-based diet, and standard reflux precautions were equally as effective in reducing the reflux symptom index (RSI) than reflux precautions and PPI therapy [14]. For patients who are unable to comply with dietary and lifestyle modifications, we currently favor 6–8 weeks of therapeutic trial with diagnostic testing reserved for nonresponders [10, 12].

pH Monitoring

There are a variety of ambulatory pH monitoring technologies available to evaluate patients with reflux-related upper aerodigestive tract disorders. These include single- or double-probe catheter-based systems, multichannel intraluminal impedance

(MIIpH), wireless telemetry pH capsules, and oropharyngeal monitoring. Katz suggested that monitoring was indicated in patients who failed empiric therapy or in whom the diagnosis of GERD or LPR was suspected [15].

Single- or double-probe catheter-based pH monitoring is useful to accurately define acid exposure in both distal and proximal esophagus. Their utility remains problematic because of the potential role of non- or weakly acidic reflux producing symptoms similar to LPR. In addition, catheter-based pH testing requires nasal intubation and is poorly received by patients. However, positive pH studies coupled with suggestive RSI and RSF scores are predictive of success of anti-reflux therapy. Intraluminal impedance testing in the esophagus measures directional bolus movement. In combination with pH testing, impedance can help categorize reflux events into acid, weakly acid, or nonacid [16]. However, even though multi-luminal impedance testing (MIIpH) may identify more refluxers and better categorize them, Sanagapalli et al. demonstrated no clear evidence that extrapolates into better treatment for these patients [17]. Again, there is no gold standard diagnostic test to compare. MIIpH is fraught with technical issues such as catheter placement, pH sensor placement, and interpretation. Esophageal parameters are typically reported using the DeMeester score which does not correlate well with oropharyngeal pH events and symptoms. Additionally, acidic changes within the oropharynx are influenced by oral intake of foods and liquids as well as nasal drainage which can influence the oropharyngeal pH measurement.

The wireless pH capsule provides a safe, effective non-catheter-based system that is inserted endoscopically. The capsule remains in place for up to 96 hours and in general is well tolerated. The capsule detaches and passes through the GI tract. There are significant limitations for the diagnosis of LPR including the inability to detail proximal acid exposure, the necessity for endoscopy, the ability to detail only strongly acidic events of pH less than 4, and the inability to provide impedance data limit this technology's utility. The pH capsule may be a useful tool in assessing patients with both typical and atypical GERD symptoms. It has limited value in patients with suspected LPR without classic GERD symptom etiology.

One of the most recent developments in pH testing is the oropharyngeal pH probe (Restech DX-pH probe, Respiratory Technology Corporation, Houston, TX, USA). The procedure involves the trans-nasal placement of a small-diameter catheter in the posterior oropharynx. This tube monitors liquids and aerosolized acid and connects wirelessly to a monitor worn by or in close proximity to the patient. Several studies have demonstrated the reliability of this technique in demonstrating oropharyngeal reflux events [18, 19]. The Ryan score, created by Dr. Tom Ryan DeMeester, is proprietary to the Restech software and defines normal values while identifying patients with abnormal pharyngeal pH environments. It is a composite that is generated by measuring the percent time pH below 5.5 while upright and below 5.0 while supine, the number of episodes where pH droops below the thresholds, and the duration of the longest reflux episode. A positive Ryan score is diagnostic of significant oropharyngeal reflux [20].

However, Weiner et al. showed a poor correlation of oropharyngeal testing when compared to multichannel intraluminal impedance and pH monitoring [18, 19]. Friedman concluded that there were no pretest indicators of positive or negative testing suggesting the frequent need for objective evaluation [21]. Also, it has been demonstrated that oropharyngeal acid exposure does not predict symptom response to PPI therapy [22]. Again, the lack of a gold standard and typical comparison to DeMeester score and esophageal findings as well as small sample size limit the power of these studies. Given the overlap of laryngopharyngeal symptoms of LPR with other upper aerodigestive diseases including states of hypersensitivity, reflux symptom scores are often overinflated leading to misdiagnosis of LPR as the cause of the symptom complex. Oropharyngeal pH testing is instrumental in measuring acidic conditions within the oropharynx. In situations of elevated symptom scores but a negative oropharyngeal pH measurement, neurosensory changes with localized hypersensitivity should be entertained, as is often the case with chronic neurogenic cough. In the situation of an elevated symptom score with positive Ryan score with strong correlation of symptoms to reflux events, LPR is likely the cause, though both reflux and hypersensitivity states can coexist. Thus, oropharyngeal pH testing is an excellent tool to guide treatment options, especially in the patient who has seen multiple doctors from multiple specialties for their oro-laryngopharyngeal symptoms.

There is debate about whether patients who are to undergo pH testing should be tested on or off acid suppression medication. Pritchett et al. [23] evaluated 39 patients with refactory symptoms who had pH impedance monitoring on acid suppression therapy and subsequently monitored the same group of patients with pH testing off therapy. Of the patients on therapy, 25 (64%) had normal results. 28 (72%) had abnormal results off therapy. The authors concluded that pH impedance testing on therapy is preferred since it better predicts baseline acid reflux and thus provides more useful clinical information [24].

A wide range of opinions exists about the efficacy of various diagnostic tests for LPR. Many patients with LPR symptoms have neurosensory changes and hypersensitivity as a cause of their symptoms. pH testing is useful in demonstrating an absence of reflux in patients with vaguely mediated hypersensitivity as well as confirming the presence of reflux, supporting and reinforcing with patients the need for treatment. pH impedance testing is able to detect acid, nonacid, and gaseous fluid, but it is uncomfortable for patients, can be difficult to interpret, and does not predict severity of disease.

Oropharyngeal pH monitoring is better tolerated, equally sensitive, and easier to perform and interpret. pH telemetry capsule testing requires endoscopy and provides accurate data but only measures pH at the distal esophagus.

As mentioned, there is differing opinions as to which modality is preferred. Many authors have highlighted the problems with sensitivity and specificity of all diagnostic tests for LPR. We favor oropharyngeal testing as an initial approach to patients that require pH monitoring [25]. If a trial of dietary and lifestyle changes does not effect significant improvement in symptoms and symptom scores, then oropharyngeal pH testing can be useful in determining the presence of absence of acid. The technology itself is highly sensitive to changes in pH. If a test is performed and the patient is symptomatic during testing yet there is no acid present, the potential for neurosensory changes is heightened, and treatment and counseling can be appropriately directed. Conversely, a patient who is noncompliant on dietary and lifestyle changes can be presented with oropharyngeal pH data demonstrating significant episodes of acid exposure, and correlation with symptoms can either be counseled on the importance of significant dietary and lifestyle changes or be offered pharmacological interventions, with appropriate discussions of potential risks. Typically pharmacological intervention should be used as a bridge to allow time for diet and behavioral change and weight loss with an overall goal to dietary changes trending more toward a plant-based, Mediterranean-style diet. Pharmaceuticals, like alkaline water, or coating agents, such as alginates, should be viewed as more a "band-aid" than a definitive treatment, whereas dietary change should be encouraged as the cure.

Salivary Pepsin

Salivary pepsin testing is an inexpensive, noninvasive test that may represent a reasonable diagnostic alternative. Although laryngeal mucosa can be resistant to acid exposure of a pH greater than 4 [26], studies have shown that pepsin can cause laryngeal mucosal damage in mildly acidic and even alkaline environments [26, 27]. Ocak et al. showed a high specificity rate of a positive salivary pepsin test in predicting LPR; however, they demonstrated a low sensitivity rate perhaps due to sample collection frequency [26]. These findings were confirmed in subsequent studies suggesting positive salivary pepsin tests could be considered diagnostic for LPR, but a negative study does not rule this out. The latter group of patients need to undergo additional diagnostic testing [27]. Timing of testing, typically morning, and multiple testing samples throughout the day will likely provide greater sensitivity and specificity for an LPR diagnosis. Salivary testing remains a potentially promising test when combined with pH testing to further identify those patients at risk for laryngopharyngeal tissue damage and inflammation. What remain to be determined and studied are the multiple neurosensory changes that can occur resulting in altered levels of sensitivity. Changes in neuronal sensitivity mediated by upregulation of acid receptors could potentially cause symptoms even in the presence of weak levels of acid, possibly potentiated by the presence of pepsin. High levels of pepsin in the presence of an acidic environment with no significant neuronal change likely will be highly predictive of LPR. Future studies looking at the oropharyngeal pH, levels of extra- and intracellular pepsin, better characterization of neuronal sensitivity with levels of transient receptor potential, TRP channels and acid-sensing ion channel (ASIC) receptors as well as more complete characterizations of symptoms, such as the reflux symptom score (RSS), will become the gold standard in diagnosing LPR [28].

High-Resolution Manometry

In patients with known LPR whose symptoms persist despite high-dose PPI therapy, other diagnoses including but not limited to allergies, sinus disease, and asthma are considered to be causative [29]. However, reflux disease cannot adequately be ruled out by PPI treatment failure. Nonacid reflux and breakthrough acid reflux may exist [30]. Impedance testing in addition to high-resolution monitoring may be useful in evaluating these patients. Impedance testing can detect any reflux and determine the frequency and direction, while manometry can determine if the upper esophageal sphincter and lower esophageal tone are normal during activation and relaxation, as well as assess peristalsis [31]. However, it is unclear how impedance and manometry may affect management of patients with LPR who have failed high doses of PPIs. Carol et al. demonstrated nonacid reflux and breakthrough acid reflux in 74% of 54 patients with presumed LPR who failed empiric high-dose PPI therapy [29]. These diagnoses would have been missed by traditional pH testing. Furthermore, eight patients had esophageal motility as a cause of their symptoms. In patients who fail adequate dietary and behavioral change, despite aggressive education, and then fail subsequent pharmaceutical intervention, the index of suspicion for esophageal dysmotility should be raised. Many of the symptoms within the RSI can be mimicked by other diseases and neurosensory change. Post-viral vagal neuropathies can cause motor and sensory changes resulting in laryngopharyngeal hypersensitivity. As the vagus is the major motor nerve of the esophagus and stomach, these neurosensory changes can be accompanied by esophageal and gastric motor dysfunction resulting in a variety of symptoms that are poorly controlled with dietary changes or pharmaceuticals and a combination. The combination of impedance and high-resolution manometry proved valuable in the direction of therapy for all patients. Poorly controlled symptoms in patients with significant dysmotility also suggest a potential decreased outcome with surgical intervention. Further studies, perhaps with the inclusion of pharyngeal impedance, will be necessary to determine the role of impedance and manometry testing in the diagnosis of patients with LPR.

Reflux Scintigraphy

There is no clear-cut definition of gastroesophageal reflux disease (GERD). As mentioned previously, there is also no gold standard diagnostic criteria for laryngopharyngeal reflux (LPRD). We have previously discussed the advantages and limitations of a variety of pH monitoring techniques. Reflux scintigraphy is a safe, cost-effective, noninvasive technique that offers a valuable screening tool in patients with suspected LPR. To perform reflux scintigraphy, patients are positioned upright and asked to swallow a technetium-based tracer mixed with water while dynamic images are taken with a gamma camera. Falk et al. demonstrated a greater percentage of proximal reflux and aspiration in LPR than in patients with classic GERD and as expected demonstrated greater rates of reflux in both groups while patients were supine [32]. Their study was limited due to its retrospective nature and different reported standards for scintigraphy. Nevertheless, scintigraphy remains an interesting option for distinguishing patients with LPR and aspiration associated with GERD [32].

Conclusion

In conclusion, we feel that the best initial approach to most patients with suspected LPR should be a 6–8-week therapeutic trail. (Diagnostic Algorithm) We find barium esophagram could be of minimal value in further evaluation. Oropharyngeal testing despite its limitations does offer a minimally invasive, well-tolerated diagnostic technique that is usually of significant help in directing reflux therapy. Dual-channel pH monitoring with or without impedance can help categorize in better detail reflux disorders but may not offer any better direction in the selection of therapies. The telemetry capsule does provide the longest data recording but has limited value in proximal and nonacid reflux disease. Salivary pepsin and scintigraphy are interesting options that may serve as a screening or objective role in the evaluation of these patients, but more retrospective studies are needed to better assess their place in the LPR diagnostic paradigm.

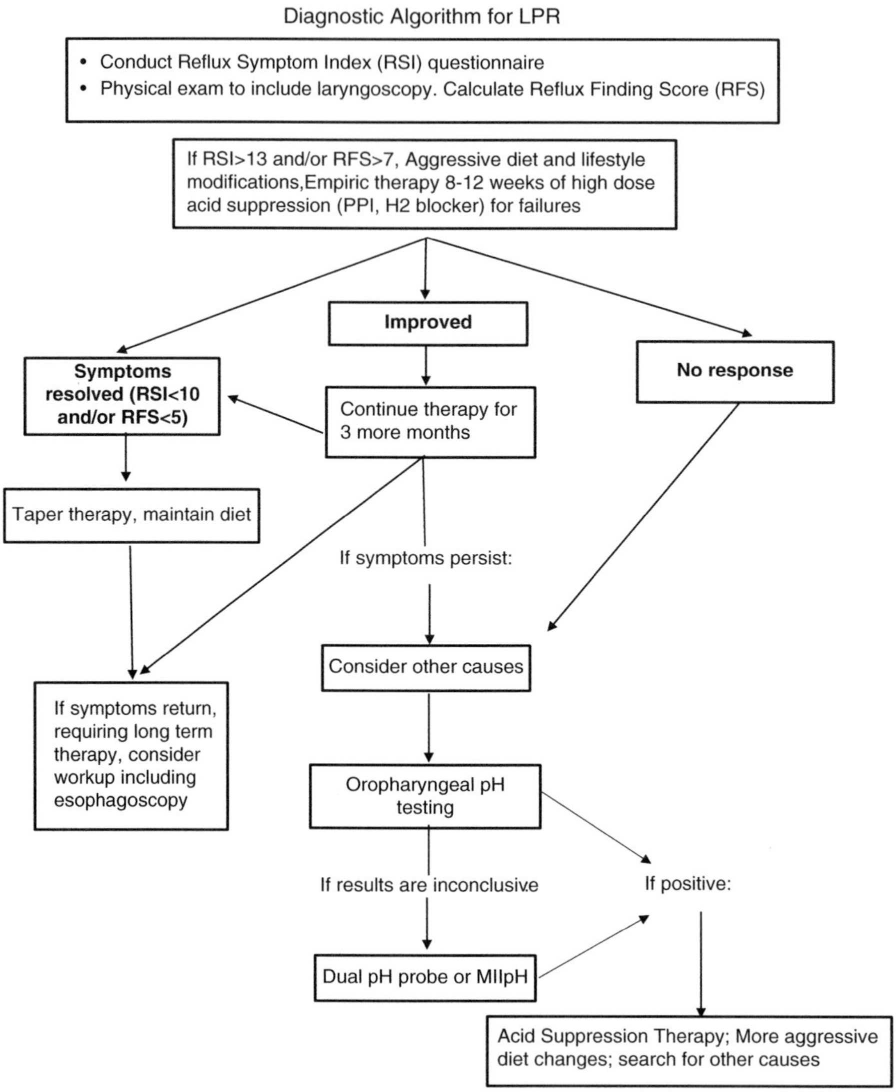

References

1. Wright MR, Sharda R, Vaezi MF. Unmet needs in treating laryngo-pharyngeal reflux disease: where do we go from here? Expert Rev Gastroenterol Hepatol. 2016;10(9):995.
2. Kimura Y, Sugiura M, Kato T, Makino N, Ohmae Y, Kishimoto S. Value of barium swallow studies in predicting the response to rabeprazole in elderly patients with laryngopharyngeal reflux disease and nonerosive reflux disease in particular. Ann Otol Rhinol Laryngol. 2017;119(9):631–5.

3. Stachler RJ, Francis DO, Schwartz SR, Damask CC, Digoy GP, Krouse HJ, McCoy SJ, Ouellette DR, Patel RR, Reavis CW, Smith LJ, Smith M, Strode SW, Woo P, Nnacheta LC. Clinical practice guideline: hoarseness (dysphonia) (update). Otolaryngol Head Neck Surg. 2018;158:S1–S42.
4. Ford CN. Evaluation and management of laryngopharyngeal reflux. JAMA. 2005;294(12):1534–40.
5. Falk GL, Vivian SJ. Laryngopharyngeal reflux: diagnosis, treatment and latest research. Eur Surg. 2016;48(2):74–91.
6. Shiraev P, Bullen A. Proton pump inhibitors and cardiovascular events: a systematic review. Heart Lung Circ. 2018;27(4):443–50.
7. Hart E, et al. Proton pump inhibitors and risk of acute and chronic kidney disease: a retrospective cohort study. Pharmacotherapy. 2019;39(4):443–53.
8. Llorente C, Jepsen P, Inamine T, et al. Gastric acid suppression promotes alcoholic liver disease by introducing overgrowth or intestinal enterococcus. Nat Commun. 2017;8:837.
9. Cheung KS, Leung WK. Long-term use of proton-pump inhibitors and risk of gastric cancer: a review of current evidence. Ther Adv Gastroenterol. 2019;12:1–11.
10. Goldstein FC, Steenland K, Zhao L, Wharton W, Levey AI, Hajjar I. Proton pump inhibitors and risk of mild cognitive impairment and dementia. J Am Geriatr Soc. 2017;65(9):1969–74.
11. Brett AS. Evidence against an alleged association between PPIs and dementia. Review of "Taipale H et al. Am J Gastroenterol 2017 Jul 11. Lochhead P et al. Gastroenterology 2017 Jul 17." NEJM Journal Watch 2017.
12. Taipale H, Tolppanen AM, Tiihonen M. No association between proton pump inhibitor use and risk of Alzheimer's disease. Am J Gastroenterol. 2017;112(12):1802–8.
13. Sidhwa F, Moore A, Alligood E. Diagnosis and treatment of the extraesophageal manifestations of gastroesophageal reflux disease. Ann Surg. 2017;265(1):63–7.
14. Zalvan C, Hu S, Greenberg B, Geliebter J, et al. A comparison of alkaline water and mediterranean diet vs proton pump inhibition for treatment of laryngopharyngeal reflux. JAMA Otolaryngol Head Neck Surg. 2017;143(10):1029–3.
15. Katz PO, Gerson LB, Vela MF. Guidelines for the diagnosis and management of gastroesophageal reflux disease. Am J Gastroenterol. 2013;108(3):308–28.
16. Boeckxstaens GE, Smout A. Systematic review: role of acid, weakly acidic and weakly alkaline reflux in gastro-oesophageal reflux disease. Aliment Pharmacol Ther. 2010;32: 334–43.
17. Sanagapalli S, Sweis R. Combined pH-impedance testing for reflux: current state of play and future challenges. Front Gastroenterol. 2017;8:154–5.
18. Golub JS, Johns MM III, Lim JH, DelGaudio JM, Klein AM. Comparison of an oropharyngeal pH probe and a standard duel pH probe for the diagnosis of laryngopharyngeal reflux. Ann Otol Rhinol Laryngol. 2009;118:1–5.
19. Wiener GJ, Tsukashima R, Kelly C, Wolf E, Schmeltzer M, Bankert C, et al. Oropharyngeal pH monitoring for the detection of liquid and aerosolized supraesophageal gastric reflux. J Voice. 2009;23:498–504.
20. Ayazi S, Lipham JC, Hagen JA, et al. A new technique for measurement of pharyngeal pH: normal values and discriminating pH threshold. J Gastrointest Surg. 2009;13(8):1422–9.
21. Friedman M, Hamilton C, Samuelson CG, Kelley K, Taylor R, Darling R, Taylor D, Fisher M, Maley A. The value of routine pH monitoring in the diagnosis and treatment of laryngopharyngeal reflux. Otolaryngol Head Neck Surg. 2012;146(6):952–8.
22. Yadlapati R, Pandolfino JE, Lidder AK, Shabeeb N, et al. Oropharyngeal pH testing does not predict response to proton pump inhibitor therapy in patients with laryngeal symptoms. Am J Gastroenterol. 2016;111:1517–24.
23. Pritchett JM, Aslam M, Slaughter JC, Ness RM, Garrett CG, Vaezi MF. Efficacy of esophageal impedance/pH monitoring in patients with refractory gastroesophageal reflux disease, on and off therapy. Clin Gastroenterol Hepatol. 2009;7(7):743–8.
24. Barry DW, Vaezi MF. Laryngopharyngeal reflux: more questions than answers. Cleve Clin J Med. 2010;77(5):327–34.

25. Martinucci I, de Bortoli N, Savarino E. Optimal treatment of laryngopharyngeal reflux disease. Ther Adv Chronic Dis. 2013;4(6):287–301.
26. Ocak E, Kubat G, Yurulmaz. Immunoserologic pepsin detection in the saliva as a non-invasive rapid diagnostic test for laryngopharyngeal reflux. Balkan Med J. 2015;32:46–50.
27. Bulmer DM, Ali MS, Brownlee IA, Detmar PW, Pearson JP. Laryngeal mucosa: its susceptibility to damage by acid and pepsin. Laryngoscope. 2010;120:777–82.
28. Lechien JR, Saussez S, Karkos PD. Laryngopharyngeal reflux disease: clinical presentation, diagnosis and therapeutic challenges in 2018. Curr Opin Otolaryngol Head Neck Surg. 2018;26(6):392–402. https://doi.org/10.1097/MOO.0000000000000486.
29. Carroll TL, Fedore LW, Aldahlawi MD. pH impedance and high-resolution manometry in laryngopharyngeal reflux disease high-dose proton pump inhibitor failures. Laryngoscope. 2012;122(11):2473–81.
30. Fass R. Proton-pump inhibitor therapy in patients with gastro-oesophageal reflex disease: putative mechanisms of failure. Drugs. 2007;67(11):1521–30.
31. Ayazi S, Hagen JA, Zehetner J, et al. The value of high-resolution manometry in the assessment of the resting characteristics of the lower esophageal sphincter. J Gastrointest Surg. 2009;13:2113.
32. Falk M, Van der Wall H, Falk GL. Differences between scintigraphic reflux studies in gastrointestinal reflux disease and laryngopharyngeal reflux disease and correlation with symptoms. Nucl Med Commun. 2015;36:625–30.

Chapter 13
Pepsin Testing

Claude Nganzeu, Jonathan M. Bock, Craig H. Zalvan, and Nikki Johnston

Pepsin as a Biomarker of Reflux and Aspiration

There is growing evidence that reflux into the airways is responsible for the etiology and the exacerbation of a range of respiratory conditions, including idiopathic pulmonary fibrosis, chronic obstructive pulmonary disease, chronic cough, cystic fibrosis, and chronic rhinosinusitis. Some groups have published extensively on the ability of pepsin to function as a biomarker of reflux in the upper airways, but data are still evolving on the association between the presence of pepsin and MII-pH

C. Nganzeu
Medical College of Wisconsin, Milwaukee, WI, USA
e-mail: cnganzeu@mcw.edu

J. M. Bock
Department of Otolaryngology & Communication Sciences, Division of Laryngology & Professional Voice, Medical College of Wisconsin, Milwaukee, WI, USA
e-mail: jbock@mcw.edu

C. H. Zalvan
ENT and Allergy Associates, LLP; Voice and Swallow Division, Tarrytown, NY, USA

The Institute for Voice and Swallowing Disorders, Phelps Hospital, Northwell Health, Sleepy Hollow, NY, USA

Professor of Otolaryngology at the Donald and Barbara Zucker School of Medicine at Hofstra/Northwell, Phelps Hospital Campus, Sleepy Hollow, NY, USA

Communication at Mercy College, Dobbs Ferry, NY, USA
e-mail: czalvan@entandallergy.com

N. Johnston (✉)
Department of Otolaryngology and Communication Sciences, Division of Laryngology and Professional Voice and Pediatric Otolaryngology, Department of Microbiology and Immunology, Milwaukee, WI, USA
e-mail: njohnston@mcw.edu

C. H. Zalvan (ed.), *Laryngopharyngeal and Gastroesophageal Reflux*,
https://doi.org/10.1007/978-3-030-48890-1_13

data. Pepsin has excellent positive and negative predictive values as a biomarker to detect reflux and is known to decrease markedly after fundoplication. Recent studies have evaluated correlations between MII-pH and salivary pepsin data and shown that pepsin and MII-pH data appear to correlate well. This correlation was shown by Hayat et al., where healthy individuals and patients with heartburn were subjected to 24-h MII-pH monitoring and simultaneous measurement of pepsin in saliva upon waking, after lunch, and after dinner. Pepsin was measured using an enzyme-linked immunosorbent assay (ELISA) [1]. Their study showed significantly more pepsin-positive saliva samples from patients with heartburn compared to healthy individuals, 40.1% and 21%, respectively. Furthermore, pepsin was more frequently detected in saliva from patients with GERD and hypersensitive esophagus than asymptomatic subjects and patients with functional heartburn. The data also showed that patients with heartburn had a significantly higher concentration of pepsin than healthy subjects and patients with functional heartburn: 75 ng/mL and 0 ng/mL, respectively. Finally, when looking at the correlation between salivary pepsin concentration and likelihood of disease, salivary pepsin greater than 210 ng/mL had a specificity and positive predictive value greater than 94.5% and the likelihood ratio of 25.1, indicating a strong association between high salivary pepsin values and the likelihood of reflux disease. In another study using 24-h MII-pH monitoring and ELISA to measure pepsin, Na et al. determined that patients with LPR had a significantly higher concentration of pepsin in saliva compared to healthy subjects, especially upon waking: 17.2 ng/mL and 20.4 ng/mL, respectively [2]. Similarly, a recent case-control study by Klimara et al. measuring pepsin in saliva from healthy reflux-free control patients and patients with LPR compared pepsin presence/levels with MII-pH data [3]. A higher number of patients with LPR had pepsin in their saliva compared to healthy individuals (11/26 and 0/13, respectively), and a significant correlation was found between salivary pepsin in waking saliva samples and MII-pH measurements, including reflux bolus duration and proximal and distal recumbent reflux episodes. These data demonstrate that pepsin in saliva could be a reliable biomarker for LPR, especially when measured in the morning upon waking. However, though data shows salivary pepsin could be a reliable biomarker for GER and LPR disease, there is a weaker correlation between salivary pepsin and other reflux-related airway inflammatory diseases. For example, in patients with chronic upper respiratory symptoms indicative of laryngeal hyperresponsiveness such as chronic cough, globus sensation, dyspnea, and episodic choking, Spyridoulias et al. found a specificity of 0.78 for the presence of salivary pepsin as a predictor for inflammatory changes on laryngoscopy but a sensitivity of only 0.53 [4]. Notably, pepsin did not significantly correlate with reflux symptom inventory scores or reflux events on MII-pH monitoring, and many patients had discordant results between various modalities. However, almost half of patients with pulmonary symptoms but minimal inflammatory changes on laryngoscopy had detectable salivary pepsin.

There are currently several diagnostic methods available to confirm or reject if reflux disease is responsible for a patient's symptoms. However, these tests are invasive and expensive and have low sensitivity and specificity. For example, symptom questionnaires have 63% sensitivity and 67% specificity, endoscopy has approximately 30% sensitivity for diagnosing reflux disease, and pH-metry has sensitivity in the region of 60%. None of these can be considered as first-line diagnostic tests. Peptest (RD Biomed Limited, UK), a noninvasive test based on lateral flow technology, was introduced to rapidly identify reflux in patients presenting with a range of reflux symptoms. Patients diagnosed with symptoms of GER, LPR, and EER including various respiratory diseases have been tested for reflux using Peptest to identify pepsin as a biomarker of reflux disease.

For a diagnostic test to be considered as a first-line test, it needs to be simple to use and noninvasive with high patient compliance, give rapid results, and be cost-effective. Peptest is being clinically validated measuring pepsin in, for example, saliva samples provided by patients at specific time points. Samples are being collected in the morning upon waking and before eating and cleaning teeth, postprandial 60 min after finishing a meal, or 15 min after experiencing symptoms. All samples are stored in a refrigerator before being analyzed for the presence of pepsin using Peptest. Peptest is a lateral flow device (LFD) with two unique anti-pepsin human monoclonal antibodies, one to capture and another to detect pepsin. The intensity of the pepsin test line within the window of the LFD is measured using a Peptest cube reader and automatically converted into the concentration of pepsin (ng/mL) present.

Unfortunately, some research studies question the clinical application of Peptest due to lack of reproducibility. Initial study of the use of pepsin salivary assay in GERD diagnosis showed a specificity of 96% and a sensitivity of 44% when comparing healthy individuals to patients with GERD [1]. In their subsequent study, to confirm their previous study's results and determine if the test sensitivity can be improved when samples from GERD patients are collected over a 72-hour period, they measured the maximal salivary pepsin concentration in patients with GERD and observed a specificity and sensitivity 60% and 37.5%, respectively for detection of pepsin. For the 72-hour salivary pepsin maximal concentration, the data resulted in a specificity and sensitivity of 42.9% and 76.7%, respectively, for GERD patients. The data showed variable specificity and sensitivity values for salivary pepsin concentration in GERD patients despite the use of identical techniques and regular recalibration but different Peptest batch [5]. Similarly, in a meta-analysis by Guo et al., looking at five studies evaluating the use of salivary pepsin assay for the diagnosis of GERD, results not only showed variable sensitivity and specificity but also lack of reproducibility among different studies [6]. In brief, these studies do not discard pepsin as a good biomarker but conclude that further study is needed before pepsin can be used as a diagnostic tool for GERD.

Pepsin was recently found to be significantly elevated in nonerosive esophagitis (NERD), corroborating earlier studies which also found higher pepsin levels in NERD patients [7–9]. Another study found that nearly 70% of samples given after symptoms of GERD or LPR were positive for pepsin and over 80% of patients with reflux confirmed by MII-pH had at least one positive sample suggesting that Peptest is a "good first-line product" [10].

Many studies utilize impedance pH testing with DeMeester scoring as the standard for "reflux," both with LPR and GERD patients. However, the intrinsic sensitivity of laryngopharyngeal tissues to acidic and pepsin-mediated damage is a significant factor that is not taken into account in these studies. pH as high as 5.5 and even 6.0 can contribute to ongoing activation of pepsin and cause direct tissue damage to mucosa not typically prone to acidic exposure, events of which would not be considered positive with DeMeester scoring.

Consideration of laryngopharyngeal sensitivity has not been included in any of the studies on the utility of pepsin testing to date. Given most studies utilize subjective scoring systems as a diagnostic tool of LPR, such as the Reflux Symptom Index (RSI), elevated sensitivity must be taken into account. In patients with hypersensitivity, likely from upregulation of acid sensing receptors and neuronal signaling channels, such as the Transient Receptor Protein (TRP) group of channels, high symptom scores may be present in the absence of any acid or pepsin. Therefore, the ultimate diagnosis of LPR should focus on a combination of pH testing, confirmation of pepsin with pepsin localization, and measurement of TRP channels and acid receptors to differentiate between hypersensitivity and true reflux events. Salivary pepsin testing will likely play a role in the diagnosis of both LPR and GERD. Increase in sampling, better understanding of the timing of pepsin secretion, and even tissue localization of pepsin will likely help to increase the diagnostic yield of pepsin as a biomarker.

References

1. Hayat JO, Gabieta-Somnez S, Yazaki E, Kang JY, Woodcock A, Dettmar P, Mabary J, Knowles CH, Sifrim D. Pepsin in saliva for the diagnosis of gastro-oesophageal reflux disease. Gut. 2015;64(3):373–80. https://doi.org/10.1136/gutjnl-2014-307049. Epub 2014/05/09.
2. Na SY, Kwon OE, Lee YC, Eun YG. Optimal timing of saliva collection to detect pepsin in patients with laryngopharyngeal reflux. Laryngoscope. 2016;126(12):2770–3. https://doi.org/10.1002/lary.26018. Epub 2016/04/15.
3. Kilimara MJ, Johnston N, Samuels TL, Blumein JH, Bock JM. Correlation of salivary and nasal lavage pepsin with MII-pH testing. Laryngoscope. 2019;130:961.
4. Spyridoulias A, Lillie S, Vyas A, Fowler SJ. Detecting laryngopharyngeal reflux in patients with upper airways symptoms: symptoms, signs or salivary pepsin? Respir Med. 2015;109(8):963–9. https://doi.org/10.1016/j.rmed.2015.05.019. Epub 2015/06/06.
5. Woodland P, Singendonk MMJ, Ooi J, Nikaki K, Wong T, Lee C, Glasinovic E, Koning R, Lutter R, Benninga MA, van Wijk MP, Sifrim D. Measurement of salivary pepsin to detect gastroesophageal reflux disease is not ready for clinical application. Clin Gastroenterol Hepatol. 2019;17(3):563–5. https://doi.org/10.1016/j.cgh.2018.05.016. Epub 2018 May 18.
6. Guo Z, Wu H, Jiang J, Zhang C. Pepsin in saliva as a diagnostic marker for gastroesophageal reflux disease: a meta-analysis. Med Sci Monit. 2018;24:9509–16. https://doi.org/10.12659/MSM.913978.
7. Wang Y, Lang XQ, Wu D, He YQ, Lan CH, Xiao X, Wang B, Zou DW, Wu JM, Zhao YB, Dettmar PW, Chen DF, Yang M. Salivary pepsin as an intrinsic marker for diagnosis of subtypes of gastroesophageal reflux disease and gastroesophageal reflux disease-related disorders. J Neurogastroenterol Motil. 2019; https://doi.org/10.5056/jnm19032. [Epub ahead of print].
8. Dulery C, Lechot A, Roman S, et al. A study with pharyngeal and esophageal 24h pH-impedance monitoring in patients with laryngopharyngeal symptoms refractory to proton pump inhibitors. Neurogastroenterol Motil. 2017;29:e12909.

9. Rasijeff AMP, Jackson W, Burke JM, Dettmar PW. PWE-172 does salivary pepsin measurement change diagnostic outcome in patients investigated by 24h pH monitoring? Gut. 2015;64:A287–8.
10. Bor S, Capanoglu D, Vardar R, Woodcock AD, Fisher J, Dettmar PW. Validation of peptest™ in patients with gastro-esophageal reflux disease and laryngopharyngeal reflux undergoing impedance testing. J Gastrointestin Liver Dis. 2019;28(4):383–7. https://doi.org/10.15403/jgld-335.

Chapter 14
Transnasal Esophagoscopy

Jacqui E. Allen

Introduction

The esophagus is a muscular tube connecting the pharynx with the stomach, delivering foodstuffs and swallowed material. This route also permits retrograde passage of material from the stomach or esophagus back toward, and sometimes into, the pharynx and larynx. Known as reflux, this process occurs in normal individuals to some extent every day; however, the extent and amount varies, and the ability of the tissue to withstand the enzymatic exposure to gastric juice also varies. In some cases, tissue integrity is affected and/or symptoms are produced. When this occurs, the term "reflux disease" is appropriate (as per the Montreal classification), and description of where the material arises and where it reaches enables us to specifically describe the reflux event [1]. For example, escape from the stomach into the esophagus is termed gastroesophageal reflux (GER), but if material is within the esophagus only and returns to the pharynx, then the term esophagopharyngeal reflux (EPR) is more appropriate. With the rise in obesity, proliferation of convenience food, and epidemic of diabetes within the Western society, prevalence of reflux disease continues to rise. Dysfunction or obstruction of the esophagus may also lead to complaint of dysphagia. Usually this symptom requires a comprehensive and multidisciplinary assessment. The otolaryngologist is part of this team and with availability of transnasal esophageal examination can play an even more integral role in patient management.

This chapter outlines a method of esophageal evaluation and therapy delivery that will enable us to deal with the increasing numbers of individuals who will present with manifestations of pharyngoesophageal disease. This technique is transnasal esophagoscopy (TNE) and is faster, cheaper, and safer while being equally accurate in diagnosing and managing most common pharyngoesophageal disorders. It must

J. E. Allen (✉)
University of Auckland, Auckland, New Zealand
e-mail: jeallen@voiceandswallow.co.nz

C. H. Zalvan (ed.), *Laryngopharyngeal and Gastroesophageal Reflux*,
https://doi.org/10.1007/978-3-030-48890-1_14

become part of our armamentarium and be considered an integral part of patient management, in the same way as flexible nasendoscopy has become.

Anatomic Considerations

The esophagus is an integral part of the gut and the site of transition from skeletal muscle to the smooth muscle found throughout the rest of the enteric system. The layered design of the esophagus accommodates its dual purpose of shortening to envelop bolus and rhythmicity to massage the bolus forward. To this end, the enteric nervous system (ENS) identified within layers of the esophageal muscle is critical to these functions and indeed further contains specialized neural cells and tissue to enable the sequential functioning of the organ and of the gut as a whole. Coordination of esophageal contractions with sphincter control is essential and is accomplished through a variety of gut-airway reflexes, to ensure that bolus does not inappropriately move in a retrograde fashion and threaten the airway.

Upper and lower esophageal sphincters are specialized zones of higher pressure, designed to delimit the esophageal lumen from the laryngopharynx and from the stomach. Airway protection is a primary driver of upper esophageal sphincter (UES) behavior given the close proximity of the airway to the UES valve. The UES is comprised of 40% elastic and connective tissue and 60% muscle fibers, which are primarily slow twitch type and in a state of tonic contraction [2]. During deglutition, these fibers cease contracting, allowing the hyolaryngeal complex to distract open the UES (through its counterclockwise anterosuperior motion arc) and the tongue to provide propulsive force in addition to the hydrostatic pressure exerted by the bolus, thus resulting in bolus transit into the esophagus. Additionally, the UES works to prevent swallowing of air which can inadvertently trigger reflex arcades including the esophago-UES relaxation reflex wherein fast distension of the esophagus triggers relaxation at the UES while slow distension typically results in a UES contractile (protective) response [2–4]. Interestingly, studies suggest that acid/refluxate exposure in the esophagus may alter these UES responses desensitizing the esophagus to the appropriate reflex [3, 5, 6]. While a UES-relaxation response is important and necessary during belch, vomiting, and regurgitation (hence it relaxes to rapid filling), it is also possible for ingested material to be released into the pharynx and threaten the airway. Slower esophageal distension, often with liquid, generally results in augmentation of UES pressures to mitigate slow drift of unintended refluxate into the mid- to proximal esophagus [2, 3, 6]. Cough episodes also augment UES pressure, again to prevent inadvertent escape of material from esophagus to the pharynx [7].

The lower esophageal sphincter (LES), on the other hand, is working to protect the esophagus itself by limiting retrograde gastric flow into the esophageal lumen. Given the caustic nature of gastric refluxate due to the presence of substances including hydrochloric acid, pepsin, bile acids, and hydrolytic digestive enzymes and the known role that reflux plays in the development of esophageal adenocarcinoma, normal LES function also plays a critical protective role.

Reflux Disease and Implications

As detailed in the rest of this book, reflux disease results in damage and dysfunction of gut and airway. Overexposure of mucosal surfaces to caustic agents results in damage which can range from pain sensations and nonerosive esophagitis (NERD) to erosive esophagitis (ERD) (Fig. 14.1), laryngopharyngitis, or chronic wound healing responses and fibrosis. Reflux disease has been implicated in ear disease, chronic cough, voice disorders (Fig. 14.2), nasal congestion, asthma and lower respiratory disease, and development of malignancy. Reavis and colleagues reported that the most common symptoms associated with adenocarcinoma of the esophagus were cough and pharyngeal-related symptoms (not classical reflux symptoms) [8]. Recently, Nouraei et al. reported the presence of esophagogastric malignancy in 27% of 177 patients with swallow symptoms localized only to the pharynx [9] underlining the need to examine the whole system to provide true reassurance to the patient.

Figure 14.1 Endoscopic view of distal esophagus demonstrating Grade C (LA classification) esophagitis.

Figure 14.2 Laryngeal inflammatory changes seen in many conditions including laryngopharyngeal reflux, snore trauma, postnasal drainage, inhalant irritation, or a combination of these factors.

Carcinoma of the esophagus is a disease often characterized by late presentation and dismal survival (Fig. 14.3). This is due in large part to the paucity of symptoms in early carcinoma and the ability for these symptoms to mimic or match symptoms

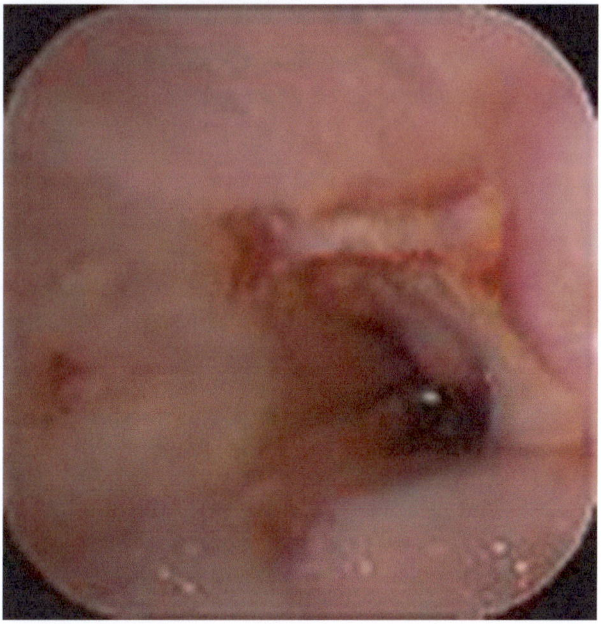

Fig. 14.1 Endoscopic image of Grade C (confluent areas of erosion across several rugal folds) esophagitis in the distal esophagus

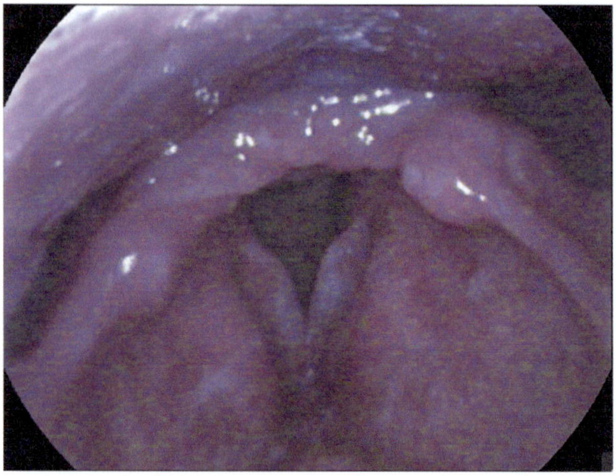

Fig. 14.2 Endoscopic image of the larynx exhibiting edema and irregularity of the vocal folds, interarytenoid mucosal redundancy, and prominent false vocal folds – all signs of laryngeal inflammation and often linked to laryngopharyngeal reflux

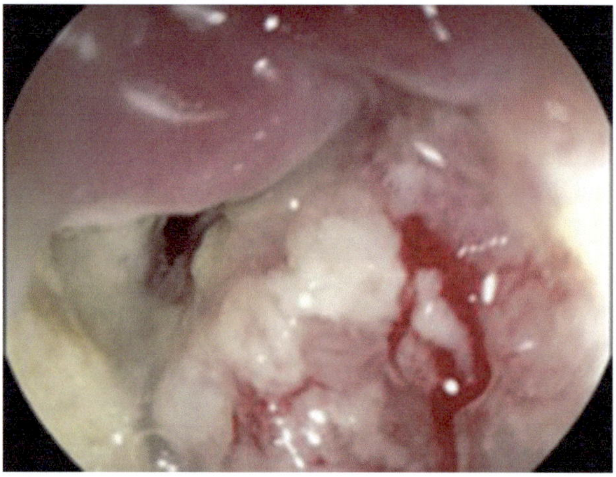

Fig. 14.3 Endoscopic image of gastroesophageal junctional carcinoma, with irregular margins and luminal narrowing

of less dangerous pathology such as reflux disease, infective esophagitis, hiatal hernia, nonmalignant rings and strictures, and even allergic disease (Fig. 14.4). Treatment is readily available for these benign conditions, and if identified early, curative treatment is possible for esophageal malignancy. TNE gives us the power to search for and find precursors to adenocarcinoma, such as Barrett's metaplasia (BM), and to identify these earlier, with minimal risk, lower costs, and equivalent accuracy. However, if we do not look, we will not find, and it is this simple point that underpins the need to adopt the technique of transnasal office-based esophagoscopy (TNE).

Figure 14.3 Endoscopic image of gastroesophageal junction carcinoma.

Figure 14.4 Endoscopic image of trachealized esophagus typically seen in eosinophilic esophagitis.

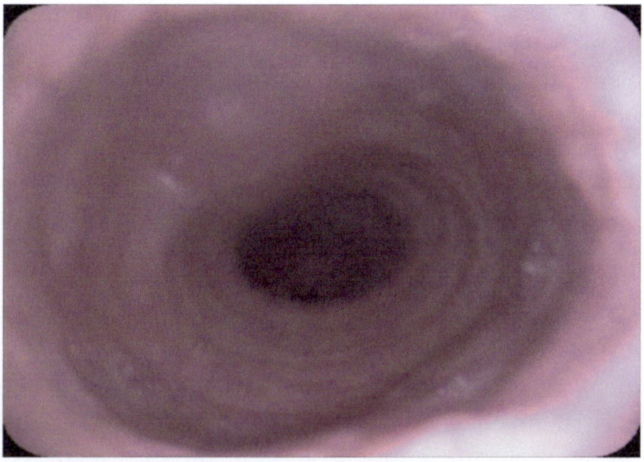

Fig. 14.4 Endoscopic image of mid-esophagus demonstrating trachealization typical of eosinophilic esophagitis

Why Use Transnasal Esophagoscopy?

Screening of the esophagus for cancer or precursor conditions (such as Barrett's metaplasia) would require extensive resources. Large-scale studies have been performed previously examining the benefit and cost-effectiveness of sedated screening gastroscopy to identify adenocarcinoma [10–13]. These works did not support population screening, finding that costs outweighed the number of identified tumors. Large international societies such as the British Society of Gastroenterology, American Gastroenterology Association, and American College of Gastroenterology therefore do not recommend population screening. However, these studies did not evaluate the office-based transnasal technique [10–12] where risk is lower, costs are substantially lower, and performance of the procedure is considerably shorter and less onerous. As previous work confirms excellent sensitivity (98%) and specificity (100%) of transnasal endoscopic evaluation of BM [14, 15] and there are also additional enhancing strategies such as real-time confocal laser endoscopy, narrow band imaging, acetic acid application, or chromoendoscopy that may be applied to esophageal evaluation, rate of detection is likely to be at least equivalent to a sedated gastroscopy [10, 16–18]. Although other methods for detection of metaplastic esophageal change are being explored, such as surface brush sampling [19–25], endoscopy provides the benefit of visual identification and specificity in biopsy site selection. Wider surface area sampling such as semi-abrasive transepithelial brush biopsies allows increased numbers of cells to be examined increasing the yield in detecting metaplastic change or possible malignancy. Initial work in 2011 reported a dramatic increase in identifiable BM (70% increase compared to forceps biopsies) and dysplasia (87% increase number of detections compared to forceps biopsies) when using abrasive brush biopsy techniques [23]. In addition, Vennalaganti et al. reported increased interrater agreement of cytology specimens obtained from wide-area transepithelial brush biopsy compared to forceps biopsies, with inter-rater agreement average of kappa = 0.86 (range 0.61–0.99) [24]. Recently, Mariano et al. compared cytological brush biopsy findings to histopathological examination in 123 patients, reporting the sensitivity and specificity of brush biopsy as 98% and 96%, respectively, when compared to histology [25]. They did not report whether cytology identified additional abnormal cases compared to histological exam. As brush biopsies are less time consuming and cover more tissue, they may provide a better option in screening populations.

In an office-based setting, the cost of screening is reduced as there is no need for sedation, anesthesia input, recovery room staff, or equipment. Many more procedures can be completed within the same time frame making cost per procedure much lower. When distal pathology is identified, then referral to gastroenterology may be indicated, to allow definitive treatment to be undertaken particularly if the distal esophagus or stomach is the site of disease. Gastroenterology review will also address abdominal symptoms, malabsorption, bowel-related dysfunction, and direct further distal endoscopy if needed. A good working relationship between otolaryngology and gastroenterology services is beneficial to the patients and services overall, with each complementing the other in terms of service provision. TNE screening examinations may assist in preventing unnecessary sedated examinations clogging up the gastroenterology suite, enabling the GI suite to provide tertiary care of identified pathology. Routine long-term surveillance screening for conditions such as BM and post-radiotherapy esophagitis and posttreatment (e.g., dilatation, carcinoma, Heller's myotomy) assessments are all ideally suited to non-sedated TNE. This does not take work from one service to another but rather allows best allocation of resource to the needed service provision. Collaborative care pathways that span across specialties are needed to ensure timely evaluation and avoid patients "slipping through the cracks." They also engender upskilling and learning within each specialty, with flow of ideas and greater skill mix enhancing patient care.

In 2008, the American Bronchoesophagological Association (ABEA) published a position statement supporting the equivalence of TNE with traditional esophagoscopy in image quality and diagnostic capability but also highlighting the additional benefit that TNE offers in difficult access patients, speed, and reduced costs [26]. Work has been published comparing accuracy of TNE with traditional sedated gastroscopy (EGD) in diagnosis of Barrett's metaplasia, with comparable results [14, 15, 27, 28]. Sensitivity and specificity of TNE compared to sedated esophagogastroscopy (EGD) as a gold standard sits at 98–100% and 100%, respectively, for endoscopic diagnosis and 66.7% sensitivity and 100% specificity for histological diagnosis of BM [14, 15]. Histological diagnosis is affected by sampling bias and error, particularly as TNE working channels are narrow caliber and therefore biopsy forceps are usually only 1 mm diameter. This may indicate need for a greater number of biopsies to be taken during TNE compared with EGD or for use of global sampling tools such as a cytology brush. Further work has evaluated patient tolerance of the TNE procedure compared to sedated EGD, with preference given to the transnasal route [14, 29]. From a cost-effectiveness standpoint, the significantly reduced cost of office-based unsedated esophagoscopy improves the utility substantially. Procedural safety is enhanced through avoidance of sedation medication, even if procedural work (biopsies, dilation, injection) is required in the esophageal lumen. Patients tolerate a wide variety of interventions with topical anesthetic application alone – ideal for the office setting.

The flexibility of transnasal esophagoscopy lends itself to frequent application with an increasing range of patients. There is a true advantage in being able to decide to examine the esophagus of the patient before you, on the spot, at the first visit, without need to reschedule another date or compete for GI suite time. Within a single patient encounter, the history and examination from mouth to the pylorus may be undertaken, and meaningful, well-informed treatment decisions made. Recorded video of the examination is hugely beneficial when viewed with the patient to allay fear, to explain mechanical distortion such as a patulous lower esophageal sphincter, and to engender compliance to treatment advice, especially when encouraging dietary change in the setting of reflux disease. There is no substitution for seeing it with one's own eyes!

What Is Transnasal Esophagoscopy?

Transnasal esophagoscopy is the passage of a thin-caliber flexible endoscope via the nasal cavity to access and evaluate the nasopharynx, oropharynx, hypopharynx, larynx, UES, esophagus, LES, and a portion of the stomach. It is an extended esophagogastroscopy, probably rightly described as a pharyngolaryngoesophagoscopy (PLE) via a transnasal route.

If you are working with a 120 cm endoscope, it is also possible to reach the duodenum! Described in 1991 by gastroenterologists, it was taken up in earnest by otolaryngologists in the late 1990s [30, 31]. Even with endoscopes as thin as 5.5 mm in diameter, it is possible to incorporate a working channel of 2 mm, allowing for irrigation, insufflation, biopsy, and interventions, e.g., flexible injection, passing of guidewire for balloon dilation, and laser fiber passage (Fig. 14.5) [30, 32]. Portability of endoscope systems has also improved, as has the quality of illumination and durability of the endoscope. Therefore, TNE is both a diagnostic and therapeutic procedure, sometimes within the same examination.

Figure 14.5 Photograph of the distal tip of a flexible videoendoscope demonstrating the light outlets, suction channel, and image capture lens.

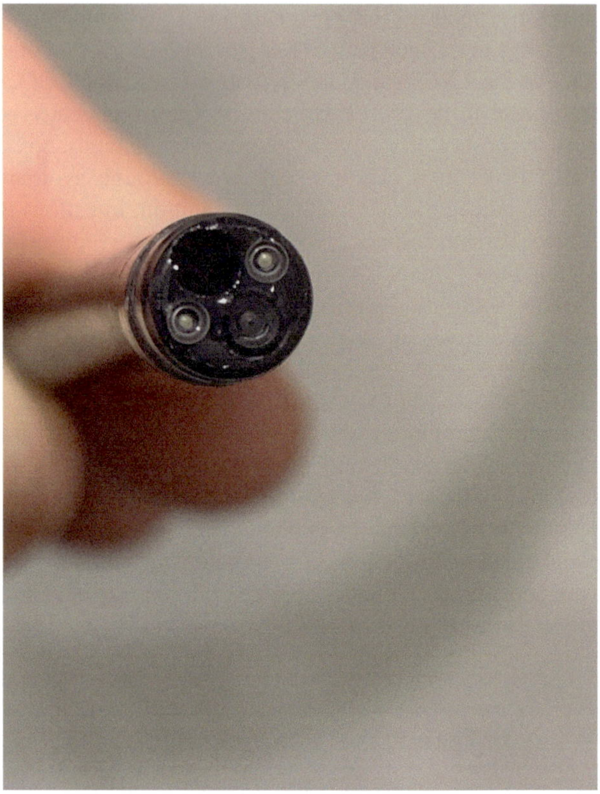

Fig. 14.5 Image of distal tip end of a transnasal esophagoscopy (Pentax, EE-1580 K shown) showing the dual light sources, camera lens, and working channel

How Can I Do Transnasal Esophagoscopy?

Practical Performance of TNE

Transnasal esophagoscopy is generally performed in the awake patient, in an upright position, as one would be for eating and most wakeful activities, providing a realistic view of sphincter tone and position during wakefulness. This may be particularly useful at the gastroesophageal junction in identifying sliding hiatal hernia and patulous LES. Topical anesthesia to the nasal cavity is typically provided for comfort, and additional swallowed anesthetic gel can also be given if a strong gag reflex is present. Successful completion of TNE occurs in approximately 96–97% of cases, with the most common cause of non-completion being nasal anatomy precluding passage of the endoscope [29, 31, 33, 34].

Passage through the nose is often easiest via the middle meatus and aided by gel lubrication of the endoscope. The postnasal space anatomy is noted, and palatal movement can be assessed. The oropharynx and hypopharynx are then examined, followed by the laryngeal complex. Biopsies can be taken if needed within the pharynx. Liquid anesthetic may also be directed through the working channel of the endoscope to specific areas, for example, the glottis if one is undertaking laryngeal work or wishes to perform tracheobronchoscopy. Alternatively, the endoscope is directed through the upper esophageal sphincter (UES) in conjunction with the subject swallowing. This can be aided by insufflation but usually this is not necessary. The UES is sensitive to dilation and may generate a gag reflex, of which the subject should be warned. To ease this response, the subject is advised to use a controlled breathing pattern (in the nose and slowly out through pursed lips). Beware a hypopharyngeal pseudodiverticulum (Zenker's diverticulum) which is situated posteriorly and is usually easier to pass into than the true lumen of the esophagus. Inadvertent pouch entry may theoretically result in perforation, although the smaller size of the TNE endoscopes somewhat mitigates this risk and there have been few reported cases. When comfortable passage of the UES has been achieved, the endoscope is then advanced down the esophagus to the gastroesophageal junction (GEJ). The esophageal lumen is examined, but often the best views of this are achieved on retraction of the endoscope. Mass lesions, ulceration, white patches (possible acanthosis vs candidiasis vs eosinophilic microabscesses), and external compression are evaluated. The TNE is then passed into the stomach. Food material within the stomach suggests a possible motility or gastric outlet issue, as patients are instructed not to eat for at least 3 hours prior to the procedure. In addition, blood, polyps, and other lesions can be visualized often prompting an evaluation by the gastroenterologist. The endoscope is then retroflexed by a slight advancement of the scope and rotation of the angulation wheel or lever of the scope. This allows visualization of the caudal aspect of the GEJ.

After insufflation of the stomach and evaluation of the caudal GEJ, air is suctioned from the stomach to prevent post-procedure nausea and discomfort. The scope is then withdrawn into the GEJ region. Insufflation of the stomach results in reflexive decreased peristalsis allowing for a more complete evaluation and potential procedure or biopsy of the LES region.

GEJ position is noted relative to the diaphragmatic "pinch" – the site of the crural fibers that encircle the esophagus at the diaphragmatic hiatus. If the rugae of the stomach are elevated more than 2 cm above the pinch site, then a hiatal hernia is present (Fig. 14.6).

Figure 14.6 Endoscopic view of gastroesophageal junction demonstrating a hiatal hernia.

Watch reactivity of the GEJ with breathing. Sniffing should demonstrate a closure twitch of the diaphragmatic sling fibers. Next, assess the squamocolumnar junction (also called the Z-line) – is it regular or sawtooth, and are there isolated islands of darker mucosa at its margins, suggestive of Barrett's metaplasia? Biopsies may be taken here, and if BM is suspected, then quadrantic biopsies (Seattle protocol) at 1 cm vertical intervals are recommended. Alternative methods to obtain histological diagnosis include the use of brush biopsies or an abrasive sponge (Cytosponge™). The Prague classification can be used to describe the circumferential and vertical extent of Barrett's metaplasia (Fig. 14.7) [35]. In practical terms, if BM is suspected and confirmed by biopsies, then surveillance endoscopy is recommended every 2 years or sooner if associated with dysplasia or if symptoms change.

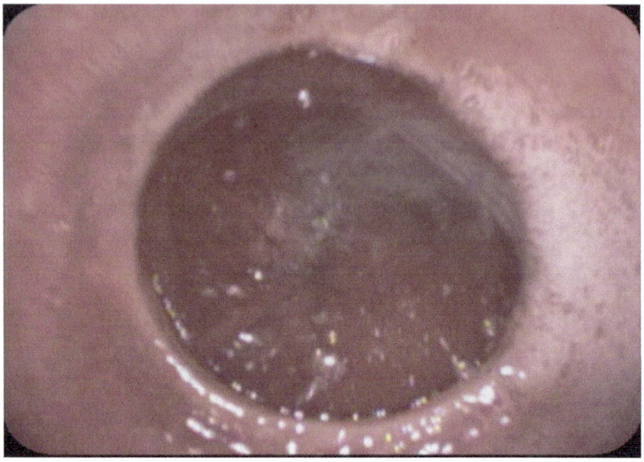

Fig. 14.6 Endoscopic image of distal esophagus demonstrating a hiatal hernia and Schatzki's ring

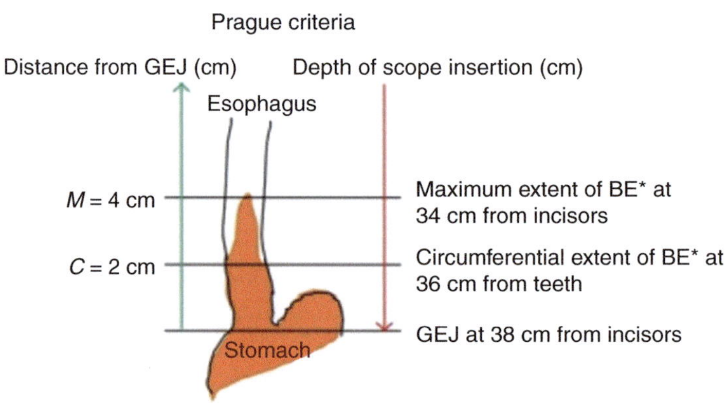

Fig. 14.7 Prague classification of Barrett's metaplasia extent. This describes the circumferential extent (C) of Barrett's metaplasia as well as the maximal proximal extension (M), anchored on where the gastroesophageal junction is in each individual. For example, if the GEJ is at 38 cm from the incisors (as shown) and circumferential BM is seen between 36 and 38 cm, then $C = 2$. If there is a further extending tongue of BM above this level, then it is measured from GEJ to its proximal extent, e.g., a further 2 cm means a total of 4 cm from the GEJ and hence $M = 4$. The classification would be C2M4 [Sharma, Dent, Armstrong et al., 2006]. (Figure courtesy of Dr. David McGouran, MRCP)

In the case of high-grade dysplasia, then presentation at a multidisciplinary tumor board meeting is recommended for consideration of definitive treatment, usually submucous resection.

A retroflex maneuver within the esophagus (usually a technique performed in the stomach) has been described by Zalvan as a method for examining the undersurface of the UES [Zalvan CH personal communication, manuscript in preparation]. When the endoscope is being withdrawn prior to reaching the UES, a retroflex maneuver is performed to study the caudal side of the UES. At the same time, insufflation toward the UES can be undertaken which should demonstrate reflexive contraction of the UES with a triggered peristaltic wave distally. Zalvan terms this the volume induce peristaltic reflex (VIPR). In subjects with disordered motility, this response appears to be lacking. The ability to identify motility problems during endoscopic examination aids decision-making in whom should be further investigated by either fluoroscopy or manometry.

How to Make the Transition

Otolaryngologists are familiar with the anatomy of the laryngopharynx and even the esophagus from a rigid endoscopic perspective, and to move into viewing this region via flexible endoscopes with better illumination, magnified view, and distal chip cameras is a natural progression. Many large studies have now reported equivalent accuracy for diagnosis of common esophageal diseases such as Barrett's metaplasia (BM), esophagitis, solid masses, and carcinoma [14, 15, 36–38].

Otolaryngologists are also familiar with endoscopes. We can drive them, manipulate them, and appreciate the 2D information in a 3D construct. Stepping up to a slightly larger-caliber endoscope with an additional control wheel takes a small number of procedures to feel comfortable, but over a short time one becomes facile with manipulation of the device. The greater learning curve is in becoming comfortable with identifying findings within the esophagus and stomach, so that reporting is accurate and appropriate.

Standardization of reporting for TNE is lacking but has been suggested by proponents of TNE use. Training in use of TNE is also provided for residents in certain ORL training programs, but this remains inconsistent. In some countries, uptake has been limited by billing constraints, with coding for TNE lacking, despite the obvious advantages of this cost-saving approach [32, 39, 40]. With the focus shifting in many health environments to one of screening for serious disease (e.g., cancer) very early, the need for high-turnover methods is greater. Credentialing in TNE is on the horizon, and likely there is a need for a minimum dataset that is reported after each procedure, just as there is with traditional EGD.

Spending time with a clinician familiar with TNE or gastroscopy is a valuable way to become familiar with endoscopic examination findings, when and where to biopsy, and tips and pearls for passing the endoscope. As one becomes accustomed to normal appearances of the esophagus, LES, and gastric region, it becomes easier to identify pathology even in its early stages.

Indications

Almost anyone that comes to the otolaryngology office is a candidate for TNE [Table 14.1], and in fact a large amount of laryngeal work can also be comfortably accomplished with the 60 cm TNE endoscopes available currently. This author uses

Table 14.1 Indication for TNE examination and some common findings

Indication	Area of interest	Findings
Dysphagia	P, E, G	Anything! Can be normal through to malignancy
Foreign body sensation (globus pharyngeus)	P, L, E, G	Often normal Tight UES Patulous LES Osteophytes Heterotopic gastric mucosa (inlet patch) Elongated uvula, vallecula cyst
Lodged foreign body	P, E, G	Usually can propel item to stomach
Reflux disease (esophageal and extra-esophageal)	P, L, E, G	Vocal fold edema VF erythema Interarytenoid edema and rugosity VP granulomata Esophagitis Hiatal hernia +/– Schatzki's ring Gastritis Barrett's metaplasia Mass lesions (polyps, malignancy)
Chronic cough	P, L, E	Vagal neuropathy – strong gag response Reflux disease – laryngeal edema, erythema, rugosity Cough variant asthma – looks normal Benign vocal fold lesions – cough polyp, cough plaques Subglottic stenosis
Head and neck cancer and posttreatment	P, L, E	Xerostomia, xeropharyngia Strictures Lymphedema of the piriformis and larynx Volume loss – tongue, excised tissue VF paralysis Fibrosis – constrictors, floor of mouth, sphincters, temporomandibular joints
Barrett's esophagus (BE) surveillance	E	Barrett's metaplasia Ulceration/esophagitis Hiatal hernia, patulous LES
High-risk factor screening	P, L, E, G	Direct search for malignancy
Persistent mucus	P, L, E, G	Xerostomia and xeropharyngia Anatomical shelves/strictures
Central chest pain	E, G	Tertiary contractions of the esophagus LES patulous Esophagitis
Regurgitation	L, E, G	Laryngeal inflammation Tight UES Patulous LES/HH

Table 14.1 (continued)

Indication	Area of interest	Findings
Interventional		
Stricture dilation (anastomosis, inflammatory, malignant)	E, G	Treatment related vs inflammation (caustic, reflux) vs malignancy Eccentric vs concentric Granulation vs mature
Sphincter dilation (UES, LES)	E, G	CP hypertrophy Inflammatory peptic stricture
Biopsies – esophageal, laryngopharyngeal, gastric	L, E, G	For mucosal irregularity or mass lesions, or possible BM Keratosis, inflammation, polyps Metaplasia (intestinal/BM), dysplasia Carcinoma – squamous or adeno
Injection – botulinum toxin	E, G	Normal appearance Hypertrophy of muscle
Ablation – fiber-based laser, argon plasma coagulation	E, G	Heterotopic gastric mucosa Barrett's metaplasia Early esophageal carcinoma

Legend: *P* pharynx, *L* larynx, *E* esophagus, *G* gastric, *VF* vocal fold, *UES* upper esophageal sphincter, *LES* lower esophageal sphincter, *CP* cricopharyngeal muscle, *HH* hiatal hernia, *BM* Barrett's metaplasia

the same 60 cm endoscope for laryngeal, tracheobronchial, and esophageal work. It is invaluable in the assessment of solid food dysphagia, chronic cough, dyspepsia, throat mucus and irritation, globus sensation, dysphonia, and regurgitation but also has been used for a multitude of other purposes (see below) [32, 35, 41, 42].

In many cases, the transnasal esophagoscopy approach can be used as a rule-out rather than a rule-in. That is, because of ease of performance and lower risks, checking to see if there is pathology does not require a significant level of suspicion (to justify the cardiac risks of sedation). In turn, this means that one often finds pathology in those with minimal symptoms, allowing early intervention and prevention of development of more serious pathology. Many patients are hugely thankful to see with their own eyes that there is not a cancer housed within the throat or food pipe.

TNE has been reported for screening of esophageal cancer [37, 38, 43, 44], assessment of globus sensation [45], eosinophilic esophagitis [46], swallow function, post-radiotherapy esophageal complaints [47] and chronic cough [48], management of foreign bodies of the pharynx and esophagus [49], performance of balloon dilation of the esophagus and trachea, botulinum toxin injection of the LES/pylorus, and placement of secondary tracheoesophageal puncture, esophageal stent, or wireless pH capsule [33, 50–53]. TNE has now also been utilized in unsedated endoscopic mucosal resection of esophageal carcinoma [54].

Complications

Generally, TNE is well tolerated with very few complications or side effects. Vasovagal response to endoscopy can occur (as it can with nasendoscopy using smaller non-channeled endoscopes). This is self-limiting and treated by laying the patient flat. Negotiating the nasal cavity is often the rate-limiting step and may prevent completion of the procedure if the path is very narrowed or tortuous (3–5% rate of non-completion reported due to nasal anatomy) [31, 32, 39, 40]. Epistaxis may occur from contact with the turbinates or septum. Usually this can be managed by simple decongestants and topical dressings if needed. There is a potential risk of perforating a hypopharyngeal diverticulum if one is present, and the endoscopist should be very careful in passage of the UES, in those suspected of a pouch. Other local trauma is theoretically possible; however, as the patient is awake, it is likely that they will object to misdirection of the endoscope into inappropriate tissue spaces!

Findings

As with any tissue in the body, there is a wide range of normal variance in structure and appearance of the pharynx, larynx, esophagus, and stomach. Understanding this normal spectrum gives confidence in identifying abnormalities of anatomy or consequences of disease processes. Figures provided in this chapter illustrate some of the most common entities identified by TNE that are related to patient symptoms. One symptom may also have many causes as with globus sensation which might be generated by anything from cricopharyngeal tension heightened by anxiety to an esophageal carcinoma. Again, this illustrates the need to examine thoroughly, including endoluminally, from the oral cavity to the stomach in those who complain of symptoms above the navel. Table 14.1 details further findings by symptom. Table 14.2 lists some of the most common findings by site.

A few select observations are worthy of note.

Upper Esophageal Sphincter

When passing the UES, it is usually by feel as the sphincter snugs tight around the endoscope. It provokes a gag response in many patients, and it is generally more comfortable to pass this area quickly and smoothly, without insufflating too much air proximally immediately after passage. A more thorough view may be achieved on retraction of the endoscope at the end of the procedure, wherein the patient has accommodated to the presence of the endoscope and it is often then that inlet patches/heterotopic gastric mucosa (HGM) may be identified. Initially not

Table 14.2 Findings during TNE by site

Site	Findings
Nasal	Turbinate hypertrophy Septal deviation Polyp and inflammatory disease
Postnasal	Adenoidal tissue Velopharyngeal incompetence Malignancy
Hypopharynx	Lingual tonsillar hypertrophy Posttreatment changes (DXT/surgery) Vallecula cysts Strictures – anastomotic, post-DXT Malignancy
Larynx	Glottal incompetence Benign VF lesions and papilloma Diffuse inflammation – infective vs reflux vs voice abuse Infective laryngitis VP granulomata Malignancy
Post cricoid	Hemangiomata Fibrosis or stricture Malignancy Zenker's diverticulum
UES	Stricture, hypertrophy
Esophagus	Gastric inlet patch (heterotrophic gastric mucosa) Esophagitis – allergic, chemical, reflux, infective (candida/viral/bacterial) Stricture – peptic, caustic, malignant, iatrogenic Malignancy
Gastroesophageal junction	Hiatal herniae and patulous LES Barrett's metaplasia Polyps Esophagitis/ulceration Schatzki's ring (B ring) Muscular A ring Paraesophageal herniae
Stomach	Gastritis (check *H. pylori*) Gastric fundic (benign) polyps Ulceration Malignancy

Legend: *VF* vocal fold, *VP* vocal process, *LES* lower esophageal sphincter, *H. pylori Helicobacter pylori*, *DXT* radiotherapy

considered to be symptom causing, recent papers suggest an association of HGM with pharyngeal symptoms such as globus sensation and throat irritation, as well as improvement with treatment, both medical (acid inhibitors) and surgical (argon plasma ablation of the patch) [55–60]. Furthermore, a view of the cricopharyngeal fibers of the UES is often best at this time. A hypertrophic cricopharyngeus may be seen as a prominence of the muscle at the UES level. Endoscopically, this cannot be called a bar as that is an exclusively radiological diagnosis. A hypopharyngeal diverticulum has been previously mentioned, with its neck in the hypopharynx. Often this is not detected by flexible endoscopy; however, if the endoscope passes into this pouch, it is usually on entry to the UES. Beware the endoscope not passing freely and visibility of only epithelium.

Esophagus

Esophagitis is the most common finding and typically associated with reflux disease. Grading and extent of reflux esophagitis is described by the Los Angeles classification, with Grades A–D (from least injured to most injured). There is not direct symptom correlation with these endoscopic findings; however, more circumferential disease holds more risk for development of cicatricial strictures. Allergic eosinophilic esophagitis is recognized in children and adults as reactivity to food proteins. This produces a characteristic "trachealized" or ringed appearance of the esophageal body. There may also be small white microabscesses submucosally. Food bolus impaction is the most common complaint, but more vague symptoms may be all that is present. Infective esophagitis is most commonly candidal in origin. This has a typical appearance of white plaques adherent to mucosa and may be extensive. Biopsy can confirm hyphae and rule out dysplasia. Distally the most important finding is endoscopic appearance consistent with Barrett's esophagus. This is a darker salmon pink-colored mucosa, often variegated with interspersed patches of normal pale esophageal mucosa creating islands. Again, this may be completely asymptomatic in many individuals. As previously mentioned, the extent of BM is described by the Prague classification (Fig. 14.7) and should be recorded for monitoring. Biopsy is warranted to assess for dysplastic or malignant degeneration. Surveillance is recommended two-yearly if BM is detected, as BM represents the greatest risk factor for development of adenocarcinoma of the esophagus. Carcinomata of the esophagus are distinctive, irregular, often ulcerated, or partly obstructive. Proximally this is most commonly squamous and distally adenocarcinoma. Biopsy is essential and guides further treatment decisions.

Gastroesophageal Junction/LES/Squamocolumnar Junction

The LES should be a snug closure point, at or near the crural diaphragmatic pinch. The squamocolumnar junction (mucosal transition between esophageal and gastric mucosa) is normal a pink regular rosette at or near the GEJ. If the hiatus is lax, the cardia of the stomach may rise through the hiatus and herniate into the chest. The presence of cardia greater than 2 cm above the pinch is termed a hiatus hernia. Rugae are detected, and on insufflation there is a ballooned appearance to this region. This is distinct from a mild dilation that is the esophageal vestibule just above the true GEJ. In some cases, there is a partial compensation at the apex of the hernia – a mucosal ring (B ring), known as a Schatzki's ring. If the ring diameter is less 13 mm, there may be holdup of solid food and symptom complaint. A different type of ring (A ring) may also be seen in the distal esophagus, which is a muscular ring, likely generated by crural diaphragmatic fibers.

Gastric

Superficial gastritis appears as a speckled surface within the stomach but may also show darker discoloration or rarely changed blood. Gastritis may be atrophic or associated with *Helicobacter pylori* infection. Biopsy will differentiate, and treatment of *H. pylori* is warranted for symptom control and to reduce risk of gastric cancer development. Gastric polyps are common findings and often multiple. These fundic-type polyps are benign. Larger or irregular polyps or hemorrhagic polyps require biopsy. A retroflexed view of the underside of the LES may demonstrate poor contraction around the endoscope and is described by the Hill's grading 1–4 (normal [snuggly held endoscope], mild, moderate, severe laxity around endoscope). The presence of bile or food in the starved patient is worth noting as bilious reflux may be recalcitrant to typical medical therapy, and food presence after 4 h indicates poor gastric emptying, possibly gastroparesis. This may indicate the need for additional investigations. Most gastric findings of any concern warrant referral to gastroenterology colleagues for further review and management.

Summary

Transnasal esophagoscopy is an established diagnostic and therapeutic technique that enables full aerodigestive evaluation of our patients and the ability to perform unsedated procedures in the larynx, pharynx, and esophagus. Its utility is increasing but already validated as equivalent in screening for Barrett's esophagus and reflux disease. New maneuvers and applications continue to be reported, and it offers additional benefits in safety, costs, time to treatment, and screening programs. Otolaryngologists are uniquely equipped to embrace TNE as well as continue to promote new developments and technical advances.

References

1. Mittal RK. Motor function of the pharynx, esophagus and its sphincters. San Rafael: Morgan & Claypool Life Sciences; 2011.
2. Vakil N, van Zanten SV, Kahrilas P, Dent J, Jones R, et al. Global Consensus group. The Montreal definition and classification of gastroesophageal reflux disease: a global evidence-

based consensus. Am J Gastroenterol. 2006;101:1900–20. Abstract available as http://www.ncbi.nlm.nih.gov/pubmed/16928254

3. Lang IM, Medda BK, Shaker R. Effects of esophageal acidification on esophageal reflexes controlling the upper esophageal sphincter. Am J Physiol Gastrointest Liver Physiol. 2019;316:G45–54.
4. Lang IM, Medda BK, Shaker R. Differential activation of medullary vagal nuclei caused by stimulation of different esophageal mechanoreceptors. Brain Res. 2011;1368:119–33.
5. Babaei A, Venu M, Naini SR, Gonzaga J, Lang IM, Massey BT, Jadcherla S, Shaker R. Impaired upper esophageal sphincter reflexes in patients with supraesophageal reflux disease. Gastroenterology. 2015;149:1381–91.
6. Szczesniak MM, Williams RB, Brake HM, Maclean JC, Cole IE, Cook IJ. Upregulation of the esophago-UES relaxation response: a possible pathophysiological mechanism in suspected reflux laryngitis. Neurogastroenterol Motil. 2010;22:381–6.
7. Amaris M, Dua KS, Naini SR, Samuel E, Shaker R. Characterization of the upper esophageal sphincter response during cough. Chest. 2012;142:1229–36.
8. Reavis KM, Morris CD, Gopal DV, Hunter JG, Jobe BA. Laryngopharyngeal reflux symptoms better predict the presence of esophageal adenocarcinoma than typical gastroesophageal reflux symptoms. Ann Surg. 2004;239:849–56.
9. Nouraei SAR, Murray IA, Heathcote KJ, Dalton HR. Oesophageal causes of dysphagia localised only to the pharynx: implications for the suspected head and neck cancer pathway. Clin Otolaryngol. 2018. https://doi.org/10.1111/coa.13115 . [epub ahead of print].
10. Whiteman DC, Kendall BJ. Barrett's oesophagus: epidemiology, diagnosis and clinical management. Med J Aust. 2016;205:317–24.
11. Evans RPT, Mourad MM, Fisher SG, Bramhall SR. Evolving management of metaplasia and dysplasia in Barrett's epithelium. World J Gastroenterol. 2016;22:10316–24.
12. Schneider JL, Corley DA. A review of the epidemiology of Barrett's oesophagus and oesophageal adenocarcinoma. Best Pract Res Clin Gastroenterol. 2015;29:29–39.
13. Patel A, Gyawali CP. Screening for Barrett's Esophagus: balancing clinical value and cost-effectiveness. J Neurogastroenterol Motil. 2019;25:181–8.
14. Shariff MK, Bird-Lieberman EL, O'Donovan M, Abdullahi Z, Liu X, Blazeby J, Fitzgerald R. Randomized crossover study comparing efficacy of transnasal endoscopy with that of standard endoscopy to detect Barrett's esophagus. Gastrointest Endosc. 2012;75:954–61.
15. Shariff MK, Barghese S, O'Donovan M, Abdullahi Z, Liu X, Fitzgerald RC, di Pietro M. Pilot randomized crossover study comparing the efficacy of transnasal disposable endosheath with standard endoscopy to detect Barrett's esophagus. Endoscopy. 2016;48:110–6.
16. Richardson C, Colavita P, Dinst C, Bagnato J, Billing P, Birkenhagen K, et al. Real-time diagnosis of Barrett's esophagus: a prospective, multicentre study comparing confocal laser endomicroscopy with conventional histology for the identification of intestinal metaplasia in new users. Surg Endosc. 2019;33:1585–91.
17. Xiong YQ, Ma SJ, Hu JY, Ge J, Zhou LZ, Huo ST, Qui M, Chen Q. Comparison of narrow-band imaging and confocal laser endomicroscopy for the detection of neoplasia in Barrett's esophagus: a meta-analysis. Clin Res Hepatol Gastroenterol. 2018;42:31–9.
18. Iqbal U, Siddique O, Ovalle A, Anwar H, Moss SF. Safety and efficacy of a minimally invasive cell sampling device (Cytosponge) in the diagnosis of esophageal pathology: a systematic review. Eur J Gastroenterol Hepatol. 2018. https://doi.org/10.1097/MEG.0000000001210. Epub ahead of print.
19. Ross-Innes CS, Chettouh H, Achilleos A, Galeano-Dalmau N, Debiram-Beecham I, MacRae S, et al. Risk stratification of Barrett's oesophagus using a non-endoscopic sampling method coupled with a biomarker panel: a cohort study. Lancet Gastroenterol Hepatol. 2017;2:23–31.
20. Sami SS, Dunagan KT, Johnson ML, et al. A randomized comparative effectiveness trial of novel endoscopic techniques and approaches for Barrett's esophagus screening in the community. Am J Gastroenterol. 2015;110:148–58.

21. Zhou Z, Kalatskaya I, Russell D, Marcon N, Cirocco M, Kryzyzanowski PM, et al. Combined EsophaCap cytology and MUC2 immunohistochemistry for screening of intestinal metaplasia, dysplasia and carcinoma. Clin Exp Gastroenterol. 2019;12:219–29.
22. Offman J, Fitzgerald R. Alternatives to traditional per oral endoscopy for screening. Gastrointest Endosc Clin N Am. 2017;27:379–96.
23. Johanson JF, Frakes J, Eisen D, EndoCDx Collaborative Group. Computer-assisted analysis of abrasive transepithelial brush biopsies increases the effectiveness of esophageal screening: a multicentre prospective clinical trial by the EndoCDx Collaborative Group. Dig Dis Sci. 2011;56:767–72.
24. Vennalaganti PR, Naag Kanakadandi V, Gross SA, Parasa S, Wang KK, Gupta N, Sharma P. Transepithelial sampling with computer-assisted analysis in patients with Barrett's esophagus. Am J Gastroenterol. 2015;110:1257–60.
25. Mariano VS, Pastrez PRZ, Mafra Costa A, Guimarães DP, Cunha TR, Neto SAZ, et al. Impact of brush cytology analysis for the diagnosis of esophageal squamous cell carcinoma; the quality of liquid-based preparation of cytological slides. Acta Cytol. 2019;63:240–6.
26. Amin MR, Postma GN, Setzen M, Koufman JA. Transnasal Esophagoscopy: a position statement from the American Bronchoesophagological Association (ABEA). Otolaryngol Head Neck Surg. 2008;138:411–4.
27. Saeian K, Staff DM, Vailopoulos S, et al. Unsedated transnasal endoscopy accurately detects Barrett's metaplasia and dysplasia. Gastrointest Endosc. 2002;56:472–8.
28. Peery AF, Hoppo T, Garman KS, et al. Feasibility, safety, acceptability, and yield of office-based screening transnasal Esophagoscopy (with video). Gastrointest Endosc. 2012;75:945–53.
29. Polat B, Karahatay S, Birkent H, Gerek M. The practicability of transnasal esophagoscopy and the evaluation of patient's perception: a prospective study. Clin Exp Otorhinolaryngol. 2016;9:366–9.
30. Belafsky PC, Postma GN, Daniel E, Koufman JA. Transnasal esophagoscopy. Otolaryngol Head Neck Surg. 2001;125:588–9.
31. Postma GN, Cohen JT, Belafsky PC, Halum SL, Gupta SK, Bach KK, Koufman JA. Transnasal Esophagoscopy: revisited (over 700 consecutive cases). Laryngoscope. 2005;115:321–3.
32. Howell RJ, Pate MB, Ishman SL, et al. Prospective multi-institutional transnasal esophagoscopy: predictors of a change in management. Laryngoscope. 2016;126:2667–71.
33. Howell RJ, Schopper MA, Giliberto JP, Collar RM, Khosla SM. Office-based esophageal dilation in head and neck cancer: safety, feasibility and cost analysis. Laryngoscope. 2018;128:2261–7.
34. Allen J. Transnasal esophagoscopy: review of more than 570 cases. Presentation 2018 American Bronchoesophagological Association meeting, National Harbour, Maryland.
35. Sharma P, Dent J, Armstrong D, et al. The development and validation of an endoscopic grading system for Barrett's metaplasia: the Prague C & M criteria. Gastroenterol. 2006;131:1392–9.
36. Sabirin J, Abd Rahman M, Rajan P. Changing trends in oesophageal endoscopy: a systematic review of transnasal oesophagoscopy. ISRN Otolaryngol. 2013; https://doi.org/10.1155/2013/586973.
37. Su YY, Chen WC, Chuang HC, Guo CS, Lin YT, Luo SD, Fang FM, Chien CY. Effect of routine esophageal screening in patients with head and neck cancer. JAMA Otolaryngol Head Neck Surg. 2013;139:350–4.
38. Wang CH, Lee YC, Wang CP, Chen CC, Ko JY, Han ML, et al. Use of transnasal endoscopy for screening of esophageal squamous cell carcinoma in high-risk patients: yield rate, completion rate, and safety. Dig Endosc. 2014;26(1):24–31.
39. Wellenstein DJ, Honings J, Schutte HW, Herruer JM, van den Hoogen FJA, Marres HAM, Takes RP, van den Broek GB. Cost analysis of office-based transnasal esophagoscopy. Eur Arch Otorhinolaryngol. 2019;276:1457–63.
40. Wellenstein DJ, Schutte HW, Marres HAM, Honings J, Belafsky PC, Postma GN, Takes RP, van den Broek GB. Office-based procedures for diagnosis and treatment of esophageal pathology. Head Neck. 2017;39:1910–9.

41. Lin PH, Wang CP, Lou PJ, Ko JY, Hsiao TY, Chen TC. Evaluation of swallowing disorders by use of transnasal esophagoscopy in patients treated for head and neck cancer. Head Neck. 2016;38(Suppl 1):E1137–43.
42. Roof SA, Amin MR. Transnasal esophagoscopy in modern head and neck surgery. Curr Opin Otolaryngol Head Neck Surg. 2015;23:171–5.
43. Huang YC, Lee YC, Tseng PH, et al. Regular screening of esophageal cancer for 248 newly diagnosed hypopharyngeal squamous cell carcinoma by unsedated transnasal esophagogastroduodenoscopy. Oral Oncol. 2016;55:55–60.
44. di Pietro M, Canto MI, Fitzgerald RC. Endoscopic Management of Early Adenocarcinoma and Squamous Cell Carcinoma of the Esophagus: Screening, Diagnosis, and Therapy. Gastroenterology. 2018;154(2):421–36.
45. Sanyaolu LN, Jemah A, Stew B, Ingrams DR. The role of transnasal oesophagoscopy in the management of globus pharyngeus and non-progressive dysphagia. Ann R Coll Surg Engl. 2016;98:49–52.
46. Friedlander JA, DeBoer EM, Soden JS, Furuta GT, Menard-Katcher CD, Atkins D, et al. Unsedated transnasal esophagoscopy for monitoring therapy in pediatric eosinophilic esophagitis. Gastrointest Endosc. 2016;83:299–306.
47. Farwell DG, Rees CJ, Mouadeb DA, Allen J, Chen AM, Enepekides DJ, Belafsky PC. Esophageal pathology in patients after treatment for head and neck cancer. Otolaryngol Head Neck Surg. 2010;143:375–8.
48. Athanasiadis T, Allen JE. Chronic cough: an otorhinolaryngology perspective. Curr Opin Head Neck Surg. 2013;21:517–22.
49. Shih CW, Hao CY, Wang YJ, Hao SP. A new trend in the management of esophageal foreign body: transnasal esophagoscopy. Otolaryngol Head Neck Surg. 2015;153:189–92.
50. Borgulya M, Ell C, Pohl J. Transnasal endoscopy for direct visual control of esophageal stent placement without fluoroscopy. Endoscopy. 2012;44:422–4.
51. Rees CJ. In-office transnasal Esophagoscopy-guided botulinum toxin injection of the lower esophageal sphincter. Curr Opin Otolaryngol Head Neck Surg. 2007;15:409–11.
52. Rees CJ. In-office unsedated transnasal balloon dilation of the esophagus and trachea. Curr Opin Otolaryngol Head Neck Surg. 2007;15:401–4.
53. Doctor VS. In-office unsedated tracheoesophageal puncture. Curr Opin Otolaryngol Head Neck Surg. 2007;15:405–8.
54. Nakamura M, Shiroeda H, Tahara T, Shibata T, Arisawa T. Endoscopic submucosal dissection of an esophageal tumour using a transnasal endoscope without sedation. Endoscopy. 2014;46(Suppl 1):E115–6.
55. Chong VH, Jalihal A. Heterotopic gastric mucosal patch of the esophagus is associated with higher prevalence of laryngopharyngeal symptoms. Eur Arch Otorhinolaryngol. 2010;267:1793–9.
56. Chong VH. Cervical inlet patch: an important cause of Globus pharyngeus. Eur Arch Otorhinolaryngol. 2018;275:3101–2.
57. Yamada T, Tsuji A, Onoue S, et al. Acid suppressive therapy improved symptoms due to circumferential cervical inlet patch with proton pumps (H+/K+-ATPase). World J Clin Cases. 2017;5:403.
58. Meining A, Bajbouj M. Gastric inlet patches in the cervical esophagus: what they are, what they cause and how they can be treated. Gastrointest Endosc. 2016;84:1027–9.
59. Meining A, Bajbouj M, Preeg M, et al. Argon plasma ablation of gastric inlet patched in the cervical esophagus may alleviate globus sensation: a pilot trial. Endoscopy. 2006;38:566–70.
60. Bajbouj M, Becker V, Eckel F, et al. Argon plasma coagulation of cervical heterotopic gastric mucosa as an alternative treatment for globus sensations. Gastroenterology. 2009;137:440–4.

Chapter 15
The Role of the Speech-Language Pathologist with the Diagnosis of Dysphagia and Reflux

Andrea Bracciante-Ely and Paula Dinu

Who Are Speech-Language Pathologists (SLPs)?

Speech-language pathologists (SLPs) work to prevent, assess, diagnose, and treat speech, language, social communication, cognitive-linguistic communication, and swallowing disorders (dysphagia) in both children and adults. During the 1970s and 1980s, the role of the SLP in dysphagia evolved from their experience treating speech and voice disorders of the oral and pharyngeal musculature. In the late 1960s, Dr. George Larsen, an SLP at the Seattle VA Hospital, was challenged by the chief of neurology to help their patients with observed swallowing difficulty achieve a faster discharge. Through Dr. Larsen's research, the early foundation of the clinical assessment of swallowing and management of dysphagia was laid in the early 1970s. Dr. Jeri Logemann's postdoctoral research on the speech patterns in Parkinson's disease using videofluoroscopy led to her understanding of swallowing disorders in this group of patients. She is credited with the development of the modified barium swallow (MBS) and the author of the first text on dysphagia in 1983 [1]. Ongoing research since the 1980s has led to advancements in diagnostic assessments, both clinical and instrumental, as well as in therapeutic interventions.

As defined by Logemann, "swallowing refers to the entire act of deglutition from placement of food in the mouth through the oral and pharyngeal stages of the swallow until the material enters the esophagus through the cricopharyngeal juncture" [2]. Swallowing is divided into the following four phases with impairment possible in one or multiple phases: oral preparatory phase when a food or liquid bolus is

A. Bracciante-Ely (✉) · P. Dinu
Speech and Hearing Center, Institute for Voice and Swallowing Disorders, Phelps Hospital, Northwell Health, Sleepy Hollow, NY, USA
e-mail: abraccianteely@northwell.edu; pdinu@northwell.edu

C. H. Zalvan (ed.), *Laryngopharyngeal and Gastroesophageal Reflux*,
https://doi.org/10.1007/978-3-030-48890-1_15

manipulated and/or chewed in the mouth, the oral phase where the tongue propels the food posteriorly until the swallow reflex is imitated, the pharyngeal phase where the reflexive swallow response propels the bolus through the pharynx with a stripping wave, and the esophageal phase with the bolus passing through the pharyngo-esophageal segment with esophageal peristalsis transporting the bolus through the cervical and thoracic esophagus to the stomach [2]. Swallowing is a complicated and well-coordinated series of movements that involves over 26 muscles of the head and neck, and 6 of the 12 cranial nerves are directly engaged. It is believed a normal swallow takes 1.5 seconds and the esophageal phase can take 3–20 seconds to complete depending on the bolus thickness, viscosity, and performance of the swallow. However, a complete meal, which is higher in proteins, can take over an hour and a half for the body to digest. We swallow between 600 and 1000 times per day, approximately 250 times during a meal and about 50 times when sleeping.

According to the Agency for Health Care Policy and Research (AHCPR), over 60,000 Americans die from complications associated with swallowing impairments, with the most common being aspiration pneumonia. Aspiration pneumonia is one of the leading causes of death among the elderly. Pneumonia is the fifth leading cause of death among the elderly. It is believed that 1 in 17 people will develop some form of dysphagia in their lifetime. As we know, dysphagia is most prevalent with the elderly, and many studies suggest that 75% of nursing home residents develop some form of dysphagia. Dysphagia and its sequelae can increase healthcare costs due to readmissions, chronic ED visits, extended length of stay (LOS), need for placement in an extended long-term care facility, and possibly the need for respiratory and nutritional support. In severe cases, a tracheostomy may be necessary due to chronic respiratory compromise from chronic aspiration pneumonia, as well as the possible need for alternate means of long-term nutrition and hydration. All of these complications are expensive costs that contribute to increased healthcare costs.

Esophageal Disease and Dysphagia

Dysphagia involving the oropharyngeal component is broad, and it is usually described by a patient as a symptom including a localized sensation of a discomfort or blockage in the throat or cervical esophageal region. The recognition of these different symptoms, either reported or directly observed, truly facilitates the proper diagnosis to guide treatment and further referrals to specialists for comprehensive management. Once we are below the cricopharyngeus, we encounter a substernal form of dysphagia. These types of dysphagia involve the regions below the cricopharyngeus and within the thoracic esophageal region. The sensation of dysphagia within this region, whether functional or structural, can be related to gastroesophageal (GERD) and laryngopharyngeal reflux disease (LPR).

The gastrointestinal (GI) tract includes the oral cavity, pharynx, esophagus, and stomach along with the large and small intestine. Technically, the swallowing anatomy is one continuous tube that is controlled by a series of "valves" to transport content safely and efficiently from the mouth to the anus, as well as prevent reflux of contents in a retrograde fashion. The valves of the GI tract are primarily responsible for preventing retrograde movement of gastric contents while moving nutrients to the internal cells through the circulatory system. When the valves do not function properly, the gastric contents and/or acids within the esophagus may migrate to the level of the pharynx and larynx. When acids pool in these areas, the structures of the larynx and pharynx become irritated. This chronic and persistent irritation results in edema and increased mucus production. Patients often begin to chronically clear their throat and/or chronically cough in response to the edema and mucus. Throat clearing and coughing are abusive vocal behaviors that further irritate and perpetuate the presence of edema and mucus. Sensory changes occur causing the patient to feel a fullness in the throat or a lump in the throat, known as globus sensation. Voice changes often follow with complaints of hoarseness, lower pitch, and reduced loudness. Complaints of difficulty swallowing often accompany the voice changes and include difficulty with solids more than liquids, feeling food sticking in the throat, multiple swallows for the food to clear, and/or the need to wash foods down with liquids. These complaints lead a patient to an assessment by the SLP.

Clinical Assessment

Typically in acute care settings, rehabilitation hospitals, and long-term care facilities, patients experiencing dysphagia are referred to the SLP and are first evaluated with the *Clinical Bedside Swallowing Evaluation.* While this assessment is subjective, it is extremely useful when performed by an experienced clinician. Patients that live independently often consult their primary care physician (PCP) who will make appropriate referrals to an otolaryngologist, gastroenterologist, and/or a speech-language pathologist directly. Regardless of the setting, the evaluation begins with a medical chart review of the patient detailing the history of the present illness, past medical history, surgical history, current medications, and current diet. When available, interviews with family, caregivers, or medical staff provide additional information on observed behaviors when the patient is eating and drinking that may contribute to the current swallowing difficulty. Additionally, these parties can voice concerns, expectations, and goals at this time.

During the Clinical Bedside Swallowing Evaluation, the SLP is making observations of the patient's medical status. The patient's cognitive status is quickly assessed to determine if evaluation is appropriate at the given time. A patient should be alert and able to sustain attention for the task of eating. While orientation to person, place, time, and condition is optimal, orientation to person is the minimum requirement. The clinician checks the patient's ability to follow multiple-step directives. Baseline respiratory status is assessed with attention to baseline oxygen saturation (if available), the need for oxygen, baseline cervical breath sounds using cervical auscultation, and the presence of shortness of breath. Baseline secretion management, with observation of spontaneous swallowing frequency, is also made within the first few minutes with the patient. Most importantly, the ability of a patient to perform a volitional cough should be evaluated to assess for glottis closure. Volitional cough is elicited by the patient rather than their reflexive cough as a sensory response.

An oral peripheral exam is then completed to examine symmetry, range of motion, strength, and sensation of the lips, tongue, cheeks, velum, jaw, and larynx at rest, in sustained postures, and in movement. One's communication skills, particularly speech intelligibility and vocal quality, are noted. Based on clinician judgment, oral trials of varied solid and liquid consistencies are provided as appropriate. Each consistency is assessed for adequate oral manipulation, bolus formation and transport, swallow initiation, and signs and symptoms of overt pharyngeal tolerance. While impairments in the oral phase of swallowing, such as incomplete lip closure, prolonged mastication of solids, and poor formation of a cohesive bolus, can be readily observed, some pharyngeal symptoms are often inferred when a patient appears to be eating and drinking without difficulty but has unexplained weight loss, recurrent fevers, and frequent upper respiratory infections or recurrent pneumonia. Overt signs and symptoms of impairment in the pharyngeal stage include the following: delay in swallowing, wet vocalizations, frequent throat clearing, and/or coughing during and after eating and drinking. Clinical impressions and recommendations are one of the most important parts of the Clinical Bedside Swallow Evaluation. Clinical impressions are made based on observations that lead to the following questions: *what type of dysphagia does the patient exhibit*, and *what is causing this type of dysphagia?*

Traditionally, the SLP works up to the level of the cricopharyngeus (upper esophageal sphincter) but often will "suspect" esophageal involvement during a Clinical Bedside Swallow Evaluation. Patient complaints of food sticking in the upper chest when swallowing, more difficulty swallowing solids versus liquids, globus sensation, and increased mucus production, particularly in the morning, may lead toward the differential diagnosis of pharyngeal and/or esophageal dysphagia. If symptoms of oral, pharyngeal, and/or esophageal dysphagia are observed, during the Clinical Bedside Swallowing Evaluation, additional instrumental assessment may be warranted for objective data.

Instrumental Assessment

Accurate assessment of the activity of the oral, pharyngeal, and esophageal areas during swallowing requires the use of instrumental diagnostic imaging techniques to objectively view intrinsic physiology. The main objective instrumental techniques used by the SLP to examine swallow function are the fiber-optic endoscopic evaluation of swallowing (FEES) and the modified barium swallow (MBS), also known as videofluoroscopy. A newer, yet controversial, assessment and biofeedback tool is high-resolution manometry (HRM).

FEES

FEES was established in 1988 as a joint venture between speech-language pathology and otolaryngology at the VA-Ann Arbor, Michigan [1]. FEES, an in-office or bedside examination of the swallowing structures, provides a direct view of the structures of the velopharynx, oropharynx, pharynx, larynx, and the cricopharyngeal segment (inferior pharyngeal constrictor). Coordination between airway protection, respiration, and swallowing is directly observed [3]. Because there is a "white out" period from epiglottic retroflexion during the height of the swallow, both aspiration during the swallow and cricopharyngeal function cannot be directly observed and can only be inferred based on findings after the completion of the swallow. If cricopharyngeal dysfunction is suspected or reflux is observed, an MBS may often follow. Consequently, FEES is not the preferred examination of choice in patients with suspected cricopharyngeal dysfunction, globus sensation, and/or reflux disease.

MBS

The MBS was designed as a dynamic radiographic assessment to examine oral, pharyngeal, and cervical esophageal physiology during swallowing. It is considered to be the gold standard to assess anatomy and physiology of all phases of the swallow. MBS is the most widely used and effective instrumentation technique in dysphagia. The purpose of the MBS is to define movement patterns of the structures in the oral cavity, pharynx, larynx, and cervical esophagus; measure the speed and efficiency of the swallow; and examine the effectiveness of potential rehabilitation techniques and strategies [2].

The MBS exam is useful to objectively assess the esophagus for structural deviations, such as webs, rings, diverticulum, and masses, as well as functional motility deviations, such as esophageal dysmotility, achalasia, and tertiary contractions, which may be affecting the overall system of swallowing and contributing to the reported dysphagia. Often dysphagia is attributed to "normal aging changes," also known as *presbyphagia,* when so often it is actually related to these functional and structural deviations and disorders that are often overlooked. These deviations and disorders tend to increase with age, often contributing to the cause of the dysphagia. In the elderly population, the most underrecognized cause of nutritional and respiratory compromise is usually directly related to oropharyngeal dysphagia.

MBS Protocol

The MBS exam is traditionally performed in the radiology department of a hospital by the SLP with both a radiologist and a radiology technician present; the required presence of a radiologist during the MBS is state dependent. If the radiologist is not present during the exam, a physician is required to review the images upon completion of the assessment. While there is growing support for standardization in the administration of trial consistencies and scoring of the MBS exam, this remains facility dependent. Like the clinical bedside swallow evaluation, the patient is tested with varied food and liquid consistencies that are mixed with the contrast agent barium. As in a clinical bedside swallow evaluation, viscosities and thickness of per oral (po) trials play a large role in the timing and completion of a swallow. Thinner viscosities, such as water, are liquids that move more quickly through the body than thicker viscosities like pudding or even solids. The po trials are also affected by the property of gravity. The thinner the viscosity, the faster the po trial travels and can have an easier opportunity to prematurely migrate into an unprotected open airway and result in an aspiration event; water is the most likely consistency to be aspirated. *Aspiration* is the entry of food, liquid, and/or secretions into the airway below the level of the vocal cords and into the proximal trachea. *Penetration* is the entry of food, liquids, and/or secretions into the laryngeal vestibule which remains above the vocal cords. Both penetration and aspiration can occur *silently* which is when the events just described occur without any overt signs or symptoms. These patients may have recurrent pneumonias with a "suspiciously good swallow." Typically, once any ingesta enters into the region of the laryngeal vestibule, a cough reflex is initiated to prompt the vocal cords to close to prevent migration below the vocal cords into the lungs. In fact, a cough response is considered one of the most important indicators of penetration or aspiration, although up to 55% of patients can be silent aspirators (no overt signs or symptoms) [4]. This is when the "suspiciously good swallow" may need to be further investigated with the use of an objective test, like the MBS. There is no special preparation for the exam; patients may eat and drink normally prior to the exam. Fluoroscopy, the radiographic imaging technique, is used as the patient is swallowing each item and the video images are recorded. The patient is typically seated for the exam with views of swallowing obtained in the lateral and anterior-posterior plane. Scout films, static baseline images, are taken prior to the initiation of the food and liquid trials for baseline observations of the structures. There are anatomical and radiographic landmarks we should be aware of when we are analyzing a swallow on an MBS. These include *the lips, tongue, mandible, hard palate, soft palate/velum, base of tongue, posterior pharyngeal wall, the epiglottis, valleculae, hyoid bone, the pyriform sinuses, the posterior pharyngeal wall, the aryepiglottic folds, anterior commissure, posterior commissure, the cervical spine, the vocal cords, the larynx, the trachea, the cricopharyngeus and the cervical esophageal region.*

When scout films are taken, it is at this time that anatomical changes, such as structural deformities due to surgery, radiation, or age-related degenerative changes in the cervical spine, as well as the presence of cervical hardware can be appreciated and identified as potential contributing factors to the patient's reported dysphagia. Structural variations are formally diagnosed by the attending radiologist or physician reviewing the study after the MBS has been completed. Assessment includes presentation of food consistencies that vary from puree through higher level chewable solids and liquid consistencies ranging from thin (e.g., water like), nectar thick and honey thick liquids. The timing, coordination or lack of coordination between the swallowing structures is noted during each swallow, along with the presence or absence of bolus residue following each swallow, and airway closure.

An esophageal scan or screening of the esophagus in the anterior-posterior plane, when patient positioning permits, has become more routinely practiced. For optimal observation of esophageal and gastric emptying, the scan should be performed with the patient standing. The esophageal scan is necessary due to the connection and path between the oropharyngeal and gastric anatomy. Esophageal pathology can cause both oropharyngeal and esophageal symptoms either by direct effect on bolus travel and via referred discomfort and sensory stimulation to the pharyngeal tissues. Although the SLP does not diagnose below the cricopharyngeus, a plethora of information is often found that can solve some "atypical or asymptomatic" oropharyngeal dysphagia. MBS interpretation can help direct the patient to other professionals, such as ENT/laryngology or to GI for further management. Therefore, the SLP uses the esophageal scan for characterizing and describing observations within the esophagus, in addition to the oral and pharyngeal phases of swallowing managed by the SLP. According to Jones et al., "simultaneous disorders of the pharynx and esophagus are so frequent that the complete swallowing chain should be examined in patients with dysphagia" [5]. This study examined 40 patients with unexplained pharyngeal dysphagia and found 14 with esophageal disease and 11 with combined pharyngeal and esophageal disease. They found that reflux symptoms are often manifested by laryngeal symptoms such as coughing and hoarseness. Additionally, a cricopharyngeal prominence, often referred to as a cricopharyngeal bar by the radiologist, may be a clue to potential esophageal disease. After treatment of the disease, the cricopharyngeal prominence was no longer seen on subsequent imaging. In addition, cricopharyngeal dysfunction, as well as esophageal dysmotility, can contribute to symptoms of globus sensation, throat clearing, and swallowing dysfunction, which are often interpreted as symptoms of reflux. MBS can help differentiate true anatomical causes of these symptoms from potential reflux-induced symptomology.

A study in 1992 by Triadafilopoulus et al. [6] further supports the case for esophageal screening. This study used videofluoroscopy and manometry to examine the oropharyngeal and esophageal interrelationships in patients with nonobstructive dysphagia. The rationale was that normal swallowing involves the functional coordination of the mouth, pharynx, and esophagus; therefore, if one becomes impaired, it will be likely the others may be affected. The esophageal stage was examined in 12 patients with oropharyngeal dysphagia, and the oropharyngeal stage was examined in 29 patients with esophageal motor dysfunction. The findings revealed the oropharyngeal group had delayed peristalsis, tertiary contractions, esophageal body dilation, and poor LES relaxation; 92% were identified as having nonspecific esophageal motility disorder. In the esophageal group, they found impaired lingual peristalsis, slowed pharyngeal transit time, poor pharyngeal constriction, and laryngeal vestibular and tracheal bolus penetration. ASHA Supplement 24 states "…the SLP should recognize the need for an extended VFSS (videofluoroscopic swallowing study) with an esophageal screening, or separate esophagram" [7].

Once the bolus passes through the pharynx and then through the "gate keeper" or the cricopharyngeus muscle, also referred to as the upper esophageal sphincter (UES) or the pharyngoesophageal segment (PES), peristalsis, or wavelike contractions of the esophagus, transports the bolus through the esophagus and through the lower esophageal sphincter (LES). Globus sensation, food sticking in the throat or chest when swallowing, and the need to repeatedly wash solids down with liquids are typical symptoms of cricopharyngeal dysfunction and reflux disease. Cricopharyngeal dysfunction is one of the main causes of oropharyngeal and esophageal dysphagia. The cricopharyngeus is contracted, or closed, at rest and in between swallows. The anterior hyoid movement and upward thyroid-cricoid approximation facilitates cricopharyngeal relaxation and opening when a swallow is initiated, for passage of the bolus into the esophagus. Cricopharyngeal dysfunction may result from timing issues, with abnormal or insufficient opening, incomplete relaxation of the cricopharyngeus muscle, delayed relaxation, or insufficient duration of opening where the cricopharyngeus muscle closes too early before the swallow has been completed. A common observance during the MBS in these patients is an impression of the cricopharyngeus muscle, during the swallow that resembles a bar, referred to as a CP bar. It projects anteriorly from the posterior wall, reducing the lumen. A CP bar is a structural abnormality related to hypertonicity or fibrosis. A CP bar results in inadequate opening of the port with only some of the bolus passing through, and the balance of the bolus remains pooled bilaterally in the pyriform sinuses. The more dense and viscous the bolus becomes, the greater the difficulty of clearance with the need for multiple swallow attempts to clear and/or a liquid to wash the bolus through. Incomplete or failed UES relaxation is neutrally controlled motor disorder or reduced pharyngeal force or a combination of the two [8]. An incompetent UES is caused by hypotension of the CP muscle, with reflux and/or regurgitation as a consequence.

Common structural deviations often found in these patients with cricopharyngeal dysfunction are bony outgrowths, or *osteophytes*, which can occur throughout the vertebrae and cause compression against and into the pharynx and esophagus. Cervical osteophytes found at the level of the cricopharyngeus, typically at C5–C6, usually have the most significant effect on the swallow and can present as an aspiration risk due to reduced clearance of the bolus through the narrowed pharyngoesophageal lumen.

During the esophageal scan, the patient is placed in the AP plane and includes observing the bolus moving from the oral cavity through the LES to observe esophageal clearance. If esophageal emptying is not observed or partially observed, there is likely a structural or motility issue within the esophagus; these issues are diagnosed by the attending radiologist or physician reviewing the scans upon completion of the MBS. Motility issues can arise from scleroderma, tertiary contractions, diffuse esophageal spasms, achalasia, or abnormal pressure conditions of the esophageal musculature. Structural issues may include diverticula, rings, strictures, fistulas, webs, hiatal hernias, or tumors and may be causing symptoms of dysphagia with endoluminal obstruction or extra-esophageal compression. The most common diverticula is *Zenker's*, a herniation of mucosa proximal to the cricopharyngeus muscle, which can contribute to marked retention (depending on the size of the pouch) or regurgitation superiorly into the hypopharynx, as well as resultant aspiration. The most common ring is the *Schatzki* ring, and it is often associated with a hiatal hernia above the LES. *Esophageal strictures* can cause dysphagia, with *peptic strictures* usually a result of GERD and found at the distal esophagus. *Barrett's esophagus*, typically found at the mid-distal esophagus, usually results from a chronic history of GERD and reflux esophagitis and is considered potentially premalignant. Stricture formation may also occur from an inflammatory condition of eosinophilic infiltration of the esophagus, known as *eosinophilic esophagitis*. Strictures can cause retention and/or pressure changes and contribute to backflow/regurgitation events. *Fistulas*, or abnormal connections between two separate body parts, are not as common and usually develop as a result of a trauma, surgery, or infection. A *tracheoesophageal fistula,* an opening shared between the esophagus and the trachea, rarely occurs but can lead to subglottic silent aspiration events and often resultant suspicious recurring aspiration pneumonia particularly in infants and patients with history of tracheostomies, neck resection, and/or radiation therapy.

Regurgitation or backflow superiorly through the cricopharyngeus can be observed during the esophageal scan. It can present in patients as "water brash" or sour taste and burning within the pharynx. Aspiration through the posterior commissure from the "water brash" can be observed raising the risk of aspiration. These reflux-like symptoms often are related to reflux events whether they are gastroesophageal or laryngopharyngeal. Both events are considered normal to a degree but can develop into pathophysiological conditions with tissue irritation in the larynx, pharynx, and esophagus. These conditions can contribute to the development of laryngopharyngeal inflammation causing hoarseness, dysphagia, globus, and chronic cough, including but not limited to strictures. LPR events typically occur in the day, upright, and GERD events usually occur during the night. The esophageal scan on the MBS in these patients may reveal tertiary esophageal contractions, transient lower esophageal relaxation, delayed gastric emptying, retention in the mid to distal esophagus or poor esophageal clearance, and even reduced LES resting tone (a lack of relaxation).

When esophageal dysfunction is observed during an MBS, the patient is referred to a gastroenterologist and/or laryngologist for consultation and possibly additional testing. Due to the location involving the esophageal region, a motility exam, such as the esophagram or upper GI series, may be most helpful as the patient is awake and will be able to be observed actively swallowing the trials. An esophagogastroduodenoscopy, or EGD, examines the anatomy but not motility as the patient is usually sedated. This exam is helpful when looking at structures, such as the lining of the esophagus, stomach, and duodenum, but not for function. A barium swallow, also referred to as cine esophagram, swallowing study, or esophagography, is often ordered by the gastroenterologist to assess structural characteristics of the esophagus and its functional characteristics. It is a contrast-enhanced radiographic study that is noninvasive and can be a single test or part of a series, known as an upper GI series that examines the function of the pharynx, esophagus, and stomach. It has become a diagnostic tool to identify pathologies such as esophageal motility disorders (e.g., achalasia, diffuse esophageal spasm), strictures, and perforation, as well as hiatal hernia and gastric volvulus. When aspiration is observed at the pharyngeal level of swallowing, the patient may then be referred for a modified barium swallow [9].

Once diagnostic objective assessments have been completed, it is time to consult with the dysphagia team. These medical teams are an important component to formulate and must consist of professionals with analytical paradigms with a common purpose – how to actually fix the patient! We never want a patient who has had *chronic swallowing issues* leave an objective instrumental swallowing assessment without any answers or functional treatment plan. This even involves those cases that may be "psychogenic" in nature with no overt symptoms. In all cases, especially psychogenic cases, using the MBS exam as biofeedback tool to educate the patient, support or refute the reported symptoms, and/or support the need for patient counseling is priceless. This team may consist of SLPs, otolaryngologists, laryngologists, gastroenterologists, neurologists, dietitians, nurses, and radiologists. The feedback from all involved parties help the team formulate the best diagnosis and treatment plan for the patient. Swallowing therapy may include conventional and/or nonconventional treatments depending on the type and severity of the impairment. Traditional methods would include conventional oral motor exercises, patient education, thermal stimulation, physiologic exercises, compensatory strategies, diet alterations, and swallowing maneuvers. Newer treatments may include neuromuscular electrical stimulation (NMES) and patterned electric neuromuscular stimulation (PENS) for the reeducation of the swallow mechanism and surface electromyography (sEMG) to be used as biofeedback to measure the function of the swallowing muscle groups being addressed with exercises or strategies. As referenced earlier, HRM is used as an adjunct to MBS studies allowing the SLP to evaluate pharyngeal pressures and upper esophageal relaxation. By using HRM as an additional image providing biofeedback, the SLP can further interpret the swallow mechanism physiology and create a more effective treatment plan, particularly if related to UES involvement. When using HRM, a baseline is obtained and compared to posttreatment measurements and aid formulation of biofeedback treatment plans [10].

In conclusion, dysphagia is a multifaceted disorder influenced by a variety of environmental and acquired conditions. SLPs are integral to diagnosis and management of dysphagia. The SLP evaluation and examination, including FEES or MBS, can help identify pathology within the laryngopharynx and esophagus that can be considered the cause of the patient's symptoms. These examinations can be useful in the workup and diagnosis of reflux disease to help rule out other pathologies that can contribute to symptoms, either directly or through referred sensation. Additionally, in patients who fail dietary, behavioral, and medical treatments for reflux, objective testing can identify other pathology that may be preventing improvement or be the primary cause of the symptom presentation.

References

1. Miller RM, Groher ME. Speech-language pathology and dysphagia: a brief historical perspective. Dysphagia. 1993;8(3):180–4.
2. Logemann J. Evaluation and treatment of swallowing disorders. Austin: Pro-Ed, Austin; 1983, 1986.
3. Langmore SE, Schatx K, Olsen N. Fiberoptic endoscopic examination of swallowing safety: a new procedure. Dysphagia. 1988;2:216–9.
4. Carucci LR, Turner MA. Dysphagia revisited: common and unusual causes. Radiographics. 2015;35:1–54.
5. Jones B, Ravich WJ, Donner MW, Kramer SS, Hendrix TR. Gastrointestinal. Radiology. 1985;10(3):225–33. (ISBN: 0363–2345).
6. Triadafilopoulous G, Hallstone A, Nelson-Abbott H, Bedinger K. Oropharyngeal and esophageal interrelationships in patients with non-obstructive dysphagia. Dig Dis Sci. 1992;37(4):551–7.
7. Mendell DA, Logemann JA. A retrospective analysis of the pharyngeal swallow in patients with a clinical diagnosis of GERD compared with normal controls: a pilot study. Dysphagia. 2002;17(3):220–6.
8. Cook IJ. Clinical disorders of the upper esophageal sphincter. GI Motility online, 2006. https://doi.org/10.1038/gimo37.
9. Chen A, Tuma F. Barium swallow (updated 2019 Apr 22). In: StatPearls (internet). Treasure Island: StatPearls Publishing; 2019.
10. Knigge MA, Thibeault S, McCulloch TM. Implementation of high-resolution manometry in the clinical practice of speech language pathology. Dysphagia. 2014;29(1):2–16.

Chapter 16
The Role of Reflux Disease in Chronic Rhinosinusitis

Erick Yuen, Sarah Kidwai, Ameet Kamat, and Deya Jourdy

Introduction

Chronic rhinosinusitis (CRS), an inflammatory disease of the paranasal sinuses, is one of the most commonly encountered diseases worldwide, rivaling asthma and diabetes mellitus in prevalence [1]. Affecting an estimated 1% to 12% of the world population, CRS is associated with impaired quality of life and marked functional limitations owing to the disease's symptom profile and chronicity [2]. By definition, CRS persists for at least 12 weeks and is characterized by nasal mucopurulent drainage, nasal obstruction or congestion, facial pain, pressure or fullness, and decreased or loss of sense of smell. Due to the costs of diagnostic tests, medical and surgical treatments, and lost work productivity, a significant socioeconomic burden is incurred with annual direct and indirect costs for CRS estimated at $12.8 billion in the United States [3].

E. Yuen (✉)
Department of Otolaryngology—New York Medical College, School of Medicine, Valhalla, NY, USA
e-mail: eyuen@nymc.edu

S. Kidwai
Department of Otolaryngology—Icahn School of Medicine at Mount Sinai, New York, NY, USA
e-mail: Sarah.kidwai@mountsinai.org

A. Kamat
Sinus and Skull Base Surgery, White Plains Hospital Physician Associates, Department of Otolaryngology, NY Medical College, Valhalla, NY, USA

D. Jourdy
Rhinology, Endoscopic Sinus & Skull Base Surgery, Otolaryngology & Neurosurgery, New York Medical College, Phelps Hospital, Northwell Health, Sleepy Hollow, NY, USA

ENT and Allergy Associates, LLP, Sleepy Hollow, NY, USA

C. H. Zalvan (ed.), *Laryngopharyngeal and Gastroesophageal Reflux*,
https://doi.org/10.1007/978-3-030-48890-1_16

Pathophysiology

The pathophysiology of CRS involves inflammatory changes in the nasal and sinus mucosa, leading to mucosal edema, ostial obstruction, mucosal stasis, and subsequent infection. As a multifactorial disease, many predisposing factors operating alone or in combination have been recognized to initiate these inflammatory events, including viral, bacterial, and fungal infections, inhalation of allergens and environmental pollutants, and anatomic etiologies [4, 5].

Gastroesophageal reflux has been associated with numerous supraesophageal symptoms, under the title of laryngopharyngeal reflux (LPR) disease, and implicated in the pathogenesis of various disease processes in the head and neck, including dysphonia, benign vocal cord lesions, laryngospasm, subglottic stenosis, and rhinosinusitis [4, 5]. The relationship between the gastrointestinal tract and CRS was established when Holmes et al. in 1950 proposed a connection between sinonasal disease and gastric hypersecretion [6]. A high prevalence of LPR, also known as extraesophageal reflux (EER), in CRS patients has been reported in the literature; however, no definitive causal association has been established [5, 7–10]. The role of LPR as a potential exacerbating factor of upper airway inflammatory disease has only recently been appreciated.

Mechanisms: LPR and CRS

Although the mechanism in which LPR may contribute to CRS remains elusive, three theories have been suggested. The first of these proposes that the direct exposure of the nasopharynx and nasal cavity to the refluxate causes mucosal inflammation and impaired mucociliary clearance, thereby resulting in sinus ostial obstruction and increased incidence of infection. Alterations in pH have been shown to affect ciliary motility and morphology in respiratory mucosa [11]. In children, nasopharyngeal reflux has been demonstrated in CRS patients using 24-hour pH probe studies [12, 13]. Phipps et al. in 2000 reported that 63% of their pediatric cohort with CRS had evidence of LPR, which exceeds the prevalence of 5% observed in a normal healthy population [13]. Ozmen et al. in 2008 similarly found a higher incidence of pharyngeal acid reflux events in patients with CRS (88%) compared to control (55%). The study also demonstrated the presence of pepsin in nasal lavage fluid, providing direct evidence of gastric content reflux into the nasopharynx, in 82% of patients in the study group compared to 52% in the control group. A statistically significant correlation between the number of LPR events and pepsin-specific activity was found [4]. Furthermore, anti-reflux therapy has been observed to dramatically reduce the number of pediatric patients with CRS requiring sinus surgery [14].

A second possible mechanism involves a vagus nerve-mediated inflammatory response, in which autonomic nervous system dysfunction leads to sinonasal edema and inflammation with subsequent ostial obstruction. This phenomenon has been described in asthmatics with gastroesophageal reflux disease (GERD), where a hypervagal response may contribute to the heightened airway responsiveness secondary to esophageal acidification. Vagolytic doses of intravenous atropine have been demonstrated to partially ablate the bronchoconstrictive response to acid reflux, supporting the role of a vagally mediated reflex in the inflammatory process [15]. To investigate whether an esophageal-nasal reflex exists, Wong et al. infused normal saline and hydrochloric acid into the lower esophagus of ten healthy volunteers without GERD or sinonasal disease and analyzed nasal symptom scores, nasal inspiratory peak flow, and nasal mucus production following the esophageal challenge. The study found increased nasal mucus production, increased nasal symptom scores, and reduced peak nasal inspiratory flow after normal saline and hydrochloric acid infusion, with return to baseline within 45 minutes. The authors concluded that these results support the possibility that a neural reflex mediated by the vagus nerve exists between the esophagus and the paranasal sinuses and that this neuropathic inflammation may facilitate the development of CRS in patients with GERD [16].

A third possible mechanism implicates *Helicobacter pylori* as the facilitator of CRS in the context of reflux disease. *H. pylori*, a Gram-negative, microaerophilic bacterium known to cause stomach ulcers and gastritis, has been detected in sinonasal mucosal biopsy specimens by polymerase chain reaction in CRS patients across multiple studies. Ozdek et al. reported that *H. pylori* DNA was detected in 4 of 12 patients with CRS, whereas it was not detected in any patients without CRS. Gastroesophageal reflux-related complaints were noted in 3 of 4 patients with positive results for the bacterium [17]. Morinaka et al. observed that *H. pylori* was detected in 3 of 19 nasal and maxillary sinus specimens collected from CRS patients. However, whether *H. pylori* is a causative agent for CRS remains unknown [18] (Figs. 16.1 and 16.2).

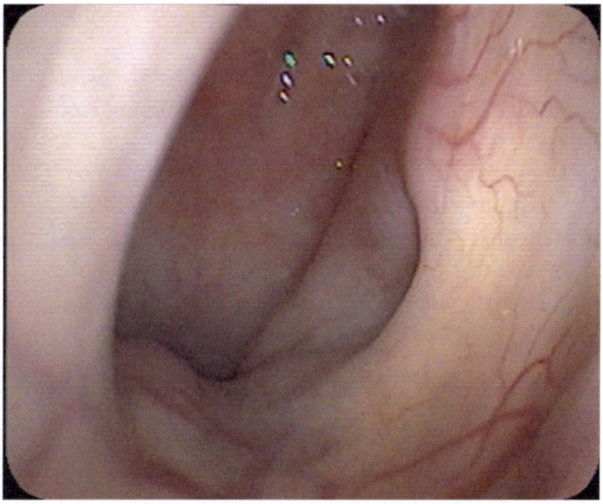

Fig. 16.1 Nasal endoscopy with view of normal Eustachian tube and sinus mucosa

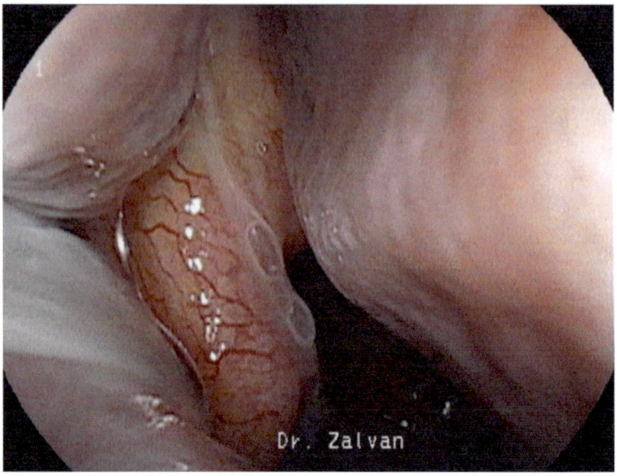

Fig. 16.2 Nasal endoscopy of acute sinusitis in setting of chronic, recurrent sinusitis with purulent drainage from the maxillary and sphenoethmoid sinuses into the nasopharynx

Management and Treatment Failure

The medical management of CRS encompasses a prolonged course of antibiotics targeting the upper respiratory flora, saline irrigation, and nasal and oral corticosteroids. Endoscopic sinus surgery (ESS) is the preferred treatment for patients with CRS who remain symptomatic despite maximal medical therapy [5]. While ESS has been shown to be an effective therapeutic option, with long-term symptomatic improvement in 98% of patients, many factors have been associated with its failure, including irreversible mucosal disease, allergy, tobacco use, and GERD [5, 19]. In a retrospective study, Chambers et al. discovered that GERD was the only historic factor that met statistical significance as a predictor of poor symptom outcome after ESS [20]. DelGaudio demonstrated using a specially designed pH probe that patients with medically and surgically refractory CRS had increased reflux at the nasopharynx, upper esophageal sphincter, and distal esophagus when compared to those without sinus disease and those with successful sinus surgery [5].

Although acid suppression therapy for the treatment of CRS seems intuitive, the use of anti-reflux medications in the management of the condition is controversial, in part due to the conflicting epidemiologic evidence linking the two disease processes together [8]. The American Academy of Otolaryngology expert panel in 2014 stated that the lack of randomized, controlled studies supporting a strong relationship between GERD and CRS in the pediatric population does not warrant empiric reflux treatment as adjunctive medical therapy [21]. The Allergy Joint Task Force concurred, stating that there is no evidence that GERD is a significant causal factor of CRS and therefore did not recommend anti-reflux therapy for refractory adult cases [22]. In the setting of ongoing controversy, national practice patterns have not favored reflux treatment for CRS [8]. Several studies have shown that the resolution of extraesophageal manifestations of reflux with proton pump inhibitors

(PPI) has been difficult to achieve. In a small prospective study, DiBaise et al. compared 11 CRS patients with 19 GERD control patients to ascertain whether aggressive anti-reflux therapy could achieve sinus symptom improvement. CRS patients alone received omeprazole 20 mg twice daily for 3 months. Modest symptom improvement was reported, but resolution occurred infrequently in the study group [23]. DelGaudio published similar findings in which only 2 of 38 patients with CRS had dramatic improvement after adequate PPI treatment was initiated [5]. In a multifactorial disease, acid suppression alone may provide partial or no relief of CRS symptoms, as reflux likely represents only one of many contributing factors. In contrast, Pincus et al. found that 14 of 15 patients who were placed on a PPI regimen demonstrated some improvement in their sinus symptoms, including 7 who reported either complete or near-complete resolution of symptoms. Due to these findings, the study concluded that anti-reflux therapy may be beneficial in the treatment of refractory CRS [24].

Conclusion

Many studies have sought to investigate the role of acid reflux in the pathogenesis of CRS, delineate the mechanisms that contribute to the disease process, and examine the efficacy of anti-reflux therapy in disease management. Due to the high prevalence of either entity, a direct relationship between CRS and GERD has been difficult to establish due to the possibility of them coexisting independently. In general, the literature suggests that there is a relationship between reflux and CRS, particularly the subtype that is refractory to medical and surgical treatments. However, the available studies often have small sample sizes, each employing different methodologies that hinder accurate interpretation of the collective data. Therefore, the evidence confirming a definitive causal association is lacking. Furthermore, the data for the effect of PPI therapy on symptom improvement in patients with CRS is conflicting, with multiple professional organizations not recommending the use of anti-reflux medications in the management of the disease. Alternatively, as part of the initial medical management for the treatment of LPR, a dietary approach consisting of alkaline water and a plant-based, Mediterranean-style diet should be attempted. Although the benefit of LPR treatment in modifying the disease course of CRS remains debatable, this diet-based approach confers a host of other health benefits, including a decreased risk of cardiovascular disease, diabetes, stroke, and cancer [25] with potential positive changes to the microbiome creating a more favorable, healthier local microenvironment. To rectify the limitations of the available literature, multicenter studies with a larger number of patients and standardized criteria for diagnosis and methodology would be beneficial.

References

1. Lin YH, Chang TS, Yao YC, Li YC. Increased risk of chronic sinusitis in adults with gastro-esophageal reflux disease: a Nationwide population-based cohort study. Medicine (Baltimore). 2015;94(39):e1642. https://doi.org/10.1097/MD.0000000000001642.
2. Xu Y, Quan H, Faris P, et al. Prevalence and incidence of diagnosed chronic rhinosinusitis in Alberta, Canada. JAMA Otolaryngol Head Neck Surg. 2016;142(11):1063–9. https://doi.org/10.1001/jamaoto.2016.2227.
3. DeConde AS, Soler ZM. Chronic rhinosinusitis: epidemiology and burden of disease. Am J Rhinol Aller. 2016;30:134–9.
4. Ozmen S, Yucel OT, Sinici I, et al. Nasal pepsin assay and pH monitoring in chronic rhinosinusitis. Laryngoscope. 2008;118:890–4.
5. DelGaudio JM. Direct nasopharyngeal reflux of gastric acid is a contributing factor in refractory chronic rhinosinusitis. Laryngoscope. 2005;115:946–57.
6. Holmes TH, Goodell H, Wolf S, Wolff HG. The nose: an experimental study of reactions within the nose in human subjects during various life experiences. Springfield: Charles C. Thomas; 1950.
7. Loehrl TA, Samuels TL, Poetker DM, Toohill RJ, Blumin JH, Johnston N. The role of extraesophageal reflux in medically and surgically refractory rhinosinusitis. Laryngoscope. 2012;122:1425–30.
8. Gilani S, Pynnonen MA, Shin JJ. National Practice Patterns of Antireflux medication for chronic rhinosinusitis. JAMA Otolaryngol Head Neck Surg. 2016;142(7):627–33. https://doi.org/10.1001/jamaoto.2016.0937.
9. Sella GC, Tamashiro E, Anselmo-Lima WT, Valera FC. Relation between chronic rhinosinusitis and gastroesophageal reflux in adults: systematic review. Braz J Otorhinolaryngol. 2017;83:356–63.
10. Bohnhorst I, Jawad S, Lange B. Prevalence of chronic rhinosinusitis in a population of patients with gastroesophageal reflux disease. Am J Rhinol Allergy. 2015;29:e70–4.
11. Holma B, Lindegren M, Morkholdt AJ. PH effects on ciliomotility and morphology of respiratory mucosa. Arch Environ Health. 1977;32:216–26.
12. Contencin P, Narcy P. Nasopharyngeal pH monitoring in infants and children with chronic rhinopharyngitis. Int J Ped Otolaryngol. 1991;22:249–56.
13. Phipps CD, Wood WE, Gibson WS, Cochran WJ. Gastroesophageal reflux contributing to chronic sinus disease in children. A perspective analysis. Arch Otolaryngol Head Neck Surg. 2000;126:831–6.
14. Bothwell MR, Parsons DS, Talbot A. Outcome of reflux therapy on pediatric chronic sinusitis. Otolaryngol Head Neck Surg. 1999;121:255–62.
15. Lodi U, Harding SM, Coghlan HC, Guzzo MR, Walker LH. Autonomic regulation in asthmatics with gastroesophageal reflux. Chest. 1997;111(1):65–70.
16. Wong IW, Rees G, Greiff L, Myers JC, Jamieson GG, Wormald PJ. Gastroesophageal reflux disease and chronic sinusitis: in search of an esophageal-nasal reflex. Am J Rhinol Allergy. 2010;24(4):255–9.
17. Ozdek A, Cirak MY, Samim E, et al. A possible role of helicobacter pylori in chronic rhinosinusitis: a preliminary re- port. Laryngoscope. 2003;113:679–82.
18. Morinaka S, Ichimiya M, Nakamura H. Detection of helicobacter pylori in nasal and maxillary sinus specimens from patients with chronic sinusitis. Laryngoscope. 2003;113:1557–63.
19. Kennedy DW. Prognostic factors, outcomes, and staging in ethmoid sinus surgery. Laryngoscope. 1992;102(Suppl 57):1–18.
20. Chambers DW, Davis WE, Cook PR, Nishioka GJ, Rudman DT. Long-term outcome analysis of functional endoscopic sinus surgery: correlation of symptoms with endoscopic examination findings and potential prognostic factors. Laryngoscope. 1997;107:504–10.
21. Brietzke SE, Shin JJ, Choi S, et al. Clinical consensus statement: pediatric chronic rhinosinusitis. Otolaryngol Head Neck Surg. 2014;151(4):542–53.

22. Peters AT, et al. Diagnosis and management of rhinosinusitis: a practice parameter update. Ann Allergy Asthma Immunol. 2014;113(4):347–85.
23. DiBiase JK, Olusola BF, Huerter JV, Quigley E. Role of GERD in chronic resistant sinusitis: a prospective, open label, pilot trial. Am J Gastroenterol. 2002;97:843–50.
24. Pincus RL, Kim HH, Silvers S, Gold S. A study of the link between gastric reflux and chronic sinusitis in adults. Ear Nose Throat J. 2006;85(3):174–8.
25. Zalvan CH, Hu S, Greenberg B, Geliebter J. A comparison of alkaline water and mediterranean diet vs proton pump inhibition for treatment of laryngopharyngeal reflux. JAMA Otolaryngol Head Neck Surg. 2017;143(10):1023–9. https://doi.org/10.1001/jamaoto.2017.1454.

Chapter 17
Pulmonary Manifestations of Reflux Disease

Steven A. Thau, Peter H. Stein, and Craig H. Zalvan

The separation of the digestive from the respiratory tract is one of the hallmarks of all land-dwelling animals. Maintaining that separation is vital to survival. Since humans and animals have a dual entry for air and food creating the aerodigestive tract, maintaining that separation becomes one of the most important homeostatic mechanisms to maintain survival of the individual and the species. In many ways, that critical separation is only defended by a few key nerves, a few millimeters of mucosa, and the thin muscles of the oropharynx and larynx. This proximity enables disorders of the digestive tract to direct and indirect effect on the respiratory tract through reflux, various feedback mechanisms, and reflexes.

In the case of gastroesophageal reflux disease (GERD), instead of the food bolus traveling from the mouth to the oropharynx into the esophagus and stomach, partially digested food and refluxate travels from the stomach into the esophagus. Food particles do not have to enter the lungs to cause respiratory complications, though the more foreign material that is inhaled into the lung, the more the patient is prone

S. A. Thau (✉)
Board Certified in Pulmonary, Critical Care, Sleep Medicine and Hospice and Palliative Care, Phelps Hospital/Northwell Health, Sleepy Hollow, NY, USA
e-mail: sthau@northwell.edu

P. H. Stein
Division of Gastroenterology, Phelps Hospital, Northwell Health, Sleepy Hollow, NY, USA
e-mail: pstein2@northwell.edu

C. H. Zalvan
ENT and Allergy Associates, LLP; Voice and Swallow Division, Tarrytown, NY, USA

The Institute for Voice and Swallowing Disorders, Phelps Hospital, Northwell Health, Sleepy Hollow, NY, USA

Professor of Otolaryngology at the Donald and Barbara Zucker School of Medicine at Hofstra/Northwell, Phelps Hospital Campus, Sleepy Hollow, NY, USA

Communication at Mercy College, Dobbs Ferry, NY, USA
e-mail: czalvan@entandallergy.com

C. H. Zalvan (ed.), *Laryngopharyngeal and Gastroesophageal Reflux*,
https://doi.org/10.1007/978-3-030-48890-1_17

to pulmonary complications. When the stomach contents, food, or swallowed nasal or sinus discharge enters the laryngopharynx, it is called laryngopharyngeal reflux (LPR). Multiple mechanisms exist to protect the laryngopharynx, and thus pulmonary system, from refluxate of these contents. Inherent anatomic protection against aspiration during feeding begins to develop in infancy. The infant larynx begins high in the neck, roughly at the level of the C3–C4 vertebrae in the neck, allowing for simultaneous feeding and breathing. As the child grows, the larynx descends to the level of C6–C7, allowing for coordination of speech with solid and liquid ingestion. The upper and lower sphincters, together with gravity and active peristalsis, are the major protective barriers to reflux. The larynx, bicarbonate secretion, local cellular protection, and multiple other mechanisms beyond the scope of this chapter combine to create a homeostatic environment with minimal refluxate entering the trachea and thus lung parenchyma. The chest cavity retains a negative pressure compared to the abdominal pressure, which is typically positive with the lower esophageal sphincter (LES) between the two regions. This thoracoabdominal pressure gradient at baseline predisposes to reflux into the esophagus in normal individuals and is minimized by proper LES tone. Pulmonary disease can result in increased respiratory effort and lower pressures, further increasing the gradient and encouraging reflux and aspiration [1]. Obesity can result in increased abdominal pressure overwhelming the LES protection and leading to worse reflux [2].

The cough reflex is the major defense of the lungs. Any foreign material, food or otherwise, will be expectorated instead of entering the respiratory tract and trachea, preventing foreign materials from reaching the bronchi, bronchioles, and ultimately the alveoli and lung parenchyma. Fortunately, should aspiration occur, there is ample respiratory reserve due to the dense packing of alveoli. The surface area of the lung is close to 70 meters squared, nearly covering the area of a football field [3]. Although this surface area allows for significant pulmonary reserve, damage to lung parenchyma does influence function. Symptoms increase as more lung volume is compromised, or if damage involves the main airways. This damage results in pulmonary distress. Inhalation of foreign material, whether it is particulate matter or toxic gases, will result in injury to at least one of the main airways, lung parenchyma, or both.

GERD and LPR present a unique challenge to maintaining lung health. In these disease processes, food particles and refluxate can present in the lung where they can quickly overwhelm cellular defense mechanisms. In addition, aspirated material tends to be acidic and can contain digestive enzymes including amylase from salivary secretions, pepsin produced by the stomach, pancreatic digestive enzymes, and bile salts. These digestive enzymes can be highly toxic to lung tissue. They can contribute to a foul taste known as "back wash," although stomach contents do not need to reach taste buds in order to create symptoms. Certain patients will experience classical GERD symptoms such as heartburn, indigestion, chest and back discomfort, eructation, and early satiety. Many patients with lung irritation will not experience classic symptoms of GERD. They may present instead with LPR-related symptoms such as a chronic cough, throat clearing, globus, dysphagia, and changes in voice. The absence of classical GERD symptoms can make challenging the acceptance of a diagnosis of reflux as a contributing or causative factor in lung disease.

Aspiration pneumonia represents the most severe form of inhalation injury to the lung, in which stomach contents or swallowed food particles are inhaled or penetrate directly into the lung. While this frequently occurs in patients whose natural cough reflexes have become diminished or nonexistent, aspiration pneumonia can occur in patients whose protective barriers have been compromised by alcohol, sedating recreational or prescription drugs, or anesthetics. To a lesser extent, aspiration can occur during normal sleep. If a patient were to lie down to sleep after a large meal, it would not be uncommon to wake up with a coughing "fit," or laryngospasm, the direct result of secretions or refluxate penetrating to the vocal folds with potential aspiration. If this occurs frequently, patients may develop a chronic cough, shortness of breath, and fevers as the inflamed lung tissue releases cytokines and pro-inflammatory mediators leading to pneumonia. In such a scenario, an infiltrate would be seen on X-ray. Many of these patients will be diagnosed with recurrent pneumonias. The use of antibiotics in patients with recurrent aspiration pneumonia has been debated. While most society recommendations recommend against the routine use of antibiotics, many clinicians will use antibiotics with good clinical response depending on the severity of presentation.

A similar physiologic response exists in the patient receiving enteral feedings through a feeding tube, both due to regurgitation of liquid food contents, and the aspiration of oral secretions. It would be expected that patients receiving enteral feedings would have an underlying inability to swallow adequately, leading to the expectation that periodic aspiration of oral secretions could occur. Routine treatment of aspiration in this patient population is not recommended; however, many clinicians will treat with a course of antibiotics if a fever, leukocytosis, elevated procalcitonin, or additional evidence of an active infection is present. In cases of severe aspiration of gastric or swallowed contents, acute respiratory distress syndrome (ARDS) can develop. Patients with ARDS will often require endotracheal intubation and mechanical ventilation with high oxygen requirements in order to avoid additional lung injury and acid-base disturbances.

Refluxed material does not need to reach the lung parenchyma in order to cause symptoms. Irritation at the level of the trachea or bronchi can be sufficient to cause airway inflammation and bronchial edema, which can lead to symptoms of cough, dyspnea, and reductions in exercise capacity. While patients with a chronic cough can occasionally respond to readily available antacid medications, many will require prescription strength medications to ameliorate their symptoms – chiefly a chronic cough. Reduction of reflux triggers, dietary and behavioral changes, and stepwise treatment of reflux discussed elsewhere in this text must be initiated in addition to pharmacological treatment. Despite adequate reflux treatment, some patients continue to have progressive coughing and dyspnea, and surgical intervention for reflux should be considered when other causes have been excluded.

Pulmonary symptoms may occur if gastric acid does not reach the lung parenchyma. For instance, if acidic or foreign material irritates the vocal cords and however is not aspirated to the trachea and bronchi, the patient may experience hoarseness, cough, or shortness of breath. In addition, irritation to the lower esophagus can lead to bronchospasm and asthma through irritation to the vagus nerve. Episodic reflux into the esophagus can be associated with oxygen desaturation which can be ameliorated with surgical therapy for reflux, suggesting a reflexive role [4]. In cases that the diagnosis of true reflux induced pulmonary dysfunction, bronchoalveolar lavage fluid (BALF) can be collected during bronchoscopy and evaluated for the presence of pepsin or bile acids which can only be present during true reflux with aspiration events [5].

Many patients will be diagnosed with asthma based on the presence of wheezing or bronchial breath sounds on exam. If a patient does not respond to conventional asthma medications, a thorough investigation of GERD is indicated to rule out aspiration and irritation as a cause of symptoms. Classic expiratory wheezing can be absent in these patients and instead, with deeper questioning, inspiratory stridor, or a "wheeze"-like sound upon inhalation, is often present in reflux-induced noisy breathing. Some patients describe the onset of acute laryngospasm episodes while asleep, resulting in bouts of severe inspiratory stridor and often brief inability to breath inward. A recent study of over 600 patients who carried a diagnosis of asthma demonstrated that over 30% of these patients did not meet diagnostic criteria for true asthma. Of these patients, 80% were taking medication for their presumed asthma. Over 90% of this group of patients were able to stop their medications without any exacerbation in pulmonary symptoms [6]. In addition, neurodegenerative diseases, stroke, and neuromuscular disorders such as Parkinson's disease and ALS may lead to decreased cough reflexes, thus leading to chronic micro-aspiration. In all the above disease processes, imaging studies are necessary to rule out aspiration. Modified barium swallow (MBS) can assess a variety of barium-coated food textures and liquid consistencies during which they are imaged fluoroscopically. This sensitive test allows for the indirect assessment of laryngeal penetration, possibly putting a patient at risk for aspiration, which can also be visualized. Even micro-aspiration can be detected with this sensitive test. Fiber-optic endoscopic evaluation of swallowing (FEES) is a more portable method that allows for direct visualization of the swallowing mechanism with a flexible laryngoscope. Food-coloring-coated food materials can then be administered and the patient monitored for penetration or aspiration as well as response to various compensatory maneuvers to help prevent the aspiration.

Patients with obstructive sleep apnea (OSA) will often have GERD. When patients have an apneic episode while sleeping, a closed glottis with respiratory effort will result in increased negative intrathoracic pressures. During normal breathing, air is pulled into the lungs through pressure gradients generated by the diaphragm contracting. Normal pressure gradients will range from -5 to -10 cm H_2O atm within the lungs. The diaphragm will attempt to pull air into the lungs; however, the closed glottis will prevent passage of air in the setting of obstructive sleep apnea, resulting in increased negative pressure that can reach -60 to -80 mmHg. This will create a vacuum-like physiologic response in the chest cavity, leading to a decrease in the protective effects of the GE junction in preventing gastric contents from refluxing into the esophagus. Refluxed gastric contents can access the esophagus with ease, leading to the potential aspiration of acidic material into the lungs, furthering lung disease in the patient with OSA [7].

GERD has been implicated as a contributing factor in numerous pulmonary diseases previously thought to be idiopathic in nature. Idiopathic pulmonary fibrosis (IPF) was previously known to be associated with GERD; however, it had been unclear as to the cause-effect relationship between these two diseases. Recent studies shed light on the etiology of IPF, with GERD being a causative factor [8, 9]. Pepsin, an enzyme present in gastric secretions, was found in elevated levels within the lung tissue of patients with IPF via bronchoalveolar lavage (BAL) compared to normal controls [10]. In addition, patients with severe GERD who concomitantly had diminished lung function showed improvement in their pulmonary function and decreased progression of pulmonary fibrosis after undergoing Nissen fundoplication surgeries [11]. Patients with asymmetric pulmonary fibrosis have also been shown to be at increased risk of GERD [12], for unclear reasons. In patients with GERD-related symptoms in whom a large hiatal hernia or dilated esophagus is present, it is reasonable to rule out concomitant pulmonary disease. In conditions such as systemic sclerosis/scleroderma, or CREST syndrome, patients will routinely have esophageal dysfunction. When patients with these syndromes have interstitial lung disease, GERD and thus LPR with aspiration should be ruled out in the initial workup.

Treatment options for pulmonary manifestations of LPR and GERD should target the underlying condition to prevent further worsening of disease. Although mostly brushed over and typically least followed, dietary and behavioral changes are paramount in controlling the short- and long-term outcome of patients with pulmonary disease from reflux. Acid-buffering compounds, such as calcium-, aluminum-, and magnesium-containing compounds, have been used commonly for decades with little efficacy. Newer alginate compounds have demonstrated promise in alleviating reflux symptoms. All of these medication types are used reactively, as "band-aids" rather than proactively, thus failing to prevent passage of acid contents into the lung. Acid-lowering medications such as H-2 blockers and proton pump inhibitors have shown increased effectiveness in improving survival for patients with IPF [13]. In patients with symptoms not responding to medications, or in those with known medication side effects or hiatal hernias, anti-reflux surgery has proven beneficial. Surgical fundoplication has been shown to decrease the rate of asthma exacerbations and reduce the amount of medications needed or asthma control [14, 15]. This surgery has been shown to slow the progression of IPF and decrease the rate of IPF exacerbations [16]. Head-to-head studies comparing surgical approaches in patients with IPF and GERD have yet to be performed. Sadly, many patients with IPF progress to pulmonary failure despite treatment. Lung transplantation remains the final treatment [17]. Reflux control through diet and medication should be considered in these circumstances to prevent continued damage to the transplanted lungs. Optimally, reflux should be diagnosed and treated with diet and behavioral intervention prior to the onset pulmonary disease, avoiding the significant morbidity and mortality associated with IPF.

Lastly, many patients with long-term LPR- or GERD-related symptoms will have undiagnosed esophageal dysmotility. Many of these patients will lack the ability to pass food quickly from the mouth into the stomach, with food stasis within the esophagus and prolonged esophageal acid exposure times. This places the patient at high risk for spillage of food particles or reflux of acidic contents and digestive enzymes into the respiratory tract. While patients with esophageal dysmotility may not have symptoms of classic GERD, esophageal dysmotility should be considered a contributing factor to pulmonary disease in difficult-to-treat situations and persistent reflux despite therapy. Other neuropathic symptoms such as chronic cough, chronic globus, chronic dysphagia, frequent regurgitation, and gastric emptying issues suggest vagal neuropathy and heighten the potential for dysmotility to contribute to recalcitrant reflux and thus pulmonary disease.

The digestive and respiratory tracts lie in proximity, sharing an initial passage from the mouth to the level of the larynx where they permanently separate. Due to this proximity, the prevention of passage of digestive contents into the respiratory tract can occasionally be compromised due to physiologic or anatomic causes. Clearly, reflux has been implicated as a major causative factor in multiple pulmonary disease processes. The astute clinician should be aware of this relationship, expediting prompt diagnosis and treatment. Patients who are nonresponsive, poorly responsive, or have chronic pulmonary disease should be considered for an LPR and GERD evaluation. Early dietary and behavioral intervention is key to prevention of progression of reflux-related pulmonary disease.

References

1. Ayazi S, DeMeester SR, Hsieh CC, Zehetner J, Sharma G, Grant KS, Oh DS, Lipham JC, Hagen JA, DeMeester TR. Thoracoabdominal pressure gradients during the phases of respiration contribute to gastroesophageal reflux disease. Dig Dis Sci. 2011;56:1718–22.
2. Pandolfino JE, El-Serag HB, Zhang Q, Shah N, Ghosh SK, Kahrilas PJ. Obesity: a challenge to esophagogastric junction integrity. Gastroenterology. 2006;130:639–49.
3. Hasleton PS. The internal surface area of the adult human lung. J Anat. 1972;112:391–400.
4. Wilshire CL, Salvador R, Sepesi B, Niebisch S, Watson TJ, Litle VR, Peyre CG, Jones CE, Peters JH. Reflux-associated oxygen desaturations: usefulness in diagnosing reflux-related respiratory symptoms. J Gastrointest Surg. 2013;17:30–8.
5. Farrell S, McMaster C, Gibson D, Shields MD, McCallion WA. Pepsin in bronchoalveolar lavage fluid: a specific and sensitive method of diagnosing gastro-oesophageal reflux-related pulmonary aspiration. J Ped Surg. 2006;41:289–93.
6. Aaron SD, Vandemheen KL, FitzGerald JM, Ainslie M, Gupta S, Lemière C, Field SK, McIvor RA, Hernandez P, Mayers I, Mulpuru S, Alvarez GG, Pakhale S, Mallick R, Boulet LP, Canadian Respiratory Research Network. Reevaluation of diagnosis in adults with physician-diagnosed asthma. JAMA. 2017;317(3):269–79. https://doi.org/10.1001/jama.2016.19627.
7. Oh JH. Gastroesophageal reflux disease: recent advances and its association with sleep. Ann N Y Acad Sci. 2016;1380(1):195–203. https://doi.org/10.1111/nyas.13143. Epub 2016 Jul 8.
8. Takahashi SM, Noth I. GERD and Idiopathic pulmonary fibrosis: cause or effect. Curr Respir Care Rep. 2013;2:260–7.

9. Stovold R, Forrest IA, Corris PA, Murphy DM, Smith JA, Decalmer S, et al. Pepsin a biomarker of gastric aspiration in lung allografts: a putative association with rejection. Am J Respir Crit Care Med. 2007;175:1298–303.
10. Lee JS, Song JW, Wolters PJ, Elicker BM, King TE Jr, Kim DS, et al. Bronchoalveolar lavage pepsin in acute exacerbation of idiopathic pulmonary fibrosis. Eur Respir J. 2019;39(2):352–8.
11. Raghu G, Yang ST, Spada C, Hayes J, Pelligrini CA. Sole treatment of acid gastroesophageal reflux in idiopathic pulmonary fibrosis: a case series. Chest. 2006;129(3):794–800.
12. Tcherakin C, Cottin V, Brillet PY, Freynet O, Naggara N, Carton Z, et al. Progression of idiopathic fibrosis: lessons from asymmetrical disease. Thorax. 2011;66(3):226–31.
13. Lee JS, Collard HR, Anstrom KJ, Martinez FJ, Noth I, et al. Anti-acid treatment and disease progression in idiopathic pulmonary fibrosis: an analysis of data from three large randomized (IPFnet) controlled trials. Lancet. 2013;1(5):369–76.
14. Silva AP, Tercioti-Junior V, Lopes LR, Coelho-Neto Jde S, Bertanha L, Rodrigues PR, Andreollo NA. Laparoscopic antireflux surgery in patients with extra esophageal symptoms related to asthma. Arq Bras Cir Dig. 2014;27(2):92–5.
15. Patel S, Dhanabalsamy N, Galvani C, Carr TF. Reduction of medication use in asthmatics following minimally-invasive Nissen fundoplication for severe GERD. Am J Respir Crit Care Med. 2017;195:A1312.
16. Raghu G, Pelligrini CA, Yow E, Flaherty KR, Meyer K, Noth I, et al. Laparoscopic anti-reflux surgery for the treatment of idiopathic pulmonary fibrosis (WRAP-IPF): a multicentre, randomised, controlled phase 2 trial. Lancet. 2018;6(9):707–14.
17. Elicker BM, Golden JA, Ordovas KG, Leard L, Golden TR, Hays SR. Progression of native lung fibrosis in lung transplant recipients with idiopathic pulmonary fibrosis. Respir Med. 2010;104:426–33.

Part III
Gastroesophageal Reflux Disease (GERD)

Co-edited by Peter H. Stein

Chapter 18
Gastroesophageal Reflux Disease (GERD) Overview and Introduction

Peter H. Stein

Gastroesophageal reflux disease (GERD) continues to plague a large number of patients seen in the practitioner's office – both that of the primary care physician and subspecialists. Consistently, proton pump inhibitor (PPI) medications rank as the most commonly prescribed medications both in the United States and abroad. Our strategy for diagnosis and management of GERD and its associated complications has changed significantly over the past decade. Most notably, our approach to treatment has shifted beyond that of prescription medications and procedural interventions. We can now shift our focus to diet as a primary strategy, as this has been repeatedly established as an effective approach. In this section of the book, an overview of GERD will be discussed.

Drs. Winston and Stein begin our section detailing the symptoms and presentation of GERD, including the spectrum of classic symptoms of heartburn and regurgitation, to those symptoms less commonly attributed to reflux disease. It is interesting to note the wide range of symptoms potentially associated with GERD, many of which the practitioner may associate with other disease processes. In addition, the subject of nonerosive reflux disease (NERD) is addressed.

Dr. Gutman follows with a comprehensive overview of functional dyspepsia. This upper abdominal discomfort can frustrate both the patient and physician, given the lack of definable biologic markers of disease, variable response to treatment, and lack of medications specifically designed to treat the disease. A comprehensive description of the diagnosis, basis of disease, treatment, and a practical approach to the patient care are provided. The overlap between functional dyspepsia and other GERD-related symptoms and consequences are significant. The currently applicable criteria for diagnosis are described, in addition to overlapping syndromes of epigastric pain.

P. H. Stein (✉)
Division of Gastroenterology, Phelps Hospital, Northwell Health, Sleepy Hollow, NY, USA
e-mail: pstein2@northwell.edu

C. H. Zalvan (ed.), *Laryngopharyngeal and Gastroesophageal Reflux*,
https://doi.org/10.1007/978-3-030-48890-1_18

Next, we delve into disease comprising complications of GERD. First, Dr. Stein discussed esophagitis, the evidence of mucosal damage in the esophagus as a result of reflux. This consequence of continued exposure of the lower esophagus to acidic gastric contents requires specific testing for diagnosis. The treatment of this disease still requires medication therapy in the vast majority of cases, although discussion and implementation of dietary changes represents a now vital role in preventing recurrence. The disease process of esophagitis lies on a spectrum with that of Barrett's esophagus – a long-term reflux-related change in the mucosa of the distal esophagus as a consequence of repeated exposure to acidic gastric contents with resultant inflammation. This topic follows that of esophagitis, with a comprehensive chapter by Dr. Stein. Barrett's esophagus diagnosis and treatment has changed dramatically in the past decade as we have accumulated new technologies and high-quality data. This rapidly changing area continues to be a focus of research given the steadily rising incidence of esophageal cancer, the dreaded consequence of Barrett's esophagus. The role of dietary changes, specifically in the treatment algorithm of Barrett's esophagus, remains an area sorely lacking in the research compendium. We support a plant-based diet in the treatment of Barrett's esophagus given the myriad benefits proven elsewhere in the treatment of GERD, although this needs confirmation through rigorous studies.

Symptoms of GERD go beyond the limited anatomic area including the esophagus and proximal stomach. Dr. Stein follows the section on Barrett's esophagus by discussing the differential diagnosis and related diseases of GERD. Unfortunately, for the practitioner, symptoms of GERD overlap with multiple other disease processes. This works in the reverse manner as well, with non-classic GERD symptoms often stumping a practitioner, potentially delaying diagnosis and appropriate treatment.

Diagnostic modalities are addressed in tandem, with Dr. Stein initially reviewing upper endoscopy and ultrasound, followed by Dr. Vakil giving an in-depth discussion on pH testing, impedance testing, and esophageal manometry. This complete review of available and up-to-date diagnostic tests describes the approach that is not only commonly employed but appropriate for the patient with suspected GERD. This testing algorithm does take both time and effort of both the physician and patient. We believe that it is not only reasonable but appropriate and imperative to begin lifestyle modifications while the workup takes place, chiefly dietary changes.

Lastly, Drs. Fuchs and Muller highlight the evolution of the DeMeester and Ryan scores. They review the use of pH measurements, identifying abnormal acid exposure within the esophagus, described as the DeMeester score. A discussion of oropharyngeal pH measurements is provided, with a detailed description of the RYAN score helping to identify patients with laryngopharyngeal reflux. Interestingly, they present data showing how, despite the DeMeester and RYAN scores representing the same parameters for esophageal and oropharyngeal acid exposure, respectively, scores on patients with GERD do not need to correlate. This completes the section on GERD, providing for a comprehensive review on the topic.

Chapter 19
GERD: Symptoms and Presentation

Diana M. Winston Comartin and Peter H. Stein

Gastroesophageal reflux is a normal physiologic process that occurs multiple times per day, typically not resulting in symptoms or mucosal damage. This differs from that of gastroesophageal reflux disease (GERD) in which contents from the stomach reflux into the esophagus creating symptoms and/or mucosal damage [1]. Our natural reflux barriers making up the complex lower esophageal sphincter allow for a degree of physiologic reflux. When those barriers are frequently compromised, physiologic reflux events can result in either symptoms or mucosal damage. Development of these symptoms or development of quantifiable mucosal injury related to this back wash of acidic contents into the esophagus defines GERD.

Patients can present with a wide range of symptoms not limited only to the esophagus. Patients occasionally manifest with symptoms in the lungs, ears, nose, and throat – topics covered elsewhere in this text. Classic GERD symptoms constitute those occurring in the esophagus, typically heartburn or regurgitation.

Heartburn is a burning feeling originating from the stomach, lower chest, or retrosternal area, radiating to the neck, throat, or back. Symptoms typically occur after meals. Symptoms can be more likely to occur after large meals or meals containing spicy foods, citrus, chocolate, alcohol, carbonation, or meals high in fat. Regurgitation is the sensation of stomach contents entering the oropharynx or mouth. Most patients will report acidic contents refluxing into the back of their throat, often with a sour or bitter taste. Many patients will perceive undigested or partially digested food contents making their way into the back of their throat during episodes of regurgitation [2].

Symptoms of GERD span well beyond that of classic heartburn and regurgitation. Patients with long-standing GERD will occasionally complain of dysphagia,

D. M. Winston Comartin (✉) · P. H. Stein
Division of Gastroenterology, Phelps Hospital Northwell Health, Sleepy Hollow, NY, USA
e-mail: dwcomartin@northwell.edu; pstein2@northwell.edu

C. H. Zalvan (ed.), *Laryngopharyngeal and Gastroesophageal Reflux*,
https://doi.org/10.1007/978-3-030-48890-1_19

difficulty swallowing food contents. This will most commonly occur with solid foods. Chronic reflux can lead to inflammation of the distal esophageal mucosal barrier. In severe cases, this can lead to Barrett's esophagus – a replacement of squamous esophageal epithelium with a columnar intestinal metaplasia. Strictures can develop due to chronic reflux as well [3]. In rare cases, patients can complain of odynophagia – pain on swallowing. The presence of odynophagia most commonly reflects the presence of severe esophagitis or an esophageal ulceration.

The presence of chest pain routinely requires ruling out cardiac causes, as GERD-related chest pain can mimic that of cardiac angina. In the absence of cardiac causes, we often attribute a burning or squeezing substernal chest pain to esophageal acid exposure. This can easily stump the clinician, as GERD symptoms can originate in the substernal area and radiate to the back, neck, jaw, or arms – alarmingly similar to the pain that would originate from cardiac etiologies. This overt pain can last anywhere from minutes to hours often with no clear exacerbating factors. It may or may not coincide with classic GERD-related symptoms of heartburn or regurgitation. If cardiac causes are ruled out, antacid therapy will help to clinch the diagnosis [4].

Patients with predominant symptoms of regurgitation will have a sour or bitter taste in the back of their mouth. Many texts will describe the "water brash" phenomenon of hypersalivation, where the presence of refluxate in the oropharynx will stimulate hypersecretion of saliva. In reality, this occurrence is quite rare although possible. Patients have reported foam forming within the mouth as a result of large amounts of saliva production, giving the appearance of a patient foaming at the mouth.

Nausea occasionally occurs as a result of reflux [5]. Although nausea can have a wide range of causes, GERD should be considered as a cause of nausea if no clear alternate explanation exists. Gastroenterologists will frequently perform an upper endoscopy early in the workup of unexplained nausea, ruling out not only GERD but additional causes such as anatomic abnormalities of the upper GI tract, peptic ulcer disease, gastritis, or infections of the upper GI tract. Often biopsies of the upper GI tract will reveal evidence of reflux disease. The finding of reflux-related changes on esophageal biopsies does not clinch the diagnosis of GERD as a cause of GERD, although it does help guide the clinician. Additional causes such as gastroparesis can result in GERD-related findings within the distal esophagus without the underlying problem being GERD in and of itself. Still, the evidence of reflux will help guide the clinician in their treatment algorithm, hopefully allowing for relief of nausea symptoms precipitating the initial workup.

Extraesophageal symptoms include asthma, a globus sensation, recurrent pneumonias, chronic cough, laryngitis, hoarseness, throat clearing, sore throat, and ear pain [6]. Many of these symptoms are covered in detail elsewhere in this text.

GERD symptoms often result in mucosal damage. This can manifest as visible esophagitis or as inflammation or mucosal damage only evident on pathology. A normal-appearing esophagus on upper endoscopy does not exclude the presence of GERD. Rather, it can confirm the diagnosis of nonerosive reflux disease (NERD). We use this term when symptoms consistent with GERD exist, with a normal EGD and normal esophageal biopsies. These patients will by and large be responsive to acid-lowering therapy. If the diagnosis remains in question after an upper endoscopy is performed, additional testing to assess for the presence of reflux and correlation with GERD symptoms should be considered as well as motility testing to rule out an underlying motility disorder, as outlined in detail elsewhere in this text.

An upper endoscopy is performed to assess for complications of GERD and to exclude other causes of the symptoms. The endoscopy may find evidence of erosive disease, which can be classified in the Los Angeles classification system or the Savary-Miller classification system [7, 8].

Rarely are symptom indices used in practice for the diagnosis of GERD. However, the two most studied symptom association measures are the symptom index (SI) [9] and the symptom association probability (SAP) [10]. Both indices have been validated with pH testing as accurate in patients who experience heartburn and are not on medical therapy. However, both indices are flawed methodologically [11] and awkward to use in clinical practice. Data reflecting the usefulness of the SI and SAP to predict treatment response is lacking. In clinical practice, there is little downside in empirically using a short one- to two-month course of acid-lowering medications if GERD is suspected, specifically proton pump inhibitors. Recent data indicates that PPI use for less than 3 years is safe [12]. A 1–2-month trial comes with minimal risk and will answer the question of whether acid-related disease, specifically GERD, is the cause of the patients' symptoms. Conversely, if the patient has reservations with regard to a medication trial, it would be reasonable to immediately institute dietary and lifestyle changes as a reasonable test as to better define the cause of symptoms. A positive response to dietary and lifestyle changes would indicate GERD as a likely source of the patients' complaints, with the added benefit of weight loss and the associated improved metabolic and physiologic consequences.

GERD can present with multiple patient complaints, well beyond the classic symptoms of heartburn and regurgitation. An astute clinician will be aware of the wide range of symptoms associated with GERD, first ruling out potentially acute or dangerous causes while maintaining acid-related disease as a likely potential culprit.

References

1. Feldman M, Friedman L et al. Sleisenger and Fordtran's gastrointestinal and liver disease pathophysiology, diagnosis, management. 9th ed.: Saunders.
2. Vakil N, van Zanten SV, Kahrilas P, et al. The Montreal definition and classification of gastroesophageal reflux disease: a global evidence-based consensus. Am J Gastroenterol. 2006;101:1900.
3. Vakil N, Traxler B, Levine D. Dysphagia in patients with erosive esophagitis: prevalence, severity, and response to proton pump inhibitor treatment. Clin Gastroenterol Hepatol. 2004;2:665.
4. Kahrilas PJ, Hughes N, Howden CW. Response of unexplained chest pain to proton pump inhibitor treatment in patients with and without objective evidence of gastro-oesophageal reflux disease. Gut. 2011;60:1473.

5. Brzana RJ, Koch KL. Gastroesophageal reflux disease presenting with intractable nausea. Ann Intern Med. 1997;126:704.
6. Martinucci I, Albano E, Marchi S, Blandizzi C. Extra-esophageal presentation of gastroesophageal reflux disease: a new understanding in a new era. Minerva Gastroenterol Dietol. 2017;63:221–34.
7. Lundell LR, et al. Endoscopist assessment of oesophagitis: clinical and functional correlation and further validation of the Los Angeles classification. Gut. 1999;45:172.
8. Ollyo JB, et al. Savary-Miller's new endoscopic grading of reflux oesophagitis: a simple reproducible, logical, complete and useful classification. Gastorenterology. 1990;98:A 100.
9. Wiener GJ, Richter JE, Copper JB, Wu WC, Castell DO. The symptom index: a clinically important parameter of ambulatory 24-hour esophageal pH monitoring. Am J Gastroenterol. 1988;83:358–61.
10. Weusten BL, Roelofs JM, Akkermans LM, Van Berge-Henegouwen GP, Smout AJ. The symptom-association probability: an improved method for symptom analysis of 24-hour esophageal pH data. Gastroenterology. 1994;107:1741–5.
11. Connor J, Richter J. Increasing yield also increases false positives and best serves to exclude GERD. Am J Gastroenterol. 2006;101:460–3.
12. Moayyedi P, Eikelboom JW, et al. Safety of proton pump inhibitors based on a large, multi-year, randomized trial of patients receiving rivaroxaban or aspirin. Gastroenterology. 2019;157:682–91.

Chapter 20
Dyspepsia: Overview and Treatment Options

David M. Gutman

Dyspepsia is among the most common conditions seen by physicians and easily among the most misunderstood. To the lay person, it is often described as indigestion with a potential array of associated upper abdominal symptoms. Truly, this is a group of conditions arising from multiple etiologies sharing a common set of symptoms, rather than a specific single disease.

Dyspepsia is defined as a syndrome characterized by chronic symptoms of upper abdominal pain, early satiety, postprandial fullness, nausea and vomiting, gas and bloating, and belching, often with heartburn as a secondary feature [1]. As with irritable bowel syndrome, it is a syndromic diagnosis. As such, dyspepsia has been confused with gastroparesis, gastroesophageal reflux disease, irritable bowel syndrome, gallbladder disease, and others. Indeed, it can also coexist or overlap the features of these disorders as well as *H. pylori* gastritis, peptic ulcer disease, biliary disease, anxiety, depression, and more. Heartburn may occur with dyspepsia, but by itself heartburn is not a dyspeptic symptom [2]. Patients may have both IBS and dyspepsia. Symptoms that improve with defecation or passing gas should not be considered dyspeptic [2]. Many consider gastroparesis to be on a spectrum with dyspepsia due to the remarkable overlap in presenting symptoms [3]. As upper abdominal pain or indigestion is among the most common reasons patients seek medical care, we will focus on the diagnostic and treatment strategies that a primary physician would choose to incorporate effectively.

D. M. Gutman (✉)
Zucker School of Medicine at Hofstra/Northwell Health, Hempstead, NY, USA
e-mail: drgutman@refluxny.com

C. H. Zalvan (ed.), *Laryngopharyngeal and Gastroesophageal Reflux*,
https://doi.org/10.1007/978-3-030-48890-1_20

Functional Dyspepsia

When a primary source of these chronic symptoms is unclear after basic diagnostic testing, we refer to the condition as functional dyspepsia, to differentiate this from the symptom complex of dyspepsia. The prior nomenclature was nonulcer dyspepsia, which is still accurate but an abandoned term. As there is no specific diagnostic test to diagnose functional dyspepsia and as the overlap of related disorders is common, the study of the cause and best treatments of dyspepsia has been challenging and controversial. The history more than any testing gives us the greatest insight as to potential root cause of dyspepsia, as well as to the subclass of functional dyspepsia. We will endeavor to highlight what is understood, especially relating to the relationship to GERD, idiopathic gastroparesis, and food, and to differentiate what is appropriate in the diagnosis and management of this common presentation.

Laboratories performed for dyspepsia will minimally include complete blood count to exclude anemia arising from blood loss and chemistries to assess for hepatobiliary dysfunction, azotemia, or hypercalcemia which can all cause dyspeptic symptoms. *H. pylori* stool antigen or breath testing may be appropriate in the initial testing. *H. pylori* serology should be abandoned as it is very often misleading both in the naïve and treated patient. Patients with pancreatobiliary symptoms such as pain radiating to the back or with abnormal liver or pancreatic enzymes may require appropriate imaging. Those with prominent nausea and vomiting may need a 4-hour solid phase gastric emptying scan or gastroparesis breath test. Endoscopy does not usually alter the management of dyspepsia but is usually the next diagnostic step as there is a general reluctance to accept the diagnosis of functional dyspepsia without ruling out ulcer or malignancy in at-risk patients. The young person taking NSAIDs and the patient with predominant heartburn symptoms may be treated empirically providing there is follow-up to assess the nonresponders. The effectiveness of this strategy is discussed later. The lack of serious findings on endoscopy in the presence of typical and chronic symptoms is diagnostic of functional dyspepsia.

Rome Criteria

When we speak of dyspepsia, we are discussing a chronic and episodic abdominal pain, rather than the acute abdominal pain of acute cholecystitis or the nausea and vomiting of a foodborne illness. The diagnosis of functional dyspepsia has evolved in recent years. The Rome Foundation has established the criteria for the clinical and research diagnosis of the functional gastrointestinal disorders (FGID) including functional dyspepsia [4], irritable bowel syndrome, and functional heartburn. The Rome III criteria of 2006 have been advanced in the Rome IV version released in 2016 to improve specificity of these diagnoses. Rome IV emphasizes that FD should no longer be considered as a single disease entity but as a spectrum (Fig. 20.1) where there is significant overlap with GERD and IBS [4]. It was also recognized

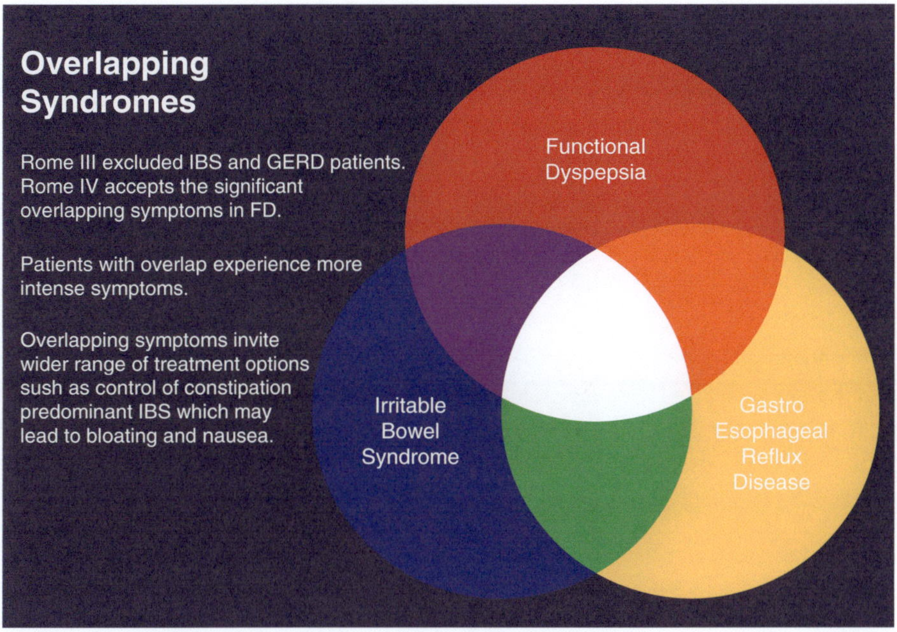

Fig. 20.1 Overlapping gastroenterological syndromes included in the Rome criteria

that patients in this overlap experienced a higher intensity and frequency of symptoms with greater impact on daily life [5]. As there are more studies utilizing Rome III than Rome IV, we shall regard them as interchangeable.

Functional dyspepsia falls into two significantly overlapping symptom complexes (Fig. 20.2) that should be differentiated as treatment effectiveness is often tied to the subgroup [5]. Postprandial distress syndrome (PDS) is characterized by bothersome postprandial fullness or early satiety [4]. There may be postprandial bloating, nausea, gas, or belching. Gastric emptying may be delayed in FD, but prominent vomiting and weight loss should lead to other diagnostic considerations including gastroparesis [3].

Epigastric pain syndrome (EPS) is characterized by bothersome epigastric burning or pain [4]. Pain may be postprandial, may be relieved by eating, or may occur during fasting. Biliary-type pain is excluded. Heartburn may coexist, as may gastroesophageal reflux disease. Heartburn is not a diagnostic criterion. While PDS is by definition postprandial, EPS does not need to be associated with eating.

Postprandial distress syndrome and epigastric pain syndrome frequently overlap. The overlap of these syndromes varies greatly depending on the community studied from one third in a referral center to one of six in community populations [3].

These symptoms are chronic occurring over at least 6 months and frequent but do not need to be daily. Rome IV emphasizes the bothersome nature of the symptoms being disruptive of usual activities. Bowel symptoms and symptoms relieved by evacuation are not part of functional dyspepsia, but there is a sizable proportion of patients with both irritable bowel syndrome and functional dyspepsia.

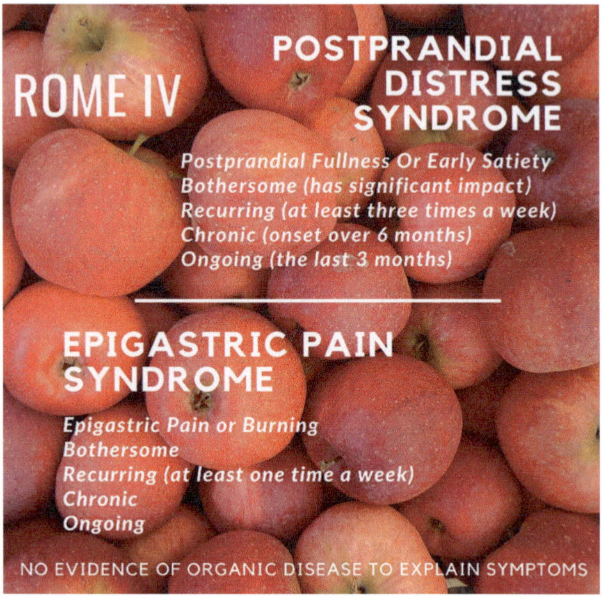

Fig. 20.2 Rome IV criteria differentiating postprandial distress syndrome from epigastric pain syndrome

Relationship of Dyspepsia to GERD and Heartburn

Patients with gastroesophageal reflux disease may have associated dyspepsia. Many patients with functional dyspepsia have associated heartburn symptoms [6]. Initially, this may not be a critical issue. Those patients that respond to PPI therapy do not necessarily benefit from specific discrimination between these two common entities. The patient with heartburn with or without dyspeptic symptoms and a normal endoscopic exam and failure to respond to proton pump inhibitor therapy can be challenging for diagnosis and treatment. They may need advanced diagnostic testing if there is sufficient disruption of quality of life that is not improved by reassurance after the normal endoscopic findings.

Patients with heartburn without findings of erosive esophagitis or at least 1 cm of Barrett's esophagus may be categorized as having nonerosive esophagitis (NERD), esophageal hypersensitivity, functional heartburn, or epigastric pain syndrome (EPS). In this time where PPI usage is very prevalent, they may have healed erosive esophagitis.

Patients with heartburn or noncardiac chest pain without severe endoscopic findings fall into three groups:

1. Nonerosive reflux disease patients are defined by a response to treatment with acid suppression, without severe endoscopic damage (defined as over 1 cm of Barrett's or esophageal erosions crossing esophageal folds – LA Grade C or D). Patients with normal endoscopy and abnormal esophageal pH testing with a high degree of esophageal acid exposure time also have nonerosive reflux disease or possibly healed erosive esophagitis.

2. Esophageal hypersensitivity is defined on pH testing by a normal acid exposure time with high symptom index or symptom association probability. That is, they have few episodes of acid reflux, but those episodes of reflux correlate with symptoms on the esophageal pH testing.
3. Functional heartburn patients and patients with functional dyspepsia with heartburn do not have excessive esophageal acid exposure nor symptom correlation. In EPS, the dominant and bothersome symptom is the epigastric pain rather than heartburn or chest pain that characterize functional heartburn.

Diagnostic Pitfalls

Gastroesophageal reflux is very common, as is functional dyspepsia. Yet the diagnosis of GERD is made many times more than FD [6]. In fact, many patients with a diagnosis of GERD truly have functional dyspepsia or functional heartburn.

Over the last 2 decades, there has been a decided shift toward diagnosis of GERD and underdiagnosis of functional dyspepsia. This bias has led, in part, to the overuse of PPI for what is deemed refractory heartburn in patients who do not have GERD [6].

Treatment

There are no US FDA- or EU EMA-approved medications for functional dyspepsia. This creates a difficult position for both primary care physicians and gastroenterologists treating this very common condition. There are several key reasons why treatments are not clearly identified for the symptom improvement in functional dyspepsia [7]:

- Treatments for EPS and PDS may be different.
- The syndromic nature of FD leaves us with no biologic markers or objective parameters of treatment efficacy [8].
- Patient-reported outcomes have not been adequately validated for FD [8].
- The overlap of GERD and IBS adds increased subjectivity to treatment response in patients with overlapping conditions.
- Excluding GERD and IBS patients from clinical trials has led to the exclusion criteria depleting the pool of candidates for clinical trials, distorts and creates bias in the study population, and reduces the power of the trial to show benefit [8].
- The patients with overlapping GERD, IBS, and FD had the greatest potential benefit of treatment due to higher severity of impactful symptoms (Fig. 20.1). Clinical trial exclusion criteria may have led to selection bias in RCT [8].
- Symptom improvement may be a better endpoint than symptom resolution due to limited efficacy of available agents [8].

There has been limited efficacy in functional dyspepsia in studies of PPI (NNT 8, RRR 0.83), prokinetic agents (NNT 12.5, RRR 0.92), and tricyclic antidepressants (TCA) (NNT 6, RRR 0.74) [8]. These limitations may reflect a lack of understanding of the cause of FD. The results could be constrained by utilizing suboptimal measures to signify a clinically significant result. Meaningful results are further obscured by pooling heterogeneous groups of FD subtypes.

For abdominal pain, TCA has had the most consistent efficacy in multiple clinical trials [2, 9]. SSRI, specifically sertraline and escitalopram, were not effective in two RCTs. While there has only been one SNRI studied, venlafaxine, there is a role for trial of SNRI for TCA-intolerant patients with EPS based on the response of abdominal pain in other functional gastrointestinal disorders (FGID) [2].

Buspirone may be effective for PDS when symptoms of early satiety, fullness, and nausea predominate. Mirtazapine is another effective treatment option for PDS when there is chronic nausea and vomiting, or weight loss, and it may also help coexisting abdominal pain [2].

Treatment Pitfalls

The mistake often made is to try to maximize the dosing of acid blockers for the patients with esophageal hypersensitivity and functional heartburn. No benefit is derived from reducing esophageal acid exposure in patients with hypersensitivity, as the esophageal acid exposure time is already low. Likewise, patients with functional heartburn, by definition, are patients where acid is not the driving force of the symptoms. Patients with functional heartburn behave therapeutically much as the patients with functional dyspepsia and are managed just as for epigastric pain syndrome. Functional dyspepsia patients often respond to acid suppression, but maximizing this with high doses or adding sucralfate does not improve outcomes.

Guidelines of the American College of Gastroenterology and Canadian Association of Gastroenterology published in 2017

The Guidelines of the ACG and CAG deserve applause for difficult conclusions in the setting of little to poor data [10]. At the same time, they deserve great scrutiny for what is below the surface of the guideline statements. We will address the most important issues and recommend the guideline and podcast for the reader to delve deeper (Fig. 20.3).

Patients with undiagnosed dyspepsia should have an *H. pylori* breath test or stool antigen test (serologic testing is no longer recommended in any setting) and have appropriate treatment as outlined in the ACG Guidelines for *H. pylori* infection [10]. Prompt endoscopy to evaluate the symptoms did not prove to be beneficial in outcomes.

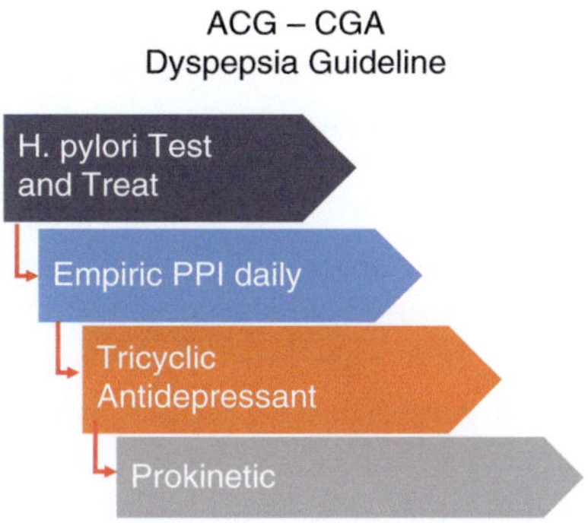

Fig. 20.3 Guidelines of the American College of Gastroenterology and Canadian Association of Gastroenterology

Alarm features in patients under 60 rarely uncovered a malignancy on endoscopy [10]. While the incidence of malignancy in patients under 60 was associated with two- to threefold relative risk of cancer, the absolute rate still was lower than 1%. There is a weak, conditional recommendation for endoscopy for patients over 60. The risk of GI malignancies may be more concerning with male gender, country of origin in Southeast Asia, or parts of South America, and other historical clues. Over 99% of dyspepsia patients do not have cancer. Biliary or pancreatic symptoms such as pain radiating to the back are best approached with imaging rather than endoscopy.

PPI empiric therapy, once daily, has been well established as safe and effective for patients after *H. pylori* eradication and is the recommended initial treatment strategy for *H. pylori*-negative patients. The flaw with this argument is that all of the data is on patients who have functional dyspepsia rather than undiagnosed dyspepsia. Again, functional dyspepsia patients have had investigation, usually endoscopy, to exclude other causes of their symptoms. With that caveat, the data is otherwise compelling that in the lower risk patient, such as those under 60, an empiric course of daily PPI with reevaluation is safe and often effective.

Tricyclic antidepressants earned a low-quality conditional recommendation as the next treatment step rather than endoscopy in undiagnosed dyspepsia patients. There are however no trials that have addressed this question directly. In patients with functional dyspepsia, TCA and not SSRI were effective in functional dyspepsia patients. It is my contention that in the face of this evidence, patients should have an established diagnosis of FD before TCA can be recommended. Whether the TCA is effective due to the central nervous system effect or the enteric nervous system effect is unknown, although I contend that the low doses required suggest a predominant ENS/motility effect. The use of TCA in older patients must require great caution and risk assessment in a disorder with no increase in mortality.

The College then recommends conditionally and with low evidence a trial of prokinetics. I would change this recommendation to no data is available to support this empiric therapy [7, 11]. Acotiamide is effective but only available in Japan and India [12]. The efficacy data available are predominantly with prokinetics not available (cisapride, tegaserod) after having been withdrawn for potential cardiac toxicities [7, 11]. The risks associated with metoclopramide and domperidone may be reasonable in patients with serious disorders as gastroparesis or scleroderma but are quite concerning for dyspepsia in the absence of any RCT. These agents available for the treatment of gastroparesis have not been studied for dyspepsia, with or without delayed gastric emptying.

The College also recommended that patients not be offered CAM. In the setting of a low-risk disease, patients are looking for a low-risk treatment. There have been many randomized clinical trials that have demonstrated statistically significant benefit of several CAM treatments. These studies are generally low quality with a high risk of bias especially due to small sample sizes. This being understood, the risks are far less than with prokinetics or with TCA in the elderly. It must be emphasized that GERD needs to be excluded clinically as peppermint oil and turmeric both significantly aggravate heartburn. To further highlight the importance of CAM in this sector, Clinicaltrials.gov notes that of the active and very recently completed interventional studies for functional dyspepsia at the time of this writing, there were 20 approaches being studied. These interventions included four herbal medications, psychotherapy, hypnosis, acupuncture, and two diets (gluten-free and artificial sweetener-free). As functional dyspepsia is a low-morbidity disorder similar to irritable bowel syndrome, treatment approaches need to be safe and focused on the improvement in not only symptoms but also quality of life.

Food and Functional Dyspepsia

Food may have a significant impact on symptoms of functional dyspepsia. A systemic review of the literature [13] found two studies where implementation of a gluten-free diet led to a reduction in dyspeptic symptoms. Six studies noted wheat as a trigger for both PDS and EPS symptoms. Dietary fat was associated with functional dyspepsia in three studies. Caffeine was associated with functional dyspepsia in four studies. Note that fat and caffeine are triggers of GERD, adding to the confounding overlap in these two common disorders. These foods may trigger duodenal eosinophilia and mast cell activation or activate inflammatory cytokines as putative mechanisms for triggering dyspepsia, but none of the studies looked at histology or immune activation [13].

FODMAPs including foods with wheat or gluten may be primary targets for intervention. When we speak of a gluten-free diet, it is important to distinguish gluten protein as an allergen in celiac disease from the fermentable oligosaccharides known as fructans. The fructans are found primarily in wheat and onions in the Western diet. The term "gluten-free diet" therefore becomes a surrogate for fructan-reduced diet. All patients should have celiac serologies prior to initiating a gluten-free diet. Testing for celiac disease after the patient has improvement in their symptoms on a gluten-free diet becomes challenging because of normalization of both the antibodies and the histological damage on small bowel biopsies. Celiac disease has significant implications beyond gastrointestinal symptoms and therefore needs to be tested in all patients before they embark on a gluten-free diet.

Organic Basis for Functional Dyspepsia

Despite a lack of proven treatment options, there have been multiple postulated treatment targets that are being studied actively. As in IBS, visceral hypersensitivity to normal stimuli has been demonstrated and is a target of neuromodulating drugs [1]. These agents often also work directly on the enteric nervous system with alterations in gastric motility, fundic accommodation, antral distension which feeds back to fundic motility, duodenal inflammation which may tie into dysbiosis of the intestinal flora, and associated antroduodenal coordination. With all these mechanisms demonstrated, we may be using obsolete terminology labeling functional dyspepsia as a functional disorder rather than an organic disorder that does not have overt endoscopic findings [3].

Among the pathophysiologic mechanisms that lead to symptoms of dyspepsia, we can break them down to psychosocial (such as anxiety), motor disturbances (impaired gastric accommodation), sensory disturbances (visceral hypersensitivity), inflammatory (postinfectious FD), and external (dietary). These are not exclusive of each other. These mechanisms make up the potential treatment avenues to explore (Fig. 20.4).

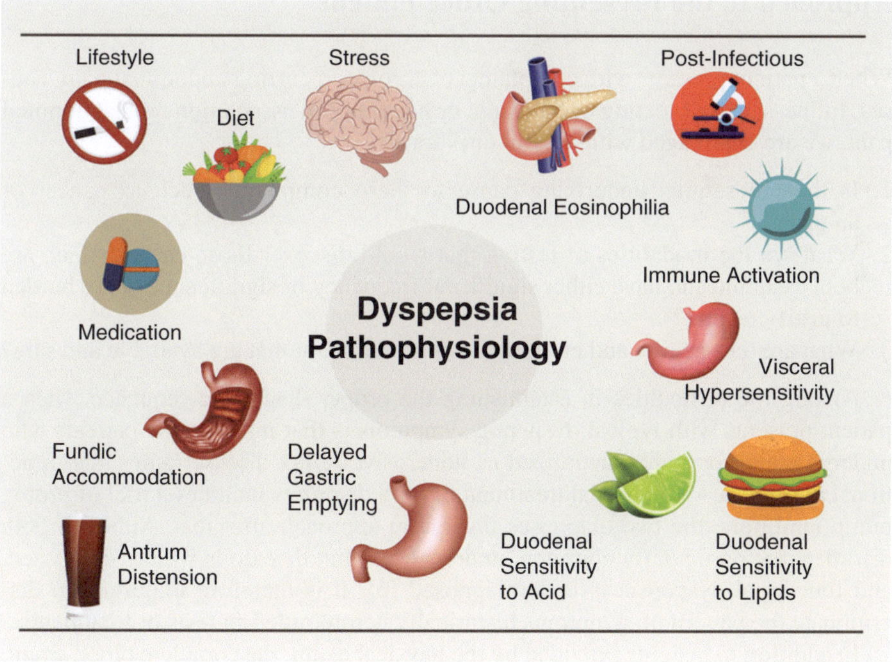

Fig. 20.4 Pathophysiology and targets for treatment

Anxiety is common in FD. Central pain processing is abnormal in many patients, although it is not clear whether the brain or the gut is the driving force of these mechanisms primarily. Anxiety and stress may lead to alterations in gastroduodenal motility, promote visceral hypersensitivity, alter immune responses of the stomach and duodenum, or delay gastric emptying [3].

Infectious gastroenteritis is known to often lead to irritable bowel syndrome and has similarly been linked to functional dyspepsia [1, 3, 5].

Duodenal inflammation and eosinophilia are associated with early satiety and pain, intestinal barrier disruption, increased intestinal permeability, and altered upper gastrointestinal microbiota [1, 5].

One third of patients with functional dyspepsia have delayed gastric emptying [1]. A large percentage of patients with gastroparesis meet criteria for FD [3].

Foods may alter gut hormonal responses or lead to an inflammatory or allergic response. This may involve cytokines including eotaxin and interleukins and mast cell and eosinophil recruitment and degranulation, with alterations in neuronal firing, intestinal permeability, and muscular contraction all leading to pain and the constellation of symptoms we describe as dyspepsia [3].

Approach to the Presenting Office Patient

When a patient presents with complaints of chronic, recurring abdominal pain, nausea, fullness, early bloating or belching, or heartburn in association with abdominal pain, we are challenged with several questions:

1. Is there a serious underlying cause to these complaints, such as cancer or an ulcer?
2. What are the modalities of testing that would discover those causes which are both treatable and have either significant frequency or significant disease burden to justify testing?
3. What are the specific and empiric forms of treatment that are available and safe?

Among the difficulties in establishing the proper diagnostic sequence when a patient presents with typical dyspeptic symptoms is that many of the patients who undergo endoscopy are categorized as nonerosive reflux disease rather than functional dyspepsia. While initial treatment of both disorders includes a trial of proton pump inhibitors, the two diagnoses diverge in approach after that. Although both disorders are particularly common, nonerosive reflux disease is widely diagnosed, and functional dyspepsia is underdiagnosed [6]. It is therefore important to discriminate the pattern of symptoms historically before ordering tests or treatments.

In addition to insights provided by the physical exam, the complete blood count, comprehensive metabolic profile, and CRP or ESR may be particularly useful. In some patients, lipase should also be ordered. Patients with anemia or liver abnormalities will require appropriate diagnostic investigations. Imaging will be needed in patients suspected of pancreatobiliary disease as the root of the dyspepsia symptoms. In patients over 60, endoscopy is appropriate, despite a low yield. Celiac testing should always be performed before advising dietary restrictions.

Younger patients should have *H. pylori* stool antigen or breath urease testing. While treatment for *H. pylori* infection when found has a limited efficacy (NNT 12), it is accepted as the one treatment which can lead to long-term benefit. The American College of Gastroenterology and Canadian Association of Gastroenterology Guidelines recommend treatment for *H. pylori* in all dyspeptic patients with infection demonstrated on biopsy, stool antigen testing, or breath testing. Serologic testing no longer has a role in modern practice. Clarithromycin regimens are associated with high resistance rates in the USA and even higher resistance in Central America, China, Iran, and South Asia and so are no longer a first- or second-line option.

In great part due to functional dyspepsia having a variable presentation and evolving syndromic definition, it has been difficult to identify consistent effective treatment strategies. Most studies are limited by high placebo response rates which increases the number needed to treat (NNT). Furthermore, despite the frequency of functional dyspepsia, there are no FDA-approved treatments available.

An empiric course of daily PPI is warranted in most patients. There is no role for high-dose PPI. Follow-up is key here, as many patients do not respond and need further evaluation or treatment. Many patients who are put on PPI never are taken off PPI despite lack of efficacy and despite guidelines which suggest that they be withdrawn every 6–12 months in patients without erosive esophagitis or Barrett's esophagus. This has led to massive oversubscription to these agents in patients who no longer are benefiting from PPI treatment.

There is significance to the designation of postprandial distress syndrome (PDS) and epigastric pain syndrome (EPS) in the choice of therapies [2].

PPI therapy is effective in one third of patients with a number needed to treat of 10. Patients with reflux symptoms (EPS) have a higher response rate. Patients with predominant nausea and bloating do not respond to PPI better than placebo. EPS patients may respond better to TCA, while PDS patients may respond better to gut-brain neuromodulators (e.g., buspirone, mirtazapine, etc.).

Whether one would recommend endoscopy to the younger (less than 60) patient after an ineffective course of PPI or following a trial of TCA as per the ACG-CAG Guidelines is an individual decision and may be based on resources available, other clinical clues, or patient preference. In my practice, patients who do not have *H. pylori* and fail PPI need the assurance of endoscopy before further empiric therapies for FD [4, 5].

As the finding of gastric cancer is low on endoscopy, the finding of nonspecific gastritis is high. Gastritis, especially chronic inactive gastritis, and chemical or reactive gastropathy without *H. pylori* rarely impact the treatment plan. That is, treatment of the gastritis does not yield clinical improvement. The exception is atrophic gastritis, which has a 3% risk of progressing to gastric carcinoma and is often associated with symptomatic motor abnormalities of gastric accommodation and motility. When severe, atrophic gastritis can be associated with achlorhydria and vitamin B12 deficiency.

Despite the ACG-CAG Guidelines, I frequently offer to patients with FD nutraceuticals including peppermint oil with caraway such as STW5, or ginger root extract. STW5, Rikkunshito, and peppermint oil with caraway have all proven efficacy in small RCTs despite the data being of low quality due to study limitations [5, 7, 14]. I only use these specific agents for PDS patients and never for EPS patients due to the potential to aggravate heartburn and associated reflux.

With proper patient selection, I have seen satisfactory results with a variety of gut-brain neuromodulating agents, especially mirtazapine, which may improve receptive fundic accommodation as a key mechanism. In several studies, the mechanisms of these gut-brain neuromodulators are independent of their central and psychological effects. The Rome Committee has thus chosen the term gut-brain neuromodulators rather than antidepressants or other terms [2]. It is key to preface the use of psychotropic medications by introducing their role on motor function of the gut in order not to be dismissed by the patient rejecting psychiatric care from the gastroenterologist. Again, in this realm, the science is good, but the data is weak.

Buspirone, a serotonin 1A agonist, is effective for improving fundic accommodation and improving symptoms of PDS and early satiety without relation to its role as an anxiolytic [1].

Amitriptyline was demonstrated to be effective for abdominal pain of EPS in patients without delayed gastric emptying, while escitalopram was not effective in this large RCT [1, 9].

The overlap with FD and gastroparesis is strong as suggested by the similarity of PDS symptoms with idiopathic gastroparesis [1, 3]. Many patients with FD have delayed gastric emptying. Diagnostic testing for gastroparesis with a 4-hour scintigraphy (avoid studies under 3 hours) or gastric emptying breath test can help predict which patients may benefit from prokinetic agents. Data is lacking for available prokinetics in functional dyspepsia [1, 10]. These medications must be used with great caution considering the risks of these medications to the basal ganglia and the heart.

Probiotics have been effective in several small RCT. Note that the studies cannot be easily extrapolated to a wide range of probiotics or a wide spectrum of patient profiles. Nonetheless, these are avenues to explore with patients in the absence of robust large RCT. Fermented milk with *Bifidobacterium bifidum* YIT10347 improved postprandial discomfort and epigastric pain but also bowel symptoms such as diarrhea and flatulence [1]. *Lactobacillus gasseri* OLL2716 was also effective over placebo. Rifaximin 400 mg t.i.d. for 2 weeks was well tolerated and superior to placebo in providing adequate relief (78% versus 52%, $P = 0.02$), especially for belching and postprandial fullness/bloating [1].

Conclusions

Dyspepsia is a heterogeneous set of upper gastrointestinal symptoms. The most common cause is idiopathic without overt organic etiology known as functional dyspepsia. This exceedingly common condition overlaps greatly with irritable bowel syndrome, idiopathic gastroparesis, and gastroesophageal reflux. Despite this being a functional gastrointestinal disorder, there are many pathologies that may characterize this condition with sensory, motor, inflammatory, and psychosocial components that make up the potential targets of therapy. Care must be taken to limit risks in the treatment of this nonthreatening disorder and focus on the bothersome and disruptive symptoms that may be ameliorated with preferably safe agents, diet, and nutraceuticals.

References

1. Tack J, Camilleri M. New developments in the treatment of gastroparesis and functional dyspepsia. Curr Opin Pharmacol. 2018;43:111–7. https://doi.org/10.1016/j.coph.2018.08.015.
2. Drossman DA, et al. Neuromodulators for functional gastrointestinal disorders (disorders of gut−brain interaction): a Rome Foundation Working Team Report. Gastroenterology. 2017;154:1140–1171.e1. https://doi.org/10.1053/j.gastro.2017.11.279.
3. Talley NJ, Ford AC. Functional dyspepsia. N Engl J Med. 2015;373:1853–63. https://doi.org/10.1056/NEJMra1501505.
4. Stanghellini V, Chan FKL, Hasler WL, et al. Rome IV – gastroduodenal disorders. Gastroenterology. 2016;150:1380–92. https://doi.org/10.1053/j.gastro.2016.02.011.
5. Koduru P, Irani M, Quigley EM. Definition, pathogenesis, and management of that cursed dyspepsia. Clin Gastroenterol Hepatol. 2018;16:467–79. https://doi.org/10.1016/j.cgh.2017.09.002.
6. Pleyer C, Bittner H, Locke GR, et al. Overdiagnosis of gastro-esophageal reflux disease and underdiagnosis of functional dyspepsia in a USA community. Neurogastroenterol Motil. 2014;26:1163–71. https://doi.org/10.1111/nmo.12377.
7. Tack J, Van den Houte K, Carbone F. The unfulfilled promise of prokinetics for functional dyspepsia/postprandial distress syndrome. Am J Gastroenterol. 2019;114:204–6. https://doi.org/10.14309/ajg.0000000000000072.
8. Vakil NB, Howden CW, Moayyedi P, Tack J. White Paper AGA: functional dyspepsia. Clin Gastroenterol Hepatol. 2017;15:1191–4. https://doi.org/10.1016/j.cgh.2017.05.013.
9. Lacy BE, Saito YA, Camilleri M, Bouras E, DiBaise JK, Herrick LM, Szarka LA, Tilkes K, Zinsmeister AR, Talley NJ. Effects of antidepressants on gastric function in patients with functional dyspepsia. Am J Gastroenterol. 2018;113:216–24. https://doi.org/10.1038/ajg.2017.458.
10. Moayyedi P, Lacy B, Andrews C, Enns R, Howden C, Vakil N. ACG and CAG clinical guideline: management of dyspepsia. Am J Gastroenterol. 2017;112:988–1013. https://doi.org/10.1038/ajg.2017.154.
11. Pittayanon R, Yuan Y, Bollegala NP, et al. Prokinetics for functional dyspepsia: a systematic review and meta-analysis of randomized control trials. Am J Gastroenterol. 2019;114:233–43. https://doi.org/10.1038/s41395-018-0258-6.
12. Tomita T, Oshima T, Miwa H. New approaches to diagnosis and treatment of functional dyspepsia. Curr Gastroenterol Rep. 2018;20:55. https://doi.org/10.1007/s11894-018-0663-4.
13. Duncanson KR, Talley NJ, Walker MM, Burrows TL. Food and functional dyspepsia: a systematic review. J Hum Nutr Diet. 2018;31:390–407. https://doi.org/10.1111/jhn.12506.
14. Fifi AC, Axelrod CH, Chakraborty P, Saps M. Herbs and spices in the treatment of functional gastrointestinal disorders: a review of clinical trials. Nutrients. 2018;10:1715. https://doi.org/10.3390/nu10111715.

Chapter 21
Erosive and Nonerosive Esophagitis

Peter H. Stein

Esophagitis is the presence of mucosal damage in the esophagus caused by the reflux of gastric contents into the esophagus. This occurs primarily as a consequence of long-standing or severe gastroesophageal reflux disease (GERD), which can be further subdivided into nonerosive reflux disease and erosive reflux disease [1].

Nonerosive reflux disease (NERD) will be discussed separately; however, this disease constitutes exactly what the name implies: reflux disease that does not cause erosions, ulcers, or endoscopically visible mucosal abnormalities. Given that no visible evidence of reflux exists in the disease process of NERD, the presence of reflux disease must be confirmed by alternate means, typically either sampling techniques such as biopsies or pH and impedance testing [2]. Further details will be addressed separately.

Erosive reflux disease exists when the patient not only experiences symptoms of GERD (heartburn, acid regurgitation, dysphagia, etc.) but in addition has the presence of esophagitis [3]. Esophagitis is by definition inflammation of the esophagus. This occurs as a result of not only the direct caustic effect of exposure to stomach contents including acid, pepsin, and bile but in addition to cytokine-mediated inflammatory cascades [4]. This can exist with endoscopically visible signs such as mucosal breaks, fissures, erosions, or ulcers. This can also exist on biopsy only, meaning no visible signs exist on endoscopy but are present on pathologic review and evaluation (Fig. 21.1).

Not all patients with symptomatic reflux will have evidence of esophagitis on endoscopy. Studies have shown that 20–60% of patients with abnormal esophageal pH testing will have evidence of esophagitis on endoscopy [5, 6]. These studies include a wide range of criteria defining esophagitis, in addition to a wide range of patients meeting study criteria for esophagitis. Given significant variability in prior studies, we should not fall into the trap of directly linking symptoms of reflux to the

P. H. Stein (✉)
Division of Gastroenterology, Phelps Hospital, Northwell Health, Sleepy Hollow, NY, USA
e-mail: pstein2@northwell.edu

C. H. Zalvan (ed.), *Laryngopharyngeal and Gastroesophageal Reflux*,
https://doi.org/10.1007/978-3-030-48890-1_21

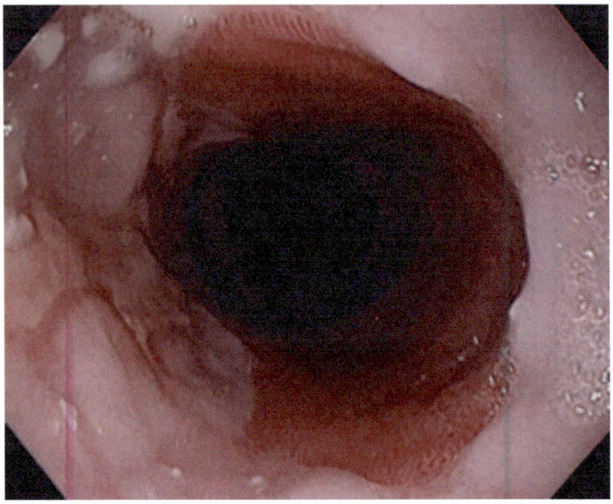

Fig. 21.1 Esophagitis with desquamated mucosa from 6 to 11 o'clock

presence or absence of esophagitis. Reflux symptoms and esophagitis are neither mutually exclusive nor always linked to one another. The take-home point is valuable; however, symptoms do not equate to quantifiable evidence of inflammation. Many patients will have symptoms of reflux in addition to abnormal pH testing; however, they will not have significant mucosal damage. Why do some patients develop mucosal damage, while others are spared? This is likely due to multiple factors which have not yet clearly been elucidated; however, a cytokine-mediated mechanism is clearly at play [4].

Erosive reflux disease, and thus esophagitis, is more prevalent in males, those over age 50, overweight patients, smokers, and patients with a hiatal hernia. These risk factors are fittingly the same as those for Barrett's esophagus, given that esophagitis is a known precursor to Barrett's esophagus [7, 8]. We do not have accurate data on the rate of progression from esophagitis to Barrett's esophagus or esophageal adenocarcinoma. This has been difficult to study, given that over 50 percent of cases of adenocarcinoma arise in patients without a previous history of GERD-related symptoms [9]. However, we do know that esophagitis is a known and established precursor to Barrett's esophagus. In addition, it is well established that Barrett's esophagus is the only known precursor lesion to esophageal adenocarcinoma, with development of dysplasia increasing the risk of progression to cancer [10]. To further support this sequence, we do have data showing reflux symptoms are associated with an increased risk of adenocarcinoma of the esophagus, most substantially in those with severe symptoms [11, 12]. If the presence of reflux symptoms, most notably severe symptoms, increases the risk of esophageal adenocarcinoma, it would be logical to surmise that the presence of esophagitis would increase this risk as well.

Upper endoscopy is the gold standard for documenting the presence and extent of esophagitis, in addition to excluding other etiologies and complications of reflux disease [5]. The earliest signs of esophagitis on endoscopy include edematous-appearing

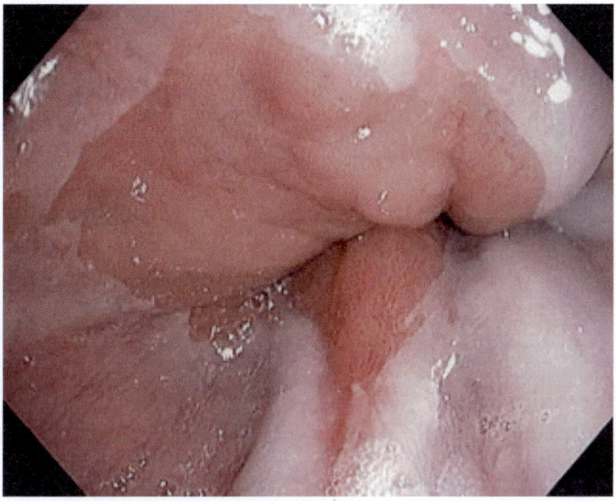

Fig. 21.2 Esophagitis with a linear erosion at 6 o'clock

mucosa and erythema. These findings are followed by friability (easy bleeding of mucosa), granularity, and red streaks. If inflammation progresses, erosions are likely to develop (Fig. 21.2). Erosions can be thought of as early or small ulcers, with shallow breaks in the mucosa. These typically are the result of prolonged acid exposure; however, these can occur with exposure to medications (pill esophagitis), infections, or heavy smoking injury likely related to microvascular insults [13, 14]. Erosions appear as a shallow break with white or yellowish exudate, surrounded by erythematous and edematous mucosa. Most commonly, erosions will begin at the GE junction along the top of esophageal mucosal folds and will appear linear extending proximally. The tops of mucosal folds are most prone to injury from acid exposure, as these mucosal areas are most likely to encounter acidic gastric contents refluxing into the distal esophagus. With severe disease, these mucosal breaks and erosions can extend long distances proximally into the mid- and proximal esophagus and can extend across mucosal folds occasionally resulting in circumferential disease. When erosions are severe and extend deeper into the mucosal and submucosal layers, they are then characterized as ulcers (Fig. 21.3).

The endoscopic grading system most commonly used for esophagitis reflects differences in extent and severity of acid-related disease. The most commonly used grading system used is termed the "LA" classification system, grading severity based on number of mucosal breaks, length, and extent. Grades range from A (mild) to D (most severe) [15]. These grades are determined visually on endoscopy; however, the true presence of esophagitis is confirmed pathologically on biopsy. The development of this grading system allowed for standardization of classification of esophagitis, with easily definable differences in number, length, and extent of mucosal breaks. Complications of reflux, such as strictures, Barrett's esophagus, or ulcers, are reported separately from the extent of esophagitis. Additional grading systems have been utilized, such as the Savary-Miller classification which was considered more ambiguous compared to the LA classification due to the inclusion of GERD-related complications [16].

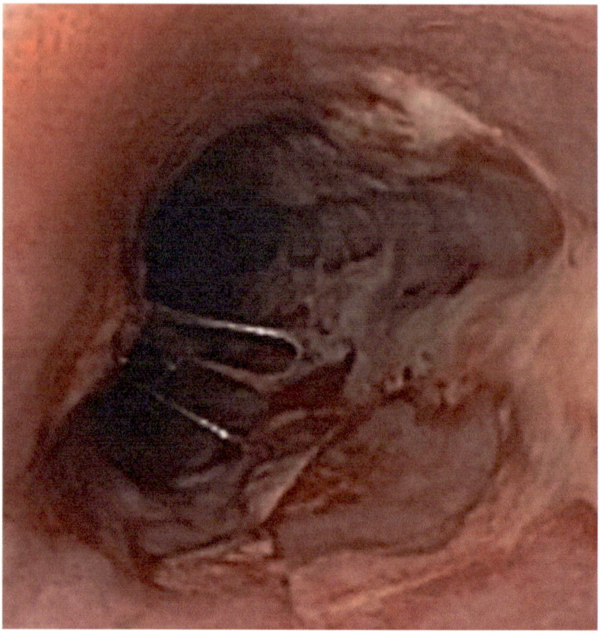

Fig. 21.3 Severe esophagitis (LA Grade D) with ulcerations extending proximally and circumferentially

Biopsy results of esophagitis will show basal cell hyperplasia and increased height of the "rete peg," two classic pathologic findings that are key words for the pathologist (Fig. 21.4) [14]. Additional findings include evidence of acute inflammation, with increased neutrophils and eosinophils. These findings can occasionally be present with normal-appearing mucosa, signifying the presence of reflux with mucosal damage despite their being endoscopically normal-appearing mucosa. Currently, additional imaging techniques, such as endoscopic sprays/stains, image processing, and advanced imaging techniques, do not play a role in the diagnosis of esophagitis.

Esophagitis is typically treated with medications. Mild esophagitis can be treated with a short course of acid-lowering medications and does not necessarily need a repeat endoscopy to confirm healing. Studies have shown that the use of a PPI at standard dosing for a period of 8 weeks will relieve symptoms of GERD and allow for healing of esophagitis in up to 86 percent of patients with documented erosive esophagitis [17, 18]. Moderate or severe esophagitis (LA Grade C or D) requires daily PPI therapy with a repeat endoscopy to rule out underlying Barrett's esophagus or esophageal cancer, normally occurring 8 weeks after starting medical therapy [5]. We treat esophagitis to prevent the formation of complications of GERD – ulcers, hemorrhage, perforation, strictures, Barrett's esophagus, and esophageal cancer. Esophagitis is a known and established precursor to Barrett's esophagus, the only known precursor to esophageal adenocarcinoma.

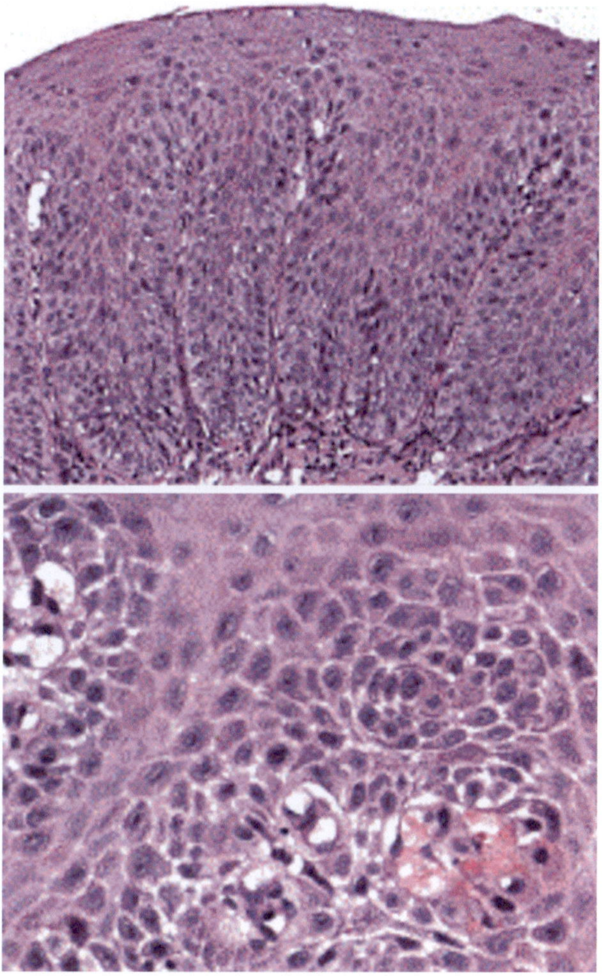

Fig. 21.4 Histologic example of an esophageal epithelium showing basal cell hyperplasia and elongation of stromal papillae

References

1. Boeckxstaens G, El-Serag HB, Smout AJ, Kahrilas PJ. Symptomatic reflux disease: the present, the past, and the future. Gut. 2014;63:1185.
2. Richter JE. Typical and atypical presentations of gastroesophageal reflux daises. The role of esophageal testing in diagnosis and management. Gastroenterol Clin North Am. 1996;25:75.
3. Kahrilas PJ. Turning the pathogenesis of acute peptic esophagitis inside out. JAMA. 2016;315:2077.
4. Souza RF, Huo X, Mittal V, et al. Gastroesophageal reflux might cause esophagitis through a cytokine-mediated mechanism rather than caustic acid injury. Gastroenterology. 2009;137:1776.
5. Katz PO, Gerson LB, Vela MF. Guidelines for the diagnosis and management of gastroesophageal reflux disease. Am J Gastroenterol. 2013;108:308.

6. Pritchett JM, Aslam M, Slaughter JC, et al. Efficacy of esophageal impedance/pH monitoring in patients with refractory gastroesophageal reflux disease, on an off therapy. Clin Gastroenterol Hepatol. 2009;7:743.
7. Castro C, Peleteiro B, Lunet N. Modifiable factors and esophageal cancer: a systematic review of published meta-analyses. J Gastroentrol. 2018;53:37.
8. Engel LS, Chow WH, Vaughan TL, et al. Population attributable risks of esophageal and gastric cancers. J Natl Cancer Inst. 2003;95:1404.
9. Bytzer P, Christensen PB, Damkier P, et al. Adenocarcinoma of the esophagus and Barrett's esophagus: a population based study. Am J Gastroenterol. 1999;94:86.
10. Qumseya BJ, Wani S, Gendy S, et al. Disease progression in Barrett's low-grade dysplasia with radiofrequency ablation compared with surveillance: systematic review and meta-analysis. Am J Gastroenterol. 2017;112:849.
11. Rubenstein JH, Taylor JB. Meta-analysis: the association of oesophageal adenocarcinoma with symptoms of gastro-oesophageal reflux. Aliment Pharmacol Ther. 2010;32:1222.
12. Lagergren J, Bergstrom R, Lindgren A, Nyren O. Symptomatic gastroesophageal reflux as a risk factor for esophageal adenocarcinoma. N Engl J Med. 1999;340:825.
13. Feldman M, Friedman LS, Brandt L. Sleisenger and Fordtran's gastrointestinal and liver disease. Philadelphia, PA: Saunders Elsevier; 2015:705–26.
14. Dent J. Microscopic esophageal mucosal injury in nonerosive reflux disease. Clin Gastroenterol Hepatol. 2007;5:4.
15. Dibaise JK. The LA classification for esophagitis: a call for standardization. Am J Gastroenterol. 1999;94:3402.
16. Monnier P, Savary M. Contribution of endoscopy to gastroesophageal reflux disease. Scand J Gastroenterol. 1984;19:26.
17. Hunt R. Acid suppression for reflux disease: "off-the-peg" or a tailored approach? Clinc Gastroenterol Hepatol. 2012;10:210.
18. Wolfe MM, Sachs G. Acid suppression: optimizing therapy for gastroduodenal ulcer healing, gastroesophageal reflux disease, and stress-related erosive syndrome. Gastroenterology. 2000;118:S9.

Chapter 22
Barrett's Esophagus

Peter H. Stein

Barrett's esophagus is a long-term complication of chronic reflux. It is a response that the esophagus undergoes as a consequence of long-term acid exposure. Barrett's esophagus is defined by the presence of abnormal columnar mucosa in the esophagus that is predisposed to malignancy – specifically esophageal adenocarcinomas [1]. Barrett's esophagus is the only known precursor to esophageal adenocarcinoma, making its diagnosis and management imperative in preventing progression to cancer.

Barrett's esophagus results from damage to the normal esophageal squamous epithelium. Prolonged exposure of the esophageal squamous mucosa to low-pH stomach acid results in recurrent and/or continuous inflammation, specifically esophagitis [2]. This may or may not be symptomatic. Many patients with Barrett's esophagus will report no prior history of significant reflux symptoms; however, many will report long-term heartburn or reflux [3]. The formation of Barrett's esophagus does not require the patient to have had symptoms of heartburn or reflux previously. In addition, Barrett's esophagus itself is asymptomatic, meaning that we cannot know the presence of Barrett's esophagus without testing for it, as many patients with Barrett's esophagus will have no current or previous symptoms associated with the disease.

As a response to long-term inflammation, the squamous mucosa in the esophagus will undergo a protective change, which over time will lead to a replacement with columnar epithelium. This is a metaplastic process, meaning that the tissue in this area changes from one type to another. The resultant abnormal columnar epithelium is termed "intestinal metaplasia," as the new epithelium appears as that of the intestinal mucosa. This represents the presence of Barrett's esophagus. The body in this instance undergoes a metaplastic change to try to protect itself from repeated bouts of inflammation [4]. Barrett's epithelial cells appear to be more resistant to acid-related

P. H. Stein (✉)
Division of Gastroenterology, Phelps Hospital, Northwell Health, Sleepy Hollow, NY, USA
e-mail: pstein2@northwell.edu

C. H. Zalvan (ed.), *Laryngopharyngeal and Gastroesophageal Reflux*,
https://doi.org/10.1007/978-3-030-48890-1_22

injury compared to that of squamous epithelium, likely due to the secretion of mucus from goblet cells and tighter mucosal junctions – much like that of intestinal mucosa that is normally exposed to stomach acid [5]. Unfortunately, the presence of this change greatly increases the risk for progression to adenocarcinoma.

Barrett's esophagus is most commonly diagnosed in those greater than 55 years old [6]. It is rare in children younger than 10 and nonexistent in those younger than 5, reflecting the nature of this disease as a result of accumulated genetic abnormalities over time [7]. Risk factors include age greater than 50, male sex, Caucasian race, obesity, family history, long-standing reflux, erosive esophagitis, and a history of smoking [8]. GERD is strongly associated with both Barrett's esophagus and esophageal adenocarcinoma, although not all patients with either condition necessarily have to have a history of GERD.

The prevalence of both Barrett's esophagus and esophageal adenocarcinoma has been steadily rising for unclear reasons [9]. One hypothesis links the declining incidence of *Helicobacter pylori* infection of the stomach as a contributing factor, as this infection decreases stomach acid. *Helicobacter pylori* incidence has been decreasing due to widespread antibiotic use and increased awareness of the infection through routine testing, with resultant appropriate treatment. Patients with untreated *Helicobacter pylori* will have decreased gastric acid production, as the bacteria act to shut off acid production to a degree, making for a more hospitable environment for bacterial replication. As a result, according to this hypothesis, decreased stomach acid would result in decreased acid exposure within the distal esophagus, thus decreasing the risk of the inflammatory sequence occurring leading to formation of Barrett's esophagus. Conversely, as we continue to decrease the incidence of *H. pylori* through appropriate antibiotic use, we are as a result increasing the gastric acid secretion in patients who otherwise may not have had their infections treated. This hypothesis would surmise that a certain number of these patients will develop reflux, increasing the risk of Barrett's esophagus and esophageal adenocarcinoma formation.

The increasing prevalence of obesity is thought to be a contributing factor as well, although the exact mechanism related to obesity has not been adequately delineated. Many hypotheses exist [10]. The increased consumption of red and processed meats in addition to other processed foods and decreased consumption of fresh vegetables, fruits, whole grains, nuts, and seeds have been thought to potentially play a role. This hypothesis extends well beyond the realm of the upper GI tract, as we now know of the importance of healthy dietary choices in our overall health.

Barrett's esophagus is currently diagnosed by endoscopy. Columnar-appearing mucosa must be endoscopically present. This appears as "salmon-colored" mucosa with a velvety texture that extends proximally starting at the GE junction into the tubular esophagus (Figs. 22.1 and 22.2).

This appears different from that of the normal esophageal mucosa, which appears paler, smoother, and slightly shiny or glossy. The length and extent of circumferential abnormal mucosa are graded endoscopically based on the Prague criteria. These criteria, originally determined by consensus guidelines, delineate the extent of

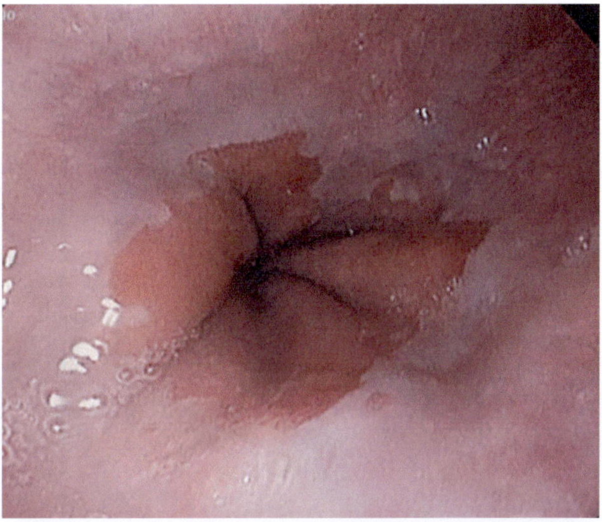

Fig. 22.1 Normal appearing GE junction with a slightly irregular/jagged Z-line

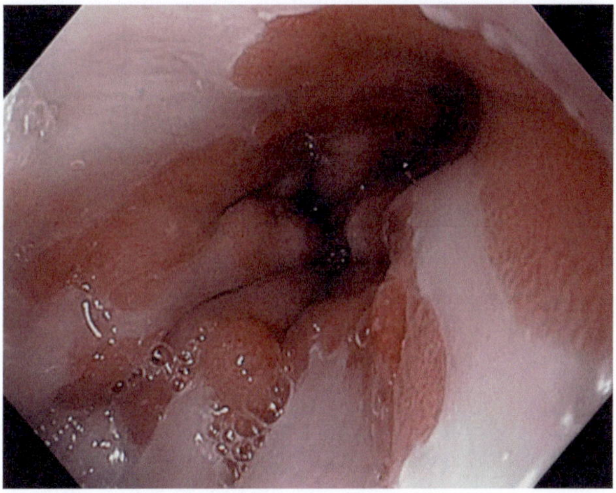

Fig. 22.2 Barrett's esophagus with salmon-colored mucosa extending proximally into the distal esophagus

circumferential Barrett's esophagus. The length of circumferential abnormal mucosa in centimeters is determined, measured from the top of the gastric folds at the GE junction proximally. The maximal length of "tongues" of abnormal mucosa extending proximal to the circumferential Barrett's esophagus is also measured. For instance, if circumferential salmon-colored mucosa extends from the GE junction 4 cm, with additional tongues of tissue extending an additional 2 cm, we would grade this as "C4M6" Barrett's esophagus. This is called the Prague C/M criteria and is widely accepted by gastroenterologists as an accurate way to describe endoscopic findings of Barrett's esophagus [11]. The presence of mucosal nodules or abnormalities, in addition to ulcers, erosions, or strictures, is noted. Any of these abnormalities increases the risk of progression to dysplastic mucosa or cancer.

Barrett's esophagus is further subdivided into short- or long-length Barrett's esophagus. Short length is considered anything less than 3 cm, while long length is considered greater than 3 cm. If the GE junction at the level of the squamocolumnar junction (the Z-line, where the esophageal mucosa transitions to gastric mucosa) appears mildly irregular or jagged but does not extend more than 1 cm, biopsies are not performed. This is due to the thought that Barrett's esophagus less than 1 cm is not clinically significant [12]. This recommendation is based on expert opinion and will likely require more high-quality data to further confirm the insignificance of an "irregular Z-line." In practice, the option to biopsy during an endoscopy becomes a judgment call based on the opinion of the performing endoscopist.

Biopsy or tissue sampling by brushing confirms the presence of intestinal metaplasia. Currently, standard of care for tissue sampling involves a "cup" or "bite" biopsy, in which a piece of tissue is removed with a forceps through the working channel of the endoscope. Recently, the addition of a brush biopsy device has been employed in an effort to increase tissue sampling and further identification of metaplastic or dysplastic epithelium [13]. This is performed using a brush that is advanced through the working channel of the endoscope, after which stiff bristles of the brush are scraped against abnormal-appearing mucosa. The tip of the brush is then removed and placed in a sterile container. Through processing of abnormal cells captured by the brush, cytologic examination can be performed allowing for determination of the presence of abnormal cells.

Nonendoscopic methods have been developed for diagnosis as well, chiefly a sponge device that can be swallowed. The patient swallows a gelatin capsule that is attached to a string. As the capsule dissolves in the stomach when exposed to gastric acid, a mesh sponge is exposed which is then withdrawn through the esophagus, thus collecting superficial cells of the esophagus. An immunohistochemical marker is then used to identify Barrett's epithelium compared to normal esophageal mucosa [14]. Initial studies have been encouraging, showing a sensitivity greater than 90 percent and a specificity greater than 94 percent for patients with Barrett's esophagus greater than 2 cm [14]. This test relies greatly on patient participation, with the understanding that many patients may not agree to this type of test.

Barrett's esophagus pathologically is subdivided into dysplastic or non-dysplastic mucosa. Dysplasia represents the presence of a series of architectural abnormalities that go beyond the scope of this text. However, the presence of dysplasia constitutes a step further toward esophageal adenocarcinoma and is due to genetic alterations that accumulate over time, leading to potentially dangerous morphologic changes. The diagnosis and grading of dysplasia into low-grade dysplasia vs. high-grade dysplasia have been controversial, as it is difficult for pathologists to adequately distinguish [15]. This typically requires the opinion of an expert GI pathologist. It is standard to confirm the presence of Barrett's esophagus with dysplasia with a second opinion pathology evaluation. High-grade dysplasia increases the risk of progression to esophageal adenocarcinoma greater than that of low-grade dysplasia [16, 17]. Unfortunately, dysplasia does not have characteristic endoscopic characteristics, making tissue sampling the only well-established and accepted means of diagnosis.

If Barrett's esophagus is seen on endoscopy, the endoscopist traditionally performs four-quadrant biopsies of the affected area of the esophagus over 1–2 cm. These biopsies are somewhat random, resulting in a significant risk of sampling error. If visible nodules, masses, or ulcers are present, the endoscopist would typically perform specific sampling of these affected areas with a biopsy forceps. If a nodule is present, it would be appropriate to perform wider sampling termed "endoscopic mucosal resection," which is the same technique used to remove large colonic polyps. The endoscopist should remove the entire area of mucosa with the defined nodule or modularity, preferably in one uninterrupted piece of mucosa to allow for adequate pathologic evaluation.

Multiple advanced imaging techniques have been developed to address the problem of sampling error. Chromoendoscopy requires the endoscopist to spray or lavage the area of Barrett's esophagus with a dye that aides in identification of dysplastic or abnormal areas (Fig. 22.3). Autofluorescence, magnification imaging, and narrow-band imaging use image processing through the endoscope or image processor to enhance visual abnormalities. Often, the junction between normal esophageal and gastric mucosa can subtly change. As can be seen in Fig. 22.4, narrow-band imaging allows for easy identification of this transition in a patient with a normal GE junction (Fig. 4). Confocal laser endomicroscopy, optical coherence tomography, and volumetric laser endomicroscopy are imaging techniques that visualize architectural mucosal abnormalities on the scale of micrometers to millimeters. Specifically, confocal laser endomicroscopy and volumetric laser endomicroscopy have shown great potential in identifying and marking abnormalities that should be further sampled. These imaging techniques are primarily used in tertiary centers, the details of which are beyond the scope of this text [18].

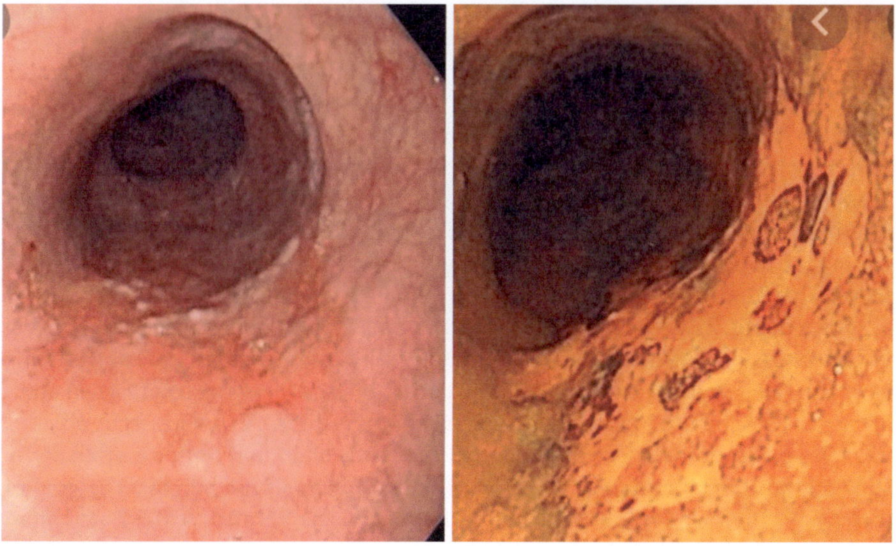

Fig. 22.3 Chromoendoscopy with indigo carmine spray highlighting subtle esophageal mucosal abnormalities. (wikimediacommons.org)

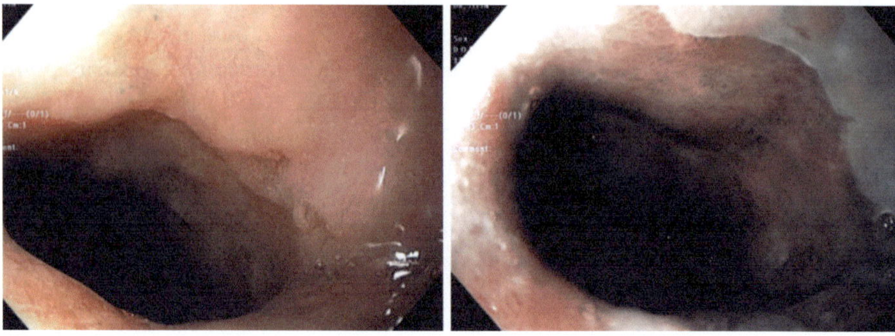

Fig. 22.4 A difficult to visualize Z-line visualized with normal white light (left) and narrow-band imaging (right)

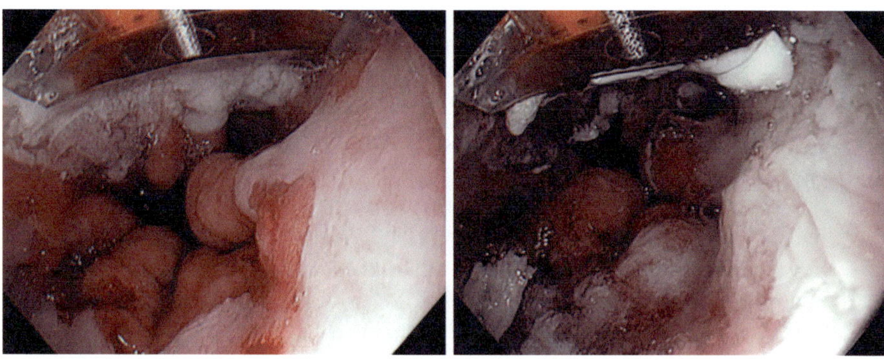

Fig. 22.5 Radiofrequency ablation (RFA) of short-segment Barrett's esophagus at the beginning of a session of RFA (left) and toward the end of a session (right)

The mainstay of treatment of Barrett's esophagus is acid suppression. Ample evidence exists showing that acid suppression protects against progression of Barrett's esophagus to a higher grade, meaning prevention of bland Barrett's esophagus to low-grade dysplasia and so on [19–21]. If dysplasia is present, endoscopic ablative therapies are recommended. Currently, we have strong supporting data for the use of radiofrequency ablation (RFA), a thermal therapy administered endoscopically [22, 23]. Figure 22.5 illustrates the same patient with Barrett's esophagus as shown in Fig. 22.2, both during initial RFA and later in the process of RFA during the same session. Cryotherapy and thermal therapy using argon plasma coagulation have also been studied, with cryotherapy currently used most frequently as an alternative to RFA or used as salvage therapy for RFA [25]. All endoscopic ablative therapies inflict tissue injury deep enough to destroy abnormal Barrett's epithelium, allowing this epithelium to be replaced with neosquamous epithelium. The goal of therapy is complete remission of intestinal metaplasia, termed "CRIM" for short [24]. Extensive endoscopic mucosal resection and surgery with resection of the affected segment have also been used and, however, have been supplanted by less invasive treatments. Currently, RFA is the preferred treatment choice due to its effectiveness and low morbidity and mortality. It is important to note that diagnosis and treatment of Barrett's esophagus are a rapidly evolving area within gastroenterology, with recommendations frequently changing to reflect new data. Current treatments have not yet focused on the importance of dietary changes. Focus on dietary changes in the setting of Barrett's esophagus should be geared toward the underlying treatment of GERD rather than Barrett's esophagus specifically, as the presence of Barrett's esophagus is due to long-term reflux. No dietary studies have as yet been performed addressing the role of diet in Barrett's esophagus. This area of research will surely be addressed in the coming years. Currently, treatment is often individualized based on age, comorbidities, life expectancy, and expert availability.

References

1. Castro C, Peleteiro B, Lunet N. Modifiable factors and esophageal cancer: a systematic review of published meta-analyses. J Gastroentrol. 2018;53:37.
2. Taylor JB, Rubenstein JH. Meta-analyses of the effect of symptoms of gastroesophageal reflux on the risk of Barrett's esophagus. Am J Gastroenterol. 2010;105:1729.
3. Gerson LB, Shetler K, Triadafilopoulos G. Prevalence of Barrett's esophagus in asymptomatic individuals. Gastroenterology. 2002;123:461.
4. Fletcher J, Wirz A, Henry E, McColl KE. Studies of acid exposure immediately above the gastro-esophageal squamocolumnar junction: evidence of short segment reflux. Gut. 2004;53:168.
5. Que J, Garman KS, Souza RF, Spechler SJ. Pathogenesis and cells of origin of Barrett's esophagus. Gastroenterology. 2019;157:349.
6. Spechler SJ. Barrett's esophagus. Semin Gastrointest Dis. 1996;7:51.
7. Hassal E. Columnar-lined esophagus in children. Gastroenterol Clin N Am. 1997;26:533.
8. Cook MB, Shaheen NJ, Anderson LA, et al. Cigarette smoking increases risk of Barrett's esophagus: an analysis of the Barrett's and Esophageal Adenocarcinoma Consortium. Gastroenterology. 2012;142:744.
9. Spechler SJ, Souza RF. Barrett's esophagus. N Engl J Med. 2014;371:836.
10. Kamat P, Wen S, Morris J, Anandasabapathy S. Exploring the association between elevated body mass index and Barrett's esophagus: a systematic review and meta-analysis. Ann Thorac Surg. 2009;87:655.
11. Alvarez Herrero L, Curvers WL, van Vilsteren FG, et al. Validation of the Prague C&M classification of Barrett's esophagus in clinical practice. Endoscopy. 2013;45:876.
12. Spechler SJ. Intestinal metaplasia at the gastroesophageal junction. Gastroenterology. 2004;126:567.
13. Goldlum JR, Shaheen NJ, Vennalaganti PR, Sharma P, Lightdale CJ. WATS for Barrett's surveillance. Gastrointest Endosc. 2018;88:201.
14. Kadri SR, Lao-Sirieix P, O'Donovan M, et al. Acceptability and accuracy of a non-endoscopic screening test for Barrett's oesophagus in primary care: cohort study. BMJ. 2010;341:c4372.
15. Vennalaganti P, Kanakadandi V, Goldblum JR, et al. Discordance among pathologists in the United States and Europe in diagnosis of low-grade dysplasia for patients with Barrett's esophagus. Gastroenterology. 2017;152:564.
16. Qumseya BJ, Wani S, Gendy S, et al. Disease progression in Barrett's low-grade dysplasia with radiofrequency ablation compared with surveillance: systematic review and meta-analysis. Am J Gastroenterol. 2017;112:849.

17. Rugge M, Fassan M, Cavallin F, Zaninotto G. Re: risk of malignant progression in Barrett's esophagus patients: results from a large population based study. J Natl Cancer Inst. 2012;104:1771.
18. Spechler SJ, Katzka DA, Fitzgerald RC. New screening techniques in Barrett's esophagus: great ideas or great practice? Gastroenterology. 2018;154:1594.
19. Singh S, Garg SK, Singh PP, et al. Acid-suppressive medications and risk of esophageal adenocarcinoma in patients with Barrett's oesophagus: a systematic review and meta-analysis. Gut. 2014;63:1229.
20. Nguyen DM, El-Serag HB, Henderson L, et al. Mediation usage and the risk of neoplasia in patients with Barrett's esophagus. Clin Gastroenterol Hepatol. 2009;7:1299.
21. Kastelein F, Spaander MC, Steyerberg EW, et al. Proton pump inhibitors reduce the risk of neoplastic progression in patients with Barrett's esophagus. Clin Gastroenterol Hepatol. 2013;11:382.
22. Shaheen NJ, Sharma P, Overholt BF, et al. Radiofrequency ablation in Barrett's esophagus with dysplasia. N Engl J Med. 2009;360:2277.
23. Orman ES, Li N, Shaheen NJ. Efficacy and durability of radio frequency ablation for Barrett's esophagus: systematic review and meta-analysis. Clin Gastroenterol Hepatol. 2013;11:1245.
24. Gosain S, Mecer K, Twaddell WS, et al. Liquid nitrogen spray cryotherapy in Barrett's esophagus with high-grade dysplasia: long-term results. Gastrointest Endosc. 2013;78:260.

Chapter 23
GERD: Differential Diagnosis and Related Diseases

Peter H. Stein

Gastroesophageal reflux disease (GERD) is a spectrum of disease that culminates as a result of gastric contents refluxing into the esophagus. It is important to note that gastroesophageal reflux, meaning the retrograde passage of gastric contents into the esophagus, is not a disease in and unto itself. This is a normal physiologic phenomenon that occurs throughout the day in all individuals [1]. When this normal physiologic process manifests with symptoms or other related diseases, we then term this GERD [2].

The most common symptoms of gastroesophageal reflux are heartburn and regurgitation, both considered classic reflux symptoms [2]. It is estimated that approximately 10–20 percent of the Western world will have symptoms of GERD, with most of these patients experiencing either heartburn or regurgitation [3]. Patients with heartburn will typically complain of a burning feeling in their stomach just below the diaphragm or within the chest along that anatomic location of the esophagus. Symptoms can occur along the entirety of the esophagus up to the cervical esophagus; however, it is common for patients to have symptoms in distinct areas that do not encompass the entirety of the esophagus (Table 23.1). Symptoms can worsen after eating, specifically with spicy foods, citrus, acidic foods, chocolates, carbonated beverages, caffeine, coffee or tea (decaffeinated as well as caffeinated), and alcohol. Cigarette smoking is a common exacerbating factor, as are weight gain and pregnancy [4] (Table 23.2). Many patients will report exacerbation of symptoms when laying down, requiring them to sleep upright or on an incline. Regurgitation can be exacerbated by the same triggers as for heartburn and constitutes the sensation of acidic fluid or food contents spontaneously traveling from the stomach to the mid or proximal esophagus and the back of the mouth. Additional symptoms can include dysphagia (difficulty swallowing), a sour taste in the back of the mouth called "water brash," odynophagia (pain on swallowing), burping, chest/

P. H. Stein (✉)
Division of Gastroenterology, Phelps Hospital, Northwell Health, Sleepy Hollow, NY, USA
e-mail: pstein2@northwell.edu

C. H. Zalvan (ed.), *Laryngopharyngeal and Gastroesophageal Reflux*,
https://doi.org/10.1007/978-3-030-48890-1_23

Table 23.1 Symptoms of GERD

Symptoms	
Heartburn	Nausea
Regurgitation	Hoarseness
Chest pain	Wheezing
Globus sensation	Dysphagia
Chronic cough	Odynophagia
Water brash (sour taste)	Burping
Epigastric pain	

Table 23.2 Exacerbating factors of GERD

Exacerbating factors	
Postprandial state	Overeating
Spicy foods	Acidic foods/citrus
Chocolate	Carbonated beverages
Caffeine	Coffee and tea (caffeinated and decaffeinated)
Alcohol	Nicotine
Lying down	Pregnancy
Weight gain	

epigastric pain, and nausea [5]. Symptom descriptions and exacerbating factors can vary widely; heartburn symptoms are by no means consistent across multiple patients. Because of the wide variability in patient symptoms, the practitioner evaluating patients for GERD must keep an open mind and cast a wide net.

It is important to note that the underlying causes of GERD are not necessarily the same as common exacerbating factors. For instance, a patient may complain of worsening symptoms after eating certain acidic foods. The food that they are ingesting has not caused the underlying anatomic or physiologic abnormality leading to underlying GERD, but rather exacerbates their previously existing condition. This common misunderstanding leads to frequent labeling of certain foods as causes of the underlying disease, with avoidance of certain otherwise perfectly healthy foods. The physician and patient are best served focusing on the underlying cause while still avoiding any foods or other factors that may lead to patient distress or discomfort.

Symptoms of GERD may be mimicked by other diseases [2] (Table 23.3). Achalasia and other motility disorders can cause heartburn, regurgitation, and chest discomfort. A Zenker's diverticulum or other esophageal diverticula can cause a sense of regurgitation due to food contents accumulating, in addition to causing significant halitosis. Gastroparesis will commonly cause heartburn due to increased volume and the prolonged presence of gastric contents, leading to decreased lower esophageal pressure. This can result in contents refluxing into the esophagus, causing a variety of symptoms including at times severe GERD-related symptoms [6]. Peptic ulcer disease can cause epigastric burning similar to that of heartburn. Functional dyspepsia, an upper gastrointestinal form of discomfort analogous to

Table 23.3 Differential diagnosis of GERD

Differential diagnosis	
Achalasia/motility disorders	Zenker's diverticulum
Gastroparesis	Peptic ulcer disease
Functional dyspepsia	Eosinophilic esophagitis
Atypical cardiac disease symptoms	Pill esophagitis
Radiation esophagitis	Infectious esophagitis
Pregnancy	Scleroderma
Parkinson's disease	Zollinger-Ellison disease
Post-esophageal myotomy	Post-bariatric surgery

irritable bowel syndrome, can cause pain and discomfort not unlike that of acid-related disease [7]. Eosinophilic esophagitis, an inflammatory condition of the esophagus related to specific food allergies, commonly causes dysphagia [8]. However additional symptoms can overlap significantly with GERD symptoms. Lastly, atypical cardiac symptoms of angina pectoris may include burning in the lower chest that can mimic heartburn. An astute practitioner will always rule out cardiac disease prior to working up GI causes of discomfort. If a patient has risk factors for cardiac disease or additional symptoms that can be explained by a cardiac etiology such as left arm numbness/pain or shortness of breath, cardiac disease should be rule out prior to any additional gastrointestinal workup. Conversely, if a patient has no additional concerning risk factors or symptoms, it would be reasonable to proceed with a workup for GERD initially.

Harm to the esophagus can exist that will manifest the same symptoms as that of GERD and, however, is not due to reflux-related disease. These can include pill esophagitis, radiation esophagitis, and infectious causes of esophagitis [9–11]. Many pills have been implicated as a cause of irritation to the esophagus if they do not pass expeditiously into the stomach, most notably bisphosphonates, potassium supplements, and NSAIDs; however, the list of potential medications that can affect the esophagus goes well beyond these three common classes of medications [12]. Especially in the immunocompromised patient, numerous pathogens can affect the esophagus including candida and herpes [11]. Frequently, patients who are using steroid inhalers for pulmonary disease (asthma, COPD) will inadvertently swallow a portion of the steroid [13]. Endoscopy in this setting will reveal small white plaques that appear to wash or brush off with lavage or biopsy, pathognomonic for candidal esophagitis. All the above disease processes can cause heartburn or dysphagia, overlapping with symptoms of GERD.

Certain other disease processes or normal physiologic states can predispose to GERD. The most common and most easily recognizable is pregnancy. Reports vary widely as to the incidence of heartburn in pregnancy, ranging from 40 to 85% of pregnant women reporting heartburn at some point during their pregnancy [14]. This is due to a decrease in lower esophageal pressure due to estrogen and progesterone in the first trimester. Later in pregnancy, mechanical factors take precedence, with the gravid uterus exerting pressure on the stomach resulting in the frequent reflux of gastric contents. Luckily, most women report complete resolution of symptoms after delivery, making this cause self-limited [15].

Scleroderma commonly causes esophageal symptoms, with up to 90% of those afflicted with the disease experiencing GERD symptoms [16]. This is due to smooth muscle fibrosis and scarring in the distal esophagus, resulting in decreased lower esophageal pressure and the reflux of stomach contents, in addition to weak and/or absent peristalsis [16]. This results in food stasis in the lower esophagus, almost always manifesting with heartburn and dysphagia. Up to 70% of patients with scleroderma will have evidence of esophagitis [17]. Almost all of these patients will need treatment with acid-lowering medications to control symptoms given their significant and often irreversible underlying anatomic disease.

Parkinson's disease can affect the entirety of the GI tract, with decreased peristalsis. This includes the esophagus, with decreased ability to pass a food bolus successfully from the mouth to the stomach [18]. Zollinger-Ellison syndrome, the disease of markedly increased acid hypersecretion as a result of increased gastrin, almost always will result in heartburn in addition to classic findings of gastroduodenal ulcers [19]. Patients who have had a myotomy of their lower esophageal sphincter for the treatment of achalasia will often have resultant reflux symptoms [20]. Lastly, patients who undergo bariatric surgery will frequently complain of heartburn, regurgitation, and nausea. This is due to a variety of factors, including decreased gastric accommodation of food contents, neurologic and hormonal factors, and damage to the lower esophageal sphincter [21].

Regardless of cause, there are various etiologies of the symptoms of GERD. An adept practitioner will think beyond the scope of classic GERD and will consider additional causes. The true skill of the diagnostician lies in teasing out the rare causes in those with common symptoms.

References

1. Richter JE. Typical and atypical presentation of gastroesophageal reflux disease. The role of esophageal testing in diagnosis and management. Gastroenterol Clin North Am. 1996;25:75.
2. Vakil N, van Zanten SV, Kahrilas P, et al. The Montreal definition and classification of gastroesophageal reflux disease: a global evidence-based consensus. Am J Gastroenterol. 2006;101:1900.
3. Dent J, El-Serag HB, Wallander MA, et al. Epidemiology of gastro-oesophageal reflux disease: a systematic review. Gut. 2005;54:710.
4. Corley DA, Kubo A. Body mass index and gastroesophageal reflux disease: a systematic review and meta-analysis. Am J Gastroenterol. 2006;101:2619.
5. Vakil NB, Traxler B, Levine D. Dysphagia in patients with erosive esophagitis: prevalence, severity and response to proton pump inhibitor treatment. Clin Gastroenterol Hepatol. 2004;2:665.
6. Triadafilopoulos G, Nguyen L, Clarke JO. Patients with symptoms of delayed gastric emptying have a high prevalence of oesophageal dysmotility, irrespective of scintigraphic evidence of gastroparesis. BMJ Open Gastroenterol. 2017;14:4.
7. Walker MM, Potter MD, Talley NJ. Tangible pathologies in functional dyspepsia. Best Pract Res Clin Gastroenterol. 2019;40:101650.
8. Ahmad M, Soetikno RM, Ahmed A. The differential diagnosis of eosinophilic esophagitis. J Clin Gastroenterol. 2000;30:242.

9. Zografos GN, Georgiadou D, Thomas D, et al. Drug-induced esophagitis. Dis Esophagus. 2009;22:633.
10. Chowhan NM. Injurious effects of radiation on the esophagus. Am J Gastroenterol. 1990;85:115.
11. O'Rourke A. Infective oesophagitis: epidemiology, cause, diagnosis, and treatment options. Curr Opin Otolaryngol Head Neck Surg. 2015;23:459.
12. Jaspersen D. Drug-induced oesophageal disorders: pathogenesis, incidence, prevention, and management. Drug Sad. 2000;22:237.
13. Kanda N, Yasuba H, Takahashi T, et al. Prevalence of esophageal candidiasis among patents treated with inhaled fluticasone propionate. Am J Gastroenterol. 2003;98:2146.
14. Ali RA, Egan LJ. Gastroesophageal reflux disease in pregnancy. Best Pract Res Clin Gastroenterol. 2007;21:793.
15. Rey E, Rodriguez-Artalejo F, Herraiz MA, et al. Gastroesophageal reflux symptoms during and after pregnancy: a longitudinal study. Am J Gastroenterol. 2007;102:2395.
16. Marie I, Dominique S, Lévesque H, et al. Esophageal involvement and pulmonary manifestations in systemic sclerosis. Arthritis Rheum. 2001;45:346.
17. Medsger TA Jr, Masi AT, Rodnan GP, et al. Survival with systemic sclerosis (scleroderma). A life-table analysis of clinical and demographic factors in 309 patients. Ann Intern Med. 1971;75:369.
18. Kalf JG, de Swart BJ, Bloem BR, Munneke M. Prevalence of oropharyngeal dysphagia in Parkinson's disease: a meta-analysis. Parkinsonism Relat Disord. 2012;18:311.
19. Ellison EC, Johnson JA. The Zollinger-Ellison syndrome: a comprehensive review of historical, scientific, and clinical considerations. Curr Probl Surg. 2009;46:13.
20. Richards WO, Torquato A, Holzman MD, et al. Heller myotomy versus Heller myotomy with Dor fundoplication for achalasia: a prospective randomized double-blind clinical trial. Ann Surg. 2004;240:405.
21. Cedar A, Appelbaum L, Schweiger C, et al. Dilated upper sleeve can be associated with severe postoperative gastroesophageal dysmotility and reflux. Obes Surg. 2010;20:140.

Chapter 24
Esophagogastroduodenoscopy (EGD) and Esophageal Ultrasound

Peter H. Stein

Upper endoscopy comprises visualization of the oropharynx, esophagus, stomach, and proximal duodenum using an endoscope. This can be called upper endoscopy (shortened “EGD”), upper gastrointestinal (GI) endoscopy, esophagogastroduodenoscopy, or trans-nasal endoscopy (TNE). The endoscope is a thin, flexible tube with a light and a camera at the tip. Passage of the endoscope through the mouth into the upper GI tract allows for direct real-time assessment and sampling, if indicated. Multiple types of upper endoscopes exist, varying by manufacturer, size, and capabilities. A standard upper endoscope is typically around 1 cm in diameter (Fig. 24.1). Three manufacturers comprise the vast majority of endoscopes used currently, those being Olympus, Pentax, and Fujifilm. All endoscopes regardless of size or manufacturer allow for real-time assessment; however, certain endoscopes allow the endoscopist to perform various types of interventions, including tissue sampling, injection of medications or substances, placement of clips, needle aspiration, or ultrasound. Endoscopic quality standards have been well established and include appropriate patient selection and preparation prior to the procedure, adequate and appropriate use of sedation, assessment and awareness of normal versus abnormal findings including appropriate tissue sampling and therapeutic interventions, and straightforward follow-up and communication post-procedure, to name a few [1, 2].

In addition, the most standard upper endoscopes currently allow for the use of real-time optical image enhancement. Depending on the manufacturer, current technologies alter the real-time image to enhance mucosal patterns and the visibility of superficial blood vessels. Current iterations of these technologies considered “digital chromoendoscopy,” function through either filtering out specific wavelengths of light, or further processing the images through proprietary software within the

P. H. Stein (✉)
Division of Gastroenterology, Phelps Hospital, Northwell Health, Sleepy Hollow, NY, USA
e-mail: pstein2@northwell.edu

C. H. Zalvan (ed.), *Laryngopharyngeal and Gastroesophageal Reflux*,
https://doi.org/10.1007/978-3-030-48890-1_24

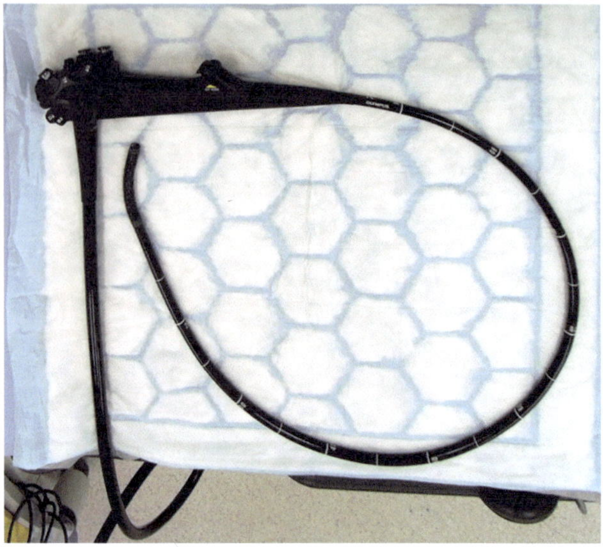

Fig. 24.1 A standard upper endoscope. (Courtesy of wikimediacommons.org)

endoscope processor. Current technologies include narrowband imaging (Olympus), flexible spectral imaging color enhancement (Fujifilm), and i-scan (Pentax Medical) [3, 4] (Fig. 24.2).

The standard upper endoscopes contain a working channel that allows passage of devices through the handheld potion of the endoscope into the area in which the tip of the endoscope is passed (Fig. 24.1). This has allowed the endoscopist to employ a host of various diagnostic and therapeutic devices, many of which are beyond the scope of this text. In short, options include tissue sampling, injection of various substances and medications, ultrasound imaging, optical coherence tomography imaging, confocal microscopy, thermal therapies, dilation, needle puncture, and endoscopic suturing devices [5–8]. All of the aforementioned diagnostic or therapeutic modalities have been developed for use through the working channel or via a distal attachment to the tip of currently available endoscopes. Device development in this realm is rapidly developing and expanding, with new tools available to the endoscopist on an ever-changing basis.

EGD is typically performed with the patient sedated in an endoscopy suite; however, it can be performed in an ambulatory setting with the patient awake in the case of trans-nasal endoscopy. This is due to the thinner nature of the TNE endoscope, which is less stimulating to the patient compared to a standard upper endoscope. For standard upper endoscopy, the patient typically lies on their left side, allowing any stomach contents or secretions (if present) to sit along the fundus and greater curvature of the stomach. This decreases the risk of aspiration of stomach contents or secretions. Of course, the patient should be free of stomach contents as they should be fasting prior to any endoscopic procedures. Occasionally, patients with gastroparesis, foreign bodies, or upper gastrointestinal bleeding will have contents present in their stomach (Fig. 24.3; normal stomach).

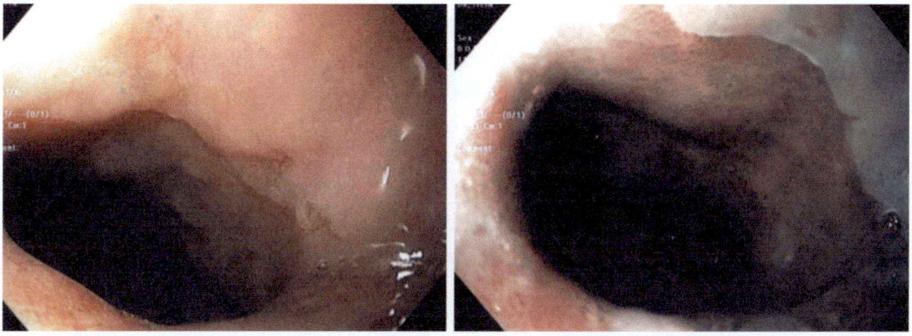

Fig. 24.2 A normal appearing GE junction view with white light (left) and narrowband imaging (right). (NBI vs. normal picture)

Fig. 24.3 A normal appearing proximal (left) and distal (right) stomach on retroflexion view. (Normal stomach with scope in view - wikimediacommons.org)

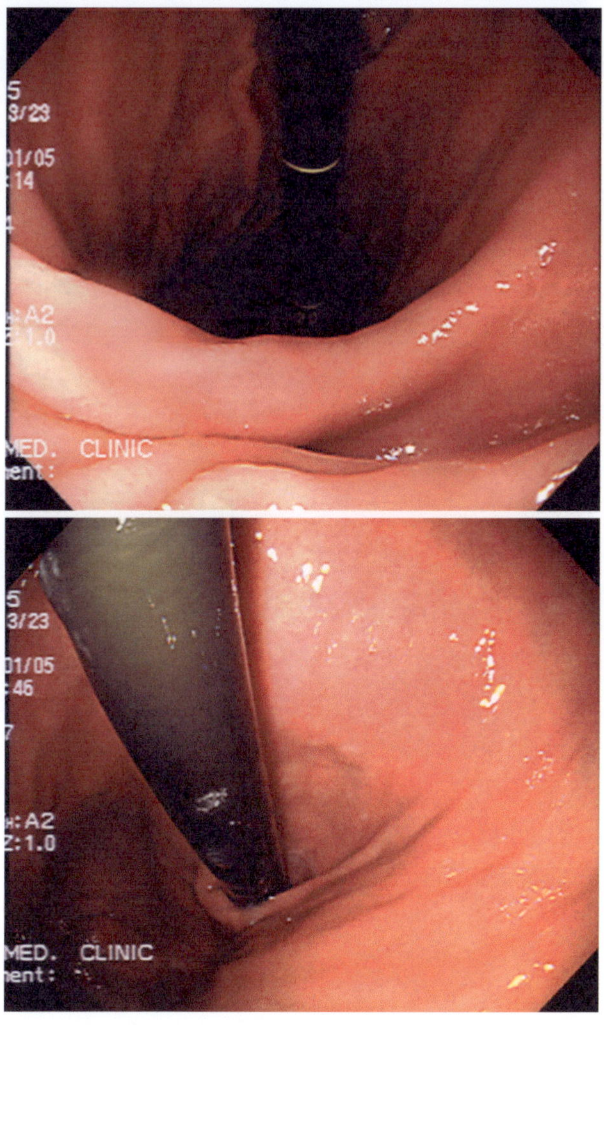

A protective bite block is placed into the patients' mouth to protect their teeth and mouth from the endoscope; the patient is given an anesthetic; and, when asleep, the endoscope is passed through their mouth into their oropharynx and upper GI tract. The upper GI tract is inflated with room air or carbon dioxide gas, distending the lumen and allowing for careful examination (Fig. 24.4). Any abnormal anatomic structures or mucosal abnormalities are then identified, leading to sampling or administration of therapies as the endoscopist deems appropriate. The length of the procedure depends on the indications and findings; however, it can take as little as a few minutes for unremarkable, diagnostic procedures.

The most common indication for upper endoscopy is gastroesophageal reflux disease (GERD) [9]. The estimated prevalence of GERD in the United States is 10–20% when defined by weekly heartburn symptoms or regurgitation [10].

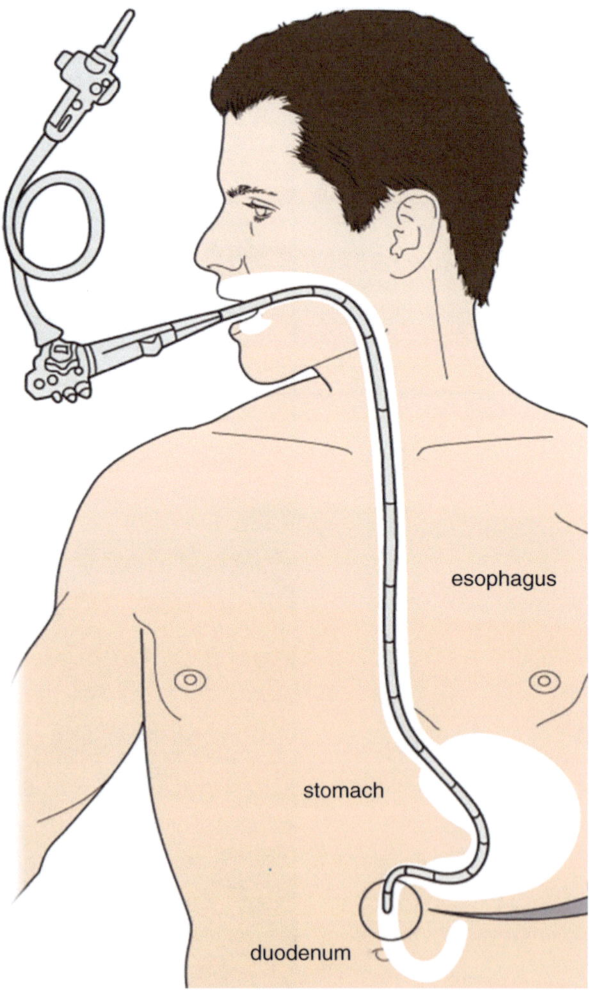

Fig. 24.4 An illustration of upper endoscopy. (wikimediacommons.org)

Prevalence would likely be higher if we included symptoms of Laryngopharyngeal Reflux (LPR) or epigastric discomfort. Many of these patients will need endoscopies eventually to confirm the cause of their symptoms and rule out GERD-related complications. This fact can lead to a staggering number of endoscopies performed yearly in the United States alone, without including non-GERD indications for endoscopy.

There are many indications for upper endoscopy. The role of upper endoscopy in GERD is to not only confirm the diagnosis but also to rule out complications of the disease, including strictures, esophagitis, Barrett's esophagus, and adenocarcinoma (1). For GERD, we can simplify the indications for endoscopy in a similar way to most medical tests; if the results are likely to influence management and empiric therapy has been unsuccessful or if therapy via endoscopy may be appropriate, then we proceed with the test. If management is unlikely to change based on the test results, then we would not proceed with the test, in this case being EGD. There is a lack of evidence that there is a benefit to performing an EGD on patients with GERD that is responsive to antisecretory therapy if additional indications or alarm signs or symptoms are not present.{table of indications} (indications: GERD, upper abdominal pain, nausea, weight loss, anemia, dysphagia, odynophagia, upper gastrointestinal bleeding, abnormal imaging of the upper GI tract, foreign body ingestion, caustic ingestion, Barrett's esophagus, gastric cancer screening ((select patients)), FAP, HNPCC).

Diagnosis of GERD can typically be made based on symptoms and confirmed by a response to antisecretory therapy (acid-lowering medications) [11]. However, if the patient has new-onset GERD symptoms after the age of 50, an endoscopy is indicated to rule out complications of GERD as discussed previously. Alarm signs or symptoms related to GERD necessitating an endoscopy include dysphagia, odynophagia, weight loss, anemia, evidence of GI bleeding, or those with multiple risk factors for Barrett's esophagus [12]. These risk factors include age of 50, male sex, obesity, a family history of Barrett's esophagus or esophageal adenocarcinoma, a smoking history, or prolonged reflux symptoms. Typically, if two or more risk factors are present, an endoscopy is recommended.

Complications of GERD all require unique and specific treatment algorithms – some endoscopic in nature. For instance, GERD-related strictures can be treated through endoscopic dilations, while Barrett's esophagus with dysplasia can be treated through endoscopically administered thermal therapy. The appropriate treatment cannot be determined if the practitioner is not aware that the disease is present, as determined through endoscopy.

Lastly, ultrasound is typically not included in the algorithm for classic GERD symptoms. This includes transabdominal and endoscopic ultrasound. Scant useful information can be gleaned from ultrasound if the patient is having symptoms of classic GERD. However, if the patient is experiencing vague or abnormal symptoms of GERD, ultrasound evaluation may be useful in ruling out other causes of symptoms. For instance, if a patient is experiencing weight loss, nonspecific abdominal pain, or jaundice or has abnormal liver enzymes in addition to GERD-related symptoms, an ultrasound would be beneficial to rule out hepatic, biliary, or pancreatic disease. In this scenario, additional three-dimensional imaging such as CT scans or

MRIs may be appropriate as well to rule out additional pathology that may be missed on upper endoscopy or ultrasound imaging, such as occult malignancies outside of the luminal gastrointestinal tract.

References

1. ASGE Standards of Practice Committee, Early DS, Ben-Menachem T, et al. Appropriate use of GI endoscopy. Gastrointest Endosc. 2012;75:1127.
2. Rizk MK, Sawhney MS, Cohen J, et al. Quality indicators common to all GI endoscopic procedures. Am J Gastroenterol. 2015;110:48.
3. Barbeiro S, Libanio D, Castro R, et al. Narrow-band imaging: clinical application in gastrointestinal endoscopy. GE Por J Gastroeneterol. 2018;26:40.
4. Gono K, Obi T, Yamaguchi M, et al. Appearance of enhanced tissue features in narrow-band endoscopic imaging. J Biomed Opt. 2004;9:568.
5. ASGE Standards of Practice Committee, Sharaf RN, Shergill AK, et al. Endoscopic mucosal tissue sampling. Gastrointest Endosc. 2013;78:216.
6. ASGE Technology Committee, Kethu SR, Banerjee S, et al. Endoscopic tattooing. Gastrointest Endosc. 2010;72:681.
7. ASGE Technology Committee, Conway JD, Adler DG, et al. Endoscopic hemostatic devices. Gastrointest Endosc. 2009;69:987.
8. ASGE Technology Committee. Confocal laser endomicroscopy. Gastrointest Endosc. 2014;80:928.
9. ASGE Standards of Practice Committee, Muthusamy VR, Lightdale JR, et al. The role of endoscopy in the management of GERD. Gastrointest Endosc. 2015;81:1305.
10. Dent J, El-Serag HB, Wallander MA, Johansson S. Epidemiology of gastro-oesophageal reflux disease: as systematic review. Gut. 2005;54:710.
11. Bytzer P, Jones R, Vakil N, et al. Limited ability of the proton-pump inhibitor test to identify patients with gastroesophageal reflux disease. Clin Gastroenterol Hepatol. 2012;10:1360.
12. Castro C, Peleteiro B, Lunet N. Modifiable factors and esophageal cancer: a systematic review of published meta-analyses. J Gastroentrol. 2018;53:37.

Chapter 25
Esophageal Manometry and Esophageal pH Testing

Nimish Vakil

Esophageal Manometry

Esophageal manometry is a physiologic test of esophageal function that complements endoscopy and provides a visual assessment of esophageal abnormalities. It measures pressures in the body of the esophagus and the lower esophageal sphincter, while pH testing quantifies acid refluxing into the esophagus.

Manometry has traditionally been performed using water-perfused catheters, which are passed through the nose and tethered at the nose while the recording is performed. By convention, ten water swallows are obtained, and the resulting pressure recordings are averaged for evaluation. In addition, a visual inspection of the recording by a trained observer detects artifacts and patterns that may not be identified by the average pressure calculations. Over the past decade, advances in technology have led to the development of high-resolution manometry using a catheter with 36 closely spaced sensors that provide a color isobaric plot of esophageal pressure and a classification of esophageal disorders [1].

Indications for Esophageal Manometry

Table 25.1 summarizes the current indications for esophageal manometry [2, 3]. Nonobstructive dysphagia is a condition where endoscopy and imaging studies such as a barium swallow reveal no evidence of an obstruction in the esophagus but the patient reports symptoms of dysphagia. The principal disorder in this category is achalasia, but other motor disorders of the esophagus such as spastic disorders can present with nonobstructive dysphagia. Preoperative evaluations are designed to

N. Vakil (✉)
University of Wisconsin School of Medicine and Public Health, Madison, WI, USA
e-mail: nvakil@wisc.edu

C. H. Zalvan (ed.), *Laryngopharyngeal and Gastroesophageal Reflux*,
https://doi.org/10.1007/978-3-030-48890-1_25

Table 25.1 : Indications for esophageal manometry

Indications
Nonobstructive dysphagia
Preoperative evaluation in reflux disease and achalasia
Evaluation of noncardiac chest pain
Prior to placement of pH and pH/impedance catheters

ensure that enough peristaltic activity exists to allow the patient to swallow after surgical treatment for reflux disease. Spastic disorders of the esophagus can present with chest pain, and manometry may be part of the evaluation of selected patients with noncardiac chest pain. Manometry is necessary to determine the correct placement of pH probes and pH impedance catheters, which depend on accurate localization of the lower esophageal sphincter. Manometry may also be useful to assess esophageal function in connective tissue disorders and scleroderma.

Method

After informed consent, catheter calibration, and application of a topical anesthetic to the patient's nostril, the manometry catheter is passed through the nose into the esophagus and is positioned by placing the distal 2–3 cm of the catheter in the stomach with the remainder of the catheter (and the multiple sensors) straddling the rest of the esophagus. After a period of acclimation, a baseline swallow-free recording is obtained followed by ten swallows of a 5-mL liquid bolus in the supine position [2].

Interpretation

The computerized printout of a high-resolution manometry includes a graphic output and summary data based on an average of the ten water swallows.

Key Concepts

The classification of esophageal motor disorders depends on an understanding of the vigor of esophageal contraction, the completeness of lower esophageal sphincter relaxation (to allow the bolus to pass through the stomach), and coordination between esophageal contraction and lower sphincter relaxation [2]. The key measures used to classify motor disorders of the esophagus are described below and are shown visually in Fig. 25.1.

Integrated relaxation pressure (IRP): The IRP is a measure of relaxation of the lower esophageal sphincter in response to swallowing and is an important measure of obstruction to flow across the gastroesophageal junction. An integrated relaxation

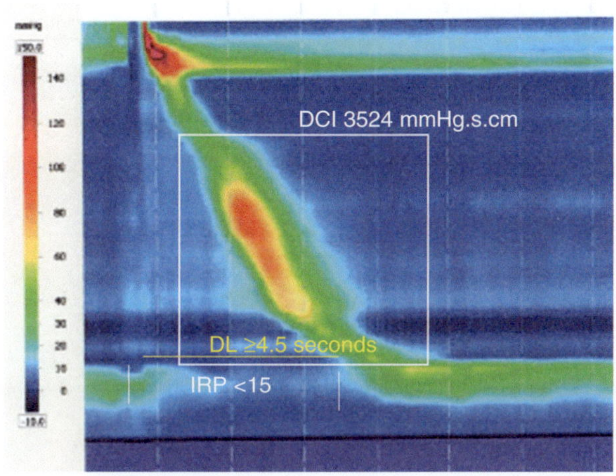

Fig. 25.1 Normal Esophageal manometry. (*DCI* distal contractile integral, *DL* distal latency, *IRP* integrated relaxation pressure)

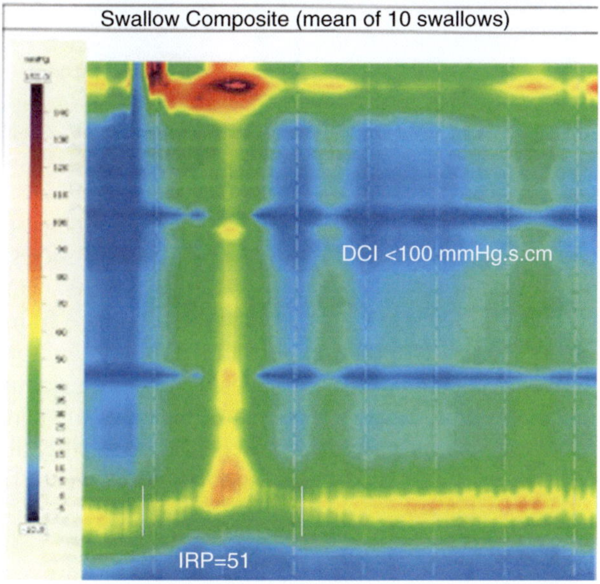

Fig. 25.2 Achalasia. The DCI is abnormal and there is no peristalsis in the esophagus. The integrated relaxation pressure is high and abnormal, and there is no relaxation of the sphincter

pressure <15 mm Hg (Fig. 25.1) is normal. Figure 25.2 shows an abnormal integrated relaxation pressure. There is no significant relaxation, and the integrated pressure remains high (>15 mm Hg). A high integrated relaxation pressure associated with aperistalsis in the esophageal body suggests a diagnosis of achalasia, while the presence of peristalsis in the esophageal body suggests an obstruction at the esophagogastric junction. Figure 25.1 shows a recording from a patient with achalasia and demonstrates the absence of peristalsis in the esophageal body and no significant relaxation of the sphincter.

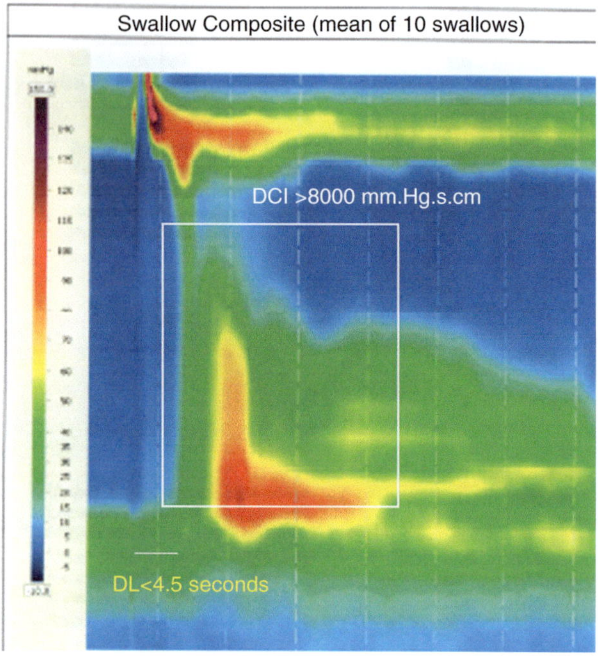

Fig. 25.3 Jackhammer esophagus. This is an example of a hypercontractile esophagus with an abnormal latency indicating a premature contraction and a high distal contractile interval indicating a hypercontractile esophagus

Distal contractile integral (DCI): The DCI is a measure of peristaltic (contractile) vigor and is used to identify hypercontractile swallows (DCI > 8000 mm Hg s cm), weak swallows (DCI < 450 mm Hg s cm), and failed peristalsis (DCI < 100 mm Hg s cm). Normal values range from 500 to 8000 mm Hg s cm. Figure 25.1 shows a normal manometry with a normal DCI. Figure 25.2 shows a recording from a patient with achalasia with no significant peristalsis. The DCI is less than 100 mm Hg s cm. Figure 25.3 shows a hypercontractile esophagus with a very high DCI indicating a hypercontractile motility disorder.

Distal Latency (DL)

The DL is the time interval (in seconds) from upper esophageal relaxation to the contractile deceleration point (CDP), the inflection point in the wave-front velocity proximal to the gastroesophageal junction. The DL evaluates for premature contractions, which form the basis for defining distal esophageal spasm and type III achalasia. The normal DL is 4.5 seconds or longer. Figure 25.3 shows a recording from a patient with a hypercontractile esophagus characterized by a premature contraction with a DL <4.5 seconds and a hypercontractile esophagus with a DCI >8000 mm Hg s cm.

Motility Disorders of the Esophagus [2]

1. Disorders of the esophagogastric outflow:
   (a) Hypotensive lower esophageal sphincter. Low pressures in the lower esophageal sphincter predispose to acid reflux.
   (b) Obstruction and the esophagogastric junction. This condition is defined by a median integrative relaxation pressure greater than 15. This may be seen in obstructions at the gastroesophageal junction, such as a stricture. When accompanied by abnormal motility in the esophageal body (100% failed swallows or 20% premature contractions), a diagnosis of achalasia is made (Fig. 25.2).
2. Major disorders of esophageal peristalsis

   These are disorders that are not seen in normal subjects and are defined as follows:

   Distal esophageal spasm (DES): More than twenty percent premature contractions defined by the distal latency. This is a disorder where premature contractions result in dysphagia and chest pain.

   Jackhammer esophagus (Fig. 25.3): High-pressure contractions in the distal esophagus (defined by two high-pressure contractions with a distal contractile integral >8000 mm Hg s cm). This disorder frequently presents with unexplained dysphagia and sometimes with chest pain.

   Absent peristalsis (Fig. 25.2): This disorder is diagnosed when there is failed peristalsis with 100% of swallow associated with impaired or absent relaxation of the lower esophageal sphincter.
3. Minor disorders of esophageal peristalsis

   A minor disorder of peristalsis is diagnosed if the integrative relaxation pressure is normal, a major disorder of peristalsis has been excluded, and either 50% of swallows are weak or failed (ineffective esophageal motility) or 50% of swallows have large peristaltic breaks (fragmented peristalsis). Both manometric findings can be seen in normal subjects and in patients with GERD and dysphagia.

   Additional images of normal and abnormal manometric recordings may be found on the Internet [3].

Importance of Esophageal Manometry in GERD

Esophageal manometry is not indicated in every patient with GERD, but it is essential in patients who are being considered for surgical or endoscopic interventions for reflux disease. Patients with major motility disorders do poorly after surgery, and identifying them before surgical intervention is important to prevent postoperative dysphagia. Manometry is a prerequisite for placement of pH/impedance catheters and pH catheters as described below.

Esophageal pH Testing

The diagnosis of GERD may be made on clinical grounds when typical symptoms of heartburn and regurgitation are present two or more times a week [4]. The diagnosis of GERD may be difficult in a subset of patients who present with laryngeal symptoms, cough, or atypical chest pain as their primary symptom. In some of these patients, typical symptoms of heartburn are absent or are negligible. Endoscopy may be normal in more than half of these patients, and a critical aspect of their management revolves around making a diagnosis of GERD. Esophageal pH testing was developed to address this need. Placement of a small sensing device in the esophagus allows a prolonged recording of pH in the esophagus and allows correlation of reflux events with meals and body position. Reflux can also be quantified allowing evaluations before and after treatment. Establishing a diagnosis of reflux disease improves the outcome of surgical treatment for reflux disease by selecting patients most likely to benefit.

Methods of pH Testing

1. Transnasal probes

   pH testing began with transnasal catheters, which have an antimony or glass electrode that measures pH. The probe is passed transnasally and anchored so that the pH-sensing tip is located 5 cm above the manometrically measured top of the lower esophageal sphincter. A 24-hour recording is obtained, and data are captured by a recorder that connects to the pH probe and is worn on a belt or strap through the period of the study. The pH catheters have been modified to allow two and four pH sensors placed at different points along the catheter to allow measurements of reflux at different points in the esophagus. The most common configuration is a dual pH probe with two electrodes positioned 15 cm apart. This allows measurement of pH in two configurations: (a) distal esophagus 5 cm above the LES and proximal esophagus, 20 cm from the upper border of the LES, and (b) intragastric pH measurement and distal esophageal recording. Values for normal subjects have been developed and validated for measurements 5 cm above the lower esophageal sphincter, and this location is always used regardless of the other sites for measurement. Table 25.2 shows the normal parameters for catheter-based pH testing [5].
2. Wireless pH testing (Bravo)

   A transnasal catheter is uncomfortable and is embarrassing for some patients to wear publicly. A wireless pH sensor was developed to address this need. In this configuration, a pH sensor is attached to the wall of the esophagus during EGD using an attachment device and a recording obtained on a data logger, which connects wirelessly to the pH probe in the esophagus. A 48-hour or 96-hour recording is possible with this device.

Table 25.2 : Catheter-based pH testing: normal values for single or dual probes

Variable	Proximal sensor	Distal sensor
Total time pH < 4 (%)	<0.9	4.2
Upright period (%)	<1.2	6.3
Recumbent period (%)	0.0	1.2

Single probes have a sensor placed 5 cm above the upper border of the lower esophageal sphincter
Dual probes have a sensor at 5 cm and 20 cm proximal to the upper border of the lower esophageal sphincter

Table 25.3 Wireless pH testing: normal values

Variable	Proximal sensor
Total time pH < 4 (%)	< 5.3
Upright period (%)	<6.9
Recumbent period (%)	<6.7

Wireless sensor is placed 5 cm above the upper border of the lower esophageal sphincter

Patients are encouraged to eat and drink normally during the recording and maintain a diary of mealtimes and periods of sleep. Each of the data recorders has a button that the patient can press to record a symptom. This places a mark in the recording, and during the analysis, symptoms can be correlated with reflux events in the esophagus. The device has been validated against other tests of reflux disease [5, 6]. Normal values are shown in Table 25.3 [7].

Interpretation of pH Studies

The following parameters are used to analyze GER for upright, supine, and total periods:

A. Percentage time pH <4 over a 24-hour period (esophageal acid exposure time or AET)
B. Total number of reflux episodes
C. Number of reflux episodes longer than 5 min
D. Longest single duration of any reflux episode
E. Mean duration of reflux episodes (acid clearance time)

Of these, the most reliable indicator of acid reflux is the esophageal acid exposure time.

A recent consensus conference proposed new criteria for pH testing in a diagnosis of GERD [8]. The consensus proposed that an AET <4% should be considered definitely normal while an AET > 6% would be definitely abnormal. The consensus proposed that >80 reflux episodes in a 24-hour period are definitely abnormal while values <40 episodes in a 24-hour period are physiologic and are normal. Values between 40 and 80 are inconclusive.

Symptom Indices

The symptom index (SI) is the percentage of symptom events preceded by reflux episodes, and the optimal threshold for the symptom of heartburn is 50% for a diagnosis of reflux. A major disadvantage of this index is that it does not consider the number of episodes of reflux, and therefore, a patient with a small number of episodes that are related by chance to symptom events that occur frequently can result in a positive symptom index.

The symptom association probability (SAP) uses statistical calculations to express the probability that symptom events and reflux episodes are associated and is considered positive if the P value of the observed association occurring by chance is <5%. It does take into account the number of reflux episodes as well as the temporal relationship of the episodes to the symptom event.

When both the SI and SAP are positive, it provides good evidence that symptoms are likely caused by reflux. Both indices are predictive of the effect of medical and surgical anti-reflux therapy. The accuracy of these tests depends to a significant degree on accurate symptom recording by the patient.

pH Impedance Studies

Impedance is a measurement of resistance to flow of a small electric current across a pair of electrodes [9, 10]. pH impedance is measured by special transnasal catheters which have a pH electrode and several impedance sensors built into the catheter. Impedance is low with a liquid bolus and high in the presence of air between electrode pairs. A significant limitation of pH monitoring as described above is that it does not detect weakly acidic or nonacidic reflux episodes. These are reflux episodes when the pH of the refluxate is between 4 and 7. Weakly acidic reflux episodes can cause esophageal symptoms and refractory esophagitis. Impedance studies can also differentiate liquid from gaseous reflux, and as a number of sensors are built along the catheter, it can detect how high the refluxate rises into the esophagus. This can be helpful in patients who have laryngeal symptoms caused by reflux. Patients who are receiving proton pump inhibitors may continue to have reflux, but the proportion of acid reflux episodes decreases, and weakly acidic reflux becomes the principal cause of symptoms. Figures 25.4, 25.5, and 25.6 illustrate normal and abnormal pH impedance recordings.

Testing on or off PPI Therapy [9, 10]

Table 25.4 describes circumstances in which pH testing is performed and illustrates conditions under which pH or pH impedance testing may be performed. The decision is often individualized based on the patient's symptoms, medication history, and the clinical question being answered. In patients in whom the test is being

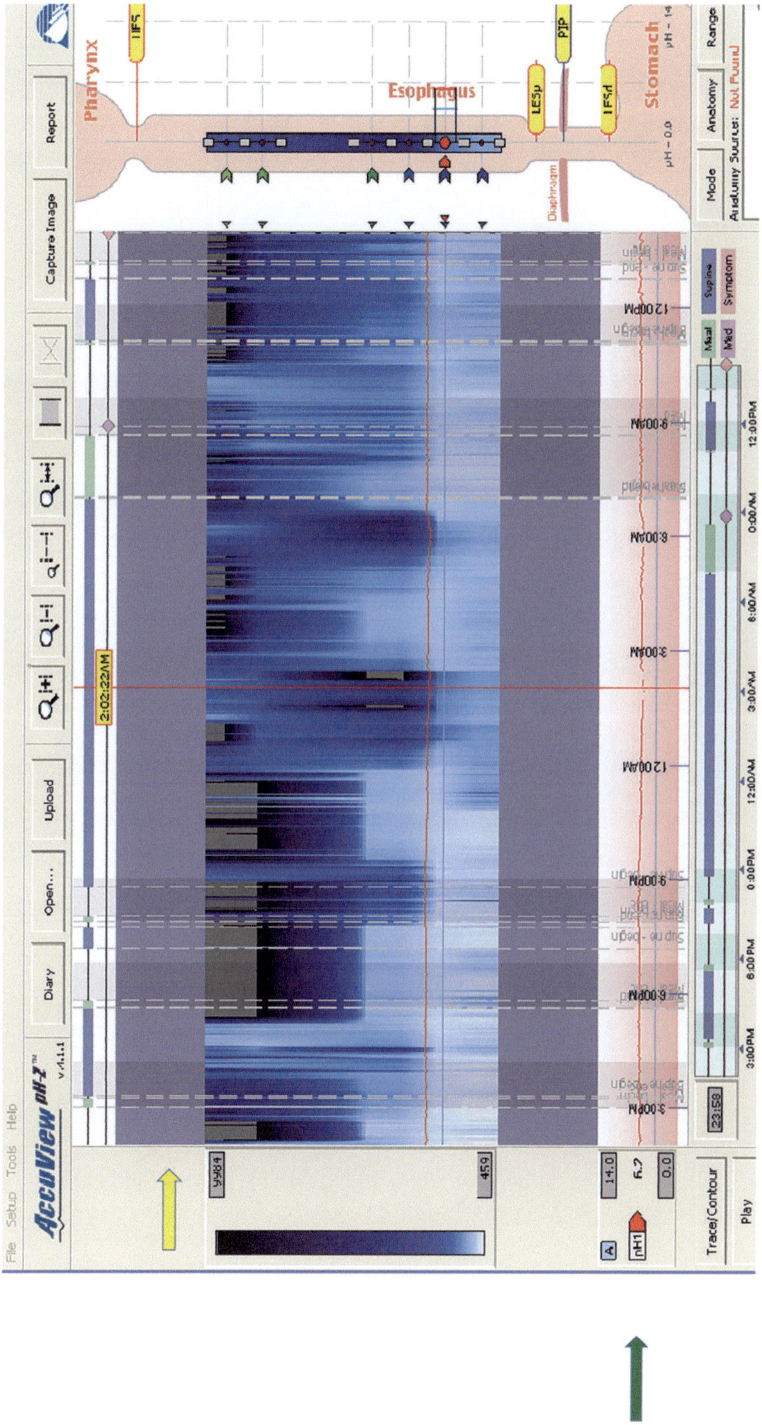

Fig. 25.4 Normal pH impedance recording. The yellow arrow points to impedance events, while the green arrow points to the pH sensor. There are no impedance events, and the distal esophageal pH is normal with no drops below the threshold of 4

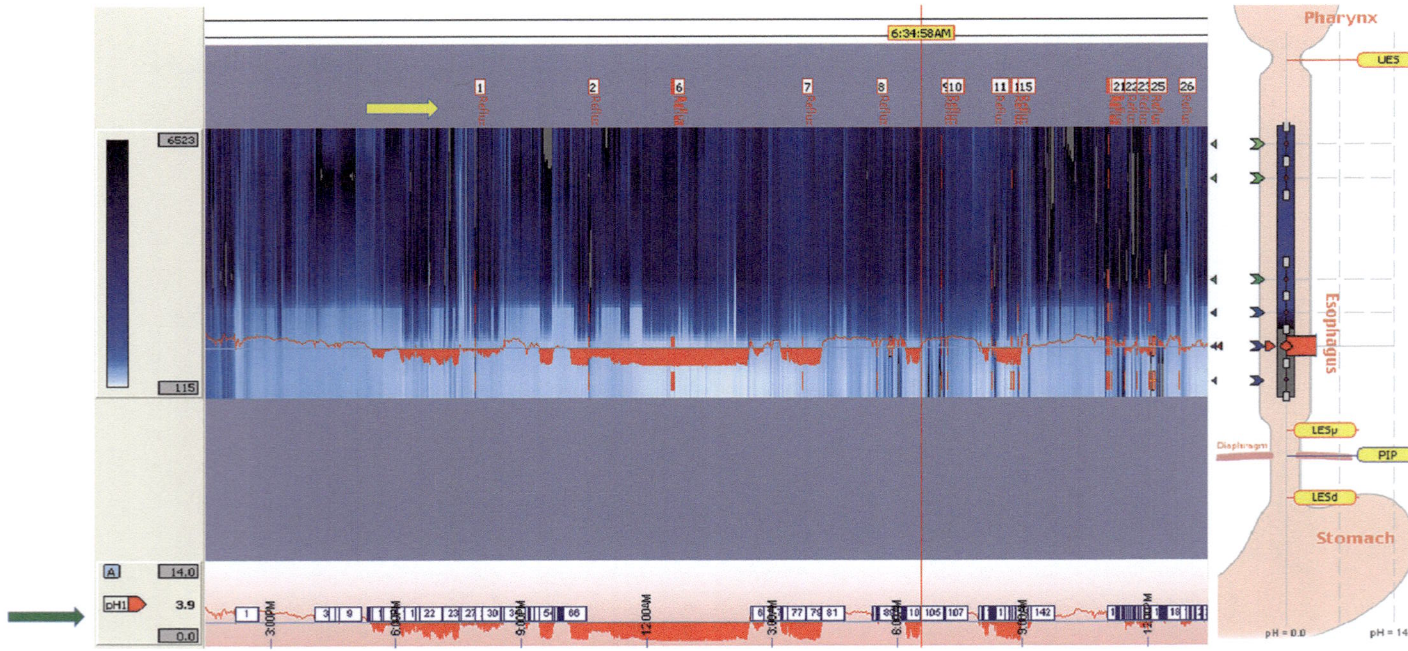

Fig. 25.5 pH impedance study showing acid reflux. The yellow arrow points to reflux events recorded by the impedance sensors. The pH recording (green arrow) demonstrates that these are acidic events because the pH drops below 4

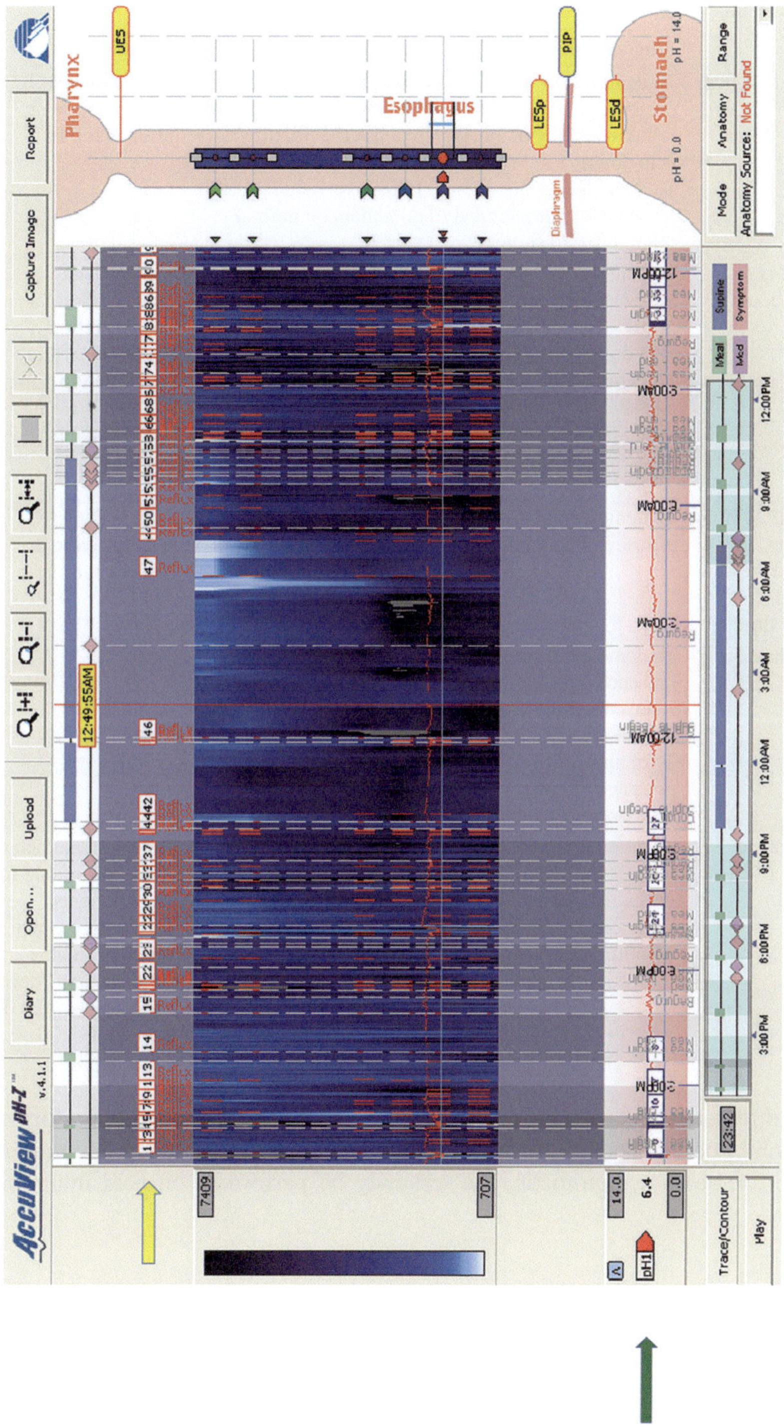

Fig. 25.6 Weakly acidic/nonacid reflux. The yellow arrow points to reflux events recorded by the impedance sensors. The pH recording (green arrow) demonstrates that these are not acidic events because the pH does not drop below 4

Table 25.4 Clinical use of pH and pH impedance testing

Test	Primary indication	Advantages	Limitations
Transnasal 24-hour pH test off all acid inhibitory drugs	To demonstrate the presence of pathological reflux when the diagnosis is in doubt To demonstrate the presence of pathological reflux prior to surgery	Dual probes can help determine if the refluxate reaches the proximal esophagus Extensively studied with good data on normal values	Fails to detect weakly acidic or gaseous reflux
Wireless pH test (48 or 96 hours)	To demonstrate the presence of pathological reflux when the diagnosis is in doubt To demonstrate the presence of pathological reflux prior to surgery	Better tolerated than transnasal catheters Extensively studied with good data on normal values Prolonged recording increases the likelihood of identifying infrequent events	Fails to detect weakly acidic or gaseous reflux Cannot determine how high the refluxate rises into the esophagus
Transnasal 24-hour pH test and wireless pH testing on all acid inhibitory drugs	To demonstrate the efficacy of acid inhibitors	Used when pH impedance is not available	Fails to detect weakly acidic or gaseous reflux
pH/impedance testing off PPI therapy	To demonstrate the presence of pathological reflux when the diagnosis is in doubt To demonstrate the presence of pathological reflux prior to surgery		
pH/impedance testing on PPI therapy	To demonstrate the presence of pathological reflux in patients who are symptomatic despite acid inhibitory therapy	The only test that can demonstrate acid, weakly acidic, and alkaline reflux as the cause of the patient's symptoms	Transnasal catheter is uncomfortable for some patients Technology is not widely available All recordings need review by a trained individual

performed to determine if reflux disease is present, the test is generally performed off acid inhibitory agents. On the other hand, when the diagnosis is not in doubt but the patient remains symptomatic, the test may be performed on acid inhibitory therapy.

Salivary Pepsin Measurements as an Indicator of Reflux Disease [11, 12]

This test is based on the principle that pepsin is not normally found in the oral cavity, and if it was, this would provide indirect evidence of gastroesophageal reflux and also of esophago-oral reflux. Initial promising results have not been replicated in more recent studies, and therefore, this test is not recommended for routine clinical work. This testing is addressed elsewhere in this textbook.

Bilitec Testing

A transnasal catheter that can sense bilirubin was used in the past to detect bile in the esophagus as a test for duodeno-gastric reflux. The test is no longer used in clinical practice, and the device is no longer available [13].

Laryngopharyngeal pH Testing

An oropharyngeal pH probe (Restech) is a catheter that was designed to meet the unmet needs of measuring oropharyngeal acid exposure events and diagnosing laryngopharyngeal reflux (LPR). This catheter is inserted transnasally and positioned in the posterior oropharynx. This pH probe can capture both liquid reflux events and aerosolized acid exposure. This technology is discussed in detail elsewhere in this book.

References

1. Kahrilas PJ, Bredenoord AJ, Fox M, et al. The Chicago classification of esophageal motility disorders, v3.0. Neurogastroenterol Motil. 2015;27:160–74.
2. Carlson D, Kahrilas P. How to effectively use high-resolution esophageal manometry. Gastroenterology. 2016;151:789–92.
3. Herbella F, Armijo P, Patti M. A pictorial presentation of 3.0 Chicago Classification for esophageal motility disorders. http://www.scielo.br/scielo.php?script=sci_arttext&pid=S1679-45082016000300439. Accessed 24 June 2019.
4. Vakil N, van Zanten SV, Kahrilas P, et al. The Montreal definition and classification of gastroesophageal reflux disease: a global evidence-based consensus. Am J Gastroenterol. 2006;101:1900–20.
5. Johnnson LF, DeMeester TR. Twenty-four-hour pH monitoring of the distal esophagus. A quantitative measure of gastroesophageal reflux. Am J Gastroenterol. 1974;62:325–32.
6. Dent J, Vakil N, Jones R, et al. Accuracy of the diagnosis of GORD by questionnaire, physicians and a trial of proton pump inhibitor treatment: the Diamond Study. Gut. 2010;59:714–21.
7. Pandolfino JE, Richter JE, Ours T, Guardino JM, Chapman J, Kahrilas PJ. Ambulatory esophageal pH monitoring using a wireless system. Am J Gastroenterol. 2003;98:740–9.
8. Gyawali CP, Kahrilas PJ, Savarino E, Zerbib F, Mion F, Smout AJPM, Vaezi M, Sifrim D, Fox MR, Vela MF, Tutuian R, Tack J, Bredenoord AJ, Pandolfino J, Roman S. Modern diagnosis of GERD: the Lyon Consensus. Gut. 2018;67(7):1351–62.
9. Hobbs P, Gyawali P. The role of esophageal pH-impedance testing in clinical practice. Curr Opin Gastroenterol. 2018;34:249–57.
10. Cho Y. How to interpret esophageal impedance pH monitoring. J Neurogastroenterol Motil. 2010;16:327–30.

11. Hayat JO, Gabieta-Somnez S, Yazaki E, Kang JY, Woodcock A, Dettmar P, Mabary J, Knowles CH, Sifrim D. Pepsin in saliva for the diagnosis of gastro-oesophageal reflux disease. Gut. 2015;64(3):373–8.
12. Vakil N. Salivary pepsin to diagnose GORD? Gut. 2015;64(3):361–2.
13. Hershcovici T, Jha LK, Cui H, Powers J, Fass R. Night-time intra-oesophageal bile and acid: a comparison between gastro-oesophageal reflux disease patients who failed and those who were treated successfully with a proton pump inhibitor. Aliment Pharmacol Ther. 2011;33(7):837–44.

Chapter 26
The Evolution of the DeMeester and RYAN Scores: Utility and Clinical Application

Dolores T. Mueller and Hans F. Fuchs

Esophageal pH-monitoring and the DeMeester Score

The European Association of Endoscopic Surgery (EAES) recommendations for the management of gastroesophageal reflux disease state that long-term pH-monitoring is one of the most important tools in the diagnostic pathway to prove the presence of GERD. It allows an objective measurement of pathologic acid exposure as well as a symptom correlation [1]. Esophageal pH-monitoring is the current gold standard. The probe is inserted either transnasally or using the BRAVO system during endoscopy and positioned 5 cm above the lower esophageal sphincter. A previous manometry is helpful to determine the exact location of the lower esophageal sphincter ensuring that the probe is placed correctly for a valid measurement.

Thresholds and parameters used to determine a pathologic acid exposure include the following:

- The percentage of time with a pH < 4 in total
- The percentage of time with a pH < 4 in upright position
- The percentage of time with a pH < 4 in supine position
- The total number of episodes of reflux per 24 hours
- The number of episodes lasting longer than 5 minutes
- The longest episode during the 24-hour interval

D. T. Mueller
Department for General, Visceral, Cancer and Transplant Surgery,
University Hospital Cologne, Kerpener Str. 62, 50937, Cologne, Deutschland
e-mail: dolores.mueller@uk-koeln.de

H. F. Fuchs (✉)
Department of General, Visceral, Cancer and Transplant Surgery,
University of Cologne, Kerpener Str. 62, 50937, Cologne, Germany
e-mail: hans.fuchs@uk-koeln.de

C. H. Zalvan (ed.), *Laryngopharyngeal and Gastroesophageal Reflux*,
https://doi.org/10.1007/978-3-030-48890-1_26

Episodes are defined as times when the esophageal pH drops below 4. Those values are combined in a composite score called the DeMeester score. Developed in 1974, studies have shown this score to have a sensitivity of 96%, a specificity of 100%, and an accuracy of 98%, still making it the current gold standard in the diagnosis of gastroesophageal reflux disease and a pathologic acid exposure. In addition, individually evaluating every single parameter leads to a more accurate and precise diagnosis of GERD [2, 3].

A DeMeester score > 14.72 shows an abnormal esophageal acid exposure. EAES recommendations state that "patients with continuous reduced quality of life, persistent troublesome symptoms, and/or progression of disease despite adequate PPI therapy in dosage and intake" may be surgical candidates [1]. In addition, an increasing number of patients present with a desire to undergo surgery to stop being dependent on medication. However, the decision for or against laparoscopic antireflux surgery should be taken with caution as 5–10% of patients may have an impaired life quality postoperatively [4–6]. A thorough evaluation of the patient, pathologic findings, and alternatives should be considered before a patient should be declared suitable for surgery. A DeMeester score > 14.72 shows a pathologic acid exposure and confirms the diagnosis of gastroesophageal reflux disease. Therefore, it is one of the most important pillars supporting the fundament of a good surgical indication [1].

Confounders and downsides of the DeMeester score mostly lay in the method itself. Those include the following:

- Changes of lifestyle during the measurement
- Hyper salivation due to the catheter
- Gastric alkalization due to *Helicobacter pylori* infection
- Continued antacid medication
- Day-to-day variation

The diagnosis of gastroesophageal reflux disease and the decision for or against antireflux surgery should not be based on a single value but rather on a combination of parameters showing pathologic patterns evaluated by different diagnostic tools. However, esophageal pH-monitoring is the current gold standard in the diagnosis of a pathologic esophageal acid exposure and therefore certainly one of the most important diagnostic tools.

Oropharyngeal pH-monitoring and the RYAN Score

For better evaluation of patients that predominantly present with atypical symptoms such as cough, globus sensation, or hoarseness, laryngopharyngeal pH measurement using the Restech device is now possible. The Restech pH measurement system allows valid measurements of pathologic acid exposure in the oropharynx due to its unique probe shape and technology [7].

The device consists of a thin probe, a transmitter, and a recorder which are connected wirelessly. The probe used to be calibrated in solutions with pH 4 and 7 before each measurement. However, since all catheters are now standardized and calibrated, only hydration of the probe is necessary prior to use. The catheter is inserted transnasally and placed above the upper esophageal sphincter in the oropharynx 5–10 mm underneath the uvula of the patient. A flashing LED light assists in finding the right location. Drinking an acidic beverage, such as soda, can also be useful in confirming the correct location.

The unique teardrop design of the tip of the catheter prevents the probe from drying out during the measurement and an accumulation of food on the catheter. The device can detect pathologic liquid and aerosolized acid exposure, and since the measuring probe is placed in the oropharynx, it might lead to more valid results in patients with suspected laryngopharyngeal reflux.

Thresholds for an abnormal acid exposure in the oropharynx differ from those in the distal esophagus. A pH value of < 5.5 upright and < 5 supine is considered pathologic compared to a pH < 4 in the lower esophagus. The initial validation study performed pharyngeal pH-monitoring in a rather low group of 55 healthy subjects to determine thresholds for this new technique. A mean pharyngeal pH of 5.6 in upright position and 4.8 in supine position was identified and rounded to discriminating thresholds of 5.5 and 5.0, respectively [7].

Three main components are used when interpreting a Restech measurement result:

- The patient report
- The patient graph
- The RYAN score

Just as with the classic pH-metry, reflux episodes during meals are excluded from the calculations. Parallel to conventional pH-monitoring, the percentage of time below threshold values for the oropharynx is used to classify abnormal acid exposure of a patient. Depending on which percentile of thresholds the pH level exceeds, patient's acid exposure can be divided into normal, mild, moderate, and severe reflux (Figs. 26.1, 26.2, 26.3).

The RYAN score, the composite score of the Restech measurement, is calculated using the following parameters:

- The percentage of time pH below threshold
- The number of reflux episodes
- The duration of the longest episode

A separate score is calculated for upright position and supine position using a threshold of pH < 5.5 for upright and pH < 5 for supine. A RYAN score of >9.4 upright and >6.8 supine shows an abnormal acid exposure [7]. Only severe acid exposure leads to a positive RYAN score. A recent study demonstrated that the new Restech device might be a valuable tool in the prediction of outcome for patients with extraesophageal atypical symptoms after laparoscopic antireflux surgery [8].

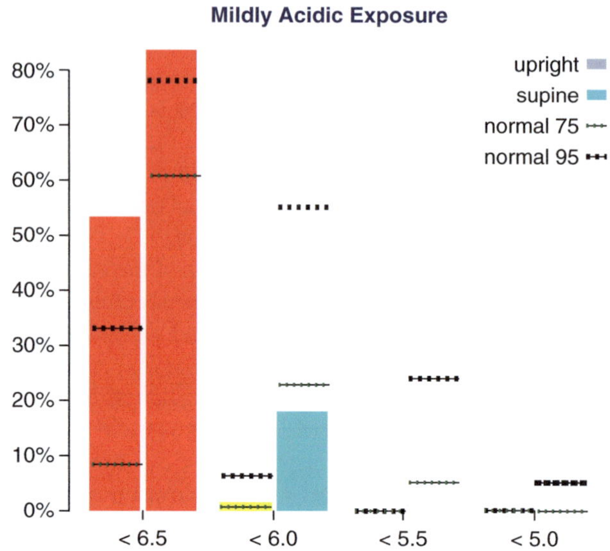

Fig. 26.1 If pH level exceeds the 95th percentile thresholds for pH 6.5 and the 75th percentile for pH 6.0, upright patient suffers from mild acid exposure

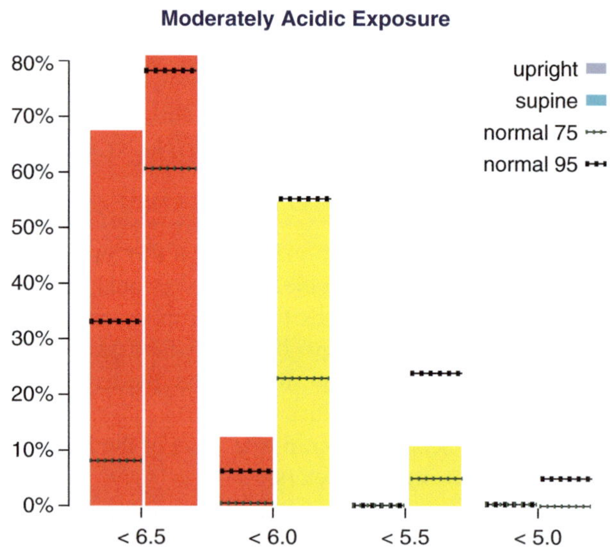

Fig. 26.2 If pH levels exceed the 95th percentile thresholds at pH 6.5 and 6.0 and the 75th percentile at pH 5.5, supine patient suffers from moderate acid exposure

The decision for or against laparoscopic antireflux surgery in patients with mainly atypical symptoms is based on gastrointestinal function testing, patient's decision, and surgeon's preference. Especially in patients with a borderline pathologic esophageal pH-metry, an additional tool can help in making the decision for or against surgery. Only patients with severe reflux and a positive RYAN score however are surgical candidates [9, 10].

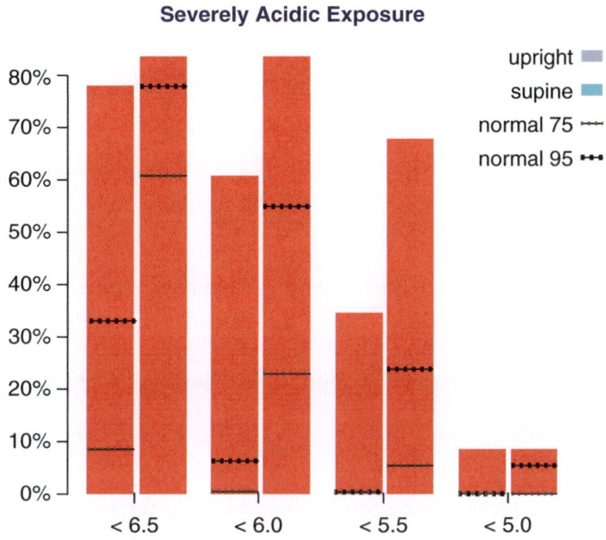

Fig. 26.3 If pH levels exceed the 95th percentile thresholds at pH 6.5, 6.0, and 5.5 and the 95th percentile at pH 5.0, upright patients suffers from severe acid exposure

Confounders and downsides of the RYAN score mostly lay in the method itself and are mostly similar to the DeMeester score. Despite the downsides of pH-metry itself, the oropharyngeal placement of the probe brings its own downsides. The Restech device is not suitable as a screening instrument for gastrointestinal reflux disease as the catheter might not measure reflux episodes that do not reach the oropharynx. An abnormal RYAN score also just represents patients with severe acid exposure but does not include patients with mild or moderate reflux.

Since laryngopharyngeal pH-monitoring is a relatively new reflux testing device, it certainly needs more validation. Our recent study with 101 patients with suspected laryngopharyngeal reflux showed that Restech is a great addition to the diagnostic pathway in patients with mainly atypical symptoms [10]. In addition to that, previous studies have shown that patients after esophagectomy can ideally serve as a human reflux model [11]. Using this thesis, further evaluation and validation of laryngopharyngeal pH-metry are currently being performed.

Discussion

The DeMeester score and the RYAN score represent the same parameters for esophageal and oropharyngeal acid exposure using different thresholds for the calculation of the actual score. However, the DeMeester score is a composite score calculated to display the results of the whole measurement, whereas two RYAN scores are calculated being able to discriminate between pathologic acid exposure in upright and supine position. In addition to that, the RYAN score misses “the number of reflux episodes ≥5 minutes” in its calculation. Table 26.1 displays the parameters used for the calculation of the different scores.

Table 26.1 Parameters used for the calculation of the DeMeester and the RYAN score

Esophageal pH-monitoring	Restech pH-monitoring, upright	Restech pH-monitoring, supine
Percentage of time with a pH < 4, total	Not used	Not used
Percentage of time with a pH < 4, upright	Percentage of time with a pH < 5.5	–
Percentage of time with a pH < 4, supine	–	Percentage of time with a pH < 5.0
Total number of episodes of reflux per 24 hours	For upright period	For supine period
Number of episodes ≥5 minutes	Not used	Not used
Longest episode during 24-hour interval	For upright period	For supine period
DeMeester score	*RYAN score upright*	*RYAN score supine*

The DeMeester score, when >14.72, shows an abnormal acid exposure, and a negative DeMeester score states that the patient has no pathologic reflux [2, 3]. This is different for the RYAN score where only severe acid exposure leads to a positive score. Mild and moderate reflux are not reflected in the RYAN score so that patients with a negative RYAN score might still have an abnormal acid exposure. A current study showed Restech to have a sensitivity of 69% and a specificity of 100% for the responsiveness to medical therapy in patients with laryngopharyngeal reflux making it a valuable tool in the diagnostic pathway [12].

However, there is currently no definition of laryngopharyngeal reflux (LPR), and with the pathophysiology of it being a multifactorial process, reflux could be an amplifying factor or a triggering cause. Due to this problem, diagnosis and clarification of the exact etiology of extraesophageal symptoms are major diagnostic challenges [13, 14].

Our current study showing the correlation between conventional pH-metry and the Restech pH measurement demonstrated that different reflux scenarios exist and that those can be evaluated using the great variety of tools in gastrointestinal function testing [10]. We included 101 patients with suspected GERD and extraesophageal symptoms such as coughing, hoarseness, or globus sensation in our study. Variations of symptoms were not specific to any different reflux scenario. Especially, atypical symptoms can be part of any scenario and a great challenge in diagnosis of their origin. According to our results, we created four subgroups (Groups A–D) reflecting different reflux scenarios:

- Group A – abnormal esophageal pH-metry/normal Restech measurement
- Group B – normal esophageal pH-metry/abnormal Restech measurement
- Group C – both abnormal
- Group D – both normal

Thirty-nine percent of patients with an abnormal esophageal pH-metry showed a normal Restech measurement (Group A). Twenty-three percent of patients with a normal esophageal pH-metry showed an abnormal Restech measurement (Group B). The other two groups (C and D) showed correlating results. Group A can be easily explained by reflux episodes that do not reach the oropharynx and therefore are not measured by the Restech catheter. Group B, however, is harder to understand from a physiologic standpoint. Patients in Group B showed a borderline abnormal DeMeester score and some reflux episodes in the esophageal pH-metry. In addition, subjects showed significantly higher scores and a greater acid exposure compared to patients with a complete negative workup (Group D, both measurements negative) suspecting a reflux-related origin of abnormal RYAN score in this group. Especially in patients with mainly atypical symptoms, the Restech measurement played a leading role in the decision-making for or against laparoscopic antireflux surgery. Twenty-five percent in Group B underwent surgery compared to 7.4% in Group D with normal results.

Our study showed that the new Restech measurement and conventional pH-metry do not necessarily need to correlate with each other. The current level of evidence using the Restech device especially in a surgical environment is rather low as previous studies included only a rather low number of subjects and did not perform both measurements simultaneously. Due to day-to-day variation and changes of lifestyle, no valid comparison of those two techniques could be done.

In patients with a borderline abnormal esophageal pH measurement, the Restech measurement can help support the decision for or against laparoscopic antireflux surgery. Further studies will show whether the Restech measurement may predict a successful surgical outcome after antireflux surgery and whether a negative Restech measurement may function as a screening instrument for GERD or LPR. Previous studies showed that patients after esophagectomy ideally serve as a human reflux model. We used this thesis to further validate the correlation between conventional pH-metry and the Restech measurement and showed a correlation of 100% of both methods in patients with a massive volume of reflux. Overall, conventional esophageal pH-metry and the Restech measurement are two different techniques for the evaluation of gastroesophageal reflux disease and laryngopharyngeal reflux disease that may supplement each other especially in patients with atypical symptoms.

References

1. Fuchs KH, Babic B, Breithaupt W, Dallemagne B, Fingerhut A, Furnee E, et al. EAES recommendations for the management of gastroesophageal reflux disease. Surg Endosc. 2014;28(6):1753–73.
2. Neto RML, Herbella FAM, Schlottmann F, Patti MG. Does DeMeester score still define GERD? Dis Esophagus. 2019;32:5.
3. Jamieson JR, Stein HJ, DeMeester TR, Bonavina L, Schwizer W, Hinder RA, et al. Ambulatory 24-h esophageal pH monitoring: normal values, optimal thresholds, specificity, sensitivity, and reproducibility. Am J Gastroenterol. 1992;87(9):1102–11.
4. Kamolz T, Granderath F, Pointner R. Laparoscopic antireflux surgery: disease-related quality of life assessment before and after surgery in GERD patients with and without Barrett's esophagus. Surg Endosc. 2003;17(6):880–5.

5. Fein M, Bueter M, Thalheimer A, Pachmayr V, Heimbucher J, Freys SM, et al. Ten-year outcome of laparoscopic antireflux surgery. J Gastrointest Surg. 2008;12(11):1893–9.
6. Galmiche JP, Hatlebakk J, Attwood S, Ell C, Fiocca R, Eklund S, et al. Laparoscopic antireflux surgery vs esomeprazole treatment for chronic GERD: the LOTUS randomized clinical trial. JAMA. 2011;305(19):1969–77.
7. Ayazi S, Lipham JC, Hagen JA, Tang AL, Zehetner J, Leers JM, et al. A new technique for measurement of pharyngeal pH: normal values and discriminating pH threshold. J Gastrointest Surg. 2009;13(8):1422–9.
8. Worrell SG, DeMeester SR, Greene CL, Oh DS, Hagen JA. Pharyngeal pH monitoring better predicts a successful outcome for extraesophageal reflux symptoms after antireflux surgery. Surg Endosc. 2013;27(11):4113–8.
9. Brown SR, Gyawali CP, Melman L, Jenkins ED, Bader J, Frisella MM, et al. Clinical outcomes of atypical extra-esophageal reflux symptoms following laparoscopic antireflux surgery. Surg Endosc. 2011;25(12):3852–8.
10. Fuchs HF, Muller DT, Berlth F, Maus MK, Fuchs C, Dubbers M, et al. Simultaneous laryngopharyngeal pH monitoring (Restech) and conventional esophageal pH monitoring-correlation using a large patient cohort of more than 100 patients with suspected gastroesophageal reflux disease. Dis Esophagus. 2018;31:10.
11. Dresner SM, Griffin SM, Wayman J, Bennett MK, Hayes N, Raimes SA. Human model of duodenogastro-oesophageal reflux in the development of Barrett's metaplasia. Br J Surg. 2003;90(9):1120–8.
12. Vailati C, Mazzoleni G, Bondi S, Bussi M, Testoni PA, Passaretti S. Oropharyngeal pH monitoring for laryngopharyngeal reflux: is it a reliable test before therapy? J Voice. 2013;27(1):84–9.
13. Koop H, Fuchs KH, Labenz J, Lynen Jansen P, Messmann H, Miehlke S, et al. S2k guideline: gastroesophageal reflux disease guided by the German Society of Gastroenterology: AWMF register no. 021-013. Z Gastroenterol. 2014;52(11):1299–346.
14. Vakil N, van Zanten SV, Kahrilas P, Dent J, Jones R. The Montreal definition and classification of gastroesophageal reflux disease: a global, evidence-based consensus paper. Z Gastroenterol. 2007;45(11):1125–40.

Part IV
Treatment of Reflux Disease: LPR and GERD

Co-edited by Peter H. Stein

Chapter 27
Overview of the Treatment of Reflux Disease

Craig H. Zalvan

Treatment for reflux, both gastroesophageal reflux disease (GERD) and laryngopharyngeal reflux (LPR), has been part of the armamentarium of healers for millennia. Initially based on outcomes from trial and error, medicine has evolved with a plethora of pharmacological intervention, procedures, and surgical manipulation of the GI tract to alleviate symptoms and improve outcomes in patients with reflux disease. In this section of the book, an overview of treatment will be discussed.

This section of the book begins with an overview of the modern, Western society treatments that have arisen over the last half century in the treatment of reflux disease. This overview sets the stage for a more detailed dive into the various dietary, behavioral, pharmacological, and procedural interventions that have evolved in the armamentarium of reflux treatment.

Most patients with reflux have a general understanding of the types of foods and behaviors that can trigger their symptoms and exacerbate their disease. Standard precautions, avoidances, and behavioral interventions are explored by Drs. Berzofsky and Sandhaus. An overview of pharmacological intervention is followed by descriptions of these standards as well as alternative treatments for reflux, including herbal, botanical, and homeopathic approaches. The pharmacological options for treatment are then explored by Drs. Jodorkovksy and Blackett. In addition to outlining a pharmacological approach tiered toward severity presentation, they also outline some of the newer and upcoming potential treatments.

C. H. Zalvan (✉)
ENT and Allergy Associates, LLP, Tarrytown, NY, USA

The Institute for Voice and Swallowing Disorders, Phelps Hospital, Northwell Health, Sleepy Hollow, NY, USA

Professor of Otolaryngology at the Donald and Barbara Zucker School of Medicine at Hofstra/Northwell, Phelps Hospital Campus, Sleepy Hollow, NY, USA

Communication Speech Department at Mercy College, Dobbs Ferry, NY, USA
e-mail: czalvan@entandallergy.com

C. H. Zalvan (ed.), *Laryngopharyngeal and Gastroesophageal Reflux*,
https://doi.org/10.1007/978-3-030-48890-1_27

Given the considerable media attention to proton pump inhibitor (PPI) therapy, Dr. Jaworak presents a comprehensive analysis of the PPI literature. In this chapter, he dissects the multiple large-scale studies linking PPI use to multiple chronic diseases. PPI, like other medications, are tools that should be used as an adjunct treatment. Dietary and behavioral changes ultimately should be the focus with medication used as a bridge to symptom resolution.

Pharmacological intervention is followed by chapters explaining the interventional approaches. Endoscopic and surgical approaches have been developed to curtail symptoms and improve outcomes in patients with chronic reflux-linked disease. Dr. Triadafilopoulos reviews the endoscopic delivery of radiofrequency energy to the gastroesophageal junction, the Stretta procedure. Drs. Testoni, Testoni, Mazzoleni, and Fanti then review a different endoscopic approach, transoral fundoplication for treatment of gastroesophageal reflux disease (GERD), or transoral incisionless fundoplication (TIF). Completing the interventional approach, Dr. Rohan outlines the various types of surgical procedures utilized in the treatment of GERD. The different fundoplication approaches will be detailed addressing the indications, diagnostic requirements, and approaches. In addition, one of the newest modalities of treatment, the LINX procedure, or magnetic bead sphincter augmentation for treatment of reflux, will be described.

Concluding this section, Dr. Benson reviews the literature describing treatments results and outcomes in laryngopharyngeal reflux (LPR). Similarly, Dr. Clarke reviews the data on treatment for GERD.

Chapter 28
Western Treatment of Reflux Disease

John O. Clarke

Introduction

Gastroesophageal reflux disease (GERD) is a common condition in the Western world, believed to affect approximately 20% of American adults on a weekly basis and over half the population of the United States on an annual basis [1]. Prevalence is similar in other Western countries and appears to be increasing over the past several decades, likely related to a combination of factors including the obesity epidemic and potentially changes in *Helicobacter pylori* prevalence [2]. While there is recognition that multiple potential mechanisms for reflux pathogenesis are at play, traditional Western therapies have focused primarily on the suppression of gastric acid and augmentation of the esophagogastric junction [3]. Recently, there has been a focus on diagnostics to better define individual patient pathophysiology for patients refractory to standard therapy in the hopes of improving their symptom control – and this has led to the utilization of more tailored therapy for precision GERD treatment [4]. This chapter will briefly highlight the key therapies utilized in Western medicine to treat GERD. Each section will be reviewed only briefly as separate chapters will follow providing more depth on each subsection.

Western Therapies

Utilizing a pyramid approach to treatment and the idea that "less is more," treatment is often from the bottom-up, starting with low-risk options that may improve symptoms and progressing to options with reward but potentially higher risk. With this

J. O. Clarke (✉)
Esophageal Program, Division of Gastroenterology & Hepatology, Stanford University, Redwood City, CA, USA
e-mail: john.clarke@stanford.edu

C. H. Zalvan (ed.), *Laryngopharyngeal and Gastroesophageal Reflux*,
https://doi.org/10.1007/978-3-030-48890-1_28

framework, options such as diet and lifestyle modification often are utilized first, followed by more invasive options such as surgery in most cases only when more conservative options have been unsuccessful.

Diet and Lifestyle

This is often the first-line approach for treatment of GERD, although data are limited in comparison to pharmaceutical options such as proton pump inhibitors (PPIs). Standard recommendations including weight loss, smoking cessation, avoiding meals late at night, and elevating the head of the bed [5]. Restriction diets are less-robustly studied but also appear to be effective based on the limited data available [6].

Medical Therapy

Western medical therapy has focused on reduction in gastric acid production since the advent of the histamine receptor antagonists (HRAs) in the 1970s. While these agents have modest efficacy and can be associated with tachyphylaxis, they are an excellent option for intermittent symptoms or as an add-on to PPI therapy. The focus on acid suppression became even more profound with the release of proton pump inhibitors (PPIs) in the 1980s. These are the most effective medical options available in the Western world for acid suppression and have shown the greatest efficacy of medical options for treatment of erosive esophagitis. However, these are not perfect medications, and symptom relief is generally not as successful as mucosal healing. In addition, there are potential safety concerns that have flooded the media in recent years [7, 8]. Other medical options can be utilized on an as-needed basis in patients who require additional add-on therapy in conjunction with PPI use, patients with mild disease who do not wish to take PPI therapy, or in specific clinical subsets. These adjunct therapies include sucralfate, alginates, baclofen, and prokinetics. For all four of these medical options, relative efficacy is modest, but they may have a role in play in specific phenotypes.

Endoscopic Therapy

Endoscopic options for GERD have been in use for the past two decades; however, only two options at present are available in the United States. Radiofrequency ablation and transoral incisionless fundoplication are both FDA-approved options; however, data are inconsistent [9–11], and these techniques are likely best utilized in patients with uncomplicated GERD who desire nonmedical therapy, preferably in conjunction with clinical trials and in the hands of an experienced provider.

Surgical Therapy

Surgery for GERD in Western medicine has focused on augmentation of the esophagogastric junction. The traditional antireflux surgery (ARS) has been the fundoplication, developed by Dr. Rudolf Nissen in the 1950s. This has been performed laparoscopically since the early 1990s with good outcome data that rivals that of the PPIs. In a recent landmark study published in *New England Journal of Medicine*, ARS was superior to maximal medical therapy for treatment of patients with confirmed GERD with symptoms refractory to PPI therapy; however, only a minority of the patients screened for study enrollment qualified to undergo the procedure [12].

In the past few years, magnetic sphincter augmentation has entered the arena with excellent emerging data similar to fundoplication [13, 14]. Finally, bariatric surgery, and in particular gastric bypass, is an excellent option for the obese GERD patient refractory to medical intervention.

Conclusion

Western therapy has focused primarily on reduction of gastric acid production and augmentation of the antireflux barrier. Recognition that GERD is a heterogeneous group comprised of multiple clinically relevant phenotypes with discrete mechanisms of symptom pathogenesis that may differ from the above – plus patient concern regarding long-term PPI use – may lead to future changes in care of the reflux patient in the Western world. In addition, patient interest in complementary and alternative therapies may lead to alternative approaches even from traditional Western practitioners – only time will tell.

Conflicts of Interest None.

Funding None.

References

1. Locke GR 3rd, Talley NJ, Fett SL, et al. Prevalence and clinical spectrum of gastroesophageal reflux: a population-based study in Olmsted County, Minnesota. Gastroenterology. 1997;112:1448–56.
2. Boeckxstaens G, El-Serag HB, Smout AJ, et al. Symptomatic reflux disease: the present, the past and the future. Gut. 2014;63:1185–93.
3. Gyawali CP, Fass R. Management of gastroesophageal reflux disease. Gastroenterology. 2018;154:302–18.
4. Triadafilopoulos G, Clarke JO, Hawn M. Precision GERD management for the 21st century. Dis Esophagus. 2017;30:1–6.
5. Ness-Jensen E, Hveem K, El-Serag H, et al. Lifestyle intervention in gastroesophageal reflux disease. Clin Gastroenterol Hepatol. 2016;14:175–82.e1–3.

6. Triadafilopoulos G, Korzilius JW. Zikos T, et al. Dig Dis Sci: Ninety-six hour wireless esophageal pH study in patients with GERD shows that restrictive diet reduces esophageal acid exposure; 2019.
7. Vaezi MF, Yang YX, Howden CW. Complications of proton pump inhibitor therapy. Gastroenterology. 2017;153:35–48.
8. Freedberg DE, Kim LS, Yang YX. The risks and benefits of long-term use of proton pump inhibitors: expert review and best practice advice from the American Gastroenterological Association. Gastroenterology. 2017;152:706–15.
9. Lipka S, Kumar A, Richter JE. No evidence for efficacy of radiofrequency ablation for treatment of gastroesophageal reflux disease: a systematic review and meta-analysis. Clin Gastroenterol Hepatol. 2015;13:1058–67.e1.
10. Fass R, Cahn F, Scotti DJ, et al. Systematic review and meta-analysis of controlled and prospective cohort efficacy studies of endoscopic radiofrequency for treatment of gastroesophageal reflux disease. Surg Endosc. 2017;31:4865–82.
11. Huang X, Chen S, Zhao H, et al. Efficacy of transoral incisionless fundoplication (TIF) for the treatment of GERD: a systematic review with meta-analysis. Surg Endosc. 2017;31:1032–44.
12. Spechler SJ, Hunter JG, Jones KM, et al. Randomized trial of medical versus surgical treatment for refractory heartburn. N Engl J Med. 2019;381:1513–23.
13. Ganz RA, Edmundowicz SA, Taiganides PA, et al. Long-term outcomes of patients receiving a magnetic sphincter augmentation device for gastroesophageal reflux. Clin Gastroenterol Hepatol. 2016;14:671–7.
14. Ganz RA, Peters JH, Horgan S. Esophageal sphincter device for gastroesophageal reflux disease. N Engl J Med. 2013;368:2039–40.

Chapter 29
The Treatment of Reflux Disease: Standard and Alternative Approach

Craig Berzofsky and Henya Sandhaus

GERD, like LPR, involves reflux of gastric contents into the esophagus. However, while GERD is frank regurgitation, typically presents with heartburn, and is often accompanied by esophagitis, gastric components contributing to symptoms in LPR have been noted to be from aerosolized acid, bile salts, pepsin, and pancreatic proteolytic enzymes in addition to acidic liquid and even frank food materials [3]. LPR tends to present during the daytime with reflux episodes occurring mostly while upright. In contrast, reflux events contributing to GERD are more frequent at night and while supine. In addition, only approximately 10% of patient with LPR are also diagnosed with GERD [2, 4]. As such, LPR is sometimes referred to as atypical reflux or extra-esophageal reflux.

Etiology of Reflux

In patients with hoarseness, chronic cough, and other laryngeal symptoms, conditions of greater morbidity should first be ruled out. Yet, when LPR is in the differential, it may be prudent to reconsider its etiology. As stated previously, reflux of gastric contents includes pepsin, a digestive enzyme that requires acid for activation. Research on laryngeal biopsies demonstrated pepsin bound to the laryngeal epithelium of nearly all LPR patients along with a decrease of carbonic anhydrase III, potentially removing protective bicarbonate locally [5]. At gastric pH of 2.0, pepsin is 100% active. Research demonstrates laryngeal damage occurring at a pH

C. Berzofsky (✉)
Center for Voice and Swallowing, White Plains Hospital, White Plains, NY, USA
e-mail: cberzofsky@wphospital.org

H. Sandhaus
Otolaryngology - Head and Neck Surgery, Southern Illinois University, Springfield, IL, USA
e-mail: hsandhaus21@siumed.edu

C. H. Zalvan (ed.), *Laryngopharyngeal and Gastroesophageal Reflux*,
https://doi.org/10.1007/978-3-030-48890-1_29

of 5.0 [6]. With pepsin retaining proteolytic activity potentially causing cellular damage up to a pH of 6.5, reflux and activation of pepsin, not just gastric acid, may be the true culprit of laryngeal damage in LPR [6].

Pepsin and acid may not be the only causative factor for symptoms of LPR. New research suggests not only reflux causes symptoms but also a complex system of reflexes, upon stimulation, can result with LPR-related symptoms. Innervation of the esophagus and larynx occurs via different branches of the vagus nerve. In the esophagus, the vagus nerve only contains excitatory neurons that cause contraction [7]. When the esophageal excitatory neurons are stimulated, a reflexive feedback mechanism to the superior laryngeal branch of the vagus nerve of the cough center in the medulla can be triggered via chemoreceptors and nociceptors [1]. This then activates efferent nerves to stimulate a reflexive cough. The mechanism of cough involves complete vocal fold closure creating increased pressure followed by expulsion of noxious material. Therefore, chronic cough undoubtedly causes vocal cord irritation, which cascades to symptoms of hoarseness, globus sensation, and evidence of edema and erythema as seen on laryngoscopy. These symptoms repeatedly incite the cough reflex, perpetuating the problem in a cyclical manner.

Neurogenic cough occurs in the absence of any noxious stimuli and is a form of sensory neuropathy due to heightened brainstem reflex. Patients who have a neurogenic cough are subject to similar symptoms of hoarseness, globus sensation, and pharyngitis [8]. Inter-arytenoid pachydermia, erythema, and edema of the vocal cords are also apparent on laryngoscopy. Similarly, distal esophageal stimulation can result in a variety of symptoms proximally through a variety of reflexes. Cough, laryngospasm, bronchospasm, acute dysphonia, globus, and discomfort are just a few of the laryngopharyngeal symptoms that can occur with esophageal stimulation. Reflux hypersensitivity can occur in the presence of normal acid exposure and produce symptoms of heartburn, globus, and discomfort identical to those seen in nonerosive reflux disease (NERD) [9].

Almost counterintuitive would be to consider hypochlorhydria as a contributing factor to symptoms of LPR. In one study comparing GERD symptoms between male and female subjects, females, with higher rates of hypochlorhydria, tended to have increased symptoms severity [10]. In fact, hypochlorhydria symptoms, such as bloating and heartburn, may be easily mistaken as secondary to hyperchlorhydria [11]. Proton pump inhibitor (PPI) overuse is a significant contributor to hypochlorhydria. PPIs are more frequently used off-label, above the standard dose, and for prolonged periods of time. One study in 2015 reported a 456% increase in PPI use since the 1990s, and it continues to be listed in the top 10 most prescribed medications in the United States [12]. In the hospital setting, PPIs are prescribed prophylactically, yet the majority of these patients do not have a justifiable reason for the medication. Additionally, these patients are habitually discharged on a PPI as clinicians fail to review their need. Furthermore, when patients attempt to stop PPI use, they can be met with rebound acid hypersecretion, which can occur after taking the medication for as little as 8 weeks [12]. Kines et al. suggest a hydrochloric acid (HCl) challenge when hypochlorhydria is suspected, composed of one capsule of betaine/HCL/pepsin starting at 650 mg taken with a protein meal. The dose can be increased until the patient becomes asymptomatic and should be continued at the highest asymptomatic dose. Contraindications would include patients with active gastritis, esophagitis, or duodenitis [11]. This protocol does not give a dose maximum; therefore, it is important to keep in mind the maximum normal amount of gastric acid secreted is 1.5 L daily.

Current Standard of Care

PPI and Histamine (H2) Antagonists PPIs were first utilized in the 1980s and function via protonation followed by binding to the α-subunit H^+K^+-ATPase to suppress acid secretion. Because of the need for protonation prior to binding, they are most effective in an acidic environment and therefore should be taken 1 hour prior to breakfast for maximal results [13]. The overall safety profile for PPIs is generally good for short-term use, while long-term patients are at risk for rebound acidosis, osteoporosis, pneumonia, and possibly *Helicobacter pylori* infection. Recent analysis of long-term use data suggests a potential increase in the risk of heart disease, cerebrovascular disease, kidney and liver disease, stomach and esophageal cancers, and death from all causes [14–17]. Discontinuation of PPIs should be slow and titrated first decreasing to a single dose per day and then one dose every other day to avoid potential rebound hypersecretion.

The nonspecific diagnostic techniques for LPR make empiric therapy with PPI a diagnostic measure used frequently. Patients are instructed to take a PPI in the morning along with an H2 receptor antagonist (H2RA) before bedtime for 1–2 months. If patients improve, they are assumed to have had LPR as their diagnosis [18]. Patients who do not respond to a single PPI in the morning are instructed to increase the dose to twice daily. However, a 2006 study shows that PPI therapy offers no significant symptom reduction relative to placebo [19]. A Cochrane Review in 2006 also showed no improvement of LPR symptoms with PPIs [20]. Those studies that did show clinically significant improvement with PPIs did not show changes with respect to LPR. Therefore, it is more likely that LPR patients who appear to improve may be decreasing acid exposure and removing triggers in an overly sensitive laryngopharynx or have concomitant GERD and do better than those without GERD.

H2 blockers work through inhibition of the histamine-driven acid secretion and gastrin-induced acid secretion [13]. They have a slower onset of action and provide only temporary relief. This is typically an add-on for nocturnal breakthrough acid or as replacement for PPI use. Tolerance to H2RAs has an onset after 1–2 weeks of therapy. A 2007 review of patients with reflux esophagitis demonstrated clinically significant benefits to those patients taking H2RAs versus placebo [21]. Interestingly, in many of the studies suggesting potential risks of long-term PPI use, H2RA use in the same population of patients did not appear to confer the same risks, suggesting a safer alternative to PPIs.

Diet Modification Western medicine has traditionally focused on the use of medication to treat disease. Yet despite the billions spent yearly, chronic diseases are on the rise. Reflux disease continues to increase and is being seen more frequently in younger populations. Additionally, the rise in esophageal cancer is raising the alarm. Recently, literature has arisen using diet rather than medicine for treatment of reflux disease. Given the high cost of medication, potential for interaction, and the benefit of diet with other chronic diseases, the focus on treatment is trending toward a more holistic, diet-based approach which has shown to be as effective as, if not better than, medication [22–24]. However, there is still controversy on whether these changes have a measurable effect on GERD. Specific to LPR, there is a lack of research on the true benefits of diet modification particularly for those without typical GERD symptoms. Most dietary interventions focus on behaviors, foods, and drinks that are more likely triggers than actual cause of reflux disease. Much of this lack of evidence results from poor standardization of testing, absence of a true gold standard in diagnosis, varied dietary interventions, and poorly controlled studies. An extensive literature review showed no evidence indicating dietary changes improved reflux symptoms or pH profiles in GERD [25]. However, The Geneva Workshop Report suggests that most reflux is postprandial, and therefore, dietary measures can be therapeutic [25, 26].

Caffeine avoidance is often recommended as a diet modification. It can be found in such foods as coffee, tea, and chocolate. Caffeine is considered an indirect precipitant of reflux through decreasing pressures of the LES and decreasing sphincter tone, leading to an increase in esophageal exposure to acid [25]. While one study showed increased GERD in caffeine drinkers, participants had to drink between four and seven cups per day to notice this difference [3]. Caffeine is, therefore, likely a trigger of reflux disease, rather than a causative factor.

Carbonated beverages similarly are understood to decrease LES pressure and sphincter tone. In healthy individuals, carbonated beverages can cause 30%–50% reduction of resting pressure, abdominal length, and overall length of the LES, thus contributing to reflux disease [27]. Additionally, as gas comes out of solution, increased gastric pressure can possibly promote reflux of gastric contents through a weakened sphincter. Aerosolized refluxate is thought to be a major factor in LPR onset and propagation. In one large prospective cohort study, consumption of carbonated soft drinks was found to be a large predictor of GERD during sleep and early morning symptoms [28]. Therefore, to decrease episodes of reflux, it is recommended to avoid carbonated beverages. Spicy foods have been recognized as an exacerbating factor of GERD symptoms due to direct irritation of previously inflamed esophageal mucosa. Additionally, these foods alone can contribute to reflux or affect the LES. Thought to cause increased gastric acid production, pepsin production, or mucosal irritation, the exact mechanism of inducing heartburn and other reflux symptoms is unknown [29]. In one study assessing a number of foods for provocation of reflux symptoms, hot-spicy foods caused symptoms in greater than half the patients with no difference in age, gender, and BMI. Additionally, many patients are likely to experience perceived reflux events when they eat spicy foods [30]. Capsaicin, the active ingredient in spicy foods, has been used as provocation tests in reflux and chronic cough. Interestingly, while immediate exposure to capsaicin can induce a wide range of reflux symptoms, continued exposure seems to reduce symptoms suggesting a potential treatment role, especially in the setting of laryngopharyngeal and esophageal hypersensitivity [31]. The potential for capsaicin to decrease reflux symptoms indicates that spicy foods are likely triggers rather than direct causes of reflux disease.

Another type of food implicated in inducing reflux symptoms is tomato-based or acidic foods such as citrus fruits and juices. Little data is available regarding the effect of these foods as a causative factor or trigger of reflux. However, they are understood to add insult to injury with the additional dose of acidic exposure to the mucosa. Furthermore, in patients with LPR who are considered to have pepsin-positive mucosa, even weak acids at pH of 5 can activate pepsin, causing damage and thus symptoms [6]. Even without pepsin present, acids with pH of 4 can damage mucosa, triggering symptoms of cough and hoarseness.

More recent theories on acid reflux suggest that a Western diet consists of food, vegetables, and water processed using nitrates, nitrites, and other preservatives. It has been hypothesized that this increase in nitrates is linked to the increased prevalence of GERD [32]. Nitrates are converted to nitrites in the oral cavity. One study determined that nitrate reductase activity is higher in patients with GERD symptoms suggesting that any increase in nitrate provides substrate to be converted to nitrite stimulating GERD at the LES [32]. Foods such as cabbage, lettuce, celery, and radishes have high nitrate content. Interestingly, they also have a more alkaline pH, and nitrate reductase activity is greater at higher pH levels suggesting a possible role in alleviating reflux symptoms [33]. Nitrates as medication relax smooth muscle and decrease LES pressure and impair esophageal clearance potentially leading to worse reflux presentation [34, 35].

High-fat foods have been implicated in reducing LES pressure and delaying gastric emptying similar to foods such as chocolate and caffeine, leading to an increase in reflux symptoms [3]. Similarly, low-carbohydrate diets have been shown to improve GERD symptoms. However, in these studies, patients were also reported to have restricted caffeine and alcohol intake. These studies reduced simple sugars in the diet, known to reduce weight and inflammation, whereas increasing fiber and complex carbohydrates to the diet appears to improve symptoms of reflux disease. No large-scale studies have been done on either low-fat diet or low-carbohydrate diet effects on LPR and GERD [3, 25].

Contradictory data is available regarding the relationship between alcohol and reflux disease. Beer and wine were able to induce symptoms only in the first hour after ingestion [36]. Interestingly, research available showed that the amount of alcohol consumed did not affect symptoms. In a study by Pehl in 2006, there was no difference between white wine and beer in the induction of reflux in patients with and without GERD [37]. In contrast, Chen et al. noted an inverse relationship between ingestion of beer and reflux disease. There also appeared to be a difference in effect depending on whether the patient had erosive or nonerosive reflux, with less effect in those patients with nonerosive GERD [38]. Thought to decrease LES pressure as a primary mechanism, direct exposure of mucosa to alcohol also likely plays a role as a trigger of reflux symptoms. Therefore, it is suggested that patients with reflux disease avoid alcoholic beverages.

Tobacco Cessation While studies suggest smokers have a 70% greater risk of reflux, causation has not definitively been determined [3]. It has been hypothesized that smoking increases acid reflux likely due to decreased salivary production and increased acid clearance time as well as lowered pressure of the LES [39, 40]. One Scandinavian study assessed that smoking cessation increases overall salivary bicarbonate, thus assisting in acid clearance [41]. Through conflicting studies, nicotine has also been implicated in increased reflux symptoms through mechanisms of increased acid and pepsin secretion, blockade of H2RA treatment, impaired blood flow, and mucous production. Timely, the increasing use of vaping of nicotine potentially has a role in increasing reflux symptoms and onset of reflux disease. The addition of alcohol to smoking can potentiate reflux by similar mechanisms of decreased LES pressure, increased acid exposure time, and direct mucosal injury from both the alcohol and many byproducts of smoking. Smoking has a moderate causal association with reflux, whereas alcohol is more likely a trigger. However, both can potentiate symptoms and possibly lead to greater complications of reflux disease, including malignant transformation [42].

Sleep Modification Sleep and body position during sleep have been studied for its effect on reflux severity. Freidin et al. showed that during sleep, mechanisms to prevent reflux, such as LES pressure, are depressed and there are varying increases in relaxation of the LES based on the sleep stage [43]. Additionally, acid clearance of the esophagus appears to be prolonged during sleep as opposed to during waking hours leading to longer exposure times of the esophagus to damaging acid and pepsin [3]. To assist in decreasing acid exposure time, elevation of the head of the bed has been suggested as a simple, early step. Although increasing the number of pillows can accomplish head elevation, typically, this does not last throughout the night. Instead, a wedge under the mattress or blocks under the frame of the bed are a more effective approach. Elevation of the head of the bed has been shown to be beneficial in those with laryngeal symptoms of reflux [44].

Another sleep position notable for its effect on GERD is left lateral recumbent (LLR). Specifically, transient LES relaxation and delayed gastric emptying have greater improvement in the LLR position rather than the right lateral recumbent position (RLR) [45]. One study combined the left lateral recumbency with the head of bed elevation using a MedCline Acid Reflux Relief System (MedCline, San Diego, CA) (Fig. 29.1) to assess the collective effects on GERD. Results confirmed that the head of bed elevation and LLR positioning significantly reduced esophageal acid exposure. An interesting result of this study showed that RLR positioning in sleep had the highest acid exposure, even greater than lying flat. This is likely due to food resting in the dependent portion of the stomach with only gas available at the LES when LLR. In contrast, RLR allows food and acid to rest at the entrance of the LES and easily reflux into the esophagus [46]. Additionally, the diaphragmatic

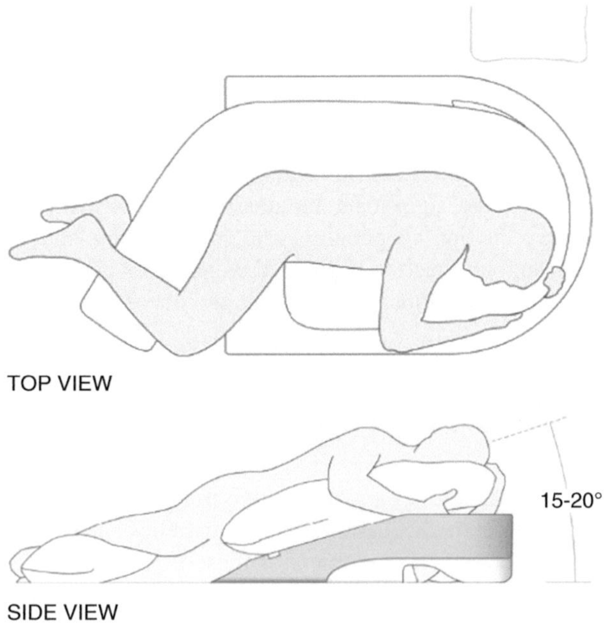

Fig. 29.1 MedCline Acid Reflux Relief System – top view and side view

pinch at the LES region likely adds to the closure of the LES in the LLR position with the opposite effect of greater opening in the RLR position.

Obstructive sleep apnea is potentially associated with increased reflux events, both GERD and LPR. Similar causative factors such as obesity and poor diet play a role in the overlap of reflux symptoms and severity; however, the negative pressures generated during obstructive events can increase reflux independently, leading to worsening acid exposure times of the esophagus and laryngopharynx [47]. In addition, nighttime reflux events can lead to poor sleep quality, increased awakenings, and worsening symptomatology. Coughing during sleep is most commonly associated with nocturnal reflux events. Reflexive laryngospasm and coughing with esophageal exposure as well as direct laryngotracheal exposure to refluxate are mechanisms that contribute to coughing and episodic stridor during sleep [47].

In the assessment of multiple factors affecting GERD including sleep position, short dinner-to-bedtime interval was found to significantly impact recurrence of reflux events in all types of reflux. Particularly, eating within 3 hours of lying down appears to have the greatest effect on reflux events. It is recommended for patients with reflux to therefore delay lying down after eating for at least 3 hours [48]. Patients with decreased peristalsis or delayed gastric emptying, both vagally mediated, are at higher risk for reflux symptoms. Having the last meal of the day be the smallest, increasing fiber content, liquid washes while eating, and remaining upright longer may be helpful in mitigating symptoms.

Weight Loss/Clothing Central obesity and enlarged abdominal girth have been implicated in amplifying the risk of reflux development, likely secondary to increased intra-abdominal pressure, the development of hiatal herniation, and shared mechanisms of onset, namely, poor diet. Similarly, intra-abdominal pressure can be elevated in those wearing tight-fitting pants or belts, and comparative effect on the LES is often seen [49]. One longitudinal study demonstrated that general weight loss could improve symptoms of GERD although decreased waist circumference had no effect on reflux [50]. A far larger study with over 15,000 patients demonstrated significant reduction in reflux symptoms with weight loss and/or waist reduction in patients who had existing abdominal obesity. A monitored, coaching approach to organized weight loss can result in substantial resolution of symptoms of reflux in overweight and obese subjects.

Alternative Treatment

For thousands of years, alternative treatments in the form of botanicals have been used to treat medical ailments of all varieties and severities. In fact, modern medication is derived from extracts of these botanicals and spices. In their herbal form, many of these supplements are not well controlled, and their dosing and strength are not standardized. There is a lack of oversight and many potential risk factors and drug interactions in both potentiating and inhibiting effects, and self-treatment can be dangerous. Numerous botanicals can be used in treating GERD and LPR under the appropriate guidance. Symptoms should be monitored and further investigated by a trained healthcare professional as needed. A brief overview of possible alternative treatments for GERD and LPR is noted in Table 29.1.

Turmeric Curcumin, which contributes to the yellow pigment of the household spice turmeric and is derived from *Curcuma longa* root, is widely known in Ayurvedic medicine as an antioxidant and anti-inflammatory. Additionally, it has been shown to have antineoplastic effects in the oral cavity and esophagus [51]. Curcumin is the active ingredient in turmeric. However, the overall composition of turmeric only contains 2–8% of curcumin. Nevertheless, it has still demonstrated the ability to increase gastrin, secretin, and bicarbonate secretion and act as an anti-inflammatory and antioxidant [52, 53]. Frequently thought to be due to caustic injury, an animal model study showed mucosal injury to be more likely due to an inflammatory reaction to acid exposure rather than direct mucosal injury by acid [54]. In studies designed to test acid exposure in GERD patients, curcumin prevented expression of inflammatory cytokines such as IL-6 and IL-8 in esophageal tissue. Human esophageal cells (HET-1A) were isolated and exposed to acidic pH with and without the presence of curcumin. IL-6 and IL-8 secretion was measured, and cells that were pre-treated with curcumin showed inhibition of IL-6 and IL-8 secretion [55]. While in vivo animal model studies comparing curcumin to lansoprazole (a common PPI) indicated curcumin to be less potent than a PPI in acid reflux esophagitis, it was found superior to PPI in mixed acid-bile reflux [56]. While human studies using curcumin have not been completed, it may be reasonable to

Table 29.1 Overview of alternative treatments for GERD/LPR

Treatment	Example	Mechanism of action
Turmeric		Antioxidant Anti-inflammatory
Botanicals	STW-5	Relax proximal stomach Increase distal motility
	Lonicerae (Chinese honeysuckle)	Unclear. Possible antioxidant
	Curania tricuspidata (mandarin melon berry)	H2 receptor blocker
Mucilage	*Althea officinalis* (marshmallow)	Temporary protective coating
Tea	*Matricaria,recutita* (chamomile)	Analgesic
	Salvia officinalis (sage)	Breaks cough reflex cycle
Homeopathy	Argenticurn nitricum	Reduces coughing
	Hepar sulphuricum	Reduces globus sensation due to cough and belching
Motility agents	Metoclopramide	Increases LES pressure
	Melatonin	Stimulates gastrin Decreases gastric acid secretion
	Rikkunshito (Japanese kampo)	Decreases sensory stimulation Increases acid clearance
Psyllium/fiber		Decreases intra-abdominal pressure
Alginate	Gaviscon	Raft forming
	Reflux Gourmet	Barrier to reflux at LES
Acupuncture	Points to calm and regulate stomach	Decreases bile and acid reflux
Alkaline water		Irreversibly inactivate pepsin

deduce from animal studies that curcumin ingestion prior to and during food intake may help decrease acid-induced inflammation.

Gum Chewing Gum chewing works on the supposition of GERD patients having nocturnal reflux and LPR patients having daytime reflux [57]. Saliva is composed of 99.5% water and 0.5% electrolytes including sodium, potassium, and bicarbonate. In fact, there are 25 mmol/L of bicarbonate in saliva. Gum chewing has been shown to increase salivary production and salivary bicarbonate concentration. Furthermore, the increase in bicarbonate concentration was based on quantity and length of gum chewing [58]. Based on this concept, Koufman and Smoak set out to assess if chewing gum could be used to increase pH and decrease symptoms in patients with LPR. They found that both esophageal and laryngeal pH increased with gum chewing. Still, those who chewed bicarbonate gum had an adjunctive anti-reflux effect compared to subjects who chewed regular gum. Additionally, no reflux events occurred at all during gum-chewing periods with a noted pH-buffering effect twice as long during chewing periods [59].

In addition to the bicarbonate effect of saliva from chewing gum, increased saliva may clear acid in a washout method via a combination of the liquid in saliva and increased swallowing, thus increasing peristalsis and decreasing acid exposure time

Table 29.2 Herbal constituents of Iberogast

Botanical Latin name	Common name	Part used	Amount (per 100 mL)
Matricaria recutita	German chamomile	Flower	20 mL
Iberis mara	Clown's mustard (bitter candy)	Tuft	15 mL
Anelica archangelica	Garden angelica	Root and rhizome	10 mL
Carum carvi	Caraway	Fruit	10 mL
Melissa officinalis	Lemon balm	Leaf	10 mL
Chelidonium maius	Greater celandine	Aerial part	10 mL
Glycyrrhiza glabra	Licorice	Root	10 mL
Silybum marianum	Milk thistle	Fruit	10 mL
Mentha piperita	Peppermint	Leaf	5 mL

Patrick [25]

[60]. However, the effect of gum chewing on increased swallow and increased peristalsis has not yet been studied.

Botanicals Numerous herbs have been found to improve symptoms of acid reflux, majority being STW 5, *Iberogast* botanical derivatives which have been used in Germany for many years. There are a total of nine Iberogast botanicals commonly used in combination including *Mentha piperita* (peppermint oil), *Glycyrrhiza glabra* (licorice root), *Melissa officinalis* (lemon balm leaf), and *Carum carvi* (caraway fruit) [25, 61] (Table 29.2). Iberogast botanicals affect different portions of the stomach differently. They increase relaxation of the proximal stomach and increase motility of the distal stomach [62]. In one meta-analysis, *Iberogast* was found to have a 60% success rate in decreasing symptoms of GERD from severe to mild or absent [63].

Peppermint has been found to relax smooth muscle and, therefore, decrease the resting LES pressure. This same relaxation of smooth muscles leads to an accelerated early phase gastric emptying and prolonged relaxation time of the pyloric sphincter [64]. Therefore, the effect of peppermint may worsen reflux in some individuals. However, in regard to LPR symptoms, peppermint has been found to have antinociceptive and anti-inflammatory properties, which may improve symptoms [65].

While *Glycyrrhiza glabra*, licorice root, has not been studied with particular respect to LPR, it has been studied for its soothing properties in sore throats. In one randomized, double-blinded study, patients who gargled licorice root just prior to intubation had significantly reduced (by 50%) cough and sore throat post extubation [66]. These mollifying affects can likely be extrapolated as a treatment for the cough and sore throat in LPR. Care must be taken when ingesting licorice root as it may act as a diuretic or interfere with numerous medications.

Mucilages are very hydrophilic gelatin-like phytochemicals derived from herbs such as *Althaea officinalis* (marshmallow) and *Ulmus fulva* (slippery elm). Mucilages have been known to coat and lubricate irritated upper digestive tract and oropharyngeal mucosa, particularly caused by cough [67, 68]. According to *Principles and Practice of Phytotherapy*, mucilages can be taken after meals for reflux esophagitis [69]. Mucilages can also form a temporary protective barrier against inflammation. Both herbs have extremely low toxicity and have been found to be safe and effective in relieving GERD symptoms [68]. Marshmallow leaves should be collected just before flowering for highest mucilage. Both marshmallow and slippery elm can be infused into water overnight for a sweet soothing drink. Early studies into *Althaea officinalis* lozenges have been done on mice to determine their disintegration and drug release time [67]. Further studies would be needed to determine optimal dosing.

Cudrania tricuspidata, or mandarin melon berry, can effectively block H2 receptors leading to a significant decrease in gastric acidity potentially leading to a decline in acid production and thus reflux symptoms [70].

Lonicera (Chinese honeysuckle), a widely used herb in Chinese formulas, is known as a heat-dissipating herb often used for sore throats [71]. It has been studied for its affects on GERD in rats. Rats that were given honeysuckle-powdered water were found to have significantly improved esophageal mucosa. While the exact mechanism was unclear, evidence appeared to point to antioxidant properties since tissues were found to have increased glutathione and lower levels of myeloperoxidase [72]. Unfortunately, no human studies are currently available.

Psyllium/Fiber Psyllium is a medicinal plant used in treatment of constipation through increasing bowel peristalsis. Chronic constipation is commonly a result of insufficient dietary fiber and fluids and is associated with GERD in nearly 30% of cases with a female predominance [73]. One study compared the effect of psyllium and PPI in GERD patients who concomitantly suffered from constipation. The difference in symptom resolution was not clinically significant showing psyllium to be just as effective as PPIs in the treatment of GERD symptoms in those who have chronic constipation [73].

Tea Studies regarding the relationship between tea and GERD have been controversial, with some reporting a positive correlation and some reporting no correlation at all [74]. In theory, theophylline products in tea are considered to decrease LES pressure. However, not all tea is processed from the same leaves. Teas derived from the *Matricaria recutita*, chamomile, plant show great analgesic as well as antibacterial properties. A similar plant used in teas, *Achillea millefolium* (yarrow), is often used for gastrointestinal symptoms of GERD [75]. Chamomile in particular is used to soothe sore throats. *Salvia officinalis*, sage, is a common cooking herb that can be instilled into teas. Multiple studies have proven the beneficial effects of sage as a tea and as an herbal supplement on pharyngitis [76, 77]. Having considered that LPR may indeed be a reflex rather than a reflux, an assuaging tea may break the cycle of cough and hoarseness.

Alginates Alternatively known as raft-forming agents, alginates have a unique mechanism of acid reflux prevention. In the presence of gastric acid, alginates form a gel. When bicarbonate is formulated with alginate, it is converted to carbon dioxide that becomes trapped in the gel as bubbles. This provides a lighter density for the gel to float to the surface of the junction of the esophagus and proximal stomach and act as a raft barrier for reflux prevention [25]. Alginate-based therapy was studied in comparison to placebo, antacids, and PPI treatments. Alginates were preferred over a placebo or antacids; however, they were found to be less effective when compared to PPI therapy. Nonetheless, a meta-analysis of studies comparing alginate therapy to PPI found the decrease in effectiveness to be clinically insignificant [78]. Alginate therapy has been shown to be effective specifically in LPR when taken in liquid preparation [3]. Overall, alginates are a safe, effective initial treatment for LPR. Once patients begin a more Mediterranean-style, plant-based diet, symptoms begin to abate. Alginates can help during symptom exacerbation and flare-ups or during dietary indiscretions during this transitional period. In addition, once patients making dietary changes start to lose weight and have symptoms abate, alginates can be used as a bridge to weaning of PPI use.

Acupuncture Patients who fail single-dose PPI use are typically prescribed a double dose. Yet, some patients do not improve even on this double dose. One study compared the addition of acupuncture to single-dose PPI versus a double-dose PPI for those who failed single-dose PPI treatment. Acupuncture treatment of five points selected specifically to calm and regulate the stomach given over a 4-week period was shown to improve symptoms of daytime and nighttime heartburn, acid regurgitation, dysphagia, and chest pain significantly as opposed to the double-dose PPI group with only daytime heartburn symptom improvement [25]. Other studies have proven that four acupuncture points (CV 12, ST36, SP6, PC6) stimulated daily for 6 weeks significantly reduce esophageal acid and bile reflux as well as GERD-related symptoms [79].

Alkaline Water Patients with LPR demonstrate increased tissue-bound pepsin which was previously thought to be inactive at pH greater than 4.4. However, recent studies establish human pepsin to be activated even at pH of 6.5, and it only becomes denatured above a pH of 8.0 [6]. According to the US FDA regulations put in place in 1973, all bottled and canned food and beverages aside from water are required to have a pH of 4.6 or less to prevent bacterial contamination [80, 81]. pH testing of numerous companies of bottled water showed an average pH of 6.7–7.4 and does not include bicarbonate [6].

While pH of 6.7–7.4 will minimally activate pepsin, it will not lead to its deactivation. Alkaline water with a pH of 8.8 has been shown to irreversibly denature pepsin in vitro. In fact, one study showed that pepsin diluted in water with a pH of 7.0 retained near maximal activity when exposed to acid. However, pepsin in alkaline water, pH 8.8, remained irreversibly inactivated even when followed by acidic contact. Additionally, alkaline water required double the amount of HCL than non-alkaline water in order to reach equivalent pepsin activity [6]. Another study comparing alkaline water and a Mediterranean diet versus standard PPI in the treatment of LPR found no clinically significant difference in the treatment [22]. This data suggests that alkaline water, in conjunction with a mostly plant-based diet, not only may be beneficial in patients with LPR but also can potentially eliminate the need for PPI use with the inherent side effects associated with pharmacotherapy.

Apple Cider Vinegar While a lot of information is available in the form of anecdotal evidence, there is little scientific evidence for the use of apple cider vinegar (ACV) as a treatment for any form of acid reflux. Vinegar itself is an acid and in undiluted amounts can cause harm to the laryngeal and esophageal mucosa. Some of the evidence for ACV use for sore throats is based on the difficulty for bacteria to grow in high-acidic environments. Theoretically, lowering the pH in the stomach can potentially lead to decreased gastrin release, thus leading to decrease in endogenous HCl and pepsin release mitigating symptoms of GERD. However, by drinking ACV, direct exposure to the laryngopharyngeal tissues could hypothetically activate tissue-bound pepsin and cause direct caustic damage as well as chemosensory stimulation. ACV is not recommended for the treatment of LPR, and further randomized, placebo-controlled studies should be undertaken prior to recommendation for any symptom of reflux.

Homeopathy According to the *Repertory of the Homeopathic Materia Medica*, there are several different remedies that can be used for sore throats. Each remedy is used for different causes of sore throats [82]. However, each remedy fits a different personal constitution to help determine which may best fit a particular individual at a specific time. Remedies such as aconite, argentum nitricum (Arg Nit), Bryonia (Bry), silica (Sil), hepar sulphuricum (Hep Sulph), and kali bichromicum (Kali Bich) are just a few that are specific for sore throats. Among these, Arg Nit is used specifically for a lost voice, while Hep Sulph is for voice loss with morning cough. Additionally, Arg Nit is noted to be useful for gastrointestinal problems and belching, a symptom of reflux. Bryonia, while noted to be for dry and painful cough, is best used by those whose cough is worsened after foods such as cabbage or beans and in the evening. The globus sensation often caused by acid reflux can likely be treated with Hep Sulph, a remedy typically used for sensation of something caught in the back of the throat [82, 83]. These remedies have been poorly studied for their use in acid reflux treatment and are not regulated. They should only be used under the guidance of a healthcare professional.

Motility Agents Decreased esophageal motility has been studied as a primary disorder in patients with GERD and may play a role in patients with LPR. Therefore, prokinetic agents have been used as secondary treatment for reflux disease. Metoclopramide, a motility agent often used as an antiemetic, has been shown to significantly increase both LES resting pressure and esophageal contractility without affecting compliance of the esophagus [84]. Multiple studies as far back as 1973 have shown similar increase in the resting pressure of LES leading to a decrease in reflux events and esophageal and potentially laryngopharyngeal exposure [84].

Table 29.3 Daily dosage of melatonin with additional nutritional supplementation

Supplement	Dosage
Melatonin	6 mg
Folic acid	10 mg
Vitamin B6	25 mg
Vitamin B12	50 mg
Betaine	100 mg
Methionine	100 mg
L-Tryptophan	200 mg

Patrick [25]

A Japanese Kampo medicine consisting of eight herbs, rikkunshito, is a gastric motility agent that has been used to treat a variety of gastrointestinal conditions such as chronic dyspepsia, anorexia, and nausea [85]. Recent studies show that it has also been useful in treatment of esophageal acid reflux symptoms in children. Using pH probe testing, children given rikkunshito were determined to have decreased frequency of symptoms, while actual acid remained unchanged, potentially from decreased sensory stimulation. Additionally, these studies show relief of symptoms and distal esophageal acid secondary to improved acid clearance [86].

Melatonin, widely associated with production in the pineal gland, is actually produced 500 times more in the intestinal tract. Melatonin levels in the gut mucosa increase by 100–400 times the amount in peripheral blood after a person eats [25]. The increased production of melatonin has been identified as a gut motility agent. There is a significant amount of melatonin-binding sites in the esophageal mucosa. Melatonin has also been noted to inhibit gastric acid secretion and stimulate gastrin, which increases contractility of the LES [25]. Daytime serum melatonin levels in patients with GERD are 50% lower than controls [87]. Pereira found that after 40 days, 100% of patients taking melatonin combined with nutritional supplementation were reflux symptom-free, while only 40% of those taking a PPI were symptom-free, potentially suggesting melatonin use as an adjunct treatment [88] (Table 29.3).

References

1. Francis DO, Vaezi MF. Should the reflex be reflux? Throat symptoms and alternative explanations. Clin Gastroenterol Hepatol. 2015;13:1560–6.
2. Koufman JA. The otolaryngologic manifestations of gastroesophageal reflux disease (GERD): a clinical investigation of 225 patients using ambulatory 24-hour pH monitoring and an experimental investigation of the role of acid and pepsin in the development of laryngeal injury. Laryngoscope. 1991;101(Suppl 53):1–78.
3. Marinucci I, de Bortoli N, Savarino E, NAcci A, Romeo SO, Bellini M, Vavarino V, Fattori B, Marchi S. Optimal treatment of laryngopharyngeal reflux disease. Ther Adv Chronic Dis. 2013;4(6):287–301.
4. Carroll TL, Werner A, Nahikian K, Dezube A, Roth DF. Rethinking the laryngopharyngeal reflux treatment algorithm: evaluating an alternate empiric dosing regimen and considering up-front, pH-impedance, and manometry testing to minimize cost in treating suspect laryngopharyngeal reflux disease. Laryngoscope. 2017;127:s1–s13.

5. Johnston N, Knight J, Dettmar PW, Lifely MO, Koufman J. Pepsin and carbonic anhydrase isoenzyme III as diagnostic markers for laryngopharyngeal reflux disease. Laryngoscope. 2004;114:2129–34.
6. Koufman JA, Johnston N. Potential benefits of pH 8.8 alkaline drinking water as an adjunct in the treatment of reflux disease. Ann Oto Rhinol Laryn. 2012;121(7):431–4.
7. Lee S, Jin Oh C, Seon JW. Sympathetic nerve entrapment point injection as an antireflux procedure for refractory laryngopharyngeal reflux: a first case report of innovative anatomic regulation. Innov Clin Neurosci. London; UK. 2016;13:32–6.
8. Altman KW, Noordzii JP, Rosen CA, Cohen S, Sulica L. Neurogenic cough. Laryngoscope. 2015;125:1675–81.
9. Yamasaki T, Fass R. Reflux hypersensitivity: a new functional esophageal disorder. J Neurogastroenterol Motil. 2017;23(4):495–503. https://doi.org/10.5056/jnm17097.
10. Iwai W, Abe Y, Iijima K, Koike T, Uno K, Asano N, Imatani A, Shimosegawa T. Gastric hypochlorhydria is associated with an exacerbation of dyspeptic symptoms in female patients. J Gastrenterol. 2013;48(2):214–21.
11. Kines K, Krupczak T. Nutritional interventions for gastroesophageal reflux, irritable bowel syndrome, and hypochlorhydria: a case report. Integr Med. 2016;15(4):49–53.
12. Ksiadzyna D, Szelag A, Paradowski L. Overuse of proton pump inhibitors. Polish Archiv Med. 2015;125(4):289–98.
13. Schubert ML, Peura DA. Control of gastric acid in health and disease. Gastroenterology. 2008;134:1842–60.
14. Hart E, Dunn TE, Feuerstein S, Jacobs DM. Proton pump inhibitors and risk of acute and chronic kidney disease: a retrospective cohort. Pharmacotherapy. 2019;39(4):443–53.
15. Xie Y, Bowe B, Li T, Xian H, Yan Y, Al-Aly Z. Risk of death among users of Proton Pump Inhibitors: a longitudinal observational cohort study of United States veterans. BMJ Open. 2017;47(6):e015735. https://doi.org/10.1136/bmjopen-2016-015735.
16. Cheung KS, Leung WK. Long term risk of proton pump inhibitors and risk of gastric cancer: a review of current evidence. Ther Adv Gastroenterol. 2019;12:1–11. https://doi.org/10.1177/1756284819834511.
17. Sukhovershin RA, Cooke JP. How may proton pump inhibitors impair cardiovascular health? Am J Cardiovasc Drugs. 2016;16(3):153–61. https://doi.org/10.1007/s40256-01600160-9.
18. Asaoka D, Nagahara A, Matsumoto K, Hojo M, Watanabe S. Current perspectives on reflux laryngitis. Clin J Gastroenterol. 2014;7:471–5.
19. Qadeer MA, Phillips CO, Lopez AR, Steward DL, Noordzij JP, Wo JM, Suurna M, Havas T, Howden CW, Vaezi MF. Proton pump inhibitor therapy for suspected GERD-related chronic laryngitis: a meta-analysis of randomized controlled trials. Am J Gastroenterol. 2006;101:2646–54.
20. Hopkins C, Yousaf U, Pedersen M. Acid reflux treatment for hoarseness. Cochrane Database Syst Rev. 2006;1:CD005054.
21. Khan M, Santana J, Donnellan C, Preston C, Moayyedi P. Medical treatments in the short term management of reflux oesophagitis. Cochrane Database Syst Rev. 2007;2:CD003244.
22. Zalvan CH, Hu S, Greenberg B, Geliebter J. Comparison of alkaline water and Mediterranean diet vs proton pump inhibition for treatment of laryngopharyngeal reflux. JAMA Otolaryngol Head Neck Surg. 2017;143(10):1023–9. https://doi.org/10.1001/jamaoto.2017.1454.
23. Koufman JA. Low-acid diet for recalcitrant laryngopharyngeal reflux: therapeutic benefits and their implications. Ann Otol Rhinol Laryngol. 2011;120:281–7.
24. Yang J, Dehom S, Sanders S, Murry T, Krishna P, Crawley BK. Treating laryngopharyngeal reflux: evaluation of an anti-reflux program with comparison to medications. Am J Otolaryngol. 2018;39(1):50–5. https://doi.org/10.1016/j.amjoto.2017.10.014. Epub 2017 Oct 31.
25. Patrick L. Gastroesophageal Reflux disease (gerd): a review of conventional and alternative treatments. Altern Med Rev. 2011;16(2):116–33.
26. Dent J, Brun J, Fendrick A, Fennerty M, Janssens J, Kahrilas P, Lauritsen K, Reynolds J, Shaw M, Talley N. An evidence-based appraisal of reflux disease management – the Geval Workshop Report. Gut. 1999;44(Suppl 2):S1–S16.

27. Hamoui N, Lord RV, Hagen JA, Theisen J, Demeester TR, Crookes PF. Response of the lower esophageal sphincter to gastric distention by carbonated beverages. J Gastrointest Surg. 2006;10(6):870–7.
28. Fass R, Quan S, O'Connor G, Ervin A, Iber C. Predictors of heartburn during sleep in a large prospective cohort study. Chest. 2005;127:1658–66.
29. Milke P, Diaz A, Valdovinos MA, Moran S. Gastroesophageal reflux in healthy subjects induced by two different species of chilli (capsicum annum). Dig Dis. 2006;24:184–8.
30. Choe JW, Joo MK, Kim HJ, Lee BJ, Kim JH, Yeon JE, Park JJ, Kim JS, Byun KS, Bak YT. Foods inducing typical gastroesophageal reflux disease symptom in Korea. J Neurogastroenterol Motil. 2017;23(3):363–9.
31. Pace F. Influence of capsaicin infusion on secondary peristalsis in patients with gastroesophageal reflux disease. World J Gastroenterol. 2016;22(45):10045–52. https://doi.org/10.3748/wjg.v22.i45.10045.
32. Nasseri-Moghaddam S, Nokhbeh-Zaeem H, Saniee P, Pedramnia S, Sotoudeh M, Malekzadeh R. Oral nitrate reductase activity and erosive gastro-esophageal reflux disease: a nitrate hypothesis for GERD pathogenesis. Dig Dis Sci. 2012;57:413–8.
33. Xu J, Xu X, Verstraete W. Quantitative measurements of the nitrate reductase activity in the human oral cavity. Foo Chem Toxicol. 2001;39:393–400.
34. Spence AD, Busby J, Murchie P, Kunzmann AT, UC MM, Coleman HG, Johnston BT, O'Rorke MA, Murray LJ, Iversen L, Lee AJ, Cardwell CR. Medications that relax the lower oesophageal sphincter and risk oesophageal cancer: an analysis of two independent population-based databases. Int J Cancer. 2018;143:22–31.
35. Mungan Z, Simsek BP. Which drugs are risk factors for the development of gastroesophageal reflux disease. Turk J Gastroenterol. 2017;28(1):S38–43.
36. Surdea-Blaga T, Negrutiu DE, Palage M, Dumitrascu DL. Food and Gastroesophageal reflux disease. Curr Med Chem. 2017; https://doi.org/10.2174/0929867324666170515123807.
37. Pehl C, Wendl B, Pfeiffer A. White wine and beer induce gastro-oesophageal reflux in patients with reflux disease. Aliment Pharmacol Ther. 2006;23:1581–6.
38. Chen S, Wang J, Li Y. Is alcohol consumption associated with gastroesophageal reflux. J Zhejiang Univ Sci B. 2010;11(6):423–8.
39. Dennis GW, Castell DO. Inhibitory effect of smoking on the lower esophageal sphincter. N Engl J Med. 1971;284(20):1136–7.
40. Kahrilas PJ, Gupta RR. The effect of cigarette smoking on salivation and esophageal acid clearance. J Lab Clin Med. 1989;114(4):431–8.
41. Trudgill NJ, Smith LF, Kershaw J, Riley SA. Impact of smoking cessation on salivary function in healthy volunteers. Scand J Gastroenterol. 1998;33(6):568–71.
42. Ness-Jensen E, Lagergren J. Tobacco smoking, alcohol consumption and gastro-oesophageal reflux disease. Best Pract Res Clin Gastroenterol. 2017;31(5):501–8. https://doi.org/10.1016/j.bpg.2017.09.004. Epub 2017 Sep 7.
43. Freidin N, Fisher MJ, Taylor W, Boyd D, Surratt P, McCallum R, Mittal R. Sleep and nocturnal acid reflux in normal subjects and patients with reflux oesophagitis. Brit Med J. Gut. 1991;32:1275–9.
44. Khoury R, Camacho-Lobato L, Katz P, Mohiuddin M, Castell D. Influence of spontaneous sleep positions on nighttime recumbent reflux in patients with gastroesophageal reflux disease. Am J Gastroenterol. 1999;94:2069–73.
45. Loots C, Smits M, Omari T, Bennink R, Benninga M, Van Wik M. Effects of lateral positioning on gastroesophageal reflux (GER) and underlying mechanisms in GER disease (GERD) patients and healthy controls. Neurogastroenterol Motil. 2013;25:222–e162.
46. Person E, Rife C, Freeman J, Clark A, Castell DO. A novel sleep positioning device reduces gastroesophageal reflux. J Clin Gastroenterol. 2015;49(8):655–9.
47. Lim KG, Morgenthaler TI, Katzka DA. Sleep and nocturnal gastroesophageal reflux: an update. Chest. 2018;154(4):963–71. https://doi.org/10.1016/j.chest.2018.05.030. Epub 2018 May 31.

48. Yang JH, Kang HS, Lee SY, Kim JH, Sung IK, Park HS, Jin CJ. Recurrence of gastroesophageal reflux disease correlated with a short dinner-to-bedtime interval. J Gastroenterol Hepatol. 2014;29(4):730–5.
49. Park SK, Lee T, Yang HJ, Park JH, Sohn CI, Ryu S, Park DI. Weight loss and waist reduction is associated with improvement in gastroesophageal disease reflux symptoms: a longitudinal study of 15,295 subjects undergoing health checkups. Neurogastroenterol Motil. 2017;29:e13009.
50. Mitchell DR, Derakhshan MH, Wirz AA, Ballantyne SA, McColl KEL. Abdominal compression by waist belt aggravates gastroesophageal reflux, primarily by impairing esophageal clearance. Gastroenterology. 2017;152:1881–8.
51. Huang MT, Lou YR, Ma W, Newmark HL, Reuhl KR, Conney AH. Inhibitory effects of dietary curcumin on forestomach, duodenal, and colon carcinogenesis in mice. Cancer Res. 1994;54:5841–7.
52. Thavor K, Mamdani MM, Straus SE. Efficacy of turmeric in the treatment of digestive disorders: a systematic review and meta-analysis protocol. Syst Rev. 2014;3:71–6.
53. Ammon HP, Wahl MA. Pharmacology of Curcuma longa. Planta Med. 1991;57:1–7.
54. Souza RF. From reflux esophagitis to esophageal adenocarcinoma. Dig Dis. 2016;34(5):483–90. https://doi.org/10.1159/000445225.
55. Rafiee P, Nelson VM, Manley S, Wellner M, Floer M, Binion DG, Shaker R. Effects of curcumin on acidic pH-induced expression of IL-6 and IL-8 in human esophageal epithelial cells (HET-1A): role of PKC, MAPKs and NF-kappaB. Am J Physiol Gastrointe Liver Physiol. 2009;296:G388–98.
56. Mahattanadul S, Radenahmad N, Phadoongsombut N, Chuchom T, Panichayupakaranant P, Yano S, Reanmongkoi W. Effects of curcumin on reflux esophagitis in rats. J Nat Med. 2006;60(3):198–205. https://doi.org/10.1007/s11418-006-0035-4. Epub 2006 Apr 28.
57. Koufman JA, Sataloff RT, Toohill R. Laryngopharyngeal reflux: consensus conference report. J Voice. 1996;10:215–6.
58. Rosenhek M, Macpherson MD, Dawes C. The effects of chewing-gum stick size and duration of chewing on salivary flow rate and sucrose and bicarbonate concentrations. Arch Oral Biol. 1993;38:885–91.
59. Koufman JA, Smoak BR. Effects of gum chewing on pharyngeal and esophageal pH. Ann Otol Rhinol Laryngol. 2001;110:1117–9.
60. Helm JF. Esophageal acid clearance. J Clin Gastroenterol. 1986;8(1):5–11.
61. Dossett ML, Cohen EM, Cohen J. Integrative medicine for gastrointestinal disease. Prim Care. 2017;44(2):265–80.
62. Braden B, Caspary W, Borner N, Vinson B, Schneider ARJ. Clinical effects of STW 5 (Iberogast) are not based on acceleration of gastric emptying in patient with functional dyspepsia and gastroparesis. Neurogastroenterol Motil. 2009;21:632–25. https://doi.org/10.1111/j.1365-2982.2008.01249.x.
63. Melzer J, Rosch W, Reichling J, Brignolis R, Saller R. Meta-analysis: phytotherapy of functional dyspepsia with the herbal drug preparation STW 5 (Iberogast). Aliment Pharacol Ther. 2004;20:1279–87.
64. Inamori M, Akiyama T, Akimoto K, Fujita K, Takahashi H, Yoneda M, Abe Y, Kubota K, Saito S, Ueno N, Nakajima A. Early effects of peppermint oil on gastric emptying: a crossover study using a continuous real-time ^{13}C breath test (Breath ID system). J Gastroenterol. 2007;42:539–42.
65. Atta AH, Alkofahi A. Anti-nociceptive and anti-inflammatory effects of some Jordanian medicinal plant extracts. J Ethnopharmacol. 1998;60(2):117–24.
66. Ruetzler K, Fleck M, Nabecker S, Pinter K, Landskron G, Lassnigg A, You J, Sessler DI. A randomized, double-blind comparison of licorice versus sugar-water gargle for prevention of postoperative sore throat and postextubation coughing. Anesth Analg. 2013;117(3):614–21.

67. Benbassat N, Kostova B, Nikolova I, Rachev D. Development and evaluation of novel lozenges containing marshmallow root extract. Pak J Pharm Sci. 2013;26(6):1103–7.
68. Yarnell E, Abascal K. Herbs for gastroesophageal reflux disease. Altern Complement Ther. 2010;16(6):344–6.
69. Mills S, Bone K. Herbal approaches to system dysfunction. In: Principles and practice of phytotherapy. 2nd ed. London: Churchill Livingstone; 2013. p. 183–207.
70. Kim JY, Jang SS, Lee JL, Sim JH, Shim JJ. Cudrania tricuspidata extract protects against reflux esophagitis by blocking H2 histamine receptors. Prev Nutr Food Sci. 2019;24(2):159–64. https://doi.org/10.3746/pnf.2019.24.2.159. Epub 2019 Jun 30.
71. Maclean W. Clinical handbook of Chinese herbs: desk reference, revised edition: Singing Dragon; London; 2017.
72. Ku SK, Seo BI, Park JH, Park GY, Seo YB, Kim JS, Lee HS, Roh SS. Effects of Lonicerae flos extracts on reflux esophagitis with antioxidant activity. World J Gastroenterol. 2009;15:4799–805.
73. Hosseni M, Salari R, Akbari Rad M, Salehi M, Birjandi B, Salari M. Comparing the effect of psyllium seed on gastroesophageal reflux disease with oral omeprazole in patients with functional constipation. J Evid Based Integr Med. 2018;23:1–6.
74. Cao H, Huang X, Zhi X, Han C, Li L, Li Y. Association between tea consumption and gastroesophageal reflux disease: a meta-analysis. Medicine. 2019;98(4):e14173.
75. Jesione W, Ott PG, Moricz AM, Kocsis B, Horvath G, Choma IR. TLC-direct bioautography and LC/MS as complementary methods in identification of antibacterial agents in plant tinctures form the asteraceae family. J AOAC Intl. 2015;98(4):857–61.
76. Wasch SG, Tinzoh LN, Zimmermann BF, Stuhlinger W, Lachemeier DW. Antioxidant capacity and polyphenolic composition as quality indicator for aqueous infusion of salvia officinalis L. (sage tea). Front Pharmacol. 2011;2:79.
77. Hubbert M, Sievers H, Lehnfeld R, Kehrl W. Efficacy and tolerability of a spray with Salvia officinalis in the treatment of acute pharyngitis, a randomized, double-blind, placebo-controlled study with adaptive design and interim analysis. Eur J Med Res. 2006;11(1):20–6.
78. Leiman DA, Riff BP, Morgan S, Metz DC, Falk GW, French B, Umscheid CA, Lewis JD. Alginate therapy is effective treatment for GERD symptoms: a systematic review and meta-analysis. Dis Esophagus. 2017;30:1–9.
79. Zhang CX, Qin YM, Guo BR. Clinical study on the treatment of gastroesophageal reflux by acupuncture. Chin J Integr Med. 2010;16(4):298–303. https://doi.org/10.1007/s11655-010-0516-y.
80. Acidified foods. Code of Federal Regulations – Title 21 – Food and Drugs; Chapter I, Department of Health and Human Services; Subchapter B – Food for Human Consumption Part 114. United Stated Food and Drug Administration. Arlington: Washington Business Information; 2019.
81. Generally recognized as safe food additives: FDA Database of Selected GRAS Substances. United States Food and Drug Administration. Springfield: National Technical Information Service; 2018.
82. Kent JT. Repertory of the homeopathic materia medica and a word index. 6th ed. New Delhi: B. Jain Publishers; 2002.
83. Hammond C. The complete family guide to homeopathy: an illustrated encyclopedia of safe and effective remedies. London: Element Books Ltd.; 1999.
84. Mikami H, Ishimura N, Fukazawa K, Okada M, Izumi D, Shimura S, Okimoto E, Aimi M, Ishihara S, Kinoshita Y. Effects of metoclopramide on esophageal motor activity and esophagogastric junction compliance in healthy volunteers. J Neurogastroenterol Motil. 2016;22(1):112–7.
85. Mochiki E, Yanai M, Ohno T, Kuwano H. The effect of traditional Japanese medicine (Kampo) on gastrointestinal function. Surg Today. 2010;40:1105–11.

86. Kawahara H, Kubota A, Hasegawa T, Okuyama H, Ueno T, Ida S, Fukuzawa M. Effects of rikkunshito on the clinical symptoms and esophageal acid exposure in children with symptomatic gastroesophageal reflux. Pediatr Surg Int. 2007;23:1001–5.
87. Pereira RS. Regression of gastroesophageal reflux disease symptoms using dietary supplementation with melatonin, vitamins, and amino acids; comparison with omeprazole. J Pineal Res. 2006;41:195–200.
88. Kandil TS, Mousa AA, El-Gendy AA, Abbas AM. The potential therapeutic effect of melatonin in gastro-esophageal reflux disease. BMC Gastroenterol. 2010;10:7.

Chapter 30
Pharmacologic Treatments for Gastroesophageal and Laryngopharyngeal Reflux Disease

Daniela Jodorkovsky and John W. Blackett

Mild or Intermittent Symptoms

Patients with mild or intermittent reflux symptoms (fewer than two episodes a week, no compromise in lifestyle, no related complications, and no erosive esophagitis) can often be successfully treated by a combination of lifestyle modifications and over-the-counter (OTC) agents, including antacids, surface agents, and alginates, H2RAs, and low-dose proton pump inhibitors. If these prove unsuccessful, then step-up therapy with daily dosing of H2RA in combination with mucosal protection and other OTC agents is encouraged while dietary and lifestyle changes are further discussed. If symptoms persist or worsen or any complications of LPR or GERD develop, prescription agents, particularly proton pump inhibitors, are usually warranted.

Lifestyle Modifications

Lifestyle modifications such as avoidance of dietary triggers, weight loss, elevation of head of the bed, and eating at least 2 hours prior to sleeping can be helpful for mild reflux and are safe. Nocturnal postures such as elevation of the head of the bed and sleeping in the left lateral decubitus position have been shown to decrease the amount of esophageal acid exposure and GERD symptoms, and can be implemented relatively easily [1–3]. These postural changes can help patients with LPR at night, typically presenting with chronic coughing at night. Posture plays less of a role during the daytime when most people experience LPR. Obesity can lead to increased

D. Jodorkovsky (✉) · J. W. Blackett
Division of Digestive and Liver Diseases, Columbia University Medical Center, New York, NY, USA
e-mail: Dj2470@cumc.columbia.edu; Jwb2158@cumc.columbia.edu

C. H. Zalvan (ed.), *Laryngopharyngeal and Gastroesophageal Reflux*,
https://doi.org/10.1007/978-3-030-48890-1_30

intra-abdominal pressure and higher incidence of hiatal hernia, leading to increased GERD symptoms [4]. Weight loss in overweight and obese patients also decreases acid exposure and symptoms [1]. While cigarette smoking and alcohol consumption are associated with reflux, there is a lack of evidence that tobacco or alcohol cessation improves symptoms, though it is still recommended [5]. Nonetheless, lifestyle and dietary modifications should be the first step in patients with mild or infrequent symptoms without erosive disease. Detailed and thorough education through handouts, literature, online, and text references, and enlistment of a nutritionist are key at this early stage in treatment to obtain short-term improvement and long-term prevention of chronic disease.

Antacids

Over-the-counter antacids include aluminum hydroxide, magnesium hydroxide or trisilicate, calcium carbonate, and sodium bicarbonate. They are available as chewable or dissolvable tablets or liquids. Antacids work to neutralize gastric acid, thus decreasing esophageal acid exposure during periods of reflux [6]. They also act as a coating agent in the pharynx and esophagus to buffer direct mucosal contact of acid and pepsin. They provide fast relief of heartburn, but the effects typically only last 30–60 minutes. They are useful when taken as needed for occasional reflux, but are not effective in preventing symptoms [7]. Antacids are safe and affordable but taken in excess can have adverse effects. Magnesium antacids can cause diarrhea. Aluminum antacids can cause hypophosphatemia by binding intestinal phosphate when taken in high doses [8]. Case reports have reported the development of osteomalacia in patients taking long-term aluminum hydroxide therapy in doses ranging from 2.3 g per day for 30 months to 20 g per day for 5 years [9]. The susceptibility likely depends in large part on dietary phosphate intake as well. In patients with renal impairment, they can cause neurotoxicity and anemia [10]. Calcium antacids taken in excess can cause milk alkali syndrome, resulting in hypercalcemia, metabolic alkalosis, and renal dysfunction [11, 12]. Antacids can also interfere with the absorption of medications taken concomitantly, so administration should be separated by at least 2 hours in general [13]. Antacid interactions are particularly common with quinolone, tetracycline, and cephalosporin antibiotics, oral glucocorticoids, and nonsteroidal anti-inflammatory drugs (NSAID) [14].

Surface Agents and Alginates

Sucralfate is a sulfated polysaccharide complexed with aluminum hydroxide. It forms a protective coating that protects the gastric lining from acid, pepsin, and bile salts. It has an affinity for injured tissue, helping protect ulcers and other damaged tissue from further injury [15–17]. Sucralfate has few adverse effects. It can bind to other medications taken at the same time, and in patients with renal failure, it can lead to aluminum toxicity. It can also sometimes cause constipation [18]. It is more effective than placebo for GERD but less so than PPIs, and thus its use is generally limited to pregnant patients with nonerosive disease or patients intolerant to PPIs [19].

Sodium alginate is a polysaccharide derived from seaweed, which forms a viscous gel 'raft' when it contacts stomach acid. This floats on top of food in the postprandial acid pocket to prevent acid reflux [20–22]. It is frequently formulated in combination with antacids such as sodium bicarbonate and calcium carbonate. Adverse effects are rare, but include constipation, abdominal distention, nausea, and flatulence [9]. Products in which sodium alginate is the primary ingredient are only available in the United Kingdom but can be purchased online.

Histamine 2 Receptor Antagonists

H2RAs inhibit the histamine 2 receptor on gastric parietal cells, and thereby decrease the secretion of gastric acid. Drugs in this class include cimetidine, famotidine, ranitidine, and nizatidine. Their onset of action is slower compared to antacids, peaking at 2.5 hours, but lasts 4–10 hours [23]. They are more effective than antacids and placebo for treating nonerosive and milder erosive esophagitis but have limited efficacy in severe erosive esophagitis [24, 25]. They are less effective than proton pump inhibitors in healing erosive esophagitis [26]. H2 blockers are also limited in long-term treatment of GERD due to the onset of tachyphylaxis after 2–6 weeks [27, 28]. H2 blockers, in particular famotidine, have also been associated with the development of hematopoietic side effects including anemia, thrombocytopenia, neutropenia, and pancytopenia [29–33]. Cimetidine has also rarely been associated with gynecomastia and impotence in men taking it for prolonged periods [34]. In general, H2 blockers are useful for patients with mild chronic GERD whose symptoms can be controlled without proton pump inhibitors. Their role in patients with LPR remains in question, as no specific study has demonstrated significant improvement in LPR symptoms over placebo alone, likely due to the lack of a true gold standard by which to compare results. However, while instituting lifestyle changes, they can be helpful in alleviating symptoms of GERD and some symptoms of LPR. Given their safety profile, they are often utilized during this transition. H2RAs also provide an option for medical treatment when trying to wean off PPI therapy and can be used for breakthrough symptoms during episodes of dietary indiscretion.

Severe or Frequent Symptoms, or Erosive Esophagitis

Patients with severe symptoms or evidence of erosive esophagitis typically require prescription medications, with proton pump inhibitors as first line therapy. Patients who do not respond to proton pump inhibitors may be treated with combination PPI and H2 blockers. Some patients with GERD, especially those with comorbid motility disorders, may benefit from promotility agents. Potassium-competitive acid blockers are a promising new therapy that may provide faster onset and similar efficacy as PPIs, but are not yet available in the United States. In general, patients with severe GERD with erosive esophagitis may require long-term maintenance acid suppression. In patients without severe erosive esophagitis, PPIs should be continued at the lowest dose that provides symptomatic relief and attempts to discontinue the medication should be considered periodically. In patients who are on PPIs for over 6 months, they should be tapered and use of on-demand PPI can be given for recurrent symptoms.

Proton Pump Inhibitors

Proton pump inhibitors include omeprazole, pantoprazole, esomeprazole, rabeprazole, lansoprazole, and dexlansoprazole. PPIs irreversibly bind and inhibit the hydrogen-potassium ATPase pump on gastric parietal cells, thereby blocking acid secretion. They are most effective when the parietal cells are stimulated by a meal and should be taken 30 minutes prior to eating [35, 36]. They take several days to reach full effect [37]. PPIs are superior to H2 blockers in healing esophagitis and peptic ulcer disease [38, 39]. In patients with erosive esophagitis, symptomatic relief can be expected in 27% of patients on placebo, 60% on H2 blockers, and 83% on PPIs [40]. Esophagitis heals in 24% of patients on placebo, 50% on H2 blockers, and 78% on PPIs [40].

The adverse effects of proton pump inhibitors are an area of controversy and are discussed in detail in another chapter. Areas of concern include the risk of infections such as pneumonia and those caused by *Clostridium difficile*, small intestinal bacterial overgrowth, osteoporosis and fractures, vitamin deficiencies, acute and chronic kidney injury, and dementia [41, 42]. Most of the data on adverse effects of PPIs come from observational and retrospective studies, and the absolute risk of adverse effects is small. A recent large double-blind randomized controlled trial of patients taking rivaroxaban or aspirin assigned to receive either pantoprazole or placebo found that there was no difference in safety events including pneumonia, cardiovascular outcomes, dementia, cancer, hospitalizations, fractures, chronic kidney disease, or all-cause mortality during the 3-year follow-up period [43]. Patients on pantoprazole did have a higher number of enteric infections than the placebo group, though the absolute risk difference was low (1.4% vs. 1.0%).

PPIs are metabolized via the hepatic cytochrome P450 system, which can lead to drug interactions in some patients. Use of PPIs may inhibit activation of clopidogrel and other thienopyridines due to shared hepatic metabolism, thus attenuating the antiplatelet effect [44–46]. While observational studies have shown small but significant associations between PPIs and antiplatelet agents, the only randomized controlled trial comparing omeprazole vs. placebo in patients taking clopidogrel showed no difference in cardiovascular outcomes [47]. Thus, the US Food and Drug Administration recommends that patients taking clopidogrel should consult with their physician prior to taking a PPI. Omeprazole and esomeprazole cause more cytochrome P450 inhibition than other PPIs, and the FDA recommends that pantoprazole, lansoprazole, and dexlansoprazole should be considered in patients taking clopidogrel who require a PPI [48–50].

PPIs can also decrease the efficacy of some protease inhibitors used for HIV due to gastric acid-dependent absorption. PPIs are contraindicated in patients taking rilpivirine, and atazanavir should be avoided in patients requiring a PPI dose higher than 20 mg of omeprazole [51, 52]. H2 blockers may be used if they are dosed at a separate time from the protease inhibitor.

Within-class differences among PPIs are few. All PPIs are similarly effective in healing esophagitis and symptomatic relief when given at equivalent doses [53]. Dexlansoprazole has a novel dual delayed release delivery system allowing for a single daily dose to provide 24-hour coverage [54]. In general, PPIs should be used in patients who fail H2 blockers, have erosive esophagitis, or have severe/frequent symptoms that interfere with their quality of life. They are more effective when taken daily compared to "on demand," though taking as needed may be preferred by patients and acceptable in those without erosive esophagitis [55, 56].

The use of combined PPI and H2 blockers can be useful in order to limit exposure to PPIs in those concerned about adverse effects. PPIs are less effective at controlling nocturnal symptoms [57]. H2 blockers are particularly effective when used in the evening to block the nocturnal histamine surge in patients not controlled on PPIs alone [58].

Potassium Competitive Acid Blockers (P-CABs)

Potassium competitive acid blockers are a promising new acid suppression alternative to proton pump inhibitors. P-CABs include vonoprazan, revaprazan, tegoprazan, and other drugs currently in development. P-CABs compete for potassium on the luminal side of parietal cells, and reversibly inhibit hydrogen-potassium ATPase pumps [59]. They are not yet available in the US and are primarily used in Asia currently. Compared to PPIs, P-CABs have a more rapid onset of action (1 day vs. 3–5 days), and relief can often be felt after a single dose [60]. Other advantages of P-CABs over PPIs are the ability to take without food, improved nocturnal efficacy, and lack of cytochrome P450 metabolism. A randomized trial comparing vonoprazan against lansoprazole, and another comparing tegoprazan against esomeprazole, found that the P-CABs were noninferior to the PPIs in healing erosive esophagitis [61, 62]. Another study found that vonoprazan achieved significantly faster relief of symptoms compared to lansoprazole, with 31% of patients experiencing complete relief on day 1 of vonoprazan compared to 13% of patients on lansoprazole [63]. Adverse effects include nasopharyngitis, diarrhea, constipation, upper respiratory tract inflammation, falls, gastroenteritis, and eczema [60]. Long-term adverse effects may be similar to those of acid suppression in PPIs but are not well known due to the novelty of the drugs. Studies evaluating long-term safety are ongoing. No studies have looked at the use of P-CABs in the treatment of LPR. However, much like PPIs and H2RAs, they potentially can contribute to symptom control in those with true LPR.

Promotility Agents

Defects in gastric emptying, LES incompetence, and esophageal dysmotility can contribute to GERD [40]. Thus, promotility agents are sometimes used in patients with refractory GERD and are especially helpful in patients with comorbid motility disorders.

Metoclopramide (Reglan) is a dopamine receptor and serotonin receptor antagonist. It increases gastric emptying and LES tone. It can be helpful in patients with GERD in addition to delayed gastric emptying. Metoclopramide can reduce reflux but is less effective than PPIs, and is rarely used for GERD alone given its side effect profile [64]. Adverse effects include drowsiness, extrapyramidal side effects, and tardive dyskinesia if used for more than 3 months (including an FDA black box warning against use for more than 12 weeks), and QTc prolongation.

Domperidone is a peripheral dopamine blocker, similar to metoclopramide but without the central nervous system side effects as it minimally crosses the blood–brain barrier. It is not available in US currently but can be obtained with an investigational new drug application from the FDA or specialty compounding pharmacies. The efficacy for GERD is similar to metoclopramide. A small study showed that domperidone had benefits comparable to H2 blockers in the treatment of reflux esophagitis [65]. The primary adverse effect is QTc prolongation and regular EKG monitoring is recommended.

Acotiamide is an anticholinesterase primarily used for functional dyspepsia, which may improve gastric motility and accommodation [66, 67]. Developed in Japan, it is not yet available in the US. A small randomized controlled trial of 70 patients showed that adding acotiamide to PPI significantly improved symptoms in patients with nonerosive GERD, but not erosive disease [68]. More studies are needed to determine whether it may be an effective adjunctive therapy. Adverse effects include nausea, abdominal distention, and constipation.

Prucalopride is a 5-HT4 receptor agonist and prokinetic drug, typically used for constipation as it stimulates colonic motility. A small randomized controlled trial of 21 male patients showed that it decreased esophageal acid exposure and increased gastric emptying [69]. More evidence is needed to determine whether it is effective before it can be recommended for routine use in GERD. Adverse effects include headache, abdominal pain, nausea, and diarrhea.

Bethanechol stimulates the parasympathetic nervous system, as well as esophageal and gastric motility. It is more commonly used for urinary retention, but small studies have shown some efficacy compared to placebo in reflux symptoms and endoscopic findings [70, 71]. It is rarely used for GERD due to the availability of more efficacious drugs such as PPIs. Adverse effects include flushing, diaphoresis, tachycardia, and hypotension.

Baclofen is a GABA agonist, which reduces transient LES relaxations. Small studies have shown that it can decrease the amount of esophageal reflux time and symptoms, but no effect on healing of erosive esophagitis has been demonstrated [72–74].

Other Agents

A number of antiulcer medications available in Asia have been studied in patients with reflux disease. Rebamipide is a mucosal protectant antiulcer agent, not commonly used for reflux, but has been shown in a small study to be effective when combined with PPIs in preventing recurrence of symptoms in patients who are PPI-responsive, with no adverse effects reported [75]. It does not appear to be effective in patients who have PPI refractory reflux [76]. Similarly, irsogladine is an antiulcer medication used primarily in Japan, China, and Korea, which facilitates gap junctional intercellular communication [77]. A small trial found that patients with nonerosive esophageal reflux disease had improved quality of life on irsogladine combined with PPI compared to PPI alone [78]. Teprenone, another mucosal protectant antiulcer agent, was inferior to omeprazole in a randomized controlled trial of patients with upper GI symptoms including GERD in achieving symptom control [79], so is not recommended for reflux. Ecabet is an antiulcer medication with antipepsin effects as well as mucosal protectant effect that has been shown to improve experimentally induced esophagitis in rats. There are no human studies evaluating its efficacy for reflux, so is not generally used for this indication [80, 81]. Polaprezinc is a zinc containing mucosal protectant antiulcer agent that has shown some efficacy in preventing radiation esophagitis, but has not been studied in reflux disease [82]. Misoprostol is a prostaglandin analogue that inhibits acid secretion by gastric parietal cells, used for the prevention of NSAID-induced peptic ulcer disease [83]. It is also used to induce abortion, so it is contraindicated in women of childbearing age who are not on contraception. It has not been studied in the treatment of reflux disease.

Pharmacologic treatments for GERD

Medication	Usual dose	When to consider	Mechanism	Adverse effects
Antacids				
Aluminum hydroxide	200 mg QID	Mild or intermittent GERD	Neutralize gastric acid	Hypophosphatemia, osteomalacia
Magnesium hydroxide	200 mg QID			Diarrhea
Calcium carbonate	500–1000 mg QID			Milk alkali syndrome
Sodium bicarbonate	325–1000 mg QID			Nausea, gas
Surface agents or alginates				
Sucralfate	1 g QID	GERD in pregnant patients	Forms protective lining	Aluminum toxicity, constipation
Sodium alginate	10–20 ml QID	Post-prandial GERD	Forms viscous gel raft on top of postprandial acid pocket	Constipation, abdominal distention, nausea

(continued)

Pharmacologic treatments for GERD				
Medication	Usual dose	When to consider	Mechanism	Adverse effects
Histamine 2 receptor antagonists				
Cimetidine	200–400 mg BID	Mild or intermittent GERD	Decrease gastric acid secretion by blocking H2 receptor on parietal cells	Rarely anemia, thrombocytopenia
Famotidine	10–20 mg BID			
Ranitidine	75–150 mg BID			
Nizatidine	150 mg BID			
Proton pump inhibitors				
Esomeprazole	40 mg QD to BID	Mild GERD to erosive esophagitis	Decrease gastric acid secretion by blocking Na-K ATPase on parietal cells	Pneumonia, infections caused by *C. difficile*, osteoporosis, dementia
Omeprazole	20–40 mg QD			
Pantoprazole	40 mg QD to BID			
Lansoprazole	30 mg QD			
Dexlansoprazole	30–60 mg QD			
Rabeprazole	20 mg QD			
Potassium-competitive acid blockers				
Vonoprazan	5–40 mg QD	Mild GERD to erosive esophagitis	Decrease gastric acid secretion by blocking Na-K ATPase on parietal cells	Likely similar to PPIs but limited data
Revaprazan	150–300 mg QD			
Tegoprazan	50–100 mg QD			
Promotility agents				
Metoclopramide	5–10 mg TID	Gastroparesis	Dopamine/serotonin receptor antagonist	Tardive dyskinesia, QTc prolongation
Domperidone	10 mg TID		Peripheral dopamine receptor antagonist	QTc prolongation
Acotiamide	100 mg TID	Functional dyspepsia	Acetylcholinesterase inhibitor	Nausea, abdominal distention, constipation

Pharmacologic treatments for GERD

Medication	Usual dose	When to consider	Mechanism	Adverse effects
Prucalopride	2 mg QD	Constipation	5-HT4 receptor agonist	Abdominal pain, diarrhea, headache
Bethanechol	10–50 mg TID	Urinary retention	Stimulates parasympathetic nervous system	Flushing, diaphoresis, tachycardia, hypotension
Baclofen	10–20 mg TID	Mild GERD, hiccups	GABA agonist	Drowsiness, headache

References

1. Kaltenbach T, Crockett S, Gerson LB. Are lifestyle measures effective in patients with gastroesophageal reflux disease? An evidence-based approach. Arch Intern Med. 2006;166(9):965–71.
2. Katz LC, Just R, Castell DO. Body position affects recumbent postprandial reflux. J Clin Gastroenterol. 1994;18(4):280–3.
3. Stanciu C, Bennett JR. Effects of posture on gastro-oesophageal reflux. Digestion. 1977;15(2):104–9.
4. Murray L, Johnston B, Lane A, Harvey I, Donovan J, Nair P, et al. Relationship between body mass and gastro-oesophageal reflux symptoms: the Bristol Helicobacter Project. Int J Epidemiol. 2003;32(4):645–50.
5. Watanabe Y, Fujiwara Y, Shiba M, Watanabe T, Tominaga K, Oshitani N, et al. Cigarette smoking and alcohol consumption associated with gastro-oesophageal reflux disease in Japanese men. Scand J Gastroenterol. 2003;38(8):807–11.
6. Maton PN, Burton ME. Antacids revisited: a review of their clinical pharmacology and recommended therapeutic use. Drugs. 1999;57(6):855–70.
7. Hershcovici T, Fass R. Pharmacological management of GERD: where does it stand now? Trends Pharmacol Sci. 2011;32(4):258–64.
8. Shields HM. Rapid fall of serum phosphorus secondary to antacid therapy. Gastroenterology. 1978;75(6):1137–41.
9. Sun J, Yang C, Zhao H, Zheng P, Wilkinson J, Ng B, et al. Randomised clinical trial: the clinical efficacy and safety of an alginate-antacid (Gaviscon Double Action) versus placebo, for decreasing upper gastrointestinal symptoms in symptomatic gastroesophageal reflux disease (GERD) in China. Aliment Pharmacol Ther. 2015;42(7):845–54.
10. Kirschbaum BB, Schoolwerth AC. Acute aluminum toxicity associated with oral citrate and aluminum-containing antacids. Am J Med Sci. 1989;297(1):9–11.
11. Medarov BI. Milk-alkali syndrome. Mayo Clin Proc. 2009;84(3):261–7.
12. Beall DP, Scofield RH. Milk-alkali syndrome associated with calcium carbonate consumption. Report of 7 patients with parathyroid hormone levels and an estimate of prevalence among patients hospitalized with hypercalcemia. Medicine (Baltimore). 1995;74(2):89–96.
13. Hurwitz A. Antacid therapy and drug kinetics. Clin Pharmacokinet. 1977;2(4):269–80.
14. Sadowski DC. Drug interactions with antacids. Mechanisms and clinical significance. Drug Saf. 1994;11(6):395–407.
15. McCarthy DM. Sucralfate. N Engl J Med. 1991;325(14):1017–25.
16. Nagashima R. Mechanisms of action of sucralfate. J Clin Gastroenterol. 1981;3(Suppl 2):117–27.
17. Nagashima R. Development and characteristics of sucralfate. J Clin Gastroenterol. 1981;3(Suppl 2):103–10.

18. Fisher RS. Sucralfate: a review of drug tolerance and safety. J Clin Gastroenterol. 1981;3(Suppl 2):181–4.
19. Simon B, Ravelli GP, Goffin H. Sucralfate gel versus placebo in patients with non-erosive gastro-oesophageal reflux disease. Aliment Pharmacol Ther. 1996;10(3):441–6.
20. Hampson FC, Farndale A, Strugala V, Sykes J, Jolliffe IG, Dettmar PW. Alginate rafts and their characterisation. Int J Pharm. 2005;294(1–2):137–47.
21. Hampson FC, Jolliffe IG, Bakhtyari A, Taylor G, Sykes J, Johnstone LM, et al. Alginate-antacid combinations: raft formation and gastric retention studies. Drug Dev Ind Pharm. 2010;36(5):614–23.
22. Castell DO, Dalton CB, Becker D, Sinclair J, Castell JA. Alginic acid decreases postprandial upright gastroesophageal reflux. Comparison with equal-strength antacid. Dig Dis Sci. 1992;37(4):589–93.
23. Wolfe MM, Sachs G. Acid suppression: optimizing therapy for gastroduodenal ulcer healing, gastroesophageal reflux disease, and stress-related erosive syndrome. Gastroenterology. 2000;118(2 Suppl 1):S9–31.
24. Cloud ML, Offen WW, Robinson M. Nizatidine versus placebo in gastroesophageal reflux disease: a 12-week, multicenter, randomized, double-blind study. Am J Gastroenterol. 1991;86(12):1735–42.
25. Sabesin SM, Berlin RG, Humphries TJ, Bradstreet DC, Walton-Bowen KL, Zaidi S. Famotidine relieves symptoms of gastroesophageal reflux disease and heals erosions and ulcerations. Results of a multicenter, placebo-controlled, dose-ranging study. USA Merck Gastroesophageal Reflux Disease Study Group. Arch Intern Med. 1991;151(12):2394–400.
26. Wang WH, Huang JQ, Zheng GF, Xia HH, Wong WM, Lam SK, et al. Head-to-head comparison of H2-receptor antagonists and proton pump inhibitors in the treatment of erosive esophagitis: a meta-analysis. World J Gastroenterol. 2005;11(26):4067–77.
27. Komazawa Y, Adachi K, Mihara T, Ono M, Kawamura A, Fujishiro H, et al. Tolerance to famotidine and ranitidine treatment after 14 days of administration in healthy subjects without Helicobacter pylori infection. J Gastroenterol Hepatol. 2003;18(6):678–82.
28. Fackler WK, Ours TM, Vaezi MF, Richter JE. Long-term effect of H2RA therapy on nocturnal gastric acid breakthrough. Gastroenterology. 2002;122(3):625–32.
29. Lipsy RJ, Fennerty B, Fagan TC. Clinical review of histamine2 receptor antagonists. Arch Intern Med. 1990;150(4):745–51.
30. Compoginis JM, Gaspard D, Obaid A. Famotidine use and thrombocytopenia in the trauma patient. Am Surg. 2011;77(12):1580–3.
31. Ecker RD, Wijdicks EF, Wix K, McClelland R. Does famotidine induce thrombocytopenia in neurosurgical patients? J Neurosurg Anesthesiol. 2004;16(4):291–3.
32. Nakano T, Kuroiwa T, Tsumita Y, Kaneko Y, Hiromura K, Ueki K, et al. Aplastic anemia associated with initiation of nizatidine therapy in a hemodialysis patient. Clin Exp Nephrol. 2004;8(2):160–2.
33. Takami N, Yamamoto Y, Matsuo H, Ohtani H, Sawada Y. Agranulocytosis possibly caused by ranitidine in a patient with renal failure. Int J Clin Pharmacol Ther. 2002;40(11):520–3.
34. Jensen RT, Collen MJ, Pandol SJ, Allende HD, Raufman JP, Bissonnette BM, et al. Cimetidine-induced impotence and breast changes in patients with gastric hypersecretory states. N Engl J Med. 1983;308(15):883–7.
35. Hatlebakk JG, Katz PO, Camacho-Lobato L, Castell DO. Proton pump inhibitors: better acid suppression when taken before a meal than without a meal. Aliment Pharmacol Ther. 2000;14(10):1267–72.
36. Hatlebakk JG, Katz PO, Kuo B, Castell DO. Nocturnal gastric acidity and acid breakthrough on different regimens of omeprazole 40 mg daily. Aliment Pharmacol Ther. 1998;12(12):1235–40.
37. Cederberg C, Lind T, Rohss K, Olbe L. Comparison of once-daily intravenous and oral omeprazole on pentagastrin-stimulated acid secretion in duodenal ulcer patients. Digestion. 1992;53(3–4):171–8.
38. Khan M, Santana J, Donnellan C, Preston C, Moayyedi P. Medical treatments in the short term management of reflux oesophagitis. Cochrane Database Syst Rev. 2007;2:CD003244.

39. Walan A, Bader JP, Classen M, Lamers CB, Piper DW, Rutgersson K, et al. Effect of omeprazole and ranitidine on ulcer healing and relapse rates in patients with benign gastric ulcer. N Engl J Med. 1989;320(2):69–75.
40. DeVault KR, Castell DO, American College of Gastroenterology. Updated guidelines for the diagnosis and treatment of gastroesophageal reflux disease. Am J Gastroenterol. 2005;100(1):190–200.
41. Schoenfeld AJ, Grady D. Adverse effects associated with proton pump inhibitors. JAMA Intern Med. 2016;176(2):172–4.
42. Nehra AK, Alexander JA, Loftus CG, Nehra V. Proton pump inhibitors: review of emerging concerns. Mayo Clin Proc. 2018;93(2):240–6.
43. Moayyedi P, Eikelboom JW, Bosch J, Connolly SJ, Dyal L, Shestakovska O, et al. Safety of proton pump inhibitors based on a large, multi-year, randomized trial of patients receiving rivaroxaban or aspirin. Gastroenterology. 2019;157(3):682–691.e2.
44. Abraham NS, Hlatky MA, Antman EM, Bhatt DL, Bjorkman DJ, Clark CB, et al. ACCF/ACG/AHA 2010 expert consensus document on the concomitant use of proton pump inhibitors and thienopyridines: a focused update of the ACCF/ACG/AHA 2008 expert consensus document on reducing the gastrointestinal risks of antiplatelet therapy and NSAID use. Am J Gastroenterol. 2010;105(12):2533–49.
45. Abraham NS, Hlatky MA, Antman EM, Bhatt DL, Bjorkman DJ, Clark CB, et al. ACCF/ACG/AHA 2010 expert consensus document on the concomitant use of proton pump inhibitors and thienopyridines: a focused update of the ACCF/ACG/AHA 2008 expert consensus document on reducing the gastrointestinal risks of antiplatelet therapy and NSAID use. A report of the American College of Cardiology Foundation Task Force on Expert Consensus Documents. J Am Coll Cardiol. 2010;56(24):2051–66.
46. Abraham NS, Hlatky MA, Antman EM, Bhatt DL, Bjorkman DJ, Clark CB, et al. ACCF/ACG/AHA 2010 Expert Consensus Document on the concomitant use of proton pump inhibitors and thienopyridines: a focused update of the ACCF/ACG/AHA 2008 expert consensus document on reducing the gastrointestinal risks of antiplatelet therapy and NSAID use: a report of the American College of Cardiology Foundation Task Force on Expert Consensus Documents. Circulation. 2010;122(24):2619–33.
47. Bhatt DL, Cryer BL, Contant CF, Cohen M, Lanas A, Schnitzer TJ, et al. Clopidogrel with or without omeprazole in coronary artery disease. N Engl J Med. 2010;363(20):1909–17.
48. Ogilvie BW, Yerino P, Kazmi F, Buckley DB, Rostami-Hodjegan A, Paris BL, et al. The proton pump inhibitor, omeprazole, but not lansoprazole or pantoprazole, is a metabolism-dependent inhibitor of CYP2C19: implications for coadministration with clopidogrel. Drug Metab Dispos. 2011;39(11):2020–33.
49. Bouziana SD, Tziomalos K. Clinical relevance of clopidogrel-proton pump inhibitors interaction. World J Gastrointest Pharmacol Ther. 2015;6(2):17–21.
50. Fontes-Carvalho R, Albuquerque A, Araujo C, Pimentel-Nunes P, Ribeiro VG. Omeprazole, but not pantoprazole, reduces the antiplatelet effect of clopidogrel: a randomized clinical crossover trial in patients after myocardial infarction evaluating the clopidogrel-PPIs drug interaction. Eur J Gastroenterol Hepatol. 2011;23(5):396–404.
51. Crauwels H, van Heeswijk RP, Stevens M, Buelens A, Vanveggel S, Boven K, et al. Clinical perspective on drug-drug interactions with the non-nucleoside reverse transcriptase inhibitor rilpivirine. AIDS Rev. 2013;15(2):87–101.
52. Brath H, Mehta N, Savage RD, Gill SS, Wu W, Bronskill SE, et al. What is known about preventing, detecting, and reversing prescribing cascades: a scoping review. J Am Geriatr Soc. 2018;66(11):2079–85.
53. Ip S, Bonis P, Tatsioni A, Raman G, Chew P, Kupelnick B, et al. Comparative effectiveness of management strategies for gastroesophageal reflux disease. Rockville: AHRQ Comparative Effectiveness Reviews; 2005.
54. Sharma P, Shaheen NJ, Perez MC, Pilmer BL, Lee M, Atkinson SN, et al. Clinical trials: healing of erosive oesophagitis with dexlansoprazole MR, a proton pump inhibitor with a novel

dual delayed-release formulation—results from two randomized controlled studies. Aliment Pharmacol Ther. 2009;29(7):731–41.
55. Tsai HH, Chapman R, Shepherd A, McKeith D, Anderson M, Vearer D, et al. Esomeprazole 20 mg on-demand is more acceptable to patients than continuous lansoprazole 15 mg in the long-term maintenance of endoscopy-negative gastro-oesophageal reflux patients: the COMMAND study. Aliment Pharmacol Ther. 2004;20(6):657–65.
56. Pace F, Pallotta S, Bianchi PG. On-demand proton pump inhibitor therapy in patients with gastro-oesophageal reflux disease. Dig Liver Dis. 2002;34(12):870–7.
57. Johnson DA, Katz PO. Nocturnal gastroesophageal reflux disease: issues, implications, and management strategies. Rev Gastroenterol Disord. 2008;8(2):98–108.
58. Xue S, Katz PO, Banerjee P, Tutuian R, Castell DO. Bedtime H2 blockers improve nocturnal gastric acid control in GERD patients on proton pump inhibitors. Aliment Pharmacol Ther. 2001;15(9):1351–6.
59. Andersson K, Carlsson E. Potassium-competitive acid blockade: a new therapeutic strategy in acid-related diseases. Pharmacol Ther. 2005;108(3):294–307.
60. Oshima T, Miwa H. Potent potassium-competitive acid blockers: a new era for the treatment of acid-related diseases. J Neurogastroenterol Motil. 2018;24(3):334–44.
61. Ashida K, Sakurai Y, Hori T, Kudou K, Nishimura A, Hiramatsu N, et al. Randomised clinical trial: vonoprazan, a novel potassium-competitive acid blocker, vs. lansoprazole for the healing of erosive oesophagitis. Aliment Pharmacol Ther. 2016;43(2):240–51.
62. Lee KJ, Son BK, Kim GH, Jung HK, Jung HY, Chung IK, et al. Randomised phase 3 trial: tegoprazan, a novel potassium-competitive acid blocker, vs. esomeprazole in patients with erosive oesophagitis. Aliment Pharmacol Ther. 2019;49(7):864–72.
63. Oshima T, Arai E, Taki M, Kondo T, Tomita T, Fukui H, et al. Randomised clinical trial: vonoprazan versus lansoprazole for the initial relief of heartburn in patients with erosive oesophagitis. Aliment Pharmacol Ther. 2019;49(2):140–6.
64. Durazo FA, Valenzuela JE. Effect of single and repeated doses of metoclopramide on the mechanisms of gastroesophageal reflux. Am J Gastroenterol. 1993;88(10):1657–62.
65. Masci E, Testoni PA, Passaretti S, Guslandi M, Tittobello A. Comparison of ranitidine, domperidone maleate and ranitidine + domperidone maleate in the short-term treatment of reflux oesophagitis. Drugs Exp Clin Res. 1985;11(10):687–92.
66. Matsueda K, Hongo M, Tack J, Saito Y, Kato H. A placebo-controlled trial of acotiamide for meal-related symptoms of functional dyspepsia. Gut. 2012;61(6):821–8.
67. Tack J, Pokrotnieks J, Urbonas G, Banciu C, Yakusevich V, Bunganic I, et al. Long-term safety and efficacy of acotiamide in functional dyspepsia (postprandial distress syndrome)-results from the European phase 3 open-label safety trial. Neurogastroenterol Motil. 2018;30(6):e13284.
68. Yamashita H, Okada A, Naora K, Hongoh M, Kinoshita Y. Adding acotiamide to gastric acid inhibitors is effective for treating refractory symptoms in patients with non-erosive reflux disease. Dig Dis Sci. 2019;64(3):823–31.
69. Kessing BF, Smout AJ, Bennink RJ, Kraaijpoel N, Oors JM, Bredenoord AJ. Prucalopride decreases esophageal acid exposure and accelerates gastric emptying in healthy subjects. Neurogastroenterol Motil. 2014;26(8):1079–86.
70. Thanik KD, Chey WY, Shah AN, Gutierrez JG. Reflux esophagitis: effect of oral bethanechol on symptoms and endoscopic findings. Ann Intern Med. 1980;93(6):805–8.
71. Euler AR. Use of bethanechol for the treatment of gastroesophageal reflux. J Pediatr. 1980;96(2):321–4.
72. Cossentino MJ, Mann K, Armbruster SP, Lake JM, Maydonovitch C, Wong RK. Randomised clinical trial: the effect of baclofen in patients with gastro-oesophageal reflux—a randomised prospective study. Aliment Pharmacol Ther. 2012;35(9):1036–44.
73. van Herwaarden MA, Samsom M, Rydholm H, Smout AJ. The effect of baclofen on gastro-oesophageal reflux, lower oesophageal sphincter function and reflux symptoms in patients with reflux disease. Aliment Pharmacol Ther. 2002;16(9):1655–62.

74. Kroch DA, Madanick RD. Medical treatment of gastroesophageal reflux disease. World J Surg. 2017;41(7):1678–84.
75. Yoshida N, Kamada K, Tomatsuri N, Suzuki T, Takagi T, Ichikawa H, et al. Management of recurrence of symptoms of gastroesophageal reflux disease: synergistic effect of rebamipide with 15 mg lansoprazole. Dig Dis Sci. 2010;55(12):3393–8.
76. Adachi K, Furuta K, Miwa H, Oshima T, Miki M, Komazawa Y, et al. A study on the efficacy of rebamipide for patients with proton pump inhibitor-refractory non-erosive reflux disease. Dig Dis Sci. 2012;57(6):1609–17.
77. Akagi M, Amagase K, Murakami T, Takeuchi K. Irsogladine: overview of the mechanisms of mucosal protective and healing-promoting actions in the gastrointestinal tract. Curr Pharm Des. 2013;19(1):106–14.
78. Suzuki T, Matsushima M, Masui A, Tsuda S, Imai J, Nakamura J, et al. Irsogladine maleate and rabeprazole in non-erosive reflux disease: a double-blind, placebo-controlled study. World J Gastroenterol. 2015;21(16):5023–31.
79. Sakurai K, Nagahara A, Inoue K, Akiyama J, Mabe K, Suzuki J, et al. Efficacy of omeprazole, famotidine, mosapride and teprenone in patients with upper gastrointestinal symptoms: an omeprazole-controlled randomized study (J-FOCUS). BMC Gastroenterol. 2012;12:42.
80. Omura N, Kashiwagi H, Chen G, Yano F, Suzuki Y, Aoki T. Effects of ecabet sodium on experimentally induced reflux esophagitis. J Gastroenterol. 2000;35(7):504–9.
81. Tsuboi K, Omura N, Yano F, Kashiwagi H, Yanaga K. Effects of ecabet sodium on acute mixed reflux esophagitis in rats. Scand J Gastroenterol. 2009;44(12):1408–15.
82. Yanase K, Funaguchi N, Iihara H, Yamada M, Kaito D, Endo J, et al. Prevention of radiation esophagitis by polaprezinc (zinc L-carnosine) in patients with non-small cell lung cancer who received chemoradiotherapy. Int J Clin Exp Med. 2015;8(9):16215–22.
83. Chen MC, Amirian DA, Toomey M, Sanders MJ, Soll AH. Prostanoid inhibition of canine parietal cells: mediation by the inhibitory guanosine triphosphate-binding protein of adenylate cyclase. Gastroenterology. 1988;94(5 Pt 1):1121–9.

Chapter 31
Proton Pump Inhibitor Controversies

Aaron J. Jaworek

The first proton pump inhibitor (PPI), omeprazole, was approved by the FDA in 1989. It was an important milestone in the treatment of GERD and related conditions because for the first time, a medication could reduce acid production in the stomach for 24 hours. Given its safety profile from initial clinical trials, FDA approval for use in any age was obtained [1]. With as many as 20% of Americans suffering from GERD and with esophageal adenocarcinoma rates on the rise in the United States during the 1980s and 1990s, the need for *adequate* treatment of GERD was imperative [2]. It seemed as if this new drug could not have come at a better time. Since the introduction of omeprazole, five additional proton pump inhibitors have been made available in the United States – lansoprazole, pantoprazole, rabeprazole, esomeprazole, and dexlansoprazole.

At the beginning of the twenty-first century, however, a cultural shift occurred in how information was acquired by the public with the rising popularity of social media and other internet resources. As a result, skepticism of science and medical knowledge could be reinforced by social media posts from any source irrespective of the quality of evidence to support the claim. One consequence of this phenomenon is that receiving information from a licensed medical professional about the safety and effectiveness of a treatment can be perceived as insufficient when making a decision. That medical decision is made only when the patient, clinician, *and* (social) media sources are in agreement. A well-known example of this kind of doubt in scientific research amplified by social media is the refusal to vaccinate. The consequences can be far-reaching. In 2019, the United States has seen an unprecedented number of measles cases since the disease was declared eradicated in 2000 [3]. In a similar manner, PPI use has become entangled in controversy.

A. J. Jaworek (✉)
Drexel University College of Medicine, Department of Otolaryngology – Head and Neck Surgery, Philadelphia, PA, USA

Temple University Lewis Katz School of Medicine, Department of Otolaryngology – Head and Neck Surgery, Philadelphia, PA, USA

C. H. Zalvan (ed.), *Laryngopharyngeal and Gastroesophageal Reflux*,
https://doi.org/10.1007/978-3-030-48890-1_31

What has reinforced public opinion that PPIs may be dangerous are research studies finding associations between PPI use and outcomes like cardiovascular disease, kidney disease, dementia, and even death. News media reporting about those studies frequently exaggerate the conclusions while failing to assess quality (e.g., study design, methods, analysis). For example, the important distinction between *association* and *causation* often is minimized or ignored completely. Instead, emphasis is placed on any statistically significant relationship between PPI exposure and the outcome investigated, despite obvious limitations within the study.

Clinically, this has translated into a willingness of many healthcare professionals to accept the exaggerated interpretation rather than critically appraising the best evidence to understand whether a new discovery warrants a change in practice. Countless times, the author has had an encounter with a patient who discontinued use of his PPI following the recommendation of another clinician citing the dangers of long-term use. It becomes a one-sided debate excluding the prescribing physician who is then left with the delicate challenge of navigating damage control, being forced to explain the nuances and shortcomings of the quality of the research that led other clinicians to their decision, while avoiding severing working relationships with those same clinicians despite divergent analyses of the scientific literature.

This sentiment has been echoed within the medical literature among a growing number of review articles on the subject of PPI risks. For example, Mitchell Schubert, MD wrote:

> The sensationalized reporting of potential adverse associations of PPIs in the medical literature and lay press has influenced provider prescribing and patient adherence. The unintended consequences are that patients who require PPIs, such as those taking dual antiplatelet agents, are not being prescribed or taking these necessary medications. In addition, physicians are spending an inordinate amount of additional time placing these findings into proper perspective for their patients and reassuring them upon initiating PPI treatment as well as at every follow-up visit [4].

Similarly, Vaezi and colleagues argued:

> Multiple "false alarms" related to the safety of PPIs could ultimately lead to inappropriate discontinuation of treatment with potentially serious consequences for some patients. Investigators, the press, and, perhaps, even editors of medical and scientific journals should take responsibility to avoid subjecting the public to what Lewis Thomas called an "epidemic of anxiety" causing unintended harm. The media should take a more balanced, critical, and responsible approach in their reporting of epidemiological data so that weak and inconclusive results are not over interpreted and presented to the lay public as facts [5].

This situation closely resembles the ongoing struggle of clinicians advocating for the safety of vaccinations when the ill effects of fraudulent research concluding that they cause autism continue to resonate among a growing minority of parents. After numerous large studies have dispelled this myth, the *informed* medical community does not endorse any connection between vaccines and autism, and conversations with patients reflect this understanding [6]. Similarly, for PPI use and associated risks observed in some studies early on, subsequent higher quality studies and meta-analyses have weakened or even reversed many of those earlier findings. It is the responsibility of the medical community to educate patients on the best current evidence in order to provide the highest quality care.

Despite numerous controversies surrounding PPI use, which will be explored in more detail later in this chapter, undeniable is the fact that PPIs contribute an exorbitant amount to healthcare spending in the United States. With GERD accounting for $15–20 billion annually in overall healthcare spending in the United States, over 50% of that comes from prescriptions, primarily PPIs, contributing more than $10 billion [7]. In turn, insurance companies have initiated additional prescribing rules that include prior authorizations, prescribing *ladders* whereby one PPI must be tried before the next can be approved, and increased cost of PPI prescriptions. This has fueled shifting practice patterns by discouraging PPI prescriptions at adequate doses in favor of lower doses or abandoning PPIs altogether.

Additional insights into cost savings and PPI use have emerged. For example, Gosselin and colleagues found that patients compliant with PPI therapy had greater incremental healthcare cost savings compared with noncompliant patients (annual savings of $3261 vs $2406) [8]. On the other hand, studies have indicated that earlier reflux testing can be more cost-effective than prolonged empiric trials of PPIs for both GERD and laryngopharyngeal reflux (LPR) patients [9, 10]. Carroll and colleagues calculated an average weighted cost of $1897 per patient for up-front reflux testing (multichannel intraluminal pH impedance with dual pH probes and high-resolution manometry) vs $3033 for initial PPI twice daily and $3366 for initial PPI daily + Histamine-2 receptor blocker (H2B) at bedtime for 6 months [10]. Additionally, reflux surgeries may prove more cost-effective over time than long-term PPI use in select patients [11, 12].

Another obstacle contributing to the economic burden of PPIs remains the difficulty for some patients being able to discontinue them successfully. Weaning PPI therapy can be difficult as patients may experience rebound symptoms for many weeks after discontinuation. In 120 healthy volunteers, rebound acid hypersecretion occurred after as little as 8 weeks of PPI treatment. Forty-four percent of those in the study who were on a PPI for 8 weeks experienced acid-related symptoms 9–12 weeks after discontinuing the PPI [13].

Serum gastrin levels can be used clinically to predict the rebound acidity that occurs with long-term use of PPI. Levels commonly are increased up to four times the upper limit of normal while on PPIs. In some patients, levels can be elevated as much as 40 times the upper limit of normal (4000 ng/L). These elevated levels normalize very slowly after PPI withdrawal [14]. Two additional studies reported that increased acid production can continue more than 8 weeks post PPI discontinuation, adding to the concerns about rebound acidity and the need to wean PPIs slowly [15, 16].

While it is important to educate patients regarding this possibility, it should not deter clinicians from recommending discontinuation of PPIs when clinically indicated. The author has had success in this regard through the communication of weaning strategies with the patient and anticipatory guidance about the potential for rebound symptoms. This is not initiated unless the patient has incorporated other long-term treatment strategies such as diet and lifestyle modifications, in some cases surgery, and has confirmed absence of disease on endoscopy (laryngoscopy and esophagoscopy); this is frequently combined with the use of reflux testing (pharyngeal pH probe or multichannel intraluminal pH impedance with dual pH probes) to confirm adequate treatment prior to weaning.

Research bias remains a critical component in the PPI controversy as the majority of research on PPI risk is based on retrospective reviews and observational studies. Within those studies, modest associated risks with low incidence rates yield a very low overall risk. In nearly every study to date, hazards ratios (HR), odds ratios (OR), and relative risks (RR) remain <2, and in many cases <1.5. Observational studies may be inherently incapable of accurately discerning weak associations from null effects due to their susceptibility to systematic errors of bias, confounding, and other methodological weaknesses [17, 18]. Also, statistical significance only takes random errors related to sample size into consideration; it ignores systematic errors. Laine and colleagues reported on the difficulty in eliminating residual bias in observational studies even with statistical adjustment, because all confounding factors are not recorded or even known [19]. This may be especially important when effect sizes are small (OR, HR, RR <2), and so it may not be possible to determine whether the association is valid or the result of residual bias.

Furthermore, there may be some yet identified or uncaptured confounding relationships that contribute the risk observed in these studies. To illustrate the potential pitfalls with observational studies, Jena and colleagues employed the *falsification method* to evaluate the association of PPI use with community-acquired pneumonia (CAP) but also seemingly unrelated diseases, such as urinary tract infections [20]. In a large population-based cohort, they noted an association of PPI use with asthma, deep vein thrombosis, osteoarthritis, and rheumatoid arthritis, among other diseases. They even demonstrated a dose relationship in osteoarthritis, chest pain, and urinary tract infections.

The types of bias frequently encountered in studies on PPI risk are as follows:

1. *Channeling Bias*: Refers to the tendency of clinicians to prescribe certain medications to patients with more severe underlying illness (e.g., A PPI for patients with morbid obesity, coronary artery disease, diabetes mellitus, chronic kidney disease, etc.).
2. *Selection Bias*: Patients are chosen to receive one therapy over another due to multiple influential factors such as comorbidities, socioeconomic status, insurance status, practice patterns within a community or institution, perceived severity of disease, and specific symptoms.
3. *Protopathic Bias*: Occurs when a drug is used to treat early signs of the outcome, giving the appearance that the drug is causally related with the outcome.
4. *Strength of Methodology*: A study is only as good as its design (prospective, retrospective, control group, randomization, etc.).
5. *Confounding*: Variable of influence not accounted for in a study, which can lead to false associations. For example, if GERD is diagnosed based on symptoms alone, patients with cardiac chest pain might be included in the cohort influencing the outcome of cardiac events from PPI use.

6. *Generalizability*: Ability to extend research findings from the study population to a different population. For example, a study from one country may not be generalizable to other countries with different susceptibilities, pathophysiology, prevalence of disease, diagnostic accuracy, treatment patterns, etc. Other examples include demographics, disease states, as well as regional and dietary differences.

An important observation was made by Vaezi and colleagues regarding meta-analyses of low-quality studies.

> The application of meta-analysis to observational studies is controversial because the high risk of bias/confounding in the individual studies makes the calculation of a single summary effect estimate potentially misleading. Because the PPI safety literature consists predominantly of observational studies, published meta-analyses have focused on reporting pooled summary estimates and drawing conclusions from these. As a result, besides providing a more precise but potentially biased effect estimate, these meta-analyses have offered little value in addressing key questions regarding the causal nature of the reported associations [5].

PPI Adverse Effects

Risks of PPI use can be divided broadly into *immediate* and *delayed categories*. Immediate adverse events can be categorized further into *hypersensitivity* reactions (allergy, anaphylaxis, subacute cutaneous lupus erythematosus, etc.) and *other* immediate adverse reactions. Hypersensitivity reactions due to PPI exposure are very rare but have been reported [21]. Other immediate adverse events, which typically are mild and uncommon include headache, abdominal pain, nausea/vomiting, diarrhea/constipation, flatulence/bloating, and rebound acid regurgitation. Even less common but reported adverse events include gynecomastia and alopecia. The author has observed a case of gynecomastia and alopecia attributed to PPI use among thousands of patients treated with PPIs over the last 10 years.

Medication interactions remain an important consideration when starting a PPI. This can be due to a variety of mechanisms. One interaction is the concomitant use of medications that are metabolized by the same hepatic enzymes (CYP2C19, CYP1A2, and CYP2C9/10). Examples include clopidogrel, warfarin, fluconazole, carbamazepine, phenytoin, citalopram, diazepam, and tacrolimus. The FDA in 2009 warned against combining clopidogrel and PPIs, in particular potent CYP2C19 inhibitors such as omeprazole [22]. For CYP2C19 metabolized medications, preference for pantoprazole and esomeprazole will help to minimize this effect [23].

Another mechanism whereby PPI use can alter effectiveness of other medications is with increased gastric pH. Examples include erlotinib, nelfinavir, and rilpivirine, which are contraindicated due to their importance in HIV treatment. Concomitant use with digoxin should be avoided when possible, and digoxin levels should be monitored closely with PPI use. Use of the enteric-coated version of mycophenolate sodium can help reduce any potential interaction with PPI use. Iron supplements and levothyroxine also are at risk of reduced effectiveness in the presence of PPI, although this interaction is mild and inconsistent. Antibiotics potentially affected via this mechanism include cefuroxime, cefpodoxime, and ciprofloxacin.

Lastly, decreased renal clearance has been proposed as another mechanism for medication interactions with concomitant PPI use. One example includes methotrexate which could lead to increased levels.

Delayed adverse effects of PPI use have been the focus of much discussion, research, and controversy. Each has been listed with the most relevant and up-to-date literature in the analysis.

Cancer

Esophageal Cancer

It has been established for some time that GERD is an important risk factor for development of esophageal adenocarcinoma (EAC). Evaluating the ability of anti-reflux therapies to prevent EAC requires large-scale studies with long follow-up periods and controlling for confounding factors [2]. No RCTs have been carried out to date for these reasons and for the ethical dilemma of withholding treatment in a symptomatic population potentially at higher risk of developing esophageal cancer.

Some attention has been given to the notion that acid reflux therapy with PPI might actually *increase* risk of developing EAC rather than be protective. For example, a nationwide case–control study in Denmark evaluating 9883 patients with a new diagnosis of Barrett's esophagus found an elevated RR for high-grade dysplasia and EAC in long-term low (RR 2.2, 95% CI 0.7–6.7) and high (RR 3.4, 95% CI 1.1–10.5) adherence PPI use compared to age- and sex-matched controls [24]. A population-based cohort study of 796,492 adults in Sweden exposed to maintenance therapy with PPI revealed an overall standardized incidence ratio (SIR) for EAC of 3.93 (95% CI 3.63–4.24) on PPI [25]. This remained increased for non-GERD indications of PPI use such as with nonsteroidal anti-inflammatory drugs (NSAID) and aspirin use. The SIR also was increased for esophageal squamous cell carcinoma but to a lesser degree.

On the other hand, Krishnamoorthi and colleagues analyzed 9660 patients with Barrett's esophagus in the United Kingdom utilizing a large primary care database. When time-varying statistical models were used, PPI use was associated with a protective effect against progression to EAC (HR 0.43, 95% CI, 0.36–0.52) [26].

As EAC incidence rates have stabilized, or even declined somewhat in the last 15 years in the United States [27, 28], the number of patients taking PPIs continued to increase over that time frame [29]. Therefore, it seems unlikely that PPI use would increase risk of EAC. Additionally, channeling and protopathic biases among others are frequently cited as limitations to the available studies.

A comprehensive analysis of all available studies led to the conclusion that PPI use most likely has either a protective effect or no effect against progression to EAC. Most importantly, the best available evidence *does not* demonstrate an association with PPI use and *increased* risk of EAC. A meta-analysis of five cohort studies and two case–control studies associated a 71% decrease in risk of EAC or high-grade dysplasia with PPI use in patients with Barrett's esophagus (adjusted OR 0.29, 95% CI 0.12–0.79) [30]. A follow-up meta-analysis of those seven studies plus two additional population-based case–control studies found that the association was no longer statistically significant (unadjusted OR 0.43, 95% CI 0.17–1.08) [31]. A similar observation was found when the authors restricted analysis to five studies with higher scientific quality and adjustment for confounders (adjusted OR 0.98, 95% CI 0.46–2.10) [31].

A systematic review and meta-analysis of 12 studies indicated that anti-reflux surgery also might prevent EAC better than anti-reflux medication in patients with GERD (incidence rate ratio 0.76, 95% CI 0.42–1.39) [32]. The authors of the study, however, stated that it was not possible to make conclusions because of the limited sample size, possible bias, and confounding in the included studies.

Gastric and Neuroendocrine Tumors (NET)

Human studies have not confirmed an association between PPIs and development of gastric cancer or gastric NETs despite mixed findings. Higher quality studies (RCTs) favor no association of risk.

Association of Risk

A Dutch database of nearly 30,000 PPI users demonstrated that after 8 years of follow-up, 45 (0.16%) patients were diagnosed with gastric cancer compared with 22 (0.01%) cases among the 350,000 control subjects not using PPIs [14]. The difference among the groups was significant, thus interpreted as an increased risk among the PPI users; however, potential protopathic bias (e.g. a cancerous lesion not yet detected could have been present before PPI use) could not be excluded by the authors.

The Danish National Health-Care System was interrogated to evaluate the incidence of gastric cancer among 18,790 new PPI users between 1990 and 2003. Poulsen and colleagues found an incidence rate ratio (IRR) of 1.2, and although *Helicobacter pylori* infection and a confounding by *indication* bias may be an explanation, the *possibility* of a causal association between long-term PPI use and risk of gastric cancer was considered [33].

A meta-analysis of 11 observational studies with 5980 gastric cancer patients reported that the use of acid suppressive drugs was associated with an increased risk of gastric cancer (adjusted OR 1.42, 95% CI 1.29–1.56), although the lack of information on *H. pylori* infection again limited the results [34]. This association was present for PPI use (adjusted OR 1.39, 95% CI 1.19–1.64) and H2B (adjusted OR 1.40, 95%CI 1.24–1.59).

No Association of Risk

In a population-based study by Garcia-Rodriguez and colleagues, rates of gastric cancer were elevated fivefold in patients with GERD and similar diagnoses; in those patients, the authors concluded that treatment with PPI appeared to be a marker for cancer risk rather than a causative factor [35].

In a pooled analysis of four RCTs by Song and colleagues, PPIs were *not* associated with gastric atrophy, intestinal metaplasia, or other pre-malignant changes [36].

In the SOPRAN and LOTUS trials, 812 adults were randomized to anti-reflux surgery vs PPI and followed with serial biopsies. With up to 12 years of follow-up, there was no difference between groups in gastric pre-malignant changes or in gastric NETs [37].

Lastly, a recent FDA-mandated long-term follow-up study by Schneider and colleagues found no evidence of an increased risk of gastric cancer, other GI cancers, or any cancer with pantoprazole use [38].

Colon Cancer

Three large case–control studies have been conducted to evaluate any association between PPI use and colorectal cancer (CRC). A UK general practice research database study, based on more than 4400 CRC cases and 44,000 controls, demonstrated that long-term PPI therapy at a regular dose was not associated with a significantly increased risk of CRC for >5 years of PPI exposure [39]. Similarly, two large population-based case–control studies, one from Denmark and one from the Netherlands, also did not show any evidence of increased risk of CRC in long-term PPI users [40, 41].

Cardiac

Analysis of outcomes related to PPI use and cardiac events is difficult since multiple confounding variables often are present. Also, the overlap in symptoms of GERD and cardiac disease can make patient selection and identification difficult [42]. No significant differences in ischemic events or mortality were observed in any RCTs evaluating PPI use, and the use of PPIs in patients taking clopidogrel was associated with a significantly reduced risk of GI bleeding [43, 44]. Results seem to suggest that PPIs are a *marker* of increased risk rather than a direct cause of worse outcomes, and further studies are needed to clarify this important issue [45]. Also, lab experiments on rats suggest that PPIs and gastrin may exert a *protective* effect, not harm, on cardiac myocytes [46, 47].

In an RCT that compared patients taking clopidogrel and omeprazole versus clopidogrel and placebo, Bhatt and colleagues noted no differences between the groups in adverse cardiac events, defined as death from cardiovascular causes, acute nonfatal myocardial infarction (MI), need for revascularization, and acute stroke [48]. A cohort study including over 20,000 patients hospitalized with myocardial infarction, coronary artery revascularization, or unstable angina did not find a significant relationship between PPI use and an increased risk of serious cardiovascular disease [49]. Noteworthy is that the majority of patients in this study were receiving pantoprazole and fewer than 10% were receiving omeprazole. In a meta-analysis that included 16 studies (8 RCTs, 7 observational studies, and 1 retrospective analysis of an RCT) with a total of 447,408 subjects, the observational studies, but *not* the RCTs, showed a slight increased risk of adverse cardiovascular events with PPIs [50].

Using an administrative claims database from two insurance cohorts constituting over five million patients from 2001 to 2014, a US study by Landi and colleagues found no evidence that PPIs increase the risk of MI compared with H2B [51].

Sehested and colleagues analyzed 214,998 individuals from a Danish nationwide registry. During a median follow-up of 5.8 years, there were 5608 myocardial infarctions identified. Current PPI exposure was associated with significantly higher rates of MI (HR 1.31, 95% CI 1.23–1.39) after adjusting for age, sex, comorbidities, and concomitant medication. H2B use was not significantly associated with MI (HR 1.15, 95% CI 0.92–1.43). Long-term PPI use, compared to non-use, was associated with a 36% (CI 7-73%) greater risk of MI within a 6-month period [52].

Death

In 2017, a controversial study by the US Department of Veterans Affairs (VA) was undertaken exploring association of PPI exposure and risk of death. It was an observational cohort study of over three million patients from the VA electronic database with median follow-up of 5.7 years [53]. The population consisted mostly of older white male veterans. In that study, PPI use was associated with increased risk of death compared to H2B use (HR 1.25 (CI 1.23-1.28)), PPI use vs no PPI (HR 1.15 (CI 1.14-1.15)), and PPI use vs no PPI/no H2B (HR 1.23, CI 1.22-1.24).

Criticisms of this study:

1. Cause of death was not reported, only mortality; if a variety of causes of death was found, it would be unlikely that the mortality was due to PPI exposure.
2. The *exposure* was any patient *prescribed* PPI or H2B in the electronic health record regardless of whether the individual took the medication as prescribed or even at all.
3. Confounding variables were difficult to account for in the database (e.g., alcohol abuse and psychiatric illness), and *external adjustment* was undertaken to esti-

mate just three of the unmeasured confounders: obesity, smoking, and therapeutic agents.
4. No standardized diagnostic algorithm was applied prior to PPI prescription. This leads to heterogeneity within the subjects.
5. "There were significant baseline differences in that cohort participants who were treated with PPI were older and were more likely to have comorbid conditions, including diabetes, hypertension, cardiovascular disease, and hyperlipidemia. Cohort participants treated with PPI were also more likely to have upper GI tract bleeding, ulcer disease, *H. pylori* infection, Barrett's esophagus, achalasia, stricture, and esophageal adenocarcinoma [53]."

This study alone cannot result in any conclusion (causation or association) between PPI exposure and death. Therefore, it is important that clinical decisions regarding PPI use not be based on any possible relationship with risk of death.

In a follow-up to the original study, Xie and colleagues sought to look at the cause-specific mortality associated with PPI use using a longitudinal observational cohort study among patients treated at the US Dept of Veterans Affairs [54]. New users of PPIs ($n = 157{,}625$) and H2B ($n = 56{,}842$) were assessed for all-cause mortality and cause-specific mortality associated with taking PPIs (values reported as number of attributable deaths per 1000 patients taking PPIs). There were 45.20 excess deaths (95% CI 28.20–61.40) per 1000 patients taking PPIs. Circulatory system diseases (number of attributable deaths per 1000 patients taking PPIs = 17.47, 95% CI 5.47–28.80), neoplasms (12.94, 1.24–24.28), infectious and parasitic diseases (4.20, 1.57–7.02), and genitourinary system diseases (6.25, 3.22–9.24) were associated with taking PPIs. There was a graded relationship between cumulative duration of PPI exposure and the risk of all-cause mortality and death due to circulatory system diseases, neoplasms, and genitourinary system diseases. Analyses of sub-causes of death suggested that taking PPIs was associated with an excess mortality due to cardiovascular disease (15.48, 5.02–25.19) and chronic kidney disease (4.19, 1.56–6.58). Among patients without documented indication for acid suppression drugs ($n = 116{,}377$), taking PPIs was associated with an excess mortality due to cardiovascular disease (22.91, 11.89–33.57), chronic kidney disease (4.74, 1.53–8.05), and upper gastrointestinal cancer (3.12, 0.91 to 5.44) [54]. Formal interaction analyses suggested that the risk of death due to these sub-causes was not modified by a history of cardiovascular disease, chronic kidney disease, or upper gastrointestinal cancer. Again, similar limitations as noted from the prior study can be applied to this follow-up study.

Dementia

Perhaps the most controversial topic influencing decision-making with regard to PPI use is the potential association with risk of dementia. Initially, two studies from Germany published in 2015 and 2016 demonstrated an association with PPI use and dementia [55, 56]. This ignited an enormous debate about the safety of PPIs among clinicians and patients alike. One study used a prospective cohort of patients 75 years and older, and the other mined a database from an insurance company. The HR for both studies was 1.4 while accounting for multiple confounding variables. Notably, stroke, diabetes, age, anticholinergic drugs, and polypharmacy also were associated with increased risk of dementia in those studies.

In the first study, Haenisch and colleagues, using data from a longitudinal multicenter cohort study in Germany, assessed the association between PPI use and risk of dementia in 3,076 elderly subjects ≥75 years of age [55]. They found that patients receiving PPIs had a significantly increased risk of any dementia (38%) and of Alzheimer's disease (44%) compared with subjects not receiving PPI medication.

In the second study, a population-based observational cohort from Germany examined the incident cases of dementia in 73,679 patients over 75 years of age [56]. PPI use was analyzed over an 18-month period, divided into 3-month blocks, prior to diagnosis. Regular PPI use was defined as the patient receiving at least one prescription for PPI in each of the six 3-month blocks. Compared with the general population, the adjusted HR of developing dementia was 1.44 (95% CI, 1.36–1.52) with regular PPI use and 1.16 (95% CI, 1.13–1.19) with intermittent use (1–5 of the 3-month blocks with at least one PPI prescription).

Concerns have been raised about the validity of the conclusions from these studies [57]. In particular, the authors could not ascertain from this dataset the type of dementia, level of education, and impact of polypharmacy. In addition, PPI users were associated with all a priori covariates, thus supporting the idea that this group was generally less healthy than the broader German population. Although the authors adjusted for these covariates in their analysis, severity of the comorbidities was not incorporated, and other potentially unidentified variables create uncertainty.

The following subsequent studies have demonstrated no association with PPI use and risk of cognitive decline or dementia:

1. In a prospective cohort of 10,486 volunteers that included 2,800 PPI users in the National Alzheimer's Coordinating Center Database, Goldstein and colleagues looked at development of mild cognitive impairment and progression to Alzheimer's disease [58]. PPI use at every follow-up interview (denoted "always PPI use") was associated with *lower* risk of transition to mild cognitive impairment or dementia caused by any etiology (HR 0.73, 95% CI, 0.55–0.97). When looking at suspected Alzheimer's disease cases, there was no association with "always PPI use" status (HR 0.74, CI 0.53–1.04). In addition, intermittent PPI use also was not associated with mild cognitive impairment or dementia of any etiology.
2. A second study that questioned the association of PPI use and dementia was based on 70,718 cases of Alzheimer's disease from the Finnish National Alzheimer's Disease Registration Database (MEDALZ) [59]. In a nested case–control design, Taipale and colleagues matched cases on the basis of age, sex, and region of residence with three or four controls from the national registry. After adjusting for covariates, PPI use was *not* associated with Alzheimer's dis-

ease (adjusted OR 1.03, 95% CI 1.00–1.05). Lack of any association persisted irrespective of time on PPI (studied up to 3 years).

3. A third study evaluated the association of PPI use and cognitive function in 13,864 nurses from the Nurses' Health Study II [60]. A lengthy health questionnaire, bloodwork, and data from a self-administered computerized neuropsychological test battery were obtained. When compared with those who were "never" PPI users, PPI use of 5–14 years was associated with a modest decrease in attention and psychomotor speed (−0.06, 95% CI −0.11–0). Similarly, H2B was associated with cognitive function decline. When H2B users were eliminated from the PPI user group, the decline in cognitive function associated with PPI use was attenuated in magnitude and statistical significance.
4. After analyzing data from two large population-based studies of twins in Denmark, Wod and colleagues found no association between PPI use and cognitive decline [61]. Data were collected prospectively from surveys of middle-aged individuals 46–67 years old (the Middle Aged Danish Twin study) and older individuals (the Longitudinal Study of Aging Danish Twins) who underwent cognitive assessments (a 5-component test battery) over a 10-year period (middle-age study, n = 2346) or a 2-year period (longitudinal study of aging, n = 2475). PPI use was obtained from a nationwide prescription register in Denmark.
5. A meta-analysis by Li and colleagues that included six cohort studies concluded that there was no statistical association between PPI use and increased risk of dementia or Alzheimer's disease [62]. The pooled RR of dementia and Alzheimer's disease were 1.23 (95% CI 0.90–1.67) and 1.01 (95% CI 0.78–1.32), respectively, compared with those of non-PPI users.
6. Another meta-analysis of 12 studies (8 cohort and 4 case–control) by Hussain and colleagues found no association between PPI use and risk of dementia with a pooled RR of 1.05 (95% CI, 0.96–1.15) [63]. Subgroup analysis based on study design (cohort: P = 0.14; case–control: P = 0.14), sex (RR 1.25, 95% CI 0.97–1.60), H2B (P = 0.93), and Alzheimer's disease (RR 1.00, 95% CI 0.91–1.09) revealed no significant association between PPI use and dementia risk.
7. Ten independent studies involving 642,305 participants were included in a meta-analysis by Song and colleagues. PPI use was not associated with dementia (HR 1.04, 95% CI 0.92–1.15) and Alzheimer's disease (HR 0.96, 95% CI 0.83–1.09) [64].
8. Using a nationwide South Korean database, Park and colleagues reported that PPIs were not associated with a higher risk of dementia when compared with H2B [65, 66]. A retrospective propensity score-matched cohort study using the National Health Insurance Service-National Sample Cohort included 87,562 patients on PPIs and 87,562 patients on H2B. Subjects were defined as patients newly prescribed PPI or H2B between 2003 and 2013 without prior prescriptions of PPI/H2B or diagnosis of dementia from their history within the past 1 year. They followed up participants until dementia occurrence, death, or the end of the study, whichever occurred first. The incidence rate ratio (IRR) was 1.01 (95% CI

0.96–1.06) with 1-year lag time. These findings demonstrated that PPIs did not associate with dementia more strongly than did H2B.

9. An association of PPI use with *reduced* risk of dementia was found in a case–control study of 23,912 subjects from a database of general practice medical records in Germany by Booker and colleagues [67].

Fractures

In 2010, the FDA published a warning of the possible increased risk of fractures of the spine, wrist, and hip with high dose or long-term PPI use. By 2011, the FDA revised the update to remove the osteoporosis and fracture warning on OTC PPI (short-term, low dose) [68].

A meta-analysis of 18 observational studies, including a total of 244,109 fractures by Zhou and colleagues, reported a higher risk of hip fractures, spine fractures, and fractures at any site not only after long-term treatment but also in cases of PPI use for less than 1 year [69]. They calculated increased risk of hip fracture (RR 1.26, 95% CI 1.16–1.36). However, these findings were associated with heterogeneity across studies. In sub-analysis limited to cohort studies, the significant increase of hip fracture was maintained (RR 1.24, 95% CI 1.06–1.45). Also, in this sub-analysis, risk of any-site fracture increased (RR 1.33, 95% CI 1.15–1.54), and spine fractures increased (RR 1.58, 95% CI 1.38–1.82).

A separate meta-analysis of 24 observational studies (9 cohort and 15 case–control studies) with 2,103,800 participants (319,568 hip fracture patients) was completed by Poly and colleagues [70]. Patients on PPIs had a greater risk of hip fracture than those without PPI therapy (RR 1.20, 95% CI 1.14–1.28). An increased association was also observed in both "low" and "medium" doses of PPI taken and hip fracture risk (RR 1.17, 95% CI 1.05–1.29; RR 1.28, 95% CI 1.14–1.44), but it appeared to be even greater among the patients with "higher" dose (RR 1.30, 95% CI 1.20–1.40). Moreover, the overall pooled RR were 1.20 (95% CI 1.15–1.25) and 1.24 (95% CI 1.10–1.40) for the patients with short-term (<1 year) and long-term (≥3 years) PPI therapies, respectively, compared with PPI non-users. Intermediate (1–2 years) PPI therapy risk was similar to long-term therapy (RR 1.23). In all studies, results of hip fracture risk were adjusted to age, gender, co-medication, and comorbidity, but in more than half of the studies, results were not adjusted to smoking status, alcohol consumption, and previous history of fracture at any site. Of note, 9 of the 24 included studies showed no significant fracture risk associated with PPI use.

Nassar and Richter performed a meta-analysis of 33 studies with 2,714,502 patients [71]. Fracture incidence was 22.04% (95% CI, 16.10–27.97) in PPI users and 15.57% (95% CI, 12.28–18.86) in controls. The overall effect size of the point estimate was 1.28 (95% CI, 1.22–1.35) between PPI use and bone fracture incidence. This value was similar for subgroup analyses including OR, HR, retrospective studies, prospective studies, and fracture site (hip, spine, any site). There was a trend toward increased fracture incidence from short duration use: OR 1.29 (95% CI, 1.19–1.40), medium duration use: OR 1.33 (95% CI, 1.12–1.55), and long duration use: OR 1.62 (95% CI, 1.33–1.90). This trend was not observed with PPI dose intensity. Of note, 12 of the included studies failed to observe a significant association between PPI use and fracture incidence. Only one small RCT was included in the analysis.

Liu and colleagues performed a meta-analysis of 32 studies with 2,181,546 patients assessing risk of bone disease including fracture risk [72]. This included 17 cohort studies, 13 case–control studies, 2 cross-sectional studies, and no RCTs. Compared with patients not taking PPI, PPI use was associated with increased risk of developing any-site fractures (HR 1.30, 95% CI 1.16–1.45), hip fracture (HR 1.22, 95% CI 1.15–1.31), and spine fracture (HR 1.49, 95% CI 1.31–1.68).

In a population-based propensity-matched retrospective cohort study with 10,596 patients, using the National Health Insurance Research Database in Taiwan, PPI use after stroke was associated with a small but significant increased risk of hip fracture (HR 1.18, CI 1.00–1.38) and vertebral fracture (HR 1.33, CI 1.14–1.54) [73].

On the contrary, a Finnish nested case–control study using a nationwide database of elderly patients (mean age 84.1 years) with Alzheimer's disease and hip fracture (n = 8418) found no association between PPIs used for longer than a year and hip fracture (19,235 controls) [74]. Similar results were reported in three other studies [75–77]. Interestingly, the RR of fracture was lower with PPI use in both young and old adults suggesting that PPIs could exert a protective effect.

A retrospective cohort study by Harding and colleagues observed no association between PPI use and fracture risk among older adults [78]. They included data on 4,438 participants aged 65 years and older who had no fracture in the year prior to baseline and had ≥5 years of enrollment history. Time-varying cumulative exposure to PPIs was determined from automated pharmacy data by summing standard daily doses (SDDs) across fills; patients were categorized as no use (≤30 SDD), light use (31–540 SDD), moderate use (541–1080 SDD), and heavy use (≥1081 SDD). With a mean follow-up of 6.1 years, adjusted HRs comparing PPI users to nonusers were 1.08 (95% CI 0.83–1.40) for light users, 1.31 (95% CI 0.86–1.95) for moderate users, and 0.95 (95% CI 0.68–1.34) for heavy users. Therefore, among patients with PPI SDD >30, no increased risk of fracture was observed. One important limitation of this study was reliance on automated pharmacy data which would not include OTC PPI use in either group.

Gastric Polyps

No study has demonstrated malignant potential among non-syndromic gastric polyps formed as a result of long-term PPI exposure. In a study by Levy and colleagues with over 35,000 fundic gland polyps (FGP) evaluated, low-grade dysplasia was seen in only 0.3% [79]. High-grade dysplasia was even rarer, and no malignancy was observed. According to Cheesman and colleagues, if FGP is histologically confirmed, no dysplasia/carcinoma is identified, and there is no concern for syndromic FGPs, then no further follow-up is needed [80].

Infection

Community-Acquired Pneumonia (CAP)

In a systematic review and meta-analysis including 226,769 cases of CAP among 6,351,656 participants from 26 studies looking at acid suppression and risk of CAP, Lambert and colleagues noted an increased risk of CAP with PPI use (OR 1.49, 95% CI, 1.16–1.92) [81]. This risk increased to OR 2.10 (95% CI 1.39–3.16) during the first month of therapy. Moreover, PPI therapy also increased the risk of hospitalization for CAP (OR 1.61, 95% CI 1.12–2.31). Only 4 of the 26 studies reviewed were RCTs. More importantly, the largest of the RCTs showed *similar* rates of CAP in the experimental and control groups.

In another meta-analysis, Eom and colleagues also observed no increased risk of pneumonia with PPI use in high-quality RCTs [82]. Thirty-one studies were included: five case–control, three cohort, and twenty-three RCTs. A meta-analysis of the eight observational studies showed that the overall risk of pneumonia was higher among people using PPIs (adjusted OR 1.27, 95% CI 1.11–1.46) and H2B (adjusted OR 1.22, 95% CI 1.09–1.36). In the RCTs, only use of H2B was associated with a small elevated risk of hospital-acquired pneumonia (RR 1.22, 95% CI 1.01–1.48).

Using electronic health records in the United Kingdom, individuals aged 60 and older in the primary care setting receiving PPIs for 1 year or longer (n = 75,050) were analyzed with age- and sex-matched controls (n = 75,050) [83]. During the second year after initiating treatment, PPIs were associated with greater hazard of incident pneumonia (PERR-adjusted HR 1.82, 95% CI 1.27–2.54), after accounting for pretreatment pneumonia rates.

Of 4,238,504 new users of NSAIDs from Canada, United States, and United Kingdom, 2.3% also started a PPI [84]. The cumulative 6-month incidence of hospitalization for CAP (HCAP) was 0.17% among patients prescribed PPIs and 0.12% in unexposed patients. After adjustment, the authors found that PPIs were *not* associated with an increased risk of HCAP (adjusted OR 1.05, 95% CI, 0.89–1.25). Use of H2B yielded similar results (adjusted OR 0.95, 95% CI 0.75–1.21).

A cohort study by Othman and colleagues examined 160,000 new PPI users [85]. The adjusted Cox regression showed a risk of CAP 1.67 (95% CI, 1.55–1.79) times higher for patients exposed to PPI than for controls. In the self-controlled case series, among 48,451 PPI exposed patients with a record of CAP, the incidence rate ratio (IRR) was 1.19 (95% CI, 1.14–1.25) in the 30 days *after* PPI prescription but was even higher in the 30 days *before* PPI prescription (IRR 1.92, 95% CI, 1.84–2.00). Based on these results, the association between PPI use and risk of CAP was deemed likely to be due entirely to confounding factors.

The *OBERON* study randomized 2,426 ambulatory adults to a PPI vs placebo for 26 weeks for the purpose of ulcer prevention and found similar rates of pneumonia (0.9% with PPIs vs 1.9% with placebo) [86].

In a retrospective analysis of 24 short-term RCTs, patients were randomized to esomeprazole (n = 9602) and placebo (n = 5500) [87]. No association was found between PPI use and pneumonia with RR 0.66 (95% CI 0.36–1.22).

When only RCTs are analyzed, association between PPI use and CAP observed in studies of inferior design disappears. Multiple confounding factors appear to play a role in influencing any associations as cited in these studies. One important consideration is the observation in clinical practice that GERD, and more importantly LPR, can be associated with micro-aspiration of refluxate in some patients resulting in pulmonary diseases like reactive airway disease and pneumonia. When combined with elements of channeling, selection, and protopathic biases, one can arrive at a plausible explanation for the association between PPI use and CAP observed in a few studies.

Hospital-Acquired Pneumonia (HAP) and Ventilator-Associated Pneumonia (VAP)

In a large pharmacoepidemiologic cohort study, including 35,312 patients, MacLaren and colleagues found that PPIs were associated with higher rates of pneumonia than H2B (OR 1.2, 95% CI, 1.03–1.41) in mechanically ventilated adult patients administered either an H2B or PPI for 48 hours or more while intubated [88]. They also found higher risk of GI hemorrhage (OR 2.24, 95% CI 1.81–2.76), and *Clostridium difficile* infection (OR 1.29, 95% CI 1.04–1.64) with PPI. The authors acknowledged the unexpected results that PPI use was associated with *increased* risk of GI hemorrhage in their study, and they provide discussion into possible mechanisms and comparison of outcomes to previous studies. This again highlights the added uncertainty in observational cohort studies that should be considered when evaluating their findings.

A network meta-analysis on stress ulcer prophylaxis in the ICU explored risk of HAP with PPI use [89]. Twenty-four of the eligible RCTs included PPI use (4 PPI vs placebo). Proton pump inhibitors and H2B were associated with increased risk of pneumonia compared to sucralfate (OR 1.65, 95% CI 1.2–2.27 and OR 1.3, 95% CI 1.08–1.58, respectively), but not when compared to placebo or no prophylaxis (OR 1.52, 95% CI 0.95–2.42 and OR 1.19, 95% CI 0.8–1.78, respectively). Additionally, PPI use was associated with reduction in clinically important GI bleeding in this analysis (OR 0.24, 95% CI 0.10–0.60) contrary to the study by Maclaren and colleagues.

Clostridium difficile Infection

The strongest evidence coming closest to probable causation rather than mere association of risk with PPI use is *Clostridium difficile* infection (CDI), primarily in the hospital setting. In 2012, the FDA also issued a warning regarding risk of CDI in patients receiving PPI therapy with a recommendation to use the lowest PPI dose for the shortest duration appropriate to the condition being treated [90].

A systematic review of 37 case–control studies and 14 cohort studies by Tleyjeh and colleagues noted an adjusted pooled RR of 1.51 for CDI [91]. However, the available studies in their review were rated "very low quality" by the GRADE criteria [92].

Two meta-analyses, one with 186,033 patients by Arriola and colleagues and one with 202,965 patients by Deshpande and colleagues, showed increased risk of CDI associated with PPI use (OR 1.81 and 2.15, respectively) [93, 94]. A meta-analysis of 42 observational studies revealed an increased risk of both incident and recurrent CDI in patients treated with PPIs (OR 1.74, 95% CI 1.47–2.85 and OR 2.51, 95% CI 1.16–5.44, respectively) [95]. Although presenting less overall risk, the use of H2B *also* was associated with an increased risk for CDI, thus suggesting a role of acid suppression in the development of CDI in these patients. The included studies were nonrandomized, had significant statistical heterogeneity, and had variable PPI dose and duration of treatment.

Khanna and colleagues, by applying additional multivariate analysis, established that PPI use was *not* associated with an increase in severe, complicated CDI, treatment failure, or recurrence of CDI [96].

While considering the possible risk of CDI with PPI use in the inpatient setting may be warranted, clinical experience has demonstrated that very few, if any, instances of CDI occur with PPI use in the outpatient setting.

Microscopic Colitis

A large Danish case–control study identified 10,665 patients with a first-time diagnosis of microscopic colitis [97]. All cases were histologically confirmed in the Danish Pathology Register, and information on PPI use was obtained from the Danish Prescription Register. The study found a strong association between current PPI use and both collagenous colitis (OR 6.98, 95% CI 6.45–7.55) and lymphocytic colitis (OR 3.95, 95% CI 3.60–4.33). The association was observed with all PPIs but strongest with lansoprazole for collagenous colitis (OR 15.74, 95% CI 14.12–17.55) and lymphocytic colitis (OR 6.87, 95% CI 6.00–7.86). No clear dose–response pattern was observed.

Kidney Disease

Acute Interstitial Nephritis (AIN) and Acute Kidney Injury

Although acute interstitial nephritis (AIN) is rare, it remains the most frequently observed type of acute kidney injury in PPI users [98]. Despite this fact, the exact mechanism of injury has not been clearly established. Also, NSAIDs, which have an established association with AIN, often are taken concomitantly with PPIs, thereby introducing an important confounder [99].

Three large population-based studies, performed in Canada, United States, and New Zealand, reported a higher risk of AIN and acute kidney injury in patients prescribed PPIs. In the Canadian study that included 290,592 individuals older than 65 years on PPI therapy and an equal number of controls, the risk of acute kidney injury and AIN was 2.5- and threefold higher, respectively, in PPI users [100]. In the population-based nested case–cohort study from the United States that included 184,480 subjects ≥18 years of age, acute kidney injury was twofold higher in patients who had used PPIs compared with those who had not, and results were similar after controlling for multiple confounders [101]. In the New Zealand study, of the 572,661 patients without a history of kidney disease, the risk of AIN was fivefold higher for current PPI users compared with the entire cohort [102]. Moreover, current PPI users had higher incidence of acute kidney injury compared with past PPI users.

Nochaiwong and colleagues performed a meta-analysis of four cohort and five case–control studies with 2.6 million patients [103]. Of these, 534,003 (20.2%) were PPI users. Compared with non-PPI users, PPI users experienced a significantly higher risk of AKI (RR 1.44, 95% CI 1.08–1.91) and AIN (RR 3.61, 95% CI 2.37–5.51).

Conflicting results were obtained from two observational studies showing no risk of AIN/AKI associated with PPI use. Lee and colleagues examined risk of AKI with PPI and H2B in a cohort of 15,063 critically ill patients [104]. In the adjusted analysis, PPI use was no longer associated with AKI (OR 1.02, 95%CI 0.91–1.13). They adjusted for demographics, cardiovascular comorbidities, indications for PPI use, and severity of illness. Leonard and colleagues explored association of PPI use and risk of AIN and AKI with two retrospective case–control studies, one for each outcome [105]. For AIN, 68 cases were identified in the General Practice Research Database. Adjusted OR for PPI use was 3.20 (95% CI 0.80–12.79) with sensitivity analyses producing an adjusted OR range of 3–7.7. For AKI, 27,982 cases were identified with adjusted OR for PPI use equal to 1.05 (95% CI 0.97–1.14). Sensitivity analyses produced a range of adjusted OR from 1 to 1.1. NSAID and NSAID + PPI were associated with increased risk of AKI with adjusted OR 1.31 (95% CI 1.25–1.37) and 1.33 (95% CI 1.07–1.64) respectively. In that study, NSAIDs, but not PPIs, were significantly associated with increased risk of AKI. The authors stated that the number of cases of AIN likely was too small to detect any association with PPI use.

Chronic Kidney Disease (CKD)

Risk of chronic kidney disease (CKD) associated with PPI use has been observed in numerous low-quality studies with high risk of bias.

Ten observational studies with 1,005,899 patients contributed to a *narrative* review on CKD and PPI use [106]. Of the included studies, six used a retrospective study design, two were prospective, and two case-controlled studies. No RCTs could be included in their review. The observational studies suggested that the strength of evidence associating PPI use with CKD was weak and did not establish causality.

Five observational studies with 536,902 participants were included in a meta-analysis by Wijarnpreecha and colleagues [107]. When compared with non-PPI users, the pooled risk ratio (PRR) of CKD or ESRD in patients with PPI use was 1.33 (95% CI 1.18–1.51).

In the meta-analysis by Nochaiwong and colleagues of four cohort and five case–control studies with 2.6 million patients, compared with non-PPI users, PPI users experienced a significantly higher risk of CKD (RR 1.36, 95% CI 1.07–1.72) and ESRD (RR 1.42, 95% CI 1.28–1.58) [103].

Lazarus and colleagues studied 10,482 participants in the Atherosclerosis Risk in Communities study, and the risk of CKD in PPI users vs nonusers in analysis adjusted for demographic, socioeconomic, and clinical variables was HR 1.50 (95% CI 1.14-1.96) [108]. Analysis with PPI ever used modeled as a time-varying variable had adjusted HR 1.35 (95% CI 1.17-1.55). The association persisted when baseline PPI users were compared directly with H2B users (adjusted HR 1.39, 95% CI 1.01-1.91) and with propensity score-matched nonusers (HR 1.76, 95% CI 1.13-2.74).

Health system-wide data from the Geisinger Health System were used to assess risk of acute and chronic kidney disease with PPI use [109]. The dataset included 248,751 patients, 16,900 of whom were on PPIs. In the larger population, a propensity score matched hazard ratio (HR) of 1.29 (95% CI 1.16–1.43) and 1.16 (95% CI 1.09–1.24; AR 1.7/1000 patient-years) was noted for acute and chronic kidney disease, respectively.

A study by Arora and colleagues evaluated the association between PPI use and CKD in 71,516 veterans [110]. They found that among the 34% of veterans who developed CKD during the study, those using PPIs had a modest but significantly higher risk of CKD development (OR 1.10, 95% CI 1.05–1.16).

A study by Xie and colleagues used the national veterans database to identify 173,321 new PPI users and followed them for 5 years to evaluate the risk of renal disease [111]. PPI users compared to H2B users had an increased risk of incident CKD (HR 1.28, 95% CI 1.23–1.34). They also had a significantly elevated risk of doubling of serum creatinine level (HR 1.53, 95% CI 1.42–1.65), estimated glomerular filtration rate (eGFR) decline >30% (HR 1.32, 95% CI 1.28–1.37), and ESRD (HR 1.96, 95% CI 1.21–3.18). Furthermore, a graded association was detected with duration of PPI exposure and risk of renal outcomes among those exposed to PPI for 31–90, 91–180, 181–360, and 361–720 days compared with those exposed for ≤30 days.

A retrospective study by Klatte and colleagues using a large database of patients in Stockholm identified new users of PPIs (n = 105,305) and new users of H2Bs (n = 9, 578) [112]. Renal outcomes data were collected for a median of 2.7 years.

Users of PPIs, compared with H2Bs, were associated with an increased risk for doubled levels of creatinine (adjusted HR 1.26, 95% CI 1.05–1.51) and decrease in eGFR of 30% or more (adjusted HR 1.26, 95% CI 1.16–1.36). Risk of development of ESRD with PPI use was not statistically significant (adjusted HR 2.40, 95% CI 0.76–7.58). The authors acknowledged that PPIs were more often prescribed to older patients with more comorbidities and to patients more often consuming other medications such as NSAIDS, potentially contributing to the observed association of PPIs with CKD outcomes.

Nutrient Absorption: Vitamin B12, Calcium, Iron, and Magnesium

Vitamin B12

Studies investigating B12 deficiency with PPI use are sparse. In one of the largest studies investigating PPI use and B12 deficiency, 25,956 patients with vitamin B12 deficiency were compared with 184,199 patients without vitamin B12 deficiency showing an association between B12 deficiency and 2 or more years of PPI use (OR 1.65, 95% CI 1.58–1.73; 3–4/1000 patient years) [113]. This risk increased with higher daily intake to 1.5 or more pills/day (OR 1.95, 95% CI 1.77–2.15) and decreased after discontinuation of use. The same association was found for H2B, but to a lesser extent. Of note, this increased relative risk (RR) of B12 deficiency would increase the prevalence of B12 deficiency in this population (>50 years) from 2.3% to 3.8% adding to suspicion of confounders.

A cross-sectional study failed to demonstrate a significant difference between vitamin B12 serum levels in 125 long-term (>3 years) PPI users aged 65 years and older compared with controls [114].

A case–control study with even fewer patients aged 65 years and older with B12 deficiency (n = 53) and 212 controls found that current long-term (≥12 months) use of PPI/H2B was associated with increased risk of B12 deficiency (OR 4.45, 95% CI 1.47–13.34) [115]. No association was found between past or current short-term (<12 months) use of PPI/H2B and vitamin B12 deficiency. They controlled for age, gender, multivitamin use, and *Helicobacter pylori* infection.

From the available studies, it appears that decreased vitamin B12 levels with PPI use is likely, but it remains unclear to what extent with PPI dose and duration of therapy. Again, clinical experience treating GERD and LPR with PPIs has resulted in minimal, if any, B12 deficient patients in those who are tested. More high-quality studies are needed.

Calcium

A placebo-controlled, double-blind, crossover trial in elderly postmenopausal women older than 65 years of age found that *supplemental* calcium carbonate absorption in the fasting state decreased after 1 week of omeprazole therapy [116]. Only 18 of 23 subjects completed the study. Omeprazole 20 mg daily markedly decreased fractional calcium absorption from 9.1% (95% CI, 6.5–11.6) on placebo to 3.5% (95% CI 1.6–5.5) on omeprazole. Bisphosphonates (5 women) and diuretics (6 women) were allowed but were withheld on each study day until the afternoon. A multivitamin including 400 IU vitamin D was also taken daily during the study.

On the contrary, a study performed on 13 young male patients did not find any significant difference between the absorption of *dietary* calcium among eight patients taking omeprazole compared with five controls [117]. Despite significant changes in gastric pH on omeprazole, no change in the intestinal absorption of calcium, phosphorus, magnesium, or zinc from a standard test meal was observed. The authors suggested that changing the gastric pH alone does not modify the net intestinal absorption of several minerals from food.

Another study of 12 young adults in a placebo-controlled, double-blind, crossover study found that short-term acid suppression with esomeprazole did not significantly alter intestinal *dietary* calcium absorption [118]. There were two 3-week interventions that included a 14-day adjustment period to stabilize calcium homeostasis followed by 6 days of a diet containing 800 mg of calcium. During the last 3 days of the adjustment period and throughout the intervention period, subjects consumed esomeprazole or placebo. Neither calcium absorption nor urinary calcium differed significantly between the PPI and placebo groups.

This discrepancy of results appears to be related to the different methodologies used and to the better absorption of *dietary* calcium compared with *supplemental* calcium. One common hypothesis proposes that hypochlorhydria may interfere with absorption of calcium salts, thus leading to secondary hyperparathyroidism and subsequent bone resorption to maintain calcium levels [119]. However, the small studies aforementioned have demonstrated that there may not be meaningful impact of acid suppression with PPI on dietary calcium absorption. In cases of postmenopausal women (a population already at risk for osteoporosis) when on long-term PPI therapy, Eusebi and colleagues recommend increasing dietary calcium intake and, if necessary, selecting calcium supplements that are not influenced by gastric acid for absorption, such as calcium citrate [23].

Iron Deficiency and Anemia

Although a handful of case reports provide compelling evidence for the causation of iron deficiency anemia and PPI use in specific cases, high-quality studies are lacking, and the best studies fail to show a strong association.

In patients with Zollinger-Ellison Syndrome, 6 years of PPI exposure was *not* associated with decreased total body iron stores or with iron deficiency [120]. On the other hand, in patients with hereditary hemochromatosis, PPI use *was* associated with a significant reduction in the absorption of nonheme iron in the short term, as well as a significant reduction in annual phlebotomy requirements in the long term [121].

A retrospective cohort study of 98 patients on PPI by Sarzynski and colleagues found a significant association between the chronic use of PPI and the presence of anemia, showing a decrease of most hematological values in PPI users [122]. The authors noted a small sample size and presence of potential confounders influencing the validity of their results.

Patients enrolled in the LOTUS and SOPRAN studies were followed for 5 and 12 years, respectively [37]. Patients assigned to PPI use during that time frame saw no significant change in serologic markers, which included hemoglobin, iron studies, B12, folate, calcium, and vitamin D.

Magnesium

Hypomagnesemia may be associated with long-term use of PPIs according to some studies. This led the FDA in 2011 to communicate a similar warning [123]. In addition, the FDA has made the following recommendation:

> Healthcare professionals should consider obtaining serum magnesium levels prior to initiation of prescription PPI treatment in patients expected to be on these drugs for long periods of time, as well as patients who take PPIs with medications such as digoxin, diuretics, or drugs that may cause hypomagnesemia. For patients taking digoxin, a heart medicine, this is especially important because low magnesium can increase the likelihood of serious side effects. Healthcare professionals should consider obtaining magnesium levels periodically in these patients [123].

In a meta-analysis of nine studies – three cohort studies, five cross-sectional studies, and one case–control study with 109,798 patients investigating hypomagnesemia associated with PPI use – Cheungpasitporn and colleagues demonstrated a pooled relative risk (RR) of 1.43 (95% CI 1.08–1.88) [124]; these results increased to 1.63 (95% CI 1.14–2.23) with inclusion of studies only with high-quality GRADE criteria scores. Significant heterogeneity of the dataset was observed. Although this evidence supports an association of hypomagnesemia with PPI use, it is unclear if this was associated with increased *morbidity*, which would establish clinical relevance.

A meta-analysis by Park and colleagues including nine studies – two cohort, six cross-sectional, and one case–control with 115,455 patients – examining the relationship between PPI use and hypomagnesemia found a higher incidence of hypomagnesemia in PPI users than nonusers with pooled OR 1.775 (95% CI 1.077–2.924) [125]. Again, significant heterogeneity was identified among studies likely affecting validity of results.

In an effort to further explore the potential relationship between PPI use and hypomagnesemia, Kieboom and colleagues performed a prospective cohort study including 9,818 individuals [126]. They found that PPI use was associated with increased risk of hypomagnesemia (OR 2.00, 95% CI 1.36–2.93). PPI use with loop diuretic was associated with a further increased risk of hypomagnesemia (OR 7.22, 95% CI 1.69–30.83), and H2B use also was associated with increased risk of hypomagnesemia (OR 2.00, 95% CI 1.08–3.72).

Another observational cohort study examined risk of hypomagnesemia with PPI use in 170 patients on hemodialysis. Serum magnesium levels were significantly lower in PPI users than in nonusers (0.94 vs 1.03, $p < 0.0001$) [127]. The use of PPIs was an independent and strong predictor of lower magnesium levels even in multivariate analysis (OR 3.05, 95% CI 1.2498–7.4594).

Osteoporosis

The evidence linking PPI exposure with accelerating bone mineral density (BMD) loss and osteoporosis is weak and conflicting. Unlike for fracture risk, meta-analyses looking at BMD have been scarce owing to very few studies available for inclusion.

Liu and colleagues performed a meta-analysis of 32 studies with 2,181,546 patients assessing risk of bone disease [128]. Seven studies provided data on the risk of PPI use and osteoporosis. There was a modest increase in the risk of osteoporosis (HR 1.23, 95% CI 1.06–1.42) among PPI users with high heterogeneity found among studies. When the analysis was confined to cohort and case–control studies, the overall combined HR (HR 1.36, 95% CI 1.22–1.52) did not significantly change, and again substantial heterogeneity was reported. Only three of the studies provided data on the risk of PPI use and BMD. PPI use was not associated with increased risk of developing BMD loss in the femur (standardized mean difference 0.27, 95% CI -0.62 to 0.09) or in the spine (SMD 0.06, 95% CI -0.54 to 0.41).

Nassar and Richter performed a meta-analysis of 33 studies with 2,714,502 patients [71]. In 11 studies and data for 1,863 PPI users and 34,392 controls with treatment duration up to 8 years, there was no significant difference found in the standardized mean differences between PPI users and controls, either in cross-sectional BMD values or in the BMD change observed in longitudinal studies.

One of the best available prospective studies investigating osteoporosis risk with PPI use showed that continuous PPI use over 5 years was *not* associated with accelerated BMD loss in the hip or lumbar spine [129]. A total of 8,340 patients underwent initial BMD measurements, and 4,512 patients completed BMD testing after 10 years. No accelerated BMD loss was seen at any site during 5 and 10 years of follow-up, although lower baseline BMD was present in PPI users.

A population-based propensity-matched retrospective cohort study in stroke patients was conducted using the National Health Insurance Research Database in Taiwan [73]. Each group included 5,298 patients (PPI use and no PPI use). PPI use after stroke was associated with an increased risk of osteoporosis (adjusted HR

1.26, 95% CI 1.13–1.41). A pattern of dose effect was identified with the highest dose (>365 cumulative defined daily doses) associated with the highest risk (HR of 1.79, 95% CI 1.45–2.21).

Targownik and colleagues evaluated a sample of 52 long-term (≥5 years) PPI users matched to a similar cohort of 52 patients without PPI use in the previous 5 years [130]. All subjects underwent assessment of areal BMD using DXA, volumetric BMD using 3D-QCT, as well as markers of bone metabolism. Measures of bone strength, including buckling ratio and section modulus, were also compared. There were no differences detected in standard BMD, volumetric BMD, markers of bone metabolism, or measures of bone strength between the two groups.

A cross-sectional study of 40 daily PPI users (use ≥2 years) and 40 PPI nonusers was completed by Arj and colleagues [131]. Femur and posterior-anterior lumbar T- and Z-scores were quantified by dual-energy X-ray absorptiometry in all participants. Mean femoral T-scores were significantly different between PPI user vs nonuser groups (−0.44 ± 1.11 vs +0.19 ± 0.95, $p = 0.007$). In addition, the frequency of femoral osteoporosis and osteopenia in the exposed group was significantly more than in the control group ($P = 0.04$). Mean femoral Z-scores, lumbar spine T-score, and lumbar spine Z-score were not significantly different between PPI and nonuser groups, although femoral Z-score was close ($p = 0.05$). PPI use in subjects without risk factors of osteoporosis determined by the femoral T-score compared with the control group was associated with increased risk of developing osteoporosis and osteopenia in the femur bones (but not lumbar spine). Identified limitations included small sample size and lack of information about PPI dose.

Solomon and colleagues analyzed data from the Study of Women's Health Across the Nation (SWAN), a multicenter, multiethnic, community-based longitudinal cohort study of women across the menopause transition to determine the association between annualized BMD changes and new use of PPIs, H2B, or neither [132]. Dual-energy X-ray absorptiometry was used for BMD determination. Two-hundred and seven new users of PPIs, 185 new users of H2Bs, and 1,676 nonusers were identified. Study subjects had a mean age of 50 years and were followed up for a median of 9.9 years. Adjusted models found no difference in the annualized BMD change at the lumbar spine, femoral neck, or total hip in PPI users compared with H2B users or nonusers.

Maggio and colleagues investigated the relationship between PPI use and the parameters of bone mass (cortical and trabecular bone mineral density – vBMDc and vBMDt) and bone geometry (cortical and trabecular cross-sectional area – tCSA and cCSA) in older individuals [133]. The study population consisted of 1,038 subjects 65 years or older, selected from the InCHIANTI study, with complete information on computed tomography performed at tibial level (pQCT) and on medications. Only 36 subjects were identified as PPI users. PPI users showed age- and sex-adjusted lower vBMDt than nonusers (180.5 ± 54.8 vs 207.9 ± 59.4, $p = 0.001$). The inverse association between PPI use and vBMDt remained almost unchanged after adjustment for multiple confounders. There was no statistically significant difference in vBMDc, tCSA and cCSA between PPI users and nonusers.

In an RCT by Itoh and colleagues, 137 patients were randomized to risedronate daily, risedronate weekly, with or without rabeprazole 10 mg daily *after* breakfast for 9 months [134]. The BMD of trabecular bone without cortex at the third lumbar vertebra (L3) was measured using quantitative computed tomography. The Δ% value of increase in BMD and improvement of physical functioning in the bisphosphonate + PPI group were significantly larger than risedronate alone (24.6 +/−27.4 vs 12.4 +/−19.6, $p < 0.05$). The authors concluded that risedronate administration in combination with a PPI may be more effective not only for treating osteoporosis but also for improving physical fitness than treatment with risedronate alone. The study was limited by small sample size, high rate of discontinuation of treatment, short observation period, and unusual dose/timing of PPI (rabeprazole typically is used at 20 mg dose and before breakfast).

In a cross-sectional study using the Manitoba Bone Mineral Density Database, Targownik and colleagues determined the relationship between chronic PPI use and osteoporosis on an initial assessment of BMD and on BMD loss between successive assessments of BMD [135]. They observed that PPI use >1500 doses over the previous 5 years was not associated with having osteoporosis at either the hip (OR 0.84, 95% CI 0.55–1.34) or the lumbar spine (OR 0.79, 95% CI 0.59–1.06).

Prospective analysis of 161,806 postmenopausal women 50–79 years old, without history of hip fracture, enrolled in the Women's Health Initiative (WHI) Observational Study and Clinical Trials with a mean follow-up of 7.8 years was performed by Gray and colleagues [136]. The BMD measurements did not vary between PPI users and nonusers at baseline. Use of PPIs was associated with a *marginal* effect on 3-year BMD change at the hip ($P = 0.05$) but not at other sites. Of note, this effect actually represented a reduction in improved BMD in the PPI arm compared to non-PPI users as some women were participating in active treatment involving hormone therapy and/or calcium and vitamin D supplementation. When a time-dependent PPI use variable was used (including year 3), the difference in hip BMD was no longer significant ($p = 0.43$). The association was not present after examining longer follow-up to 6 years as well.

Yu and colleagues studied two cohorts of men and women over age 65, who were enrolled in the Osteoporotic Fractures in Men Study (MrOS) and the Study of Osteoporotic Fractures (SOF), respectively [137]. They used dual-energy X-ray absorptiometry and assessed baseline use of PPI and/or H2B in 5,755 men and 5,339 women. Medication use and bone mineral density (BMD) of the hip were assessed, and hip and other non-spine fractures were documented. On multivariate analysis, men using either PPIs *or* H2Bs had lower cross-sectional bone mass; however, this was not statistically significant for men using only PPI or men using only H2B. No significant BMD differences were observed among women. In that study, participants using PPIs and H2B tended to have higher BMIs, report more inactivity, and have poorer self-reported health as compared to nonusers. In addition, use of prescribed drugs was higher among users of PPIs and H2Bs, including a significantly higher usage of corticosteroids and NSAIDS. Additionally, initial recruitment of women occurred from 1986–1988, which was before PPIs were available,

PPI use in the cohort increased over time (from 5% to 16%), and an additional cohort of black women was recruited in 1996 adding to limitations within the study.

In a prospective, multicenter, double-blind study of 115 healthy postmenopausal women randomly assigned to dexlansoprazole 60 mg, esomeprazole 40 mg, or placebo daily for 26 weeks, there were no significant changes in markers of bone turnover (bone mineral density, true fractional calcium absorption, serum and urine levels of minerals, plasma levels of procollagen type 1 N-terminal pro-peptide, C-terminal telopeptide of type 1 collagen, and plasma levels of PTH) within the groups between baseline and week 26 [138].

Changes in bone remodeling rather than decreased bone mineral density (BMD) with PPI may provide a better explanation for the potential increased fracture risk observed in many studies. Therefore, the need for calcium and vitamin D supplementation while on PPI may not be necessary. Consideration also should be given to the GI side effects associated with treatments administered for osteoporosis [139].

1. *Bisphosphonates*: esophagitis, acid regurgitation, dyspepsia, abdominal pain, flatulence, bloating, nausea; acute renal failure has been observed with zoledronic acid, the most potent bisphosphonate
2. *Parathyroid hormone (teriparatide)*: nausea, vomiting, and dyspepsia
3. *Denosumab*: GERD, dyspepsia, flatulence, bloating, nausea, vomiting, and cough
4. *Calcitonin*: nausea, reduced appetite, diarrhea, abdominal pain, and hypocalcemia

Stroke

Currently, insufficient evidence exists to conclude any increased risk of stroke while taking PPIs.

A US study of 68,514 women enrolled in the Nurses' Health Study and 28,989 men enrolled in the Health Professionals Follow-up Study found no increased risk of stroke in PPI users [140].

Sehested and colleagues analyzed 214,998 individuals from a Danish nationwide registry [52]. During a median follow-up of 5.8 years, there were 7916 ischemic strokes identified. Current PPI exposure was associated with significantly higher rates of ischemic stroke (HR 1.13; 95% CI 1.08–1.19) after adjusting for age, sex, comorbidities, and concomitant medication. H2B use was not significantly associated with ischemic stroke (HR 1.02, CI 0.84–1.24). Long-term PPI use, compared with no use, had a 29% (CI 5%–59%) greater absolute risk of ischemic stroke within a 6-month period.

Wang and colleagues analyzed the Taiwan National Health Insurance database including 198, 148 PPI treatment courses and control periods without PPI use [141]. PPI use was associated with a higher risk of hospitalization due to ischemic stroke with a hazard ratio of 1.36 (95% CI 1.14–1.62). Based on subgroup analysis, patients aged <60 years were more susceptible ($P = 0.043$ for interaction), whereas gender, history of MI, diabetes mellitus, hypertension, use of antiplatelet agents or nonsteroidal anti-inflammatory drugs, or type of PPIs had no effect on the risk. In a nested case–control analysis, 15,378 patients hospitalized with ischemic stroke were compared with 15,378 matched controls [141]. An association between PPI use and increased cerebrovascular risks was identified, and the adjusted OR for PPI use was 1.77 (95% CI 1.45–2.18) within 30 days, 1.65 (95% CI 1.31–2.08) between 31 and 90 days, and 1.28 (95% CI 1.03–1.59) between 91 and 180 days before the onset of first-time ischemic stroke.

Weight Gain, Obesity

The author has observed in a handful of cases patient reports of unexpected weight gain shortly after initiating PPI use. It is usually described by the patient as increase in abdominal girth despite claims of eating the same diet and having a stable weight for many years.

Studies have been unable to identify statistically significant weight change with PPI use using large databases, [142] however, the observation of weight gain and change in abdominal girth may affect only specific individuals given their unique response to PPI exposure rather than represent a trend observed across entire populations groups. More research is needed to better understand this phenomenon.

RCT for PPI Risk

A source of much criticism in the PPI controversy is the shortage of high-quality RCTs investigating outcomes. When RCTs are included in a meta-analysis, they often contradict the results found in studies of inferior quality providing further support to the argument of research bias and confounding. An important RCT evaluating *multiple* long-term safety concerns related to PPI therapy was a multicenter study by Moayyedi and colleagues published in 2019 [143]. They performed a 3 × 2 partial factorial double-blind trial of 17,598 participants with stable cardiovascular disease and peripheral artery disease randomly assigned to groups given pantoprazole 40 mg daily (n = 8791) or placebo (n = 8807). Groups also were randomly assigned to aspirin, rivaroxaban, or both. Data were collected every 6 months for a median of 3 years and a maximum of 5 years on development of pneumonia, CDI, other enteric infections, fractures, gastric atrophy, chronic kidney disease, diabetes, COPD, dementia, cardiovascular disease, cancer, hospitalizations, and all-cause mortality. The authors observed no statistically significant difference between the pantoprazole and placebo groups in safety events *except* for enteric infections: 1.4% for PPI vs 1.0% for the placebo group (OR 1.33, 95% CI 1.01–1.75). Although CDI was nearly twice as common in the pantoprazole group compared to placebo, with only 13 total CDI events, this difference was not statistically significant.

This important RCT adds further support to the safety of PPIs and suggests that limiting PPI therapy because of concerns of long-term harm may not appropriate.

Alternative Therapies

As many as 50% of patients taking PPIs for nonerosive GERD are dissatisfied with their treatment due to unresolved symptoms [144]. These patients may seek alternatives to PPI and H2B therapy that have been deemed more "natural" or "safer." Examples include fermented products (e.g., apple cider vinegar, kombucha), aloe vera, turmeric, and ginger. The best studied and most effective adjunctive/alternative therapy remains alginates and other raft-forming agents like Gaviscon© and recently released Reflux Gourmet (refluxgourmet.com). They have been effective in treating postprandial, supine, and nonacid reflux in select patients. Besides the lack of regulatory oversight by the FDA and the uncertainty of composition and potency in many cases, alternative medicines intended to treat reflux are likely improving dyspepsia (indigestion) rather than actually reducing frequency and severity of reflux events. This confusion is found in numerous studies investigating alternative therapies as well as with patients' experiences with perceived benefits. The power of the placebo effect also cannot be ignored within this context. Nonetheless, a 2008 survey by the National Center for Health Statistics found that 38% of US adults report using some form of therapy that would be described as complementary alternative medicine (CAM), while results of an online survey published in 2018 suggested that the rate of dietary supplement and CAM utilization among patients with gastrointestinal disorders was as high as 85% [145].

Until CAM therapies can demonstrate equivalent or superior outcomes in high-quality RCTs compared to diet and lifestyle modifications, FDA approved pharmacotherapy, and surgery, it remains difficult to make any recommendation regarding their implementation in clinical practice. Most importantly, the potential harm with alternative therapies must be considered and discussed with the patient, including risk of adverse effects, drug interactions, and cost.

Conclusion

The controversy surrounding PPI use in the treatment of acid reflux has impacted nearly every medical specialty. What can be concluded from the investigations discussed in this chapter? The scrutiny behind the controversy is only partially justified and the response has been overinflated. This is due in part to the impact of cultural trends on the practice of medicine, such as the influence of media sources on public opinion, as well as evolving belief systems deeply rooted in distrust of science and regulatory oversight. This is a treacherous path to travel; on the other hand, it has led to one positive consequence – shifting focus onto the importance of living a healthy lifestyle as the foundation of disease prevention and treatment. Only when patients begin to take control of their life choices from the foods they consume, to regular exercise and achieving ideal weight, to improving mental health, do they begin to heal. The pharmacologic and surgical options still remain important for those who are faced with too many obstacles preventing them from achieving their goals. Each of these treatment options should not be viewed as dichotomous, but rather, as useful tools comprising an individualized program to conquer reflux-related diseases.

As the process to diagnose GERD and LPR becomes more sophisticated, a shift in approach to treatment has taken shape. Diagnostic testing up front with the use of pH and impedance sensors in the pharynx and esophagus are gaining momentum and may provide the key to lowering cost of healthcare spending for reflux management. The Mediterranean diet, low-acid diet, and elimination trials (e.g., gluten free, dairy free) along with lifestyle modifications are quickly becoming the first-line treatment, while medications such as PPI and H2B are being reserved for those who fail diet and lifestyle management. Additionally, a myriad of reflux surgeries are being pursued by patients as an effective long-term treatment strategy in lieu of medications. Undoubtedly, surgery has been successful in the treatment of reflux for many people; at the same time, a Cochrane review of the available studies in 2015 (only four of which were RCTs), concluded that there remains "considerable uncertainty in the balance of benefits versus harms of laparoscopic fundoplication compared to long-term medical treatment with proton pump inhibitors" [146]. Similar analyses for all reflux surgical options are needed.

Misdiagnosis remains a cornerstone of the PPI controversy leading to inappropriate prescribing. Emphasis on accurate diagnosis of acid reflux will allow for proper treatment to those who benefit. It is equally important to avoid unnecessary PPI exposure to those who have an alternative diagnosis. The prescribing clinician must seek a balance between the two opposing forces – PPI avoidance and over-reliance so that the pendulum does not swing too far in either direction.

An explosion of review articles on PPI risks have emerged in the last 5 years providing numerous insights into the complexity of the topic of PPI risks while attempting to summarize the latest research [4, 5, 18, 23, 42, 147, 148].

Schnoll-Sussman and Katz, in their review on PPI risks advised:

- Carefully assess the need for PPI therapy particularly in patients with GERD and dyspepsia. Consider early formal pH analysis testing to firmly establish acid reflux as the culprit, especially in patients where the diagnosis may be in question. In the absence of complications, use the lowest effective dose or discontinue them if possible.
- If PPIs are needed, discuss and consider alternatives taking careful account of both success and adverse events (e.g., surgery or endoscopic therapy for GERD) and document your conversations (specifically that related to potential adverse effects) as well as involve patients in decision-making. If PPIs are not indicated for symptom relief or prophylaxis, do not use them. If they are not working, look for alternative diagnoses and discontinue them.

- Perhaps most important, remind patients that medical management of GERD is not a substitute for a healthy lifestyle including maintaining a normal BMI, through diet and exercise, moderation of alcohol intake, and avoidance of smoking [42].

In an effort to mitigate potential adverse events, the American Gastroenterological Association (AGA) recommends an approach of thoughtful prescribing over routine supplementation and testing while on PPIs. The AGA "Best Practice Advice" on long-term use of PPIs in 2017 stated:

- *Best Practice Advice 2*: Patients with uncomplicated GERD who respond to short-term PPIs should subsequently attempt to stop or reduce them. Patients who cannot reduce PPIs should consider ambulatory esophageal pH/impedance monitoring before committing to lifelong PPIs to help distinguish GERD from a functional syndrome. The best candidates for this strategy may be patients with predominantly atypical symptoms or those who lack an obvious predisposition to GERD (e.g., central obesity, large hiatal hernia).
  - *Rationale*: Short-term PPIs are highly effective for uncomplicated GERD. Most patients with uncomplicated GERD respond to short-term PPIs and are subsequently able to reduce PPIs to less than daily dosing. Because patients who cannot reduce PPIs face lifelong therapy, we would consider testing for an acid-related disorder in this situation. However, there is no high-quality evidence on which to base this recommendation.
- *Best Practice Advice 6*: The dose of long-term PPIs should be periodically reevaluated so that the lowest effective PPI dose can be prescribed to manage the condition.
- *Best Practice Advice 7*: Long-term PPI users should not routinely use probiotics to prevent infection.
- *Best Practice Advice 8*: Long-term PPI users should not routinely raise their intake of calcium, vitamin B12, or magnesium beyond the Recommended Dietary Allowance (RDA).
- *Best Practice Advice 9*: Long-term PPI users should not routinely screen or monitor bone mineral density, serum creatinine, magnesium, or vitamin B12.
- *Best Practice Advice 10*: Specific PPI formulations should not be selected based on potential risks [149].

Baseline differences between PPI users and nonusers make it challenging to study potential PPI adverse effects retrospectively. And according to the GRADE working group classification, many studies are rated low or very low quality. When PPIs are appropriately prescribed, their benefits are likely to outweigh their risks. When PPIs are inappropriately prescribed, modest risks become important because there is no longer a potential benefit. There is currently insufficient evidence to recommend specific strategies for mitigating PPI adverse effects [149].

Supplementation of calcium and vitamin D does not conclusively decrease risk for fracture based on current understanding of the mechanism of fracture risk with PPI use. Therefore, it is unlikely that a policy of routinely supplementing long-term users of PPIs with calcium, vitamin D, or other vitamins would be of benefit. Similarly, routine BMD testing and routine monitoring of vitamin or mineral levels in long-term users of PPIs cannot be recommended.

While guidelines from leading organizations like the American Gastroenterological Association and the American College of Gastroenterology do not recommend routine laboratory monitoring of patients on PPIs, some institutions such as the Mayo Clinic have adopted their own practice parameters based on their assessment of the current literature. Patients treated with PPIs long-term at the Mayo Clinic have creatinine levels checked annually, a CBC every other year, and vitamin B12 level every 5 years [148]. According to Nehra and colleagues, it is reasonable to monitor estimated glomerular filtration rate annually, based on CKD guidelines for monitoring patients taking "potentially nephrotoxic medications" [148]. In their review, Eusebi and colleagues also concluded that caution should be used when prescribing PPIs to older subjects, especially if they present with other risk factors for renal disease [23]. They too suggested monitoring renal function in patients on long-term PPI treatment.

Following observations that a gluten-free diet can markedly reduce or even eliminate symptoms of reflux in some patients, the author has begun ordering gluten sensitivity labs on all patients diagnosed with reflux. The panel includes testing for celiac disease, non-celiac gluten sensitivity, and gluten allergy [150]. Those results can then guide decision-making regarding recommendation of a gluten-free diet trial prior to initiation of PPIs as part of the treatment plan. Many leading laryngologists and gastroenterologists are advising similar dietary recommendations to their patients with good results including a gluten-free diet and plant-based diets (e.g., Mediterranean diet and vegan diet) in order to treat reflux disease. For those who benefit from diet modifications, PPI reliance can be markedly reduced or even eliminated altogether.

Additional insights for best practice with long-term PPI use include the following:

- Work *with* colleagues on management strategies, rather than in opposition.
  Multidisciplinary teams dedicated to the treatment of reflux and upper GI disorders can foster a supportive working relationship among specialists
- Educate patients and other members of the treatment team when appropriate
- Confirm diagnosis and effectiveness of treatment with appropriate reflux testing when uncertainty exists
- Include the *well-informed* patient in the decision-making process. Also, remain sensitive to patients' desires regarding an individualized approach to reflux management
- When counseling patients on the controversies of PPI use, also discuss the *dangers* of untreated reflux – most importantly, the risk of esophageal adenocarcinoma
- Discuss *all* available treatment options including diet and lifestyle modifications, weight loss, medications, and surgery

As with any prescribed treatment, clinicians should stay up to date regarding the risks, benefits, and alternatives of PPI use. This demands frequent review of the current literature and critical appraisal of its content. Updated regularly utilizing the best available evidence, risk assessment tables, such as the one included in the review by Brisebois and colleagues [147], represent an effective way to communicate the quality of evidence associated with each outcome of interest. This can help facilitate informed decision-making by clinicians and patients alike. With any new peer-reviewed publication, one must decide if the conclusions within are sufficient to change practice. The clinician should avoid absolutes in decision-making based on an emotional response or misguided interpretation of the peer-reviewed literature. Equally important is staying up to date regarding limitations of the available studies in order to appreciate which clinical questions remain unanswered. The effort and time invested in this process is worth the reward of a patient who is grateful for adhering to a sustainable pathway leading to resolution of reflux disease.

Important Disclaimer GERD and LPR presentation and management have many distinctions. Most of the studies included in this chapter were for patients with GERD. Arguably, this makes generalizability more difficult (different study populations, overlapping symptomatology, and differential diagnosis). It is established that the most fundamental (albeit oversimplified) threshold for adequate LPR control is ≤1 pharyngeal reflux event daily, and for GERD <48 esophageal events daily (not to mention acid exposure times, weakly acid and nonacid reflux, mucosal changes, and patients' symptoms). This observation opens the door for even more needed research, not only to clarify association vs causation for the risks discussed but also to understand better the impact of PPI use on patients with LPR.

References

1. Strand DS, Kim D, et al. 25 years of proton pump inhibitors: a comprehensive review. Gut and Liver. 2017;11(1):27–37.
2. Coleman HG, et al. The epidemiology of esophageal adenocarcinoma. Gastroenterology. 2018;154:390–405.
3. Patel M, Lee AD, Clemmons NS, et al. National update on measles cases and outbreaks — United States, January 1–October 1, 2019. MMWR Morb Mortal Wkly Rep. ePub: 4 October 2019. https://doi.org/10.15585/mmwr.mm6840e2.
4. Schubert ML. Proton pump inhibitors: placing putative adverse effects in proper perspective. Curr Opin Gastroenterol. 2019;35:509–16.
5. Vaezi MF, et al. Complications of proton pump inhibitor therapy. Gastroenterology. 2017;153:35–48.
6. Bester JC. Measles and measles vaccination: a review. JAMA Pediatr. 2016;170(12):1209–15.
7. Gawron AJ, French DD, et al. Economic evaluations of gastroesophageal reflux disease medical management: a systematic review. PharmacoEconomics. 2014 Aug;32(8):745–58.
8. Gosselin A, Luo R, Lohoues H, Toy E, Lewis B, Crawley J, et al. The impact of proton pump inhibitor compliance on health-care resource utilization and costs in patients with gastroesophageal reflux disease. Value Health. 2009;12:34–9.
9. Kleiman DA, Sporn MJ, et al. Early referral for 24-hour esophageal pH monitoring may prevent unnecessary treatment with acid-reducing medications. Surg Endosc. 2013 Apr;27(4):1302–9.
10. Carroll TL, Werner A, et al. Rethinking the laryngopharyngeal reflux treatment algorithm: evaluating an alternate empiric dosing regimen and considering up-front, pH-impedance, and manometry testing to minimize cost in treating suspect laryngopharyngeal reflux disease. Laryngoscope. 2017 Oct;127(Suppl 6):S1–S13.

11. Funk LM, Zhang JY, et al. Long-term cost-effectiveness of medical, endoscopic and surgical management of gastroesophageal reflux disease. Surgery. 2015 Jan;157(1):126–36.
12. Faria R, Bojke L, et al. Cost-effectiveness of laparoscopic fundoplication versus continued medical management for the treatment of gastro-oesophageal reflux disease based on long-term follow-up of the REFLUX trial. Br J Surg. 2013 Aug;100(9):1205–13.
13. Reimer C, Sondergaard B, Hilsted L, Bytzer P. Proton-pump inhibitor therapy induces acid-related symptoms in healthy volunteers after withdrawal of therapy. Gastroenterology. 2009;137:80–7.
14. Kuipers EJ. Proton pump inhibitors and gastric neoplasia. Gut. 2006;55:1217–21.
15. Gillen D, Wirz AA, Ardill JE, McColl KE. Rebound hypersecretion after omeprazole and its relation to on-treatment acid suppression and helicobacter pylori status. Gastroenterology. 1999;116:239–47.
16. Fossmark R, Johnsen G, Johanessen E, Waldum HL. Rebound acid hypersecretion after long-term inhibition of gastric secretion. Aliment Pharmacol Ther. 2005;21:149–54.
17. Vaezi MF, Yang YX, Howden CW. Complications of proton pump inhibitor therapy. Gastroenterology. 2017;153(1):35–48.
18. Jaynes M, Kumar AB. The risks of long-term use of proton pump inhibitors: a critical review. Ther Adv Drug Saf. 2019;10:1–13.
19. Laine L, Nagar A. Long-term PPI use: balancing potential harms and documented benefits. Am J Gastroenterol. 2016;111:913–5.
20. Jena AB, Sun E, Goldman DP. Confounding in the association of proton pump inhibitor use with risk of community-acquired pneumonia. J Gen Intern Med. 2013;28:223–30.
21. Otani IM, Banerji A. Immediate and delayed hypersensitivity reactions to proton pump inhibitors: evaluation and management. Curr Allergy Asthma Rep. 2016;16:17.
22. Food and Drug Administration 2009. FDA Update to the labeling of Clopidogrel Bisulfate (marketed as Plavix) to alert healthcare professionals about a drug interaction with omeprazole (marketed as Prilosec and Prilosec OTC). http://www.fda.gov/Safety/MedWatch/SafetyInformation/SafetyAlertsforHumanMedicalProducts/ucm190848.htm.
23. Eusebi LH, et al. Proton pump inhibitors: risks of long-term use. J Gastroenterol Hepatol. 2017;32:1295–302.
24. Hvid-Jensen F, et al. Proton pump inhibitor use may not prevent high-grade dysplasia and oesophageal adenocarcinoma in Barrett's oesophagus: a nationwide study of 9883 patients. Aliment Pharmacol Ther. 2014;39(9):984–91.
25. Brusselaers N, et al. Maintenance proton pump inhibition therapy and risk of oesophageal cancer. Cancer Epidimiol. 2018;53:172–7.
26. Krishnamoorthi R, et al. Rates and predictors of progression to esophageal carcinoma in a large population-based Barrett's esophagus cohort. Gastrointest Endosc. 2016;84(1):40–6.
27. Howlader N, Noone AM, Krapcho M, Miller D, Brest A, Yu M, Ruhl J, Tatalovich Z, Mariotto A, Lewis DR, Chen HS, Feuer EJ, Cronin KA (eds). SEER cancer statistics review, 1975-2016, National Cancer Institute. Bethesda, MD, https://seer.cancer.gov/csr/1975_2016/, based on November 2018 SEER data submission, posted to the SEER web site, April 2019.
28. SEER Cancer Stat Facts: Esophageal Cancer. National Cancer Institute. Bethesda, MD, https://seer.cancer.gov/statfacts/html/esoph.html. Accessed 9 Aug 2019.
29. Kane SP. Omeprazole, ClinCalc DrugStats Database, Version 19.1. ClinCalc: https://clincalc.com/DrugStats/Drugs/Omeprazole. Updated November 24, 2018. Accessed 9 Aug 2019.
30. Singh S, Garg SK, Singh PP, et al. Acid-suppressive medications and risk of oesophageal adenocarcinoma in patients with Barrett's oesophagus: a systematic review and meta-analysis. Gut. 2014;63:1229–37.
31. Hu Q, Sun TT, Hong J, et al. Proton pump inhibitors do not reduce the risk of esophageal adenocarcinoma in patients with Barrett's esophagus: a systematic review and meta-analysis. PLoS One. 2017;12:e0169691.
32. Maret-Ouda J, Konings P, Lagergren J, et al. Antireflux surgery and risk of esophageal adenocarcinoma: a systematic review and meta-analysis. Ann Surg. 2016;263:251–7.

33. Poulsen AH, Christensen S, McLaughlin JK, et al. Proton pump inhibitors and risk of gastric cancer: a population-based cohort study. Br J Cancer. 2009;100:1503–7.
34. Ahn JS, Eom CS, Jeon CY, Park SM. Acid suppressive drugs and gastric cancer: a meta-analysis of observational studies. World J Gastroenterol. 2013;19:2560–8.
35. Garcia-Rodriguez LA, Lagergren J, Lindblad M. Gastric acid suppression and risk of oesophageal and gastric adenocarcinoma: a nested case control study in the UK. Gut. 2006;55:1538–44.
36. Song H, Zhu J, Lu D. Long-term proton pump inhibitor (PPI) use and the development of gastric pre-malignant lesions. Cochrane Database Syst Rev. 2014;12:CD010623.
37. Attwood SE, Ell C, Galmiche JP, et al. Long-term safety of proton pump inhibitor therapy assessed under controlled, randomised clinical trial conditions: data from the SOPRAN and LOTUS studies. Aliment Pharmacol Ther. 2015;41:1162–74.
38. Schneider JL, Kolitsopoulos F, Corley DA. Risk of gastric cancer, gastrointestinal cancers and other cancers: a comparison of treatment with pantoprazole and other proton pump inhibitors. Aliment Pharmacol Ther. 2016;43:73–82.
39. Yang YX, Hennessy S, Propert K, Hwang WT, Sedarat A, Lewis JD. Chronic proton pump inhibitor therapy and the risk of colorectal cancer. Gastroenterology. 2007;133:748–54.
40. Robertson DJ, Larsson H, Friis S, Pedersen L, Baron JA, Sorensen HT. Proton pump inhibitor use and risk of colorectal cancer: a population-based, case–control study. Gastroenterology. 2007;133:755–60.
41. van Soest EM, van Rossum LG, Dieleman JP, et al. Proton pump inhibitors and the risk of colorectal cancer. Am J Gastroenterol. 2008;103:966–73.
42. Schnoll-Sussman F, Katz PO. Clinical implications of emerging data on the safety of proton pump inhibitors. Curr Treat Options Gastro. 2017;15:1–9.
43. Cardoso RN, Benjo AM, DiNicolantonio JJ, et al. Incidence of cardiovascular events and gastrointestinal bleeding in patients receiving clopidogrel with and without proton pump inhibitors: an updated meta-analysis. Open Heart. 2015;2(1):e000248.
44. Melloni C, Washam JB, Jones WS, et al. Conflicting results between randomized trials and observational studies on the impact of proton pump inhibitors on cardiovascular events when coadministered with dual antiplatelet therapy: systematic review. Circ Cardiovasc Qual Outcomes. 2015;8:47–55.
45. Schoenfeld AJ, Grady D. Adverse effects associated with proton pump inhibitors. JAMA Intern Med. 2016;176:172–4.
46. Patil AS, Singh AD, Mahajan UB, et al. Protective effect of omeprazole and lansoprazole on b-receptor stimulated myocardial infarction in Wistar rats. Mol Cell Biochem. 2019;456:105–13.
47. Yang X, Yue R, Zhang J, et al. Gastrin protects against myocardial ischemia/ reperfusion injury via activation of RISK (reperfusion injury salvage kinase) and SAFE (survivor activating factor enhancement) pathways. J Am Heart Assoc. 2018;7(14):e005171.
48. Bhatt DL, Cryer BL, Contant CF, et al. Clopidogrel with or without omeprazole in coronary artery disease. N Engl J Med. 2010;363:1909–17.
49. Ray WA, Murray KT, Griffin MR, et al. Outcomes with concurrent use of clopidogrel and proton-pump inhibitors: a cohort study. Ann Intern Med. 2010;152:337–45.
50. Batchelor R, Kumar R, Gilmartin-Thomas JFM, et al. Systematic review with meta-analysis: risk of adverse cardiovascular events with proton pump inhibitors independent of clopidogrel. Aliment Pharmacol Ther. 2018;48:780–96.
51. Landi SN, Sandler RS, Pate V, Lund JL. No increase in risk of myocardial infarction in privately insured adults prescribed proton pump inhibitors vs histamine-2 receptor antagonists. Gastroenterology. 2018;154:861–73.
52. Sehested TSG, et al. Long-term use of proton pump inhibitors, dose–response relationship and associated risk of ischemic stroke and myocardial infarction. J Intern Med. 2018;283:268–81.

53. Xie Y, Bowe B, Li T, Xian H, Yan Y, Al-Aly Z. Risk of death among users of Proton Pump Inhibitors: a longitudinal observational cohort study of United States veterans. BMJ Open. 2017;7:e015735.
54. Xie Y, et al. Estimates of all-cause mortality and cause specific mortality associated with proton pump inhibitors among US veterans: cohort study. BMJ. 2019;365:l1580.
55. Haenisch B, von Holt K, Wiese B, et al. Risk of dementia in elderly patients with the use of proton pump inhibitors. Eur Arch Psychiatry Clin Neurosci. 2015;265:419–28.
56. Gomm W, von Holt K, Thome F, et al. Association of proton pump inhibitors with risk of dementia: a pharmacoepidemiological claims data analysis. JAMA Neurol. 2016;73:41–416.
57. Kuller LH. Do proton pump inhibitors increase the risk of dementia? JAMA Neurol. 2016;73:379–81.
58. Goldstein FC, et al. Proton pump inhibitors and risk for mild cognitive impairment and dementia. J Am Geriatr Soc. 2017;65(9):1969–74.
59. Taipale H, Tolppanen AM, Tiihonen M, Tanskanen A, Tiihonen J, Hartikainen S. No association between proton pump inhibitor use and risk of Alzheimer's disease. Am J Gastroenterol. 2017;112:1802–8.
60. Lockhead P, et al. Association between proton pump inhibitor use and cognitive function in women. Gastroenterology. 2017;153(4):971–9.
61. Wod M, et al. Lack of association between proton pump inhibitor use and cognitive decline. Clin Gastroenterol Hepatol. 2018;16:681–9.
62. Li M, et al. Proton pump inhibitor use and risk of dementia: systematic review and meta-analysis. Medicine. 2019;98:7.
63. Hussain S, et al. No association between proton pump inhibitor use and risk of dementia: evidence from a meta-analysis. J Gastroenterol Hepatol. 2020;35(1):19–28.
64. Song YQ, et al. Proton pump inhibitor use does not increase dementia and Alzheimer's disease risk: an updated meta-analysis of published studies involving 642,305 patients. PLoS One. 2019;14:7.
65. Park SK, Baek YH, Pratt N, et al. The uncertainty of the association between proton pump inhibitor use and the risk of dementia: prescription sequence symmetry analysis using a Korean healthcare database between 2002 and 2013. Drug Saf. 2018;41:615–24.
66. Park SK, et al. Beyond uncertainty: negative findings for the association between the use of proton pump inhibitors and risk of dementia. J Gastroenterol Hepatol. 2019;. epub ahead of print
67. Booker A, Jacob LE, Rapp M, et al. Risk factors for dementia diagnosis in German primary care practices. Value Health J Int Soc Pharm Outcomes Res. 2015;18:1–7.
68. Food and Drug Administration. FDA Drug Safety Communication: Possible increased risk of fractures of the hip, wrist, and spine with the use of proton pump inhibitors. Available at: https://www.fda.gov/drugs/postmarket-drug-safety-information-patients-and-providers/fda-drug-safety-communication-possible-increased-risk-fractures-hip-wrist-and-spine-use-proton-pump. Accessed 9 Aug 2019.
69. Zhou B, Huang Y, Li H, Sun W, Liu J. Proton-pump inhibitors and risk of fractures: an update meta-analysis. Osteoporos Int. 2016;27:339–47.
70. Poly TN, Islam MM, et al. Proton pump inhibitors and risk of hip fracture: a meta-analysis of observational studies. Osteoporos Int. 2019;30(1):103–14.
71. Nassar Y, Richter S. Proton-pump inhibitor use and fracture risk: an updated systematic review and meta-analysis. J Bone Metab. 2018;25(3):141–51.
72. Liu J, Li X, Fan L, et al. Proton pump inhibitors therapy and risk of bone diseases: an update meta-analysis. Life Sci. 2019;218:213–23.
73. Lin SM, Yang SH, Liang CC, Huang HK. Proton pump inhibitor use and the risk of osteoporosis and fracture in stroke patients: a population-based cohort study. Osteoporosis Int. 2018;29:153–62.
74. Torvinen-Kiiskinen S, Tolppanen AM, Koonen M, et al. Proton pump inhibitor use and risk of hip fractures among community-dwelling persons with Alzheimer's disease - a nested case-control study. Aliment Pharmacol Ther. 2018;47:1135–42.

75. Fedida B, Schermann H, Ankory R, et al. Fracture risk of young adults receiving proton pump inhibitors and H2-receptor antagonists. Int J Clin Pract. 2019;4:13339.
76. Lai SW, Lin CH, Liao KF. Proton pump inhibitors therapy and the risk of hip fracture in older people in Taiwan. Eur Geriatr Med. 2018;9:169–74.
77. Lai SW, Lin CL, Uao KF. Proton pump inhibitors therapy and the risk of major osteoporotic nonhip fractures in older adults in Taiwan. Eur J Gastroenterol Hepatol. 2019;31:272–3.
78. Harding BN, et al. Proton pump inhibitor use and the risk of fractures among an older adult cohort. Pharmacoepidemiol Drug Saf. 2018;27(6):596–603.
79. Levy MD, Bhattacharya B. Sporadic fundic gland polyps with low-grade dysplasia: a large case series evaluating pathologic and immunohistochemical findings and clinical behavior. Am J Clin Pathol. 2015;144(4):592–600.
80. Cheesman AR, Greenwald DA, Shah SC. Current management of benign epithelial gastric polyps. Curr Treat Options Gastro. 2017;15:676.
81. Lambert AA, Lam JO, Paik JJ, Ugarte-Gil C, Drummond MB, Crowell TA. Risk of community-acquired pneumonia with outpatient proton-pump inhibitor therapy: a systematic review and meta-analysis. PLoS One. 2015;10
82. Eom CS, Jeon CY, Lim JW, Cho EG, Park SM, Lee KS. Use of acid-suppressive drugs and risk of pneumonia: a systematic review and meta-analysis. CMAJ. 2011;183:310–9.
83. Zirk-Sadowski J, et al. Proton-pump inhibitors and long-term risk of community-acquired pneumonia in older adults. J Am Geriatr Soc. 2018;66(7):1332–8.
84. Filion KB, Chateau D, Targownik LE, et al. CNODES investigators. Proton pump inhibitors and the risk of hospitalisation for community-acquired pneumonia: replicated cohort studies with meta-analysis. Gut. 2014;63(4):552–8.
85. Othman F, et al. Community acquired pneumonia incidence before and after proton pump inhibitor prescription: population based study. BMJ. 2016;355:i5813.
86. Scheiman JM, Devereaux PJ, Herlitz J, et al. Prevention of peptic ulcers with esomeprazole in patients at risk of ulcer development treated with low-dose acetylsalicylic acid: a randomised, controlled trial (OBERON). Heart. 2011;97:797–802.
87. Estborn L, Joelson S. Frequency and time to onset of community-acquired respiratory tract infections in patients receiving esomeprazole: a retrospective analysis of patient-level data in placebo-controlled studies. Aliment Pharmacol Ther. 2015;42:607–13.
88. MacLaren R, Reynolds PM, Allen RR. Histamine-2 receptor antagonists vs proton pump inhibitors on gastrointestinal tract hemorrhage and infectious complications in the intensive care unit. JAMA Intern Med. 2014;174(4):564–74.
89. Alhazzani W, Alshamsi F, Belley-Cote E, et al. Efficacy and safety of stress ulcer prophylaxis in critically ill patients: a network meta-analysis of randomized trials. Intensive Care Med. 2018;44(1):1–11.
90. Food and Drug Administration. FDA Drug Safety Communication: Clostridium difficile associated diarrhea can be associated with stomach acid drugs known as proton pump inhibitors (PPIs). https://www.fda.gov/drugs/drug-safety-and-availability/fda-drug-safety-communication-clostridium-difficile-associated-diarrhea-can-be-associated-stomach. Accessed 9 Aug 2019.
91. Tleyjeh IM, Bin Abdulhak AA, Riaz M, et al. Association between proton pump inhibitor therapy and clostridium difficile infection: a contemporary systematic review and meta-analysis. PLoS One. 2012;7:e50836.
92. Guyatt G, Oxman AD, Akl EA, et al. GRADE guidelines: 1. Introduction-GRADE evidence profiles and summary of findings tables. J Clin Epidemiol. 2011;64(4):383–94.
93. Arriola V, Tischendorf J, Musuuza J, et al. Assessing the risk of hospital-acquired Clostridium difficile infection with proton pump inhibitor use: a meta-analysis. Infect Control Hosp Epidemiol. 2016;37(12):1408–17.
94. Deshpande A, Pant C, Pasupuleti V, et al. Association between proton pump inhibitor therapy and Clostridium difficile infection in a meta-analysis. Clin Gastroenterol Hepatol. 2012;10(3):225–33.

95. Kwok CS, Arthur AK, Anibueze CI, Singh S, Cavallazzi R, Loke YK. Risk of Clostridium difficile infection with acid suppressing drugs and antibiotics: meta-analysis. Am J Gastroenterol. 2012;107(7):1011–9.
96. Khanna S, Aronson SL, Kammer PP, Baddour LM, Pardi DS. Gastric acid suppression and outcomes in Clostridium difficile infection: a population-based study. Mayo Clin Proc. 2012;87(7):636–42.
97. Bonderup OK, Nielsen GL, Dall M, et al. Significant association between the use of different proton pump inhibitors and microscopic colitis: a nationwide Danish case-control study. Aliment Pharmacol Ther. 2018;48:618–25.
98. Moledina DG, Perazella MA. PPIs and kidney disease: from AIN to CKD. J Nephrol. 2016;
99. Faisal K, Khan MA, Miklos MZ, et al. The association between proton pump inhibitor use with acute kidney injury and chronic kidney disease. J Clin Gastroenterol. 2018;52:468–76.
100. Antoniou T, Macdonald EM, Hollands S, et al. Proton pump inhibitors and the risk of acute kidney injury in older patients: a population-based cohort study. CMAJ Open. 2015;3:E166–71.
101. Klepser DG, Collier DS, Cochran GL. Proton pump inhibitors and acute kidney injury: a nested case–control study. BMC Nephrol. 2013;14:150.
102. Blank ML, Parkin L, Paul C, Herbison P. A nationwide nested case– control study indicates an increased risk of acute interstitial nephritis with proton pump inhibitor use. Kidney Int. 2014;86:837–44.
103. Nochaiwong S, Ruengom C, et al. The association between proton pump inhibitor use and the risk of adverse kidney outcomes: a systematic review and meta-analysis. Nephrol Dial Transplant. 2018;33(2):331–42.
104. Lee J, Mark RG, Celi LA, et al. Proton pump inhibitors are not associated with acute kidney injury in critical illness. J Clin Pharmacol. 2016;56:1500–6.
105. Leonard CE, Freeman CP, Newcomb CW, et al. Proton pump inhibitors and traditional nonsteroidal anti-inflammatory drugs and the risk of acute interstitial nephritis and acute kidney injury. Pharmacoepidemiol Drug Saf. 2012;21:1155–72.
106. Cheema E. Investigating the association of proton pump inhibitors with chronic kidney disease and its impact on clinical practice and future research: a review. J Pharm Policy Pract. 2019;12:6.
107. Wijarnpreecha K, Thongprayoon C, et al. Associations of proton-pump inhibitors and H2 receptor antagonists with chronic kidney disease: a meta-analysis. Dig Dis Sci. 2017;62:2821–7.
108. Lazarus B, et al. Proton pump inhibitor use and the risk of chronic kidney disease. JAMA Intern Med. 2016;176(2):238–46.
109. Lazarus B, Chen Y, Wilson FP, et al. Proton pump inhibitor use and the risk of chronic kidney disease. JAMA Intern Med. 2011;76:238–46.
110. Arora P, Golzy M, Gupta A, Ranjan R, Carter R, Lohr J. Proton pump inhibitors are associated with increased risk of development of chronic kidney disease. J Am Soc Nephrol. 2015;26:219A.
111. Xie Y, Bowe B, Li T, Xian H, Balasubramanian S, Al-Aly Z. Proton pump inhibitors and risk of incident CKD and progression to ESRD. J Am Soc Nephrol. 2016;
112. Klatte DCF, Gasparini A, et al. Association between proton pump inhibitor use and risk of progression of chronic kidney disease. Gastroenterology. 2017;153(3):702–10.
113. Lam JR, Schneider JL, Zhao W, Corley DA. Proton pump inhibitor and histamine 2 receptor antagonist use and vitamin B12 deficiency. JAMA. 2013;310:2435–42.
114. den Elzen WP, Groeneveld Y, de Ruijter Wet al. Long-term use of proton pump inhibitors and vitamin B12 status in elderly individuals. Aliment Pharmacol Ther 2008; 27: 491–497.
115. Valuck RJ, Ruscin JM. A case-control study on adverse effects: H2 blocker or proton pump inhibitor use and risk of vitamin B12 deficiency in older adults. J Clin Epidemiol. 2004;57(4):422–8.
116. O'Connell MB, Madden DM, Murray AM, Heaney RP, Kerzner LJ. Effects of proton pump inhibitors on calcium carbonate absorption in women: a randomized crossover trial. Am J Med. 2005;118(7):778–81.

117. Serfaty-Lacrosniere C, Wood RJ, Voytko D, et al. Hypochlorhydria from short-term omeprazole treatment does not inhibit intestinal absorption of calcium, phosphorus, magnesium or zinc from food in humans. J Am Coll Nutr. 1995;14:364–8.
118. Wright MJ, Sullivan RR, Gaffney-Stomberg E, et al. Inhibiting gastric acid production does not affect intestinal calcium absorption in young, healthy individuals: a randomized, crossover, controlled clinical trial. J Bone Miner Res. 2010;25(10):2205–11.
119. Freedberg DE, Haynes K, Denburg MR, et al. Use of proton pump inhibitors is associated with fractures in young adults: a population-based study. Osteoporos Int. 2015;26:2501–7.
120. Stewart CA, Termanini B, Sutliff VE, et al. Iron absorption in patients with Zollinger-Ellison syndrome treated with long-term gastric acid antisecretory therapy. Aliment Pharmacol Ther. 1998;12:83–98.
121. Hutchinson C, Geissler CA, Powell JJ, et al. Proton pump inhibitors suppress absorption of dietary non-haem iron in hereditary haemochromatosis. Gut. 2007;56:1291–5.
122. Sarzynski E, Puttarajappa C, Xie Y, Grover M, Laird-Fick H. Association between proton pump inhibitor use and anemia: a retrospective cohort study. Dig Dis Sci. 2011;56:2349–53.
123. Food and Drug Administration. FDA drug safety communication: low magnesium levels can be associated with long-term use of proton pump inhibitor drugs (PPIs). Silver Spring, MD: Available at: http://www.fda.gov/drugs/drugsafety/ucm245011.htmUS Food and Drug Administration, 2011. Accessed 9 Aug 2019.
124. Cheungpasitporn W, Thongprayoon C, Kittanamongkolchai W, et al. Proton pump inhibitors linked to hypomagnesemia: a systematic review and meta-analysis of observational studies. Ren Fail. 2015;37:1237–41.
125. Park CH, Kim EH, Roh YH, et al. The association between the use of proton pump inhibitors and the risk of hypomagnesemia: a systematic review and meta-analysis. PLoS One. 2014;9(11):e112558.
126. Kieboom BC, Kiefte-de Jong JC, Eijgelsheim M, et al. Proton pump inhibitors and hypomagnesemia in the general population: a population-based cohort study. Am J Kidney Dis. 2015;66(5):775–82.
127. Mikolasevic I, Milic S, Stimac D, et al. Is there a relationship between hypomagnesemia and proton-pump inhibitors in patients on chronic hemodialysis? Eur J Intern Med. 2016;30:99–103.
128. Liu J, Li X, Fan L, et al. Proton pump inhibitors therapy and risk of bone diseases: an update meta-analysis. Life Sci. 2019;218:213–23.
129. Targownik LE, Leslie WD, Davison KS, et al. The relationship between proton pump inhibitor use and longitudinal change in bone mineral density: a population-based study [corrected] from the Canadian Multicentre Osteoporosis Study (CaMos). Am J Gastroenterol. 2012;107:1361–9.
130. Targownik LE, Goertzen AL, Luo Y, et al. Long-term proton pump inhibitor use is not associated with changes in bone strength and structure. Am J Gastroenterol. 2017;112(1):95–101.
131. Arj A, Razavi ZM, Yavari M, et al. Proton pump inhibitors use and change in bone mineral density. Int J Rheum Dis. 2016;19(9):864–8.
132. Solomon DH, Diem SJ, Ruppert K, et al. Bone mineral density changes among women initiating proton pump inhibitors or H2 receptor antagonists: a SWAN cohort study. J Bone Miner Res. 2015;30:232–9.
133. Maggio M, Lauretani F, Ceda GP, et al. Use of proton pump inhibitors is associated with lower trabecular bone density in older individuals. Bone. 2013;57:437–42.
134. Itoh S, Sekino Y, Shinomiya K, Takeda S. The effects of risedronate administered in combination with a proton pump inhibitor for the treatment of osteoporosis. J Bone Miner Metab. 2013;31:206–11.
135. Targownik LE, Lix LM, Leung S, Leslie WD. Proton-pump inhibitor use is not associated with osteoporosis or accelerated bone mineral density loss. Gastroenterology. 2010;138:896–904.
136. Gray SL, LaCroix AZ, Larson J, et al. Proton pump inhibitor use, hip fracture, and change in bone mineral density in postmenopausal women: results from the Women's Health Initiative. Arch Intern Med. 2010;170:765–71.

137. Yu EW, Blackwell T, Ensrud KE, et al. Acid-suppressive medications and risk of bone loss and fracture in older adults. Calcif Tissue Int. 2008;83:251–9.
138. Hansen KE, Nieves JW, Nudurupati S, et al. Dexlansopraole and esomeprazole do not affect bone homeostasis in healthy postmenopausal women. Gastroenterology. 2019;156:926–34.
139. Black DM, Rosen CJ. Clinical practice: postmenopausal osteoporosis. N Engl J Med. 2016;374(3):254–62.
140. Nguyen LH, Lochhead P, Joshi AD, et al. No significant association between proton pump inhibitor use and risk of stroke after adjustment for lifestyle factors and indications. Gastroenterology. 2018;154:1290–7.
141. Wang YF, Chen YT, Luo JC, et al. Proton-pump inhibitor use and the risk of first-time ischemic stroke in the general population: a nationwide population-based study. Am J Gastroenterol. 2017;112:1084–93.
142. Czwornog JL, Austin GL. Association of proton pump inhibitor (PPI) use with energy intake, physical activity, and weight gain. Nutrients. 2015;7:8592–601.
143. Moayyedi P, et al. Safety of proton pump inhibitors based on a large, multi-year, randomized trial of patients receiving rivaroxaban or aspirin. Gastroenterology. 2019;157:682–91.
144. Fass R, Shapiro M, Dekel R, Sewell J. Systematic review: proton pump inhibitor failure in gastro-oesophageal reflux disease-where next? Aliment Pharmacol Ther. 2005;22:79–94.
145. Yoon SL, Grundmann O, Smith KF, Mason SR. Dietary supplement and complementary and alternative medicine use are highly prevalent in patients with gastrointestinal disorders: results from an online survey. J Diet Suppl. 2018;29:1–14.
146. Garg SK, Gurusamy KS. Laparoscopic fundoplication surgery versus medical management for gastro-oesophageal reflux disease (GORD) in adults. Cochrane Database Syst Rev. 2015;5(11):CD003243.
147. Brisbois S, Merati A, et al. Proton pump inhibitors: review of reported risks and controversies. Laryngoscope investigative otolaryngology 2018. Open Access.
148. Nehra AK, et al. Proton pump inhibitors: review of emerging concerns. Mayo Clin Proc. 2018;93(2):240–6.
149. Freedberg DE, Kim LS, Yang YX. The risks and benefits of long-term use of proton pump inhibitors: expert review and best practice advice from the American Gastroenterological Association. Gastroenterology. 2017;152:706–15.
150. Jaworek AJ, Sataloff RT. Gluten sensitivity. J Singing. 2019;75(3):303–8.

Chapter 32
Stretta in the Management of Gastroesophageal Reflux Disease

George Triadafilopoulos

Introduction

If standard medical therapies for gastroesophageal reflux disease (GERD), such as proton pump inhibitors (PPIs), have shown an incomplete response, or if patients do not wish to remain on long-term antisecretory medications, endoscopic application of radiofrequency (RF) energy to the lower esophageal sphincter region (Stretta) may be beneficial by decreasing or eliminating symptoms and improving GERD-related quality of life (HRQL). Although its precise mechanisms are unclear, Stretta reduces transient lower esophageal sphincter relaxations (tLESRs) and decreases compliance of the esophagogastric junction (EGJ), thereby improving both proximal and distal esophageal acid exposure times, improving GERD-HRQL and heartburn and regurgitation. Ideal candidates for Stretta are those who experience frequent heartburn, regurgitation, or both; have either nonerosive reflux disease, LA grades A or B, or higher grades of esophagitis that have healed by PPI therapy; have total acid exposure time greater than 6% by pH monitoring, and have unsatisfactory control of GERD despite twice daily PPI. Patients are not good candidates for Stretta if they have absent peristalsis and incomplete LES relaxation – both suggestive of esophageal achalasia – or those with >3 cm long sliding hiatal hernia [1–3].

Technique

Stretta is performed under endoscopic guidance that assesses the location of the EGJ and allows placement of a special, single use, balloon/catheter. The apparatus then delivers pure sine-wave energy into the muscle of the EGJ using deployable

G. Triadafilopoulos (✉)
Stanford University School of Medicine, Stanford, CA, USA
e-mail: vagt@stanford.edu

C. H. Zalvan (ed.), *Laryngopharyngeal and Gastroesophageal Reflux*,
https://doi.org/10.1007/978-3-030-48890-1_32

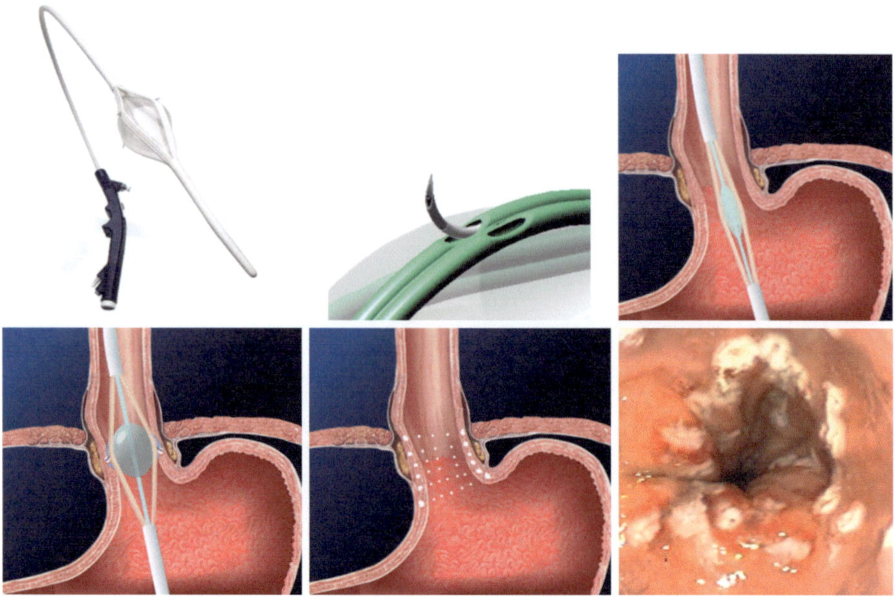

Fig. 32.1 Top left: Stretta catheter incorporating an inflatable balloon at its tip. Top middle: Magnification view of the needles that are introduced into the muscle of the EGJ. Top right: Diagram depicting the balloon placement. Bottom left: Balloon inflation at the GEJ aiming at delivering RF through the deployed needles. Bottom middles: Several applications of RF have been delivered straddling the EGJ. Bottom right: Endoscopic view of the mucosa immediately after the completion of the procedure

needles that incorporate thermocouples that modulate power output and maintain tissue temperature while minimizing mucosal temperature increases, all under impedance monitoring (Fig. 32.1). An endoscopy is performed, and the distance from the mouthguard to the EGJ is measured. The endoscope is then removed, and the RF catheter is passed over a guide wire and positioned 1–2 cm above the EGJ. After inflating a balloon near the catheter tip, four needle electrodes are deployed to 5.5 mm, delivering RF energy for 60 seconds to achieve a target (muscle) temperature of 85 °C. RF delivery is automatically stopped if mucosal temperatures or impedance values are unacceptably high. In a similar fashion, additional treatments are applied by rotating and changing the linear position of the catheter each time by 0.5–1 cm, above and below the EGJ. Retrograde treatments of the cardia are also delivered before the catheter is removed, and the EGD is repeated to assess proper location of therapy and lack of complications. The procedure typically requires 30 minutes focusing above and below the EGJ region (Fig. 32.1).

Efficacy

Many open and controlled studies have examined the efficacy of Stretta for GERD; however, there is paucity of evidence on the role of this procedure on laryngopharyngeal reflux (LPR) outcomes. In general, 50–80% of patients report GERD symptom control or cessation of PPI use in studies with follow-up periods of 1–3 years [4]. After Stretta, patients experience better symptoms and quality of life over and above that of PPI use alone (Figs. 32.2, 32.3) in both open and controlled trials. In patients with good clinical response, esophageal pH normalizes (Figs. 32.3, 32.4, 32.5). In a systematic review and meta-analysis of 28 studies of over 2400 patients with GERD, scores for health-related quality of life and heartburn were improved in patients who underwent Stretta, and the rate of PPI use was lower as compared with pre-procedure rate. Similar results have been noted when Stretta was compared with a sham treatment (Figs. 32.4, 32.5). Although Stretta reduces esophageal acid exposure time, it does not improve lower esophageal sphincter (LES) pressure. The procedure's efficacy has also been examined in a meta-analysis of 18 randomized trials, cohort studies, and reviews totaling 1441 patients where Stretta improved heartburn and GERD-related quality of life (HRQL). Esophageal acid exposure time was also lower – but did not normalize – after the procedure, as

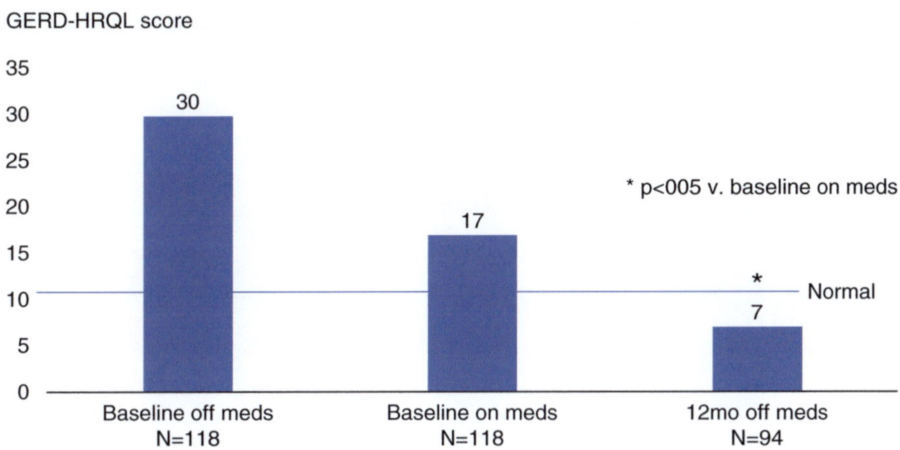

Fig. 32.2 GERD-HRQL scores before off PPI, before on PPI, and 12 months after Stretta. The procedure normalized the scores over and above the levels accomplished by PPI

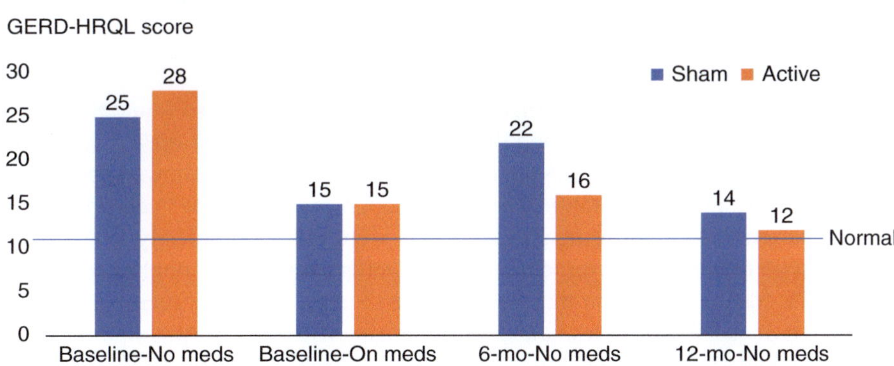

Fig. 32.3 Quality of life after either Stretta or sham procedure (off and on PPI) in a randomized trial

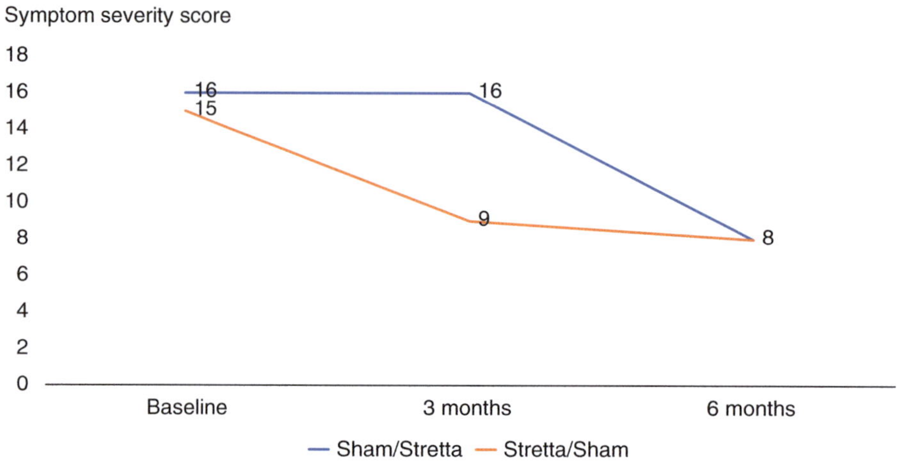

Fig. 32.4 GERD symptom severity scores after Stretta or sham treatment in a randomized, sham-controlled trial

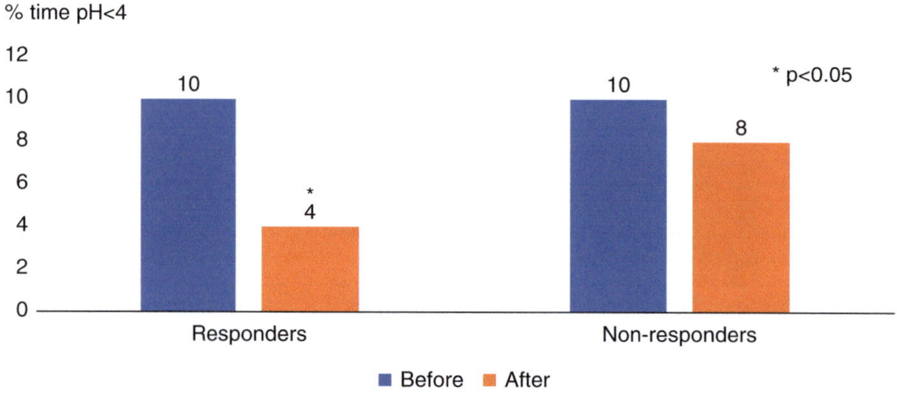

Fig. 32.5 pH control in patients who had clinically responded to Stretta compared to those who did not. The pH scores normalized in those with clinical response suggestive that the mechanism of action of the procedure is through pH control

compared with baseline. Long-term studies (8–10 years) have also found Stretta to be effective with GERD-HRQL and PPI cessation durability of 50–80% (Fig. 32.6). Another prospective study of 138 patients with refractory GERD showed decreased scores for heartburn, regurgitation, chest pain, cough, and asthma at 5 years. Further, 43% of patients were not using PPI, and 75% were either completely or partially satisfied with their GERD symptom control. Patients with GERD after laparoscopic, non-displaced fundoplication may also undergo Stretta to relieve recurrent symptoms and reduce PPI use. In a small study of patients with refractory symptoms after Nissen fundoplication followed for up to 10 years, Stretta improved GERD–health-related quality of life, patient satisfaction, and reduced medication use [5, 6].

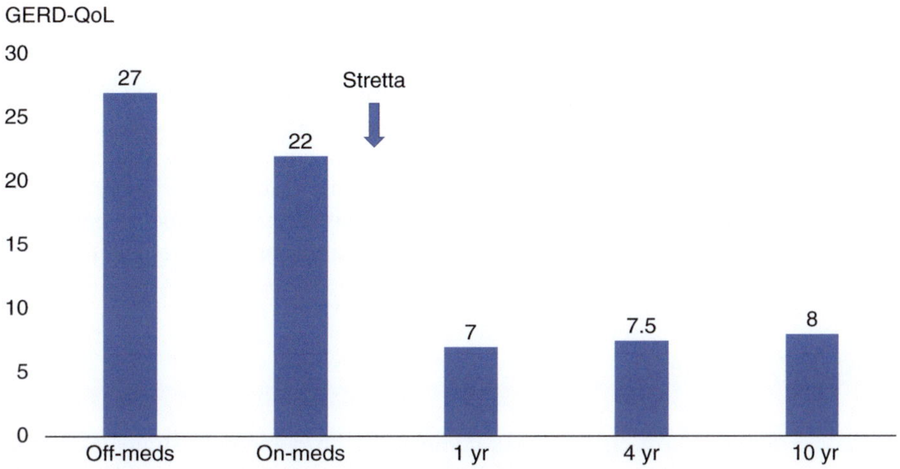

Fig. 32.6 Long-term results after Stretta in a prospective open trial. The quality of life is effectively normalized up to 10 years

Comparison to Fundoplication

Uncontrolled studies have compared Stretta (when feasible) with laparoscopic fundoplication for the treatment of GERD. After 6 months in one non-randomized study, quality of life was similar, and both groups were satisfied (89% with Stretta and 96% with fundoplication). In another study, the symptom control after Stretta was lower (51%) than surgery (91%). In another non-randomized cohort who underwent Stretta with an average follow-up of 53 months, 59% subsequently required anti-reflux surgery, and Stretta reduced symptoms in 40% of patients.

Use in Obesity

Obese patients – those with body mass index (BMI) > 30 – are at increased risk of failure after fundoplication. Stretta has been effective in improving GERD in some obese patients, with 60% reporting no or mild symptoms. In a retrospective study of obese patients with mean BMI 38.6 and GERD undergoing Stretta, there were fewer patients (45%) on PPI medications after the procedure than before (81%) at a mean follow-up of 1.5 years. However, in one study of patients with GERD who had previously undergone laparoscopic sleeve gastrectomy (LSG), Stretta did not improve GERD symptoms or patient satisfaction at short-term follow-up, and they experienced a high (6.7%) complication rate [7].

Adverse Events and Complications

Over 20 years of commercial post-marketing use, Stretta use has been associated with an excellent safety profile. Yet, serious complications have been described, including esophageal perforation and death. In a meta-analysis of 26 studies of over 2400 patients with GERD, the rate of adverse events associated with Stretta was 0.9%, and the most common adverse events were small erosions and mucosal lacerations, dysphagia, as well as chest and epigastric pain at overall rates less than 1%.

Cost-Effectiveness

To assess Stretta's cost-effectiveness compared with competing strategies in the long-term (5 years) management of GERD, a Markov model estimated health outcomes and costs from a public health perspective. Strategies included the daily PPI use, laparoscopic Nissen fundoplication, and Stretta. If using symptom-free months to measure effectiveness, PPI use dominated both Stretta and surgery. Stretta had favorable characteristics in terms of ease of use, efficacy, and cost [8].

Conclusions

Stretta is different from medical therapy (pH control, refractoriness), different from anti-reflux surgery (acid and volume reflux control, side effects), and remains a distinct, endoscopic option with unique mechanism(s) of action and documented clinical efficacy. The procedure is easy, repeatable, and not precluding subsequent anti-reflux surgery. Yet, its precise role for LPR requires further study.

References

1. Triadafilopoulos G. Stretta: a valuable endoscopic treatment modality for gastroesophageal reflux disease. World J Gastroenterol. 2014;20:7730–8.
2. Triadafilopoulos G, DiBaise JK, Nostrant TT, Stollman NH, Anderson PK, Wolfe MM, Rothstein RI, Wo JM, Corley DA, Patti MG, Antignano LV, Goff JS, Edmundowicz SA, Castell DO, Rabine JC, Kim MS, Utley DS. The Stretta procedure for the treatment of GERD: 6 and 12 month follow-up of the U.S. open label trial. Gastrointest Endosc. 2002;55:149–56.
3. Franciosa M, Triadafilopoulos G, Mashimo H. Stretta Radiofrequency Treatment for GERD: A Safe and Effective Modality. Gastroenterol Res Pract. 2013;2013:783815.
4. Corley DA, Katz P, Wo JM, Stefan A, Patti M, Rothstein R, Edmundowicz S, Kline M, Mason R, Wolfe MM. Improvement of gastroesophageal reflux symptoms after radiofrequency energy: a randomized, sham-controlled trial. Gastroenterology. 2003;125:668–76.

5. Perry KA, Banerjee A, Melvin WS. Radiofrequency energy delivery to the lower esophageal sphincter reduces esophageal acid exposure and improves GERD symptoms: a systematic review and meta-analysis. Surg Laparosc Endosc Percutan Tech. 2012;22:283–8.
6. Noar M, Squires P, Noar E, Lee M. Long-term maintenance effect of radiofrequency energy delivery for refractory GERD: a decade later. Surg Endosc. 2014;28:2323–33.
7. White B, Jeansonne LO, Cook M, Chavarriaga LF, Goldenberg EA, Davis SS, Smith CD, Khaitan L, Lin E. Use of endoluminal anti-reflux therapies for obese patients with GERD. Obes Surg. 2009;19(6):783–7.
8. Comay D, Adam V, da Silveira EB, Kennedy W, Mayrand S, Barkun AN. The Stretta procedure versus proton pump inhibitors and laparoscopic Nissen fundoplication in the management of gastroesophageal reflux disease: a cost-effectiveness analysis. Can J Gastroenterol. 2008;22:552–8.

Chapter 33
Transoral Fundoplication for Treatment of Gastroesophageal Reflux Disease

Pier Alberto Testoni, Sabrina Gloria Giulia Testoni, Giorgia Mazzoleni, and Lorella Fanti

Introduction

Gastroesophageal reflux disease (GERD) is a common disorder currently treated by medical, surgical, or endoscopic therapy.

Medical therapy still represents the gold standard of treatment: proton pump inhibitors relieve symptoms and improve the patient's quality of life in the majority of cases. However, continuous long-term medication is associated with multiple potential side effects. In recent years, there has been an increase in patients who are intolerant or unresponsive to proton pump inhibitors (PPIs) or need high dosages for long periods to treat symptoms or prevent recurrences of GERD. Moreover, medical therapy may be inadequate to treat symptoms occurring in the presence of weakly acidic reflux and has high cost in the long term for either patients or healthcare systems.

On the other hand, laparoscopic fundoplication, although still considered the gold-standard approach for GERD refractory to medical treatment, is associated

P. A. Testoni (✉) · L. Fanti
Vita-Salute San Raffaele University - IRCCS San Raffaele Scientific Institute, Division of Gastroenterology and Gastrointestinal Endoscopy, Milan, Italy
e-mail: testoni.pieralberto@hsr.it; fanti.lorella@hsr.it

S. G. G. Testoni
Vita-Salute San Raffaele University - IRCCS San Raffaele Scientific Institute, Division of Pancreatico-Biliary Endoscopy, Milan, Italy
e-mail: testoni.sabrinagloriagiulia@hsr.it

G. Mazzoleni
Ospedale "Treviglio-Caravaggio" di Treviglio ASST Bergamo Ovest, Treviglio (Bg), Italy
e-mail: mazzoleni.giorgia@hsr.it

C. H. Zalvan (ed.), *Laryngopharyngeal and Gastroesophageal Reflux*,
https://doi.org/10.1007/978-3-030-48890-1_33

with the risk of persisting postsurgery adverse events such as dysphagia (5–12%), inability to vomit or belch, gas/bloat syndrome (19%), excessive flatulence, diarrhea, or functional dyspepsia related to delayed gastric emptying [1–5].

Considering the risk of persistent side effects and invasiveness of surgery, patients suffering from mild GERD are, in general, reluctant to undergo surgical repair.

In the last 12 years, transoral incisionless fundoplication (TIF) has been shown to be an effective therapeutic option alternative to medical and surgical therapy. TIF reconfigures the tissue to obtain a full-thickness gastroesophageal valve from inside the stomach, by serosa-to-serosa plications which include the muscle layers: the new valve has been shown effective in controlling symptoms of GERD with fewer technique-related complications and no side effects, compared to surgery.

TIF may be performed by using the EsophyX® device (EndoGastric Solutions, Redmond, WA, USA) or the Medigus ultrasonic surgical endostapler (MUSE™, Medigus, Omer, Israel).

The TIF intervention with the greatest global experience so far is that performed by using the EsophyX® device (EndoGastric Solutions, Redmond, WA, USA), with about 20,000 procedures performed to date. EsophyX® constructs an omega-shaped valve 3–5 cm long, in a 250–300° circumferential pattern around the gastroesophageal junction, by deploying multiple nonabsorbable polypropylene fasteners through the two layers (esophagus and stomach) under endoscopic vision of the operator. TIF with this device has proved good and durable in long-term follow-up data from multiple investigators that have used the TIF-2 technique. The device has been recently updated and improved in a new-generation instrument: the EsophyX Z®.

Another TIF technique introduced in the last years uses the Medigus ultrasonic surgical endostapler (MUSE™) (Medigus, Omer, Israel). MUSE staples the fundus of the stomach to the esophagus below the diaphragm using multiple sets of metal stitches placed under an ultrasound-guided technique and creates an anterior fundoplication functionally similar to standard surgical Dor-Thal operation.

Differently from EsophyX®, the new flap valve is constructed under ultrasonic control. In the case of sliding hiatal hernia, the procedure can be performed only if the hernia can be reduced below the diaphragm.

Indications for TIF

Currently, based on the available literature data, TIF may be successfully offered as a routine alternative to surgery in patients without hiatal hernia or hiatal hernia no longer than 2.5 cm and reducible, suffering from gastroesophageal reflux disease with typical and atypical symptoms, with either erosive esophagitis (mainly grade A-B esophagitis, according to Los Angeles classification) or non-erosive esophagitis disease (NERD) diagnosed on the basis of pathological gastroesophageal reflux at 24-hour pH-impedance recording, or hypersensitive esophagus. To date, data supporting the efficacy of TIF in the treatment of severe grades of esophagitis or Barrett's esophagus are still lacking.

TIF may also be offered to patients who are intolerant to PPI therapy or require high-dose PPI maintenance therapy, or have some risk of developing persistent postsurgical side effects, as those suffering from ineffective esophageal clearing or delayed gastric emptying time, even if in these cases TIF outcomes risk to be less satisfactory, on the basis of personal experience.

Techniques for TIF

Preprocedure Evaluation

Preoperative upper gastro-intestinal (GI) endoscopy is mandatory to determine the length and reducibility of the hiatal hernia, if present, and the greatest transverse dimension of the hiatus under full gastric distension. In fact, with the current TIF techniques, only a hiatal hernia not exceeding 2.5 cm in length can be fully reduced below the diaphragm, while a plication performed in a hiatus with a transverse dimension >3.0 cm can end up in the thorax, a situation that reduces the efficacy of the newly created valve.

Prior to the procedure, all patients should undergo esophageal manometry to exclude primary motility disorders and 24-h pH-impedance recording to exclude patients with functional heartburn. High-resolution manometry should be preferred because it better recognizes esophageal motor disorders. If the MUSE™ device is used, barium swallow should be performed in cases of hiatal hernia to assess the reducibility of the hernia, because irreducibility is a contraindication to the procedure.

Transoral Fundoplication by EsophyX® Device

The EsophyX® device is composed of (a) a handle, wherein controls are located; (b) an 18-mm diameter chassis through which control channels run and a standard front view 9-mm diameter endoscope can be inserted; (c) the tissue invaginator, constituted of side holes located on the distal part of the chassis, to which external suction can be applied; (d) the tissue mold, which can be brought into retroflection and pushes tissue against the shaft of the device; (e) a helical screw, which is advanced into the tissue and permits retraction of the tissue between the tissue mold and the shaft; (f) two stylets, which penetrate through the plicated tissue and the tissue mold, over which polypropylene H-shaped fasteners can be deployed; and (g) a cartridge containing 20 fasteners. The updated device, EsophyX Z®, is characterized by a reduced crossing profile, the elimination of tissue mold elbow, and a fastener deployment similar to a surgical stapler firing mechanism.

Details of the second-generation EsophyX® devices are illustrated in Fig. 33.1.

The procedure is performed by two operators: one controls the device and the other one operates the endoscope. The device is inserted transorally with the patient

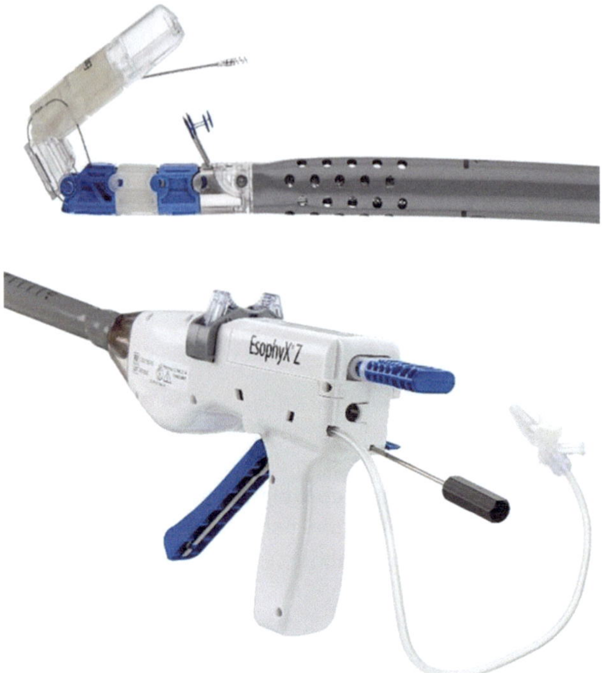

Fig. 33.1 The EsophyX® device (second generation). (Courtesy of EndoGastric Solutions, Inc., Redmond, WA, USA)

in the left lateral or supine position, under general anesthesia. Hypopharyngeal perforation has been reported in this phase of the procedure if the device is introduced without adequate caution; in difficult cases, the device can be gently rotated to pass the upper esophageal sphincter. The risk of this complication is reduced with the second-generation device, because of its smaller diameter.

Once into the stomach, air or CO_2 is insufflated to distend the gastric cavity and permits an adequate vision of the gastric fundus and esophago-gastric junction (EGJ); CO_2 is preferable, because it leads to a faster and more sustained gastric insufflation and induces less discomfort to patients. With the endoscope placed in retroflexion position, the lesser curve is located at the 12 o'clock position and the greater curve at the 6 o'clock in the patient placed in left decubitus. Once the tissue mold is retroflexed, it is closed against the EsophyX® device, rotated to 11 or 1 o'clock position (lesser curve), and pulled back to place its tip just inside the esophageal lumen. At this point, the helical screw is advanced to engage tissue under direct vision just below the Z-line, the shaft of the device is advanced caudally, the tissue mold is opened, and the helical screw cable freed from the tissue mold. Then, a tension is applied to helical retractor while a slight opening and closing of the tissue mold allows the fundus to slide through the tissue mold; in this phase, the stomach is being desufflated. Failure to desufflate the stomach during this phase of the procedure limits the size of the fundoplication.

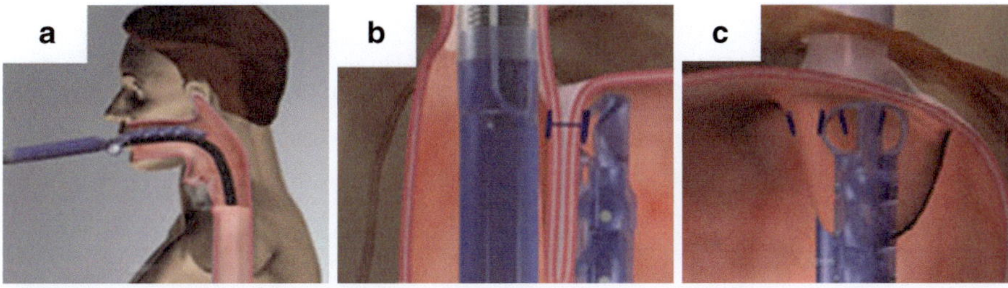

Fig. 33.2 Schematic representation of the EsophyX® procedure. (**a**) The EsophyX® device enters the esophagus through the mouth and is positioned at the gastroesophageal junction; (**b**) the device wraps the fundus around the distal esophagus and fastens a tissue fold; (**c**) this step is then repeated multiple times to reconstruct a robust tight valve (Courtesy of EndoGastric Solutions Inc., Redmond, WA, USA)

After completing this maneuver, both helical retractor and tissue mold are locked in place, suction is applied to the tissue invaginator for approximately half a minute, and the device is then advanced caudally into the stomach, which has been re-insufflated. The latter maneuver ensures that esophagogastric plication is performed in an intra-abdominal position and reduces hiatal hernia, when present.

Plication is carried out by deploying multiple polypropylene, H-shaped fasteners advanced over two stylets, one anterior and the other posterior. The fastener deployment process initiates on the far posterior and anterior sides of the esophagogastric valve adjacent to the lesser curvature, and then, it is extended to the greater curvature by rotating the tissue mold axially to slide the stomach over the esophagus, resulting in circumferential tightening and a new valve circumference of >240°. Fourteen fasteners allowing seven plications are needed to construct a satisfactory circumferential gastroesophageal valve; however, the higher is the number of fasteners deployed, the more continent is the newly created valve [6] (Fig. 33.2).

Over time, two modified techniques have been reported to create the fundoplication. The technique we used in the last years engages tissue by advancing the helical screw just below the Z line on the far posterior and anterior sides of the esophagogastric valve adjacent to the lesser curvature (11 and 1 o'clock positions). Before inserting the stylet, a torque is applied by rotation (clockwise and counterclockwise at 11 and 1 o'clock, respectively) of the tissue mold locked; such a maneuver allows part of the fundus to rotate around the esophageal wall and more tissue to be engaged by the stylet. Four fasteners for each site are deployed at 1 and 11 o'clock positions and two fasteners for each site in the middle part of the valve at 4, 6, and 8 o'clock positions to reinforce and prolong caudally the plication. This technique increased the success rate of the procedure by 30% [7].

Endoscopic pre- and postprocedural findings are reported in Fig. 33.3.

Another technique (rotational fundoplication) has been developed by Bell et al. [8]. The helical retractor is engaged at 12 o' clock, and the tissue mold is placed at 6 o' clock. The device, with the tissue mold partially closed against the fundus of the stomach, is pulled cranially by 1–3 cm into the esophagus, depending on the depth of the plication intended; tension is then applied to the helical retractor to

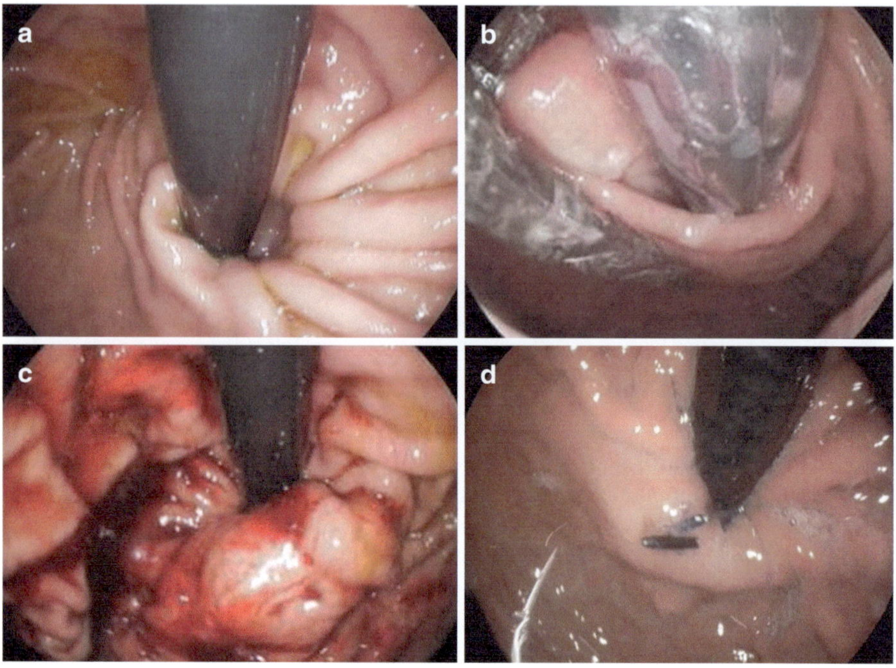

Figs. 33.3 Endoscopic findings of the gastroesophageal valve before and after the TIF procedure by EsophyX® device. (**a**) The gastroesophageal valve before the procedure by EsophyX® device; (**b**) the rotational maneuver to create the new gastroesophageal valve; (**c**) the gastroesophageal valve immediately after the EsophyX® procedure; (**d**) the gastroesophageal valve 6 months after the EsophyX® procedure. (Authors cases)

advance caudally the EGJ while the stomach is desufflated; at this time, the tissue mold locked is rotated toward the lesser curve by a radial motion of the handle of the device to the 12 o' clock position. This maneuver rolls the fundus over and around the distal esophagus to the 1 o' clock position.

Transoral Fundoplication by MUSE™

The MUSE™ device includes the endostapler and a console connected with the endostapler, containing a controller for the camera, ultrasonic range finder and various sensors, a pump for insufflation and irrigation, a suction system, power, and controls for the Light Emitting Diode (LED) (Fig. 33.4).

The endostapler has a) a handle, wherein controls are located; b) an insertion tube 15.5 mm in diameter, 66 cm long, containing the suction, insufflation/irrigation channels, and electrical and mechanical cables which operate the device; c) a rigid section 66 mm in length that contains the cartridge. Each cartridge contains five standard 4.8-mm titanium staples, the ultrasound mirror, one alignment pin funnel,

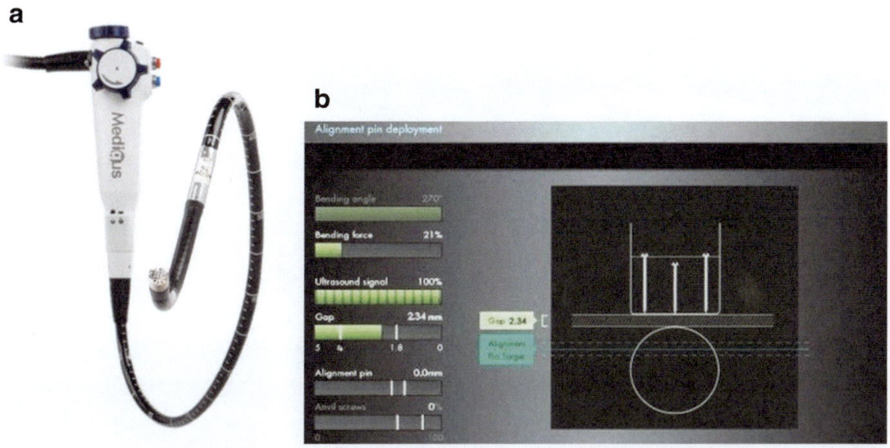

Fig. 33.4 The Medigus Surgical Ultrasonic Endostapler device (MUSE™). (Courtesy of Medigus, Omer, Israel). (**a**) The MUSE™ device; (**b**) the console connected with the endostapler, containing a controller for the camera, ultrasonic range finder, and various sensors (banding angle, banding force, alignment pin, anvil screws, gap)

and two anvil screw funnels; d) the distal tip, similar to that of an endoscope, with suction, irrigation, illumination (via LED), and visualization (via miniature camera) capabilities. The anvil, alignment pin, anvil screw, and ultrasound are all designed to ensure proper alignment and positioning of the device during stapling. The distal tip may be articulated in one direction to align with the rigid section and cartridge, with a bending radius of 26 and 40 mm. Details of the device are illustrated in Fig. 33.5.

The procedure can be performed by one operator. The patient is placed in the supine position, under general anesthesia with endotracheal intubation. Positive end-expiratory pressure (PEEP) of at least 5 mm Hg (7.5 cm H_2O) is administered. The endostapler is inserted transorally through an overtube and advanced into the stomach under direct vision; passing the rigid section across the pharyngo-esophageal junction may encounter some resistance. To avoid applying excessive force and risk of injury to the esophagus, the overtube may be withdrawn approximately 5 cm and then advanced with the endostapler as a unit. This maneuver can be repeated until the system reaches the esophageal midbody.

Once into the stomach, distended by insufflation of air or CO_2, the stapler is advanced until the tip is approximately 5 cm past the EGJ and then retroflexed by 180° to obtain an adequate vision of the gastric fundus and EGJ to select stapling location.

The most important stapling location is the leftmost location, which is typically performed first. This is the anchoring point for the fundus and should be placed as far to the left of the esophagus as possible. At times, depending on anatomy, it may be easier to perform the first stapling in a more central location. The additional stapling locations should be within 60–180° as long as the rightmost stapling should not be done on the lesser curve, because stapling in the lesser curve may attach the antrum to the esophagus and open the esophagogastric junction rather than close it. Additional staplings may be placed between the leftmost and rightmost. Once the correct location

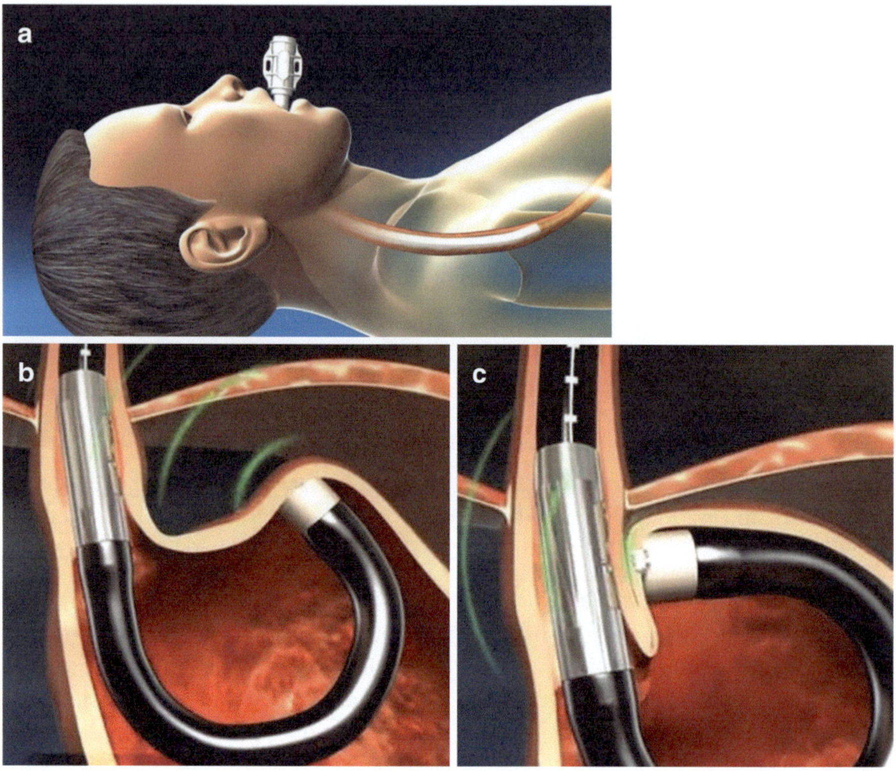

Fig. 33.5 Schematic representation of the MEDIGUS Ultrasonic Surgical Endostapler™ procedure. (**a**) The endostapler is inserted transorally through the overtube and advanced into the stomach under direct vision; (**b**) once into the stomach, distended by insufflation of CO_2, the stapler is advanced until the tip is approximately 5 cm past the EGJ and then retroflexed by 180° to obtain an adequate vision of the gastric fundus and EGJ to select stapling location. Tissue clamping and stapling are performed under ultrasonic guidance; (**c**) this step is then repeated at least twice to reconstruct a robust tight valve. The additional stapling locations should be within 60°–180° of the valve circumference. (Courtesy of Medigus, Omer, Israel)

for stapling has been identified, all the procedures are performed under ultrasound guidance. Subsequent phases of the procedure include clamping tissue, deploying alignment pin, advancing anvil screw, stapling, and retrieving anvil screws [9].

Endoscopic pre- and postprocedural findings after TIF with MUSE™ are reported in Fig. 33.6.

Postoperative Care

Antiemetic prophylaxis with at least two drugs (according to the American Society of Anaesthesiologists' (ASA) recommendations for interventions with high risk of postprocedure nausea and vomiting) and full muscle relaxation throughout the procedure are mandatory for TIF. Antiemetic prophylaxis is maintained intravenously

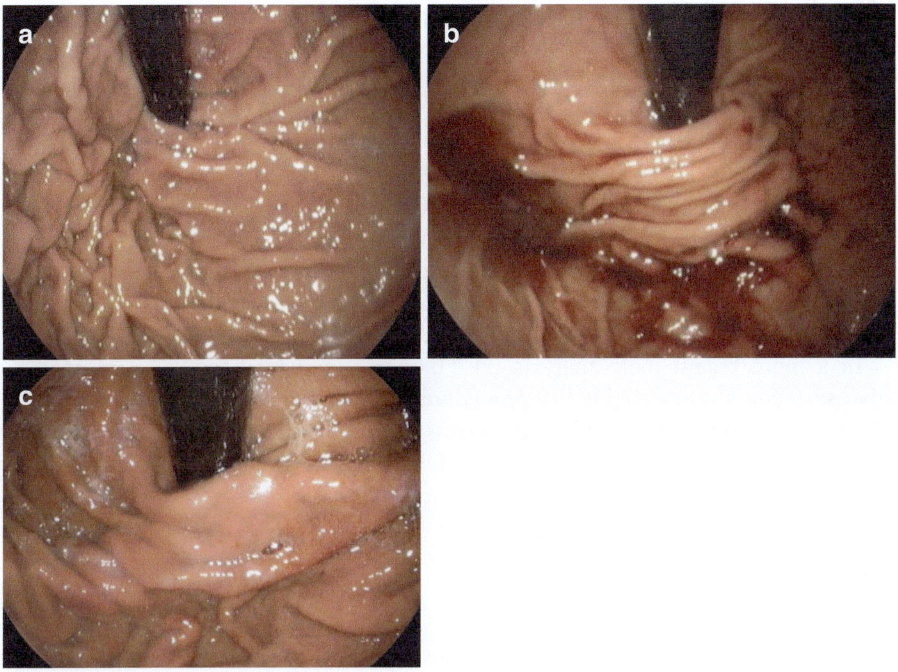

Fig. 33.6 Endoscopic findings of gastroesophageal valve before and after the TIF procedure by Medigus Ultrasonic Surgical Endostapler (MUSE™). (**a**) The gastroesophageal valve before the TIF procedure by Medigus Ultrasonic Surgical Endostapler™; (**b**) the gastroesophageal valve immediately after the TIF procedure by Medigus Ultrasonic Surgical Endostapler™; (**c**) the gastroesophageal valve 6 months after the TIF procedure by Medigus Ultrasonic Surgical Endostapler™. (Authors cases)

for 24 hours, while broad-spectrum antibiotic therapy is maintained intravenously for 48 hours, and then by oral route over a 5-day period.

Almost all patients complain of transient pharyngeal irritation, as a result of insertion and manipulation of the device, and some have mild-to-moderate epigastric pain in the 6 hours after the procedure. Pain persisting for 2–4 days may require analgesics and should be considered for esophageal or gastric leak; computed tomography (CT) scan and hydrosoluble contrast x-ray investigation should be carried out in these cases. Dysphagia or gas bloating is generally not reported by patients. At discharge, patients are instructed to follow a liquid diet for the first week and then a soft diet for the next 3 weeks. PPI can be discontinued 7–15 days after the procedure.

Complications

The overall complication rate reported in studies so far available for TIF by EsophyX® ranges from 3% to 10%. One meta-analysis including 16 studies with EsophyX reported the occurrence of severe adverse events in nineteen cases: seven cases of perforation, five cases of bleeding requiring blood transfusions, four cases of pneumothorax, and one case with severe epigastric pain [10]. Mediastinal abscess as a consequence of esophageal perforation has been reported in less than 2% of cases. Bleeding occurred at the site of the helical retractor insertion. No procedure-related deaths occurred.

The finding of free air in the abdomen immediately after the procedure is not always sign of clinically relevant complications.

In the three studies so far published on TIF by MUSE™, minor side effects such as chest pain, sore throat, transient atelectasis, shoulder pain, and belching were reported in 5.5–22% of patients. Major complications were reported in 6.2% of cases (4 out of 64 patients) and were pneumothorax, esophageal leak, and bleeding [11–13].

In a more recent meta-analysis on TIF performed by EsophyX and MUSE, adverse event was reported in 2% procedures [14].

There were no postprocedure side effects commonly seen after laparoscopic fundoplication as gas bloating, inability to belch or vomit, dysphagia, or diarrhea.

Outcomes of TIF

After more than 10 years since the introduction of TIF in clinical practice, there are sufficient data to respond to four main issues related to this new intervention: (1) Is TIF effective in controlling GERD-related symptoms, such as heartburn, regurgitation, and extra-esophageal symptoms? (2) Does TIF improve not only symptoms but also reduce gastroesophageal reflux, objectively assessed by pH-impedance recording? (3) Does symptom control obtained by TIF persist in the long-term period? (4) Are outcomes of TIF comparable to those of surgical fundoplication that can be considered the standard alternative to TIF in non-responders GERD patients or intolerant to medical therapy?

Efficacy of TIF in Controlling GERD-Related Symptoms

So far, two meta-analyses assessed the efficacy of TIF on GERD treatment.

One meta-analysis published in 2017 included 14 observational nonrandomized prospective studies and 5 randomized controlled trials on TIF performed by EsophyX® [10]. Among the observational studies, two studies provided results in 3 months (32 patients), nine in 6 months (439 patients), seven in 12 months (329 patients), three in 24 months (81 patients) and 36 months (105 patients), and only one study showed results after 4, 5, and 6 years of follow-up [15]. In all studies but three TIF was proven to discontinue antireflux medications or markedly decrease their dose; three studies raised concerns about the effectiveness of the procedure [16–18]. Six- and 12-month outcomes after TIF showed that 75–84% and 53–85% of patients had either discontinued PPI use or halved the dose of PPI therapy, respectively. Two years after TIF, daily high-dosage PPI dependence was eliminated in 75–93% of patients. Unsuccessful outcomes after TIF were reported in three studies. An open-label study comparing TIF with robot-assisted Nissen fundoplication in PPI-refractory GERD patients reported complete symptom remission and normalization of esophageal acid exposure time in 40% and 100% and in 50% an 100% of patients after TIF and Nissen fundoplication, respectively [19]. These data suggest that in a challenging clinical setting such as PPI refractoriness, Nissen fundoplication seems more effective than TIF by EsophyX®.

Another meta-analysis including 32 studies (1475 patients) on TIF performed with either EsophyX or MUSE was published in 2018 [14]. TIF success rate was 99%. GERD Health-related Quality of Life score (GERD-HRQL), Gastroesophageal Reflux Symptom Score (GERSS), and Reflux Symptom Index score (RSI) improved significantly post-TIF (mean difference 17.72, 95% CI 17.31–18.14; mean difference 23.78, 95% CI 22.96–24.60; mean difference 14.28, 95% CI 13.56–15.01; all $P < 0.001$, respectively). Hernia reduction occurred in 91% of patients (95% CI 83–98; $P < 0.001$). PPI therapy was discontinued postprocedure in 89% of patients (95% CI 82–95; $P < 0.001$).

TIF was proven effective also in controlling regurgitation and atypical GERD symptoms that generally are more difficult to manage by medical therapy, compared with heartburn. In a randomized trial with cross-over arm, regurgitation and atypical GERD symptoms were eliminated in 88% of cases at 1-year follow-up [20].

Efficacy of TIF in Controlling Gastroesophageal Reflux

In the meta-analysis published in 2017, 11 studies assessed pre- and postprocedure pH with or without impedance recordings. Overall, normalization of esophageal acid exposure, in terms of total acidic refluxes, number of refluxates, and DeMeester score, was reported in 37–89% of patients [10]. In the six randomized controlled trials (RCTs) comparing the esophageal acid exposure time with the control, TIF significantly reduced intraesophageal acid exposure time in GERD patients without PPI therapy. TIF showed similar efficacy with respect to esophageal acid exposure time, compared with PPIs, and significantly improved patients' acid exposure time compared with sham groups. Two series found worsening of distal esophageal acid exposure [18, 19].

Data from the meta-analysis published in 2018 (15 studies involving 722 patients) showed that esophageal acid exposure time (i.e., percent time with $pH < 4$) significantly improved after the TIF intervention (mean difference 3.43%, 95% CI 2.98–3.88; $P < 0.001$) and DeMeester scores improved significantly (mean difference 10.22, 95% CI 8.38–12.12; $P < 0.001$) [14]. The number of reflux episodes in a 24-hour period also significantly improved from preprocedure levels (mean difference 51.57, 95% CI 47.96–55.18; $P < 0.001$).

One multicenter study on TIF by MUSE reported statistically significant reductions in the means for percent total time and upright time pH, as well as total number

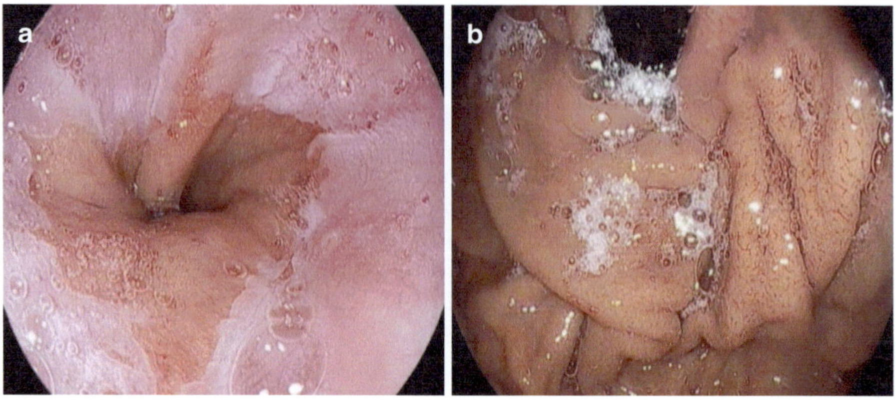

Fig. 33.7 Endoscopic findings of gastroesophageal valve from the esophagus (**a**) and from the stomach (**b**) 12 months after fundoplication by MUSE. Even if the cardiac seems to be incompetent, in retroflexed view, the neovalve persists creating a high-pressure segment that prevents reflux

of episodes [11]. The high-pressure segment created by the fundoplication appears effective in controlling gastroesophageal reflux even if at endoscopic examination cardiac incompetence seems to persist. Figure 33.7 shows long-term efficacy of TIF in controlling GERD-related symptoms.

Long-term efficacy of TIF in Controlling GERD-Related Symptoms

To date, nine studies reported long-term results up to 10 years: two studies up to 3 years [21, 22], four studies up to 4–6 years [11, 13, 15, 20, 23], and two studies up to 10 years [24, 25] (Tables 33.1, 33.2, and 33.3).

Regurgitation and atypical GERD symptoms were eliminated in 90% of cases at 2- and 3-year follow-up and in 86% of cases at 5-year follow-up [26].

In our 10-year series of TIF performed by EsophyX, the mean GERD-HRQL scores (off PPI therapy), and mean heartburn and regurgitation scores still remained significantly lower than before treatment and did not differ compared to the 2-, 3-, 5-, 7-, and 10-year scores. Similarly, as with regard to the PPI consumption, 86.7%, 84.4%, 73.5%, 83.3%, and 91.7% of patients completely stopped or halved the PPI use at 2, 3, 5, 7, and 10 years, respectively. In fact, clinical results obtained 2 years after TIF were substantially maintained up to 10 years [25] (Fig. 33.8). At the intention to treat analysis of the long-term efficacy of TIF, 10 years after TIF, 78.6% of patients had stopped or halved PPI therapy, while 35.7% had completely discontinued it. Unsuccessful outcomes of TIF occurred mainly between 6 and 12 months after the procedure, while later the results did not substantially differ. These findings show that an appropriate patient selection plays a pivotal role in achieving clinical success after TIF and confirm that factors negatively affecting postoperative outcomes play a role early in the postoperative period in most patients. Operator's experience plays an important role in TIF outcomes, too. A retrospective study in 124 unselected patients carried out in two community hospitals and reporting, respectively, 75% and 80% of patients free of typical and atypical GERD symptoms over a mean follow-up of 7 months confirmed that the operator's experience plays a major role in successful outcomes [27].

TIF and surgical fundoplication: are outcomes comparable?

Probably it is not appropriate to compare transoral fundoplication with surgical fundoplication, because the two procedures are addressed to patients with different degree of severity of GERD. TIF has been performed to date in patients with less severe grades of esophagitis (mainly grades A and B according to Los Angeles classification), without or with hiatal hernia shorter than 2.5 cm, and with hiatus with a transverse dimension <3.0 cm.

In a systematic review and network meta-analysis of trials of patients with GERD, laparoscopic Nissen fundoplication appeared to have a greater ability to improve physiologic parameters of GERD, including increased lower esophageal

Table 33.1 GERD-HRQL pre- and post-TIF in long-term follow-up studies

	Device	Follow-up (years)	Patients with complete FU	GERD-HRQL pre ON/OFF therapy (mean ± SD)	GERD-HRQL post OFF therapy (mean ± SD)	*P*
Testoni et al., 2019 [25]	Esophyx	10	12	20 ± 13 ON 46 ± 19 OFF	9.5 ± 6.1 OFF	<0.01
Chimukangara et al., 2018 [24]	Esophyx	10	23	Median 24 (15–28) ON	Median 10 (6–14)	<0.01
Trad et al., 2018 [26]	Esophyx	5	44	Median 26.4 ON Median 32.8 OFF	Median 6.8 (OFF or ON)	0.001
Stefanidis et al., 2017 [23]	Esophyx	6	44	Median 27 (2–45) ON	Median 4 (0–26) OFF	<0.001
Kim et al., 2016 [13]	MUSE	4	25	29.1 ± 5.6 OFF	5.3 ± 5.8 OFF	<0.01
Roy-Shapira et al., 2015 [11]	MUSE	4.5	13	24.2 ± 6.9 OFF	12/13 (92.3%) >50% reduction score pre	–
Muls et al., 2013 [21]	Esophyx	3	54	24.3 ± 5.9 OFF	6.4 ± 7.7 OFF (median 4, range 0–32)	<0.001
Witteman et al., 2012 [22]	Esophyx	3	19	Median 33 (7–69) ON	Median 5 (0–29) OFF	<0.0001

Table 33.2 Heartburn and regurgitation scores pre- and post-TIF in long-term follow-up studies

	Device	Follow-up (years)	Patients with complete follow-up	Patient satisfaction pre N. (%)	Patient satisfaction post N.(%)	Normalization heartburn score N. (%)	Normalization regurgitation score N. (%)	*P*
Testoni et al., 2019 [25]	Esophyx	10	12	–	–	18 ± 9 PRE 4.2 ± 3 POST	17 ± 9 PRE 3.2 ± 4.4 POST	<0.01
Chimukangara et al., 2018 [24]	Esophyx	10	23	0 (0%)	6/23 (74%)	–	–	–
Trad et al., 2018 [26]	Esophyx	5	44	1/60 (2%)	31/44 (70%)	31/39 (80%)	37/43 (86%)	<0.001
Stefanidis et al., 2017 [23]	Esophyx	5	44	21/45 (46,6%)	39/44 (88.6%)	12/21 (57.1%)	15/17 (88.2%)	0.0001
Kim et al., 2016 [13]	MUSE	4	–	–	–	–	–	–
Roy-Shapira et al., 2015 [11]	MUSE	4.5	13	–	13 (100%)	–	–	–
Muls et al., 2013 [21]	Esophyx	3	54	3/54 (6%)	38/54 (70%)	39/54 (72%)	–	<0.0001
Witteman et al., 2012 [22]	Esophyx	3	19	13/38 (34%)	13 (70%)	16/19 (86%)	16/19 (86%)	<0.0001

Table 33.3 PPI consumption pre- and post-TIF in long-term follow-up studies

	Device	Longest follow-up (years)	Patients with complete FU	Patients OFF PPIs N (%)	Patients halved/ occasionally on PPI N (%)	Patients OFF or halved/ occasionally on PPIs N (%)
Testoni et al., 2019 [25]	Esophyx	10	12	5/12 (41.7%)	6/12 (50%)	11/12 (91.7%)
Chimukangara et al., 2018 [24]	Esophyx	10	23	6/23 (27%)	–	–
Trad et al., 2018 [26]	Esophyx	5	44	20/44 (46%)	9/44 (20%)	29/44 (66%)
Stefanidis et al., 2017 [23]	Esophyx	6	44	32/44 (72.7%)	6/44 (13.7%)	38/44 (86.4%)
Kim et al., 2016 [13]	MUSE	4	36	25/36 (69.4%)	–	–
Roy-Shapira et al., 2015 [11]	MUSE	4.5	13	7/13 (53.8%)	3/13 (23.1%)	10/13 (76.9%)
Muls et al., 2013 [21]	Esophyx	3	54	35/54 (65%)	5/54 (9%)	40/54 (74%)
Witteman et al., 2012 [22]	Esophyx	3	19	8/19 (42%)	6/19 (9%)	14/19 (73.7%)

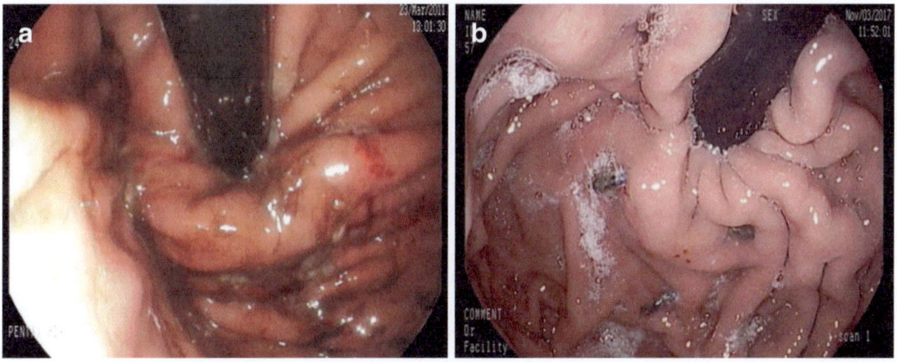

Fig. 33.8 Endoscopic findings of gastroesophageal valve immediately after (**a**) and 6 years after (**b**) the TIF procedure by EsophyX®. (Authors cases)

sphincter (LES) pressure and decreased percent time pH < 4, compared with TIF, while TIF was shown to better improve the health-related quality of life [28]. However, when the systematic review was carried out, long-lasting follow-up studies on TIF were still lacking, so the authors did not recommend TIF as a long-term alternative to PPI or surgical fundoplication for treating GERD.

In the six follow-up studies up to 4 years and more so far published on TIF, the reported patient satisfaction rate varied from 70% and 100%, the normalization of heartburns and regurgitation scores varied from 57.1% to 86% and from 86% to 88.2%, respectively. Five-year post-TIF results were substantially similar to those reported with Nissen fundoplication. A nationwide register-based follow-up study on the use of PPI after antireflux surgery reported that, at 5 years, 57.5% and 29.5% of patients still took PPI or were daily PPI-dependent [29]. In the Cochrane meta-analysis on Nissen fundoplication, the pooled analysis of long-term results showed recurrence or persistence of heartburn and reflux symptoms in 41.2% and 24.6% of cases, respectively, with persistent side effects in 14% up to 23% of cases [30]. There are very few reports of 10-year outcomes after surgical fundoplication, but, again, results are substantially comparable with our TIF findings [29–32]. In a systematic review of partial responders to PPI who had undergone laparoscopic fundoplication, 10 years after the operation, 35.8% reported heartburn and 29.1% regurgitation, with an 18.2% rate of acid-suppressive medication [31]. The nationwide register-based follow-up study on the use of PPI after antireflux surgery showed that, at 10 years, 72.4% and 41.1% of patients were taking PPI or were daily PPI-dependent [29].

Average costs associated with TIF and laparoscopic Nissen fundoplication over a 2-year follow-up, including intervention, hospital stay, office consultation, laboratory tests, pharmacy, and more, were calculated in the TIF 2.0 EsophyX vs Medical PPI Open label (TEMPO) randomized trial and were $ 71,691 for TIF and $ 92,256 for the surgical procedure [26].

Conclusions

In the past few years, TIF has become a relatively common procedure for treating pathological gastroesophageal reflux. Most of the interventions have been performed in clinical trials including patients with typical gastroesophageal reflux symptoms responsive or partially responsive to PPI therapy, without hiatal hernia, or with small hiatal hernia (<3 cm), who refused lifelong medical therapy, or were intolerant to PPIs, or required high dosage of antisecretory maintenance therapy. Patients with grade C and D esophagitis, according to Los Angeles classification, and Barrett's esophagus were excluded from these studies. However, after more than 10 years of clinical experience, there is no reason to exclude from this intervention patients with the latter conditions.

In the majority of studies, TIF was done by the EsophyX® device and was proven effective in the short term, eliminating the daily dependence from PPIs in 75–85% of patients. Similar results were obtained for TIF done with Medigus endostapler, but in few studies so far.

In the long-term studies reporting data up to 10 years, clinical results at 2–3 years have been maintained up to 10 years and were comparable with those of surgical fundoplication. Troublesome procedure-related persisting side effects were not reported in all the published studies, with both techniques.

References

1. Lundell L, Miettinen P. Continued (5 years) follow up of a randomized clinical study comparing antireflux surgery and omeprazole in GERD. J Am Col Surg. 2001;192:171–82.
2. Draaisma WE, Rijnhart-de Jong HG, Broeders IAMJ, Smout AJ, Furnee EJ, Gooszen HG. Five-year subjective and objective results of laparoscopic and conventional Nissen fundoplication. Ann Surg. 2006;244:34–41.
3. Smith CD. Surgical therapy for gastroesophageal reflux disease: indications, evaluation and procedures. Gastrointest Endoscopy Clin N Am. 2009;19:35–48.
4. Broeders JA, Draaisma WA, Bredenoord AJ, Smout AJ, Broeders IA, Gooszen HG. Long-term outcome of Nissen fundoplication in non-erosive and erosive gastro-esophageal reflux disease. Br J Surg. 2010;97:845–52.
5. Alemanno G, Bergamini C, Prosperi P, Bruscino A, Leahu A, Somigli R, Martellucci J, Valeri A. A long-term evaluation of the quality of life after laparoscopic Nissen-Rossetti anti-reflux surgery. J Minim Access Surg. 2017;13:208–14.
6. Cadiere GB, Rajan A, Germay O, Himpens J. Endoluminal fundoplication by a transoral device for the treatment of GERD: a feasibility study. Surg Endosc. 2008;22:333–42.
7. Testoni PA, Vailati C, Testoni S, Corsetti M. Transoral incisionless fundoplication (TIF 2.0) with EsophyX for gastroesophageal reflux disease: long-term results and findings affecting outcome. Surg Endosc. 2012;26:1425–35.
8. Bell RC, Cadière GB. Transoral rotational esophagogastric fundoplication: technical, anatomical, and safety considerations. Surg Endosc. 2011;25:2387–99.
9. Kauer WK, Roy-Shapira A, Watson D, Sonnenschein M, Sonnenschein E, Unger J, Voget M, Stein HJ. Preclinical trial of a modified gastroscope that performs a true anterior fundoplication for the endoluminal treatment of gastroesophageal reflux disease. Surg Endosc. 2009;23:2728–31.
10. Huang X, Chen S, Zhao H, Zeng X, Lin J, Tseng Y, Chen J. Efficacy of transoral incisionless fundoplication (TIF) for the treatment of GERD: a systematic review with meta-analysis. Surg Endosc. 2017;31:1032–44.
11. Roy-Shapira A, Bapaye A, Date S, Pujari R, Dorwat S. Trans-oral anterior fundoplication: 5-year follow-up of pilot study. Surg Endosc. 2015;29(12):3717–21.
12. Zacheri J, Roy-Shapira A, Bonavina L, Bapaye A, Kiesslich R, Schoppmann SF, Kessler WR, Selzer DJ, Broderick RC, Lehman GA, Horgan S. Endoscopic anterior fundoplication with the Medigus Ultrasonic Surgical Endostapler (MUSE) for gastroesophageal reflux: 6-month results from a multi-center prospective trial. Surg Endosc. 2015;29:220–9.
13. Kim HJ, Kwon CI, Kessler WR, Selzer DJ, McNulty G, Bapaye A, Bonavina L, Lehman GA. Long-term follow-up results of endoscopic treatment of gastroesophageal reflux disease with the MUSE™ endoscopic stapling device. Surg Endosc. 2016;30:3402–8.
14. McCarty TM, Itidiare M, Njei B, Rustagi T. Efficacy of transoral incisionless fundoplication for refractory gastroesophageal reflux disease: a systematic review and meta-analysis. Endoscopy. 2018;50:708–25.
15. Testoni PA, Testoni S, Mazzoleni G, Vailati C, Passaretti S. Long term efficacy of transoral incisionless fundoplication with Esophyx (TIF 2.0) and factors affecting outcomes in GERD patients followed for up to 6 years: a prospective single-center study. Surg Endosc. 2015;29:2770–80.
16. Demyttenaere SV, Bergman S, Pham T, Anderson J, Dettorre R, Melvin WS, Mikami DJ. Transoral incisionless fundoplication for gastro-esophageal reflux disease in an unselected patient population. Surg Endosc. 2010;24:854–8.
17. Hoppo T, Immanuel A, Schuchert M, Dubrava Z, Smith A, Nottle P, Watson DI, Jobe BA. Transoral incisionless fundoplication 2.0 procedure using EsophyX™ for gastroesophageal reflux disease. J Gastrointest Surg. 2010;14:1895–901.

18. Repici A, Fumagalli U, Malesci A, Barbera R, Gambaro C, Rosati R. Endoluminal fundoplication (ELF) for GERD using Esophyx: a 12-month follow-up in a single-center experience. J Gastrointest Surg. 2010;14:1–6.
19. Frazzoni M, Conigliaro R, Manta R, Melotti G. Reflux parameters as modified by EsophyX or laparoscopic fundoplication in refractory GERD. Aliment Pharmacol Ther. 2011;34:67–75.
20. Trad K, Fox MA, Simoni G, Shughoury AB, Mavrelis PG, Raza M, Helse JA, Barnes WE. Transoral fundoplication offers durable symptom control for chronic GERD: 3-year report from the TEMPO randomized trial with a crossover arm. Surg Endosc. 2017;31:2498–508.
21. Muls V, Eckardt AJ, Marchese M, Bastens B, Buset M, Devière J, Louis H, Rajan A, Daniel MA, Costamagna G. Three-year results of a multicenter prospective study of transoral incisionless fundoplication. Surg Innov. 2013;20(4):321–30.
22. Witteman PBL, Strijkers R, de Vries E, Toemen L, Conchillo JM, Hameeteman W, Dagnelie PC, Koek GH, Bouvy ND. Transoral incisionless fundoplication for treatment of gastroesophageal reflux diseases in clinical practice. Surg Endosc. 2012;26:3307–15.
23. Stefanidis G, Viazis N, Kotsikoros N, et al. Long-term benefit of transoral incisionless fundoplication using the Esophyx device for the management of gastroesophageal reflux disease responsive to medical therapy. Dis Esophagus. 2017;30:1–8.
24. Chimukangara M, Jalilvand AD, Melvin WS, Perry KA. Long-term reported outcomes of transoral incisionless fundoplication: an 8-year cohort study. Surg Endosc. 2019;33(4):1304–9.
25. Testoni PA, Testoni S, Distefano G, Mazzoleni G, Fanti L, Passaretti S. Transoral incisionless fundoplication with EsophyX for gastroesophageal reflux disease: clinical efficacy is maintained up to 10 years. Endoscopy International Open. 2019;07:E1–8.
26. Trad KS, Barnes WE, Prevou ER, et al. The TEMPO trial at 5 years: transoral fundoplication (TIF 2.0) is safe, durable, and cost-effective. Surg Innov. 2018;25:149–57.
27. Barnes WE, Hoddinott KM, Mundy S, et al. Transoral incisionless fundoplication offers high patient satisfaction and relief of therapy-resistant typical and atypical symptoms of GERD in community practice. Surg Innov. 2011;18:119–29.
28. Richter J, Kumar A, Lipka S, et al. Efficacy of laparoscopic Nissen fundoplication vs transoral incisionless fundoplication or proton pump inhibitors in patients with gastroesophageal reflux disease: a systematic review and network meta-analysis. Gastroenterology. 2018;154:1298–308.
29. Loedrup A, Pottegard A, Hallas J, Bytzer P. Use of proton pump inhibitors after antireflux surgery. A nationwide register-based follow-up study. Gut. 2014;63:1544–9.
30. Garg SK, Gurusamy KS. Laparoscopic fundoplication surgery versus medical management for gastro-oesophageal reflux disease (GORD) in adults. Cochrane Database Syst Rev. 2015;11:1–35.
31. Lundell L, Bell M, Ruth M. Systematic review: laparoscopic fundoplication for gastroesophageal reflux disease in partial responders to proton pump inhibitors. World J Gastroenterol. 2014;20:804–13.
32. Kelly JJ, Watson DI, Chin KF, Devitt PG, Game PA, Jamieson GG. Laparoscopic Nissen fundoplication: clinical outcomes at 10 years. J Am Coll Surg. 2007;205:570–5.

Chapter 34
Surgical Treatment for Gastroesophageal Reflux

Darren I. Rohan

Introduction

Gastroesophageal reflux disease (GERD) is one of the most common diseases involving the gastrointestinal (GI) tract. It is estimated that approximately 20% of the US population suffers from reflux episodes at least once weekly. The mainstay of treatment involves medical therapy. Proton pump inhibitors (PPIs) function by reducing the acidity in the stomach. Medications have been shown to control heartburn and reduce or eliminate esophagitis on endoscopy in about 80% of patients. Recent studies have shown that changes in diet can lead to a significant improvement of those patients that suffer from symptomatic reflux [1–3].

Many patients who achieve symptom control with medications will require prolonged use of these medications for durable effect. These patients also have a high relapse rate while on medications. This leads to frequent changes in medication regimen as well as prominent patient dissatisfaction [4]. In addition, the long-term use of proton pump inhibitors has been associated with multiple potential risks, as detailed elsewhere in this text.

Antireflux surgery works by restoring barriers that decrease the volume of gastric contents refluxing into the esophagus. Surgery includes several important maxims that lead to elimination of gastric reflux into the esophagus and a successful outcome. First, complete, tension-free repair of hiatal hernias, commonly found in patients with severe GERD, is necessary [5]. This allows for the gastroesophageal (GE) junction to be repositioned into the abdominal cavity. This is necessary to recreate the true angle of His at the GE junction, which has been shown to be important in controlling gastric reflux. In addition, fundoplication or wrapping of the fundus of the stomach around the esophagus helps to restore the valve function of

D. I. Rohan (✉)
Northwell Health, Donald and Barbara Zucker School of Medicine at Hofstra/Northwell, Hempstead, NY, USA
e-mail: drohan1@northwell.edu

C. H. Zalvan (ed.), *Laryngopharyngeal and Gastroesophageal Reflux*,
https://doi.org/10.1007/978-3-030-48890-1_34

the GE junction that allows proper swallowing while keeping gastric contents from refluxing into the esophagus [6].

Indications for Surgical Intervention in GERD

The choice to offer surgery for the treatment of reflux is usually based on the severity of symptoms. Inability to control symptoms with medication or lifestyle modification often leads to consideration of antireflux surgery in the treatment of GERD. Reflux symptoms can be classified into primarily gastrointestinal, respiratory, or laryngeal in nature. The presence of different symptomatology has been associated with differing success rates of surgery.

Gastrointestinal Symptoms

Classical symptoms of GERD are gastrointestinal in nature. The most common symptom associated with reflux is heartburn, a burning sensation in the chest associated with oral intake. Other symptoms include dysphagia, bloating, nausea, and vomiting. Patients whose symptoms significantly improve with acid suppressing medication have been shown to have better results after antireflux surgery.

Respiratory Symptoms

Many patients who experience high volume GERD experience symptoms associated with their respiratory tract. This is due to irritation of the respiratory tract secondary to reflux and aspiration of gastric contents into the respiratory tract. While medication decreases the acidity of gastric reflux, it has not been shown to decrease the amount of reflux. The most common respiratory symptom is chronic cough. Other symptoms include adult onset asthma, wheezing, hoarseness, chronic bronchitis, and frequent pneumonias. The presence of these symptoms alone is often associated with less effective medical therapy. When these symptoms are also associated with typical GI reflux symptoms, surgery has been shown to be a more effective alternative.

Laryngeal Symptoms

Laryngopharyngeal reflux (LPR) occurs when gastric contents back up into the pharynx (throat) or larynx (voice box). This causes inflammation that can lead to chronic hoarseness, reactive airway disease, persistent cough, or the feeling of a "lump" in the throat that is not relieved by swallowing. An endoscopic exam (laryngoscopy) is usually necessary to diagnose LPR. Treatment can include lifestyle and dietary changes, weight loss, or antireflux medications. For those patients who do not respond to those treatment options, antireflux surgery can be effective. However, the percentage of patients who completely respond to surgery is significantly less than those patients who undergo surgery with typical GERD symptoms.

American Gastroenterologic Association Recommendations

Most patients with GERD are treated successfully with medication or lifestyle and dietary modifications. Antireflux surgery has been shown to be effective in a selected group of patients with severe reflux. AGA, a national society of gastroenterologist, has published recommendations for those patients who should benefit from antireflux surgery based on an extensive review of the available literature [9, 10]. According to the society, surgical therapy should be considered in several groups of patients with confirmed reflux:

1. Patients who have failed medical therapy or who have intolerable side effects of medication.
2. Patients who require medication for treatment but opt for surgery in order to be able to discontinue chronic medication.
3. Patients who have complications of GERD including strictures or Barrett's esophagus.
4. Patients who frequently experience extra-esophageal manifestations of GERD that may include cough, chest pain, or adult onset asthma.

Diagnostic Studies

Several tests are performed preoperatively on patients who are being evaluated for antireflux surgery. These tests not only can identify whether patients are appropriate candidates for surgery but may also help identify which patients will benefit most from surgery [11].

Esophagogastroduodenoscopy (EGD) – Endoscopy of the stomach and esophagus can show evidence of esophageal erosions, severe esophagitis, or early evidence of cancer. In addition, endoscopy can show evidence for Barrett's esophagus, which is a change in the esophageal lining that has shown to be a precursor to esophageal cancer. Patients with severe esophagitis or Barrett's metaplasia despite maximal medical management are often considered for surgery.

Barium Swallow – An esophagram is a radiologic test performed with oral contrast that can evaluate the swallowing mechanism of the esophagus, size of hiatal hernia, and strictures. X-rays are taken as the patient is swallowing material for live evaluation of the upper GI tract. Often times, these tests show extensive reflux of gastric contents into the esophagus. This test can also show alternative diagnoses including diffuse esophageal spasm and achalasia.

pH Test –A 24 or 48-hour esophageal pH testing is used to correlate a patient's symptoms of reflux with changes in esophageal acid levels. A probe is placed in the mid esophagus that monitors pH over a one to two-day period. Patients identify symptom occurrences which are correlated with changes in esophageal acid and given a numerical score. This number is known as the DeMeester score. A higher score represents symptoms that are associated with low esophageal pH. A high DeMeester score also correlates with better surgical success for GERD [12].

Esophageal Manometry – This study evaluates the muscular function of the esophagus by monitoring muscular contractions during full swallows. Manometry is useful in preoperative evaluation. It may lead to diagnosis of other diseases for which antireflux surgery is contraindicated such as achalasia or scleroderma. Decreased muscular function of the esophagus might aid in planning the exact antireflux procedure performed. A partial wrap or loose wrap might be more appropriate for patients with decreased muscular coordination of the esophagus during swallowing.

Surgical Techniques

The surgical treatment of GERD has evolved over the years. All techniques include repair of diaphragmatic hernia with positioning of the GE junction back into the abdominal cavity as well as wrapping the stomach to form a competent valve. Surgical access to the GE Junction has been described from both the chest and abdominal cavities. In addition, many surgical procedures differ in the completeness of the stomach wrap around the GE junction.While the most common procedure performed currently is the laparoscopic Nissen 360 degree fundoplication, there are certain specific situations for using other surgical procedures described in this chapter.

Belsey Mark IV Repair

This antireflux procedure is performed through the chest cavity. It was first described in 1967 by Ronald Belsey and was the fourth iteration of a procedure that he had been perfecting for several years [13].

The procedure is approached through the left sixth or seventh interspace of the chest. The left lung is collapsed and the inferior pulmonary ligament, which lies in approximation with the esophagus, is divided. The esophagus is identified and cleared from surrounding tissue. The abdominal cavity is entered to facilitate pulling a portion of the stomach around the esophagus. The edges of the diaphragm are sewn together posteriorly. The esophagus can be lengthened if necessary, by removing a portion of the stomach. The fundus is then sewn to the esophagus creating a 240-degree partial wrap. Once the wrap is complete, the gastroesophageal junction

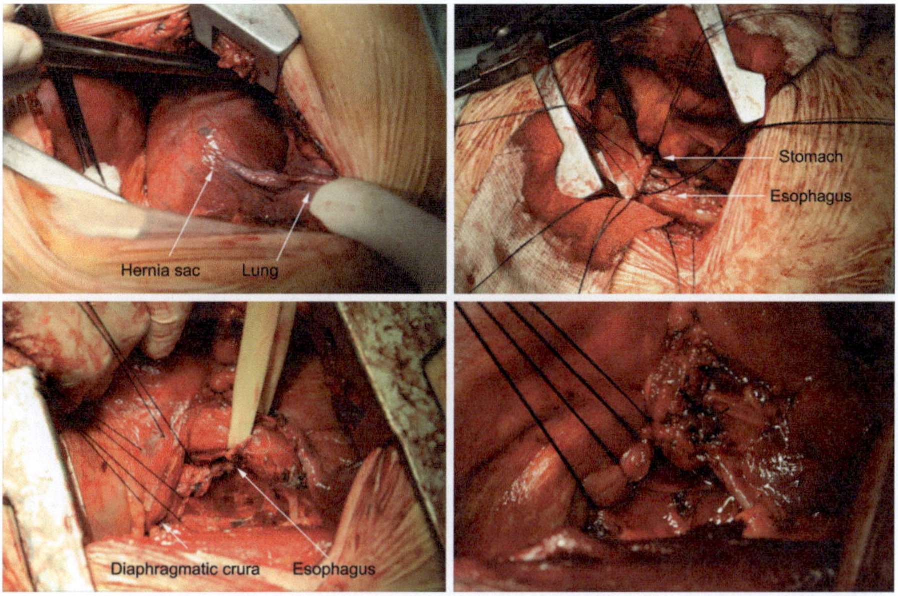

Fig. 34.1 Belsey Mark IV operation. Top left – Hernia sac adhering to lung. Bottom left- Sutures placed between the diaphragmatic crura. Top right – First row of sutures between the stomach and the esophagus. Bottom right – second row of sutures incorporating the stomach, the esophagus, and diaphragm. (Modified from Markakis et al. [25])

is placed back into the abdominal cavity, the diaphragm is approximated over the wrap, and the incisions are closed (see Fig. 34.1).

The main advantage of this procedure is allowing for the reduction in gastroesophageal reflux without effecting the swallowing functions of the esophagus. The rates of dysphagia, belching, and difficulty with vomiting are significantly less than those found in procedures that utilize a full wrap of the fundus of the stomach around the esophagus. However, recovery from open chest surgery is much more significant than that from laparoscopic abdominal surgery. Patients who have failed previous antireflux procedures are more easily approached through the chest due to the scarring in the hiatus from failed surgery. These patients may also have a shortened esophagus. For this reason, the Belsey Mark IV procedure is currently often reserved for those patients requiring a reoperative antireflux surgery. Long-term results for properly selected patients are over 80% positive at decreasing symptomatic reflux with minimal side effects [14].

Laparoscopic Partial Fundoplications

Minimally invasive partial wrap of the fundus of the stomach arround the esophagus procedures were adapted from open procedures that were first described in the 1960s. They have been converted to laparoscopic procedures with port access into the abdominal cavity in recent years. Decreased pain and morbidity of minimally invasive techniques have made laparoscopic antireflux procedures the first choice of patients who are referred for surgery. Partial wraps were originally used in patients with decreased esophageal motor function seen on manometry or barium swallow. They are found to have decreased side effects of dysphagia when compared to procedures employing complete 360 degree wraps. However, they have an increased recurrence of reflux symptoms in long-term studies. The two most common procedures were described by Dor and Toupet in the 1960s.

The Dor fundoplication is an anterior wrap of stomach over the esophagus. It requires that at least 5 cm of esophagus remains tension-free in the abdomen abdominal cavity. This is accomplished by repair of hiatal hernia, removal of the hernia sac, and mediastinal dissection of the esophageal attachments for lengthening of the esophagus in a tension-free manor. The gastric fundus is folded over anteriorly and sutured to both sides of the esophagus as well to the diaphragmatic ring with interrupted nonabsorbable sutures (see Fig. 34.2).

The Toupet fundoplication is a posterior partial 270-degree wrap leaving the anterior portion of the esophagus and gastroesophageal junction uncovered. This procedure also requires a significant amount of esophagus resting in the abdominal cavity. The short gastric vessels in the fundus of the stomach are divided. The hiatus is sutured closed posterior to the esophagus. The fundus is then brought behind the esophagus. The fundus is sutured on both sides of the esophagus and also to both crus of the diaphragm. It is essential that there is no tension on the wrap [15, 16] (Fig. 34.3).

Both procedures are currently performed with minimally invasive techniques, either laparoscopically or robotically. While these procedures are associated with less postoperative dysphagia, there is an increased rate of failure when compared to full wraps. These procedures are usually reserved for those patients with diminished esophageal motility found on manometry.

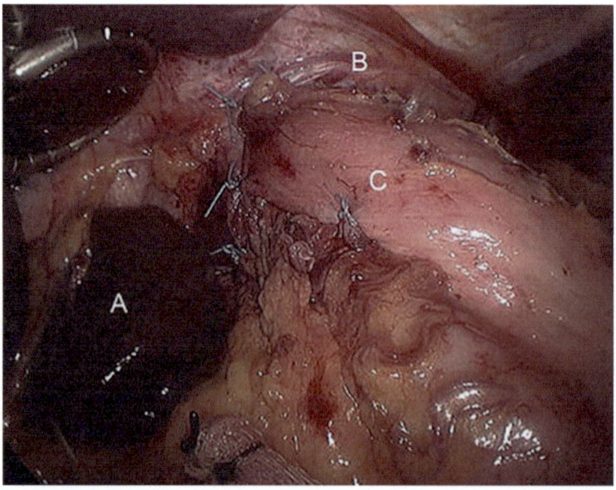

Fig. 34.2 Completed Dor fundoplication (**a**) caudate lobe of the liver, (**b**) diaphragm, (**c**) anterior fundoplication. (With permission from Palazzo et al. [26])

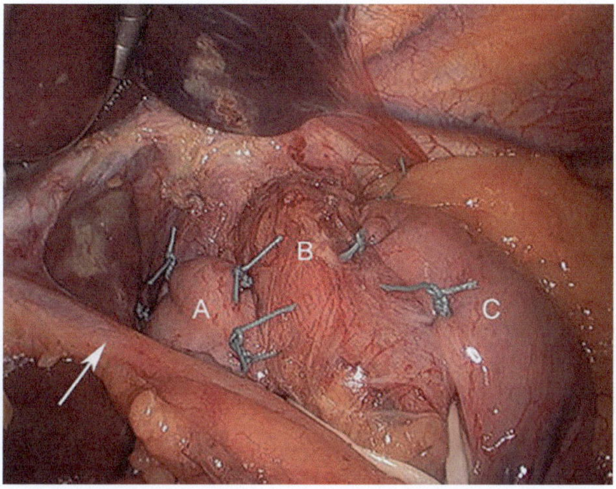

Fig. 34.3 Completed Toupet fundoplication (**a**) posterior lip of the fundoplication, (**b**) esophagus, (**c**) anterior lip of the fundoplication. (With permission from Palazzo et al. [26])

Laparoscopic Nissen Fundoplication

The Nissen fundoplication is a complete 360-degree wrap of the fundus of the stomach around the esophagus to control symptomatic reflux. Nissen originally described the open complete wrap for reflux in 1956. The laparoscopic adaptation of the procedure was first published in 1991 by Dellemagne. Currently, the laparoscopic Nissen fundoplication is the most common surgical procedure performed for symptomatic reflux with the best long-term results and patient satisfaction [17].

The procedure is performed either laparoscopically or with robotic assistance. The patient is usually supine on the operating table. Five 1-cm ports are placed in the abdomen under direct visualization. A supraumbilical port is used for the camera and the lateral right upper quadrant port is used for liver retraction. An assistant port is placed in the left lower quadrant. The two operating ports are located more medially in the right and left upper quadrants (see Fig. 34.4).

The esophagus is first mobilized and brought down into the abdominal cavity through dissection in the mediastinum. The hernia sac is dissected out of the chest with bipolar cautery or ligasure energy. Approximately, 3 cm of esophagus should be mobilized into the abdominal cavity without any tension. Next, the hiatal hernia is repaired posterior to the esophagus. Both edges of the diaphragm (crus) are dissected free with cautery. The edges are sutured together in an interrupted fashion using nonabsorbable sutures without tension. The short gastric vessels on the fundus of the stomach are divided with Ligasure (Medtronic) energy all the way to the gastroesophageal junction. The stomach attachments are cleared posteriorly with energy to allow for a full wrap without tension. The mobile fundus is then passed posteriorly behind the esophagus to the right side of the abdomen to form the wrap. A "floppy" or loose wrap is accomplished with a 56 french bougie dilator placed into the esophagus by the anesthesiologist. The rates of postoperative dysphagia are less when the wrap is allowed to be loose with no tension. The length of the wrap is between 2 and

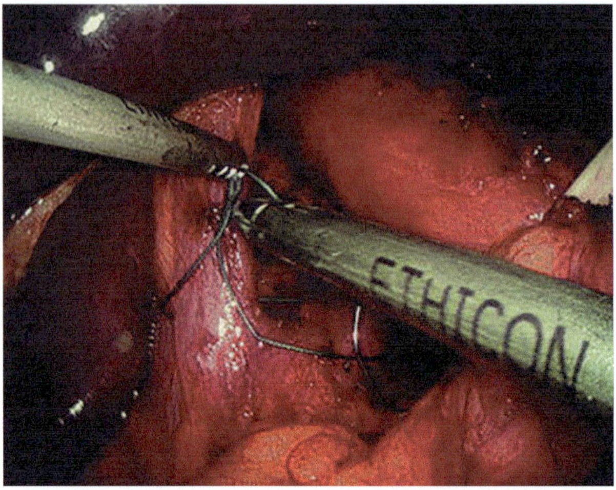

Fig. 34.4 Laparoscopic repair of the diaphragmatic crura during Nissen fundoplication (With permission from Gould [27])

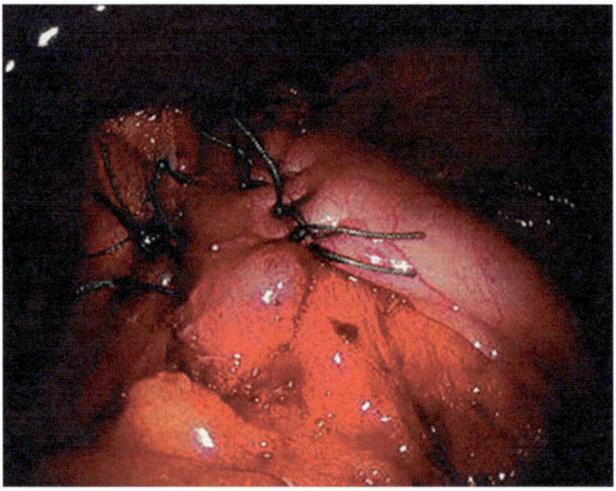

Fig. 34.5 Completed laparoscopic Nissen fundoplication showing diaphragmatic repair. (With permission from Gould [27])

3 cm over the distal esophagus. The fundus is sutured to itself anterior to the esophagus with three or four nonabsorbable interrupted sutures (see Figs. 34.5 and 34.6).

Results of Antireflux Surgery

Overall, the results of surgery for symptomatic reflux are quite good with appropriate patient selection. Best candidates for surgery have a high DeMeester score, adequate esophageal peristalsis, and a history of response to antireflux medication, especially proton pump inhibitors. Minimally invasive and robotic techniques have led to results that surpass open procedures. Proper surgical technique is essential for

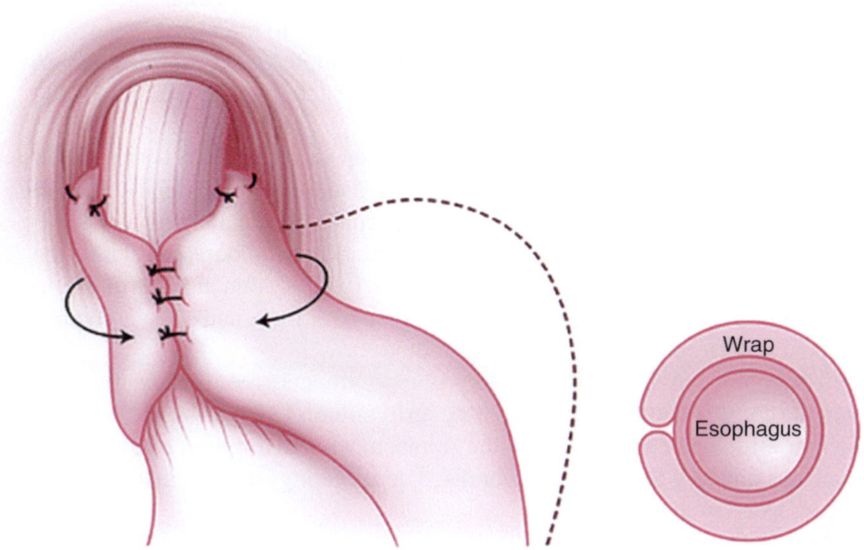

Fig. 34.6 Nissen 360-degree fundoplication around the distal esophagus. (With permission from Hinojosa and Pellegrini [28])

obtaining optimal results. Recent literature focuses on postoperative findings after laparoscopic Nissen Fundoplication.

Studies looking specifically at symptom resolution after laparoscopic Nissen surgery have found that approximately 90% of patients report significant improvement in heartburn at 1 year. Improvement for atypical symptoms of reflux, such as cough, asthma, or LPR is not as high and ranges from 60 to 80% [18]. A single-center study looking specifically at patients that presented with chronic cough as the main reflux associated symptom showed an 80% resolution in cough after surgery and for the 3-year follow-up. In addition, 75% of patients were able to stay off PPIs in the follow-up period. An objective measure of success in antireflux surgery is pH normalization as measured by esophageal pH probe. Normal pH measurements can be found in 90% of patients at 1-year follow-up. Patient satisfaction scores following the Nissen fundoplication average 80% at 5 years and are similar as far out as 15 years [7, 8]. Data for partial fundoplication show a higher PPI use in the follow-up period suggesting that partial wraps are not as durable as complete wraps.

In patients with chronic erosive esophagitis secondary to GERD, Nissen fundoplication has been shown to give superior results when compared to medical PPI treatment. Patients undergoing surgery had an 89% regression in esophagitis, compared with 53% in those patients treated with medication alone. In addition, reflux symptom scores decreased significantly in those patients who underwent surgery [16].

Patients with Barrett's esophagus secondary to severe GERD, who are treated with surgery have a lower risk of developing esophageal cancer when compared to those treated with medication alone. A recent meta-analysis confirmed a 0.76 incidence rate ratio when comparing the two groups. This study also showed a large increase risk of esophageal cancer in patients treated with surgery when compared to a background population. This is most likely due to the fact that those who are currently offered antireflux surgery have severe esophagitis. Antireflux surgery does not bring the risk of esophageal cancer down to background population [20].

Side effects of surgery include dysphagia, gas-bloat syndrome, and difficulty with vomiting. Dysphagia is reported to be approximately 10%–30% and usually resolves after a few months. Occasionally, endoscopic dilation is necessary to resolve postoperative dysphagia. Gas-bloat consists of a feeling of bloating and intestinal gas with an inability to belch, combined with increased flatulence. This may be due to delayed gastric emptying or vagal dysfunction in these patients. These symptoms are not severe, usually lessen over time, and often associated with marked improvement of symptomatic reflux.

The complication rate after surgery is approximately 5%. Herniation of the wrap into the chest is the most common long-term failure. Other anatomic complications include slipping of the wrap onto the stomach, wrap disruption, or a tight wrap that does not improve after several months. These findings usually lead to reoperation and conversion to a partial wrap.

Reflux recurrence after surgery has been a significant problem. It is most commonly responsible for the decreased use of surgery in the treatment of severe GERD. A recent cohort study with a median follow-up of 5.6 years showed that approximately 17% of patients required continued use of antireflux medication or repeat surgery. Risk factors for recurrence were advanced age, female sex, and significant comorbidities [19].

Magnetic Bead Sphincter Augmentation for Treatment of Reflux

Recent advances in technology have allowed for the reduction of reflux without changing the normal anatomy of the gastrointestinal junction. The introduction of the LINX Reflux Management System (Johnson and Johnson) has given patients who want a surgical solution to the elimination of GERD without fundoplication a viable option.

LINX contains a chain of titanium beads with magnetic cores linked together with titanium wires. When implanted around the distal esophagus, it forms a complete, flexible ring. Each bead can move independently. The magnetic force holding the beads together is approximately 27 mm Hg. Esophageal contraction associated with swallowing is usually greater than 40 mm Hg, allowing food boluses to pass without issue. The pressure created by the magnets around the esophagus creates enough force to stop reflux from the stomach into the esophagus but will still allow for vomiting or belching. Advantages of this device over previously placed foreign bodies at the gastroesophageal junction are its flexibility and anatomic movement. This allows normal motion in the esophagus during swallowing. The device was first placed on trial in 2007 and approved in the United States in 2012. The device has been studied extensively since approval [21] (see Fig. 34.7).

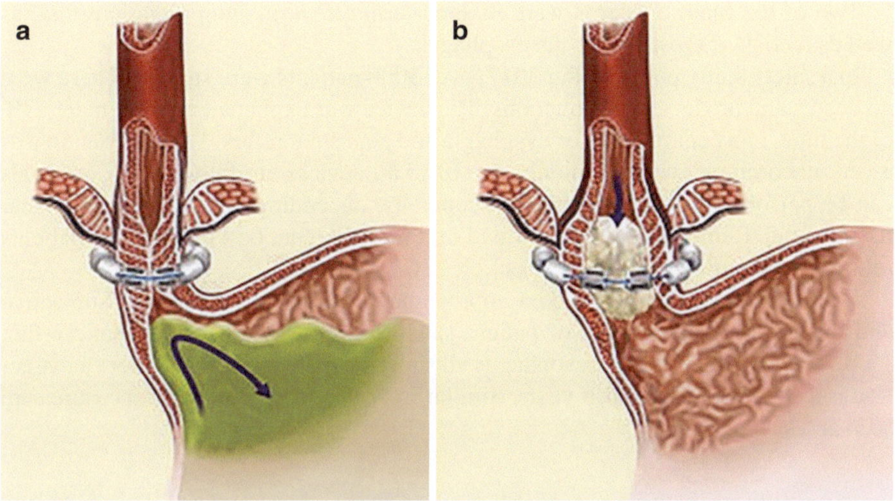

Fig. 34.7 (**a**) Device in closed state prevents reflux. (**b**) Pressure created during swallowing opens device to allow passage of food (With permission from Bonavina et al. [29])

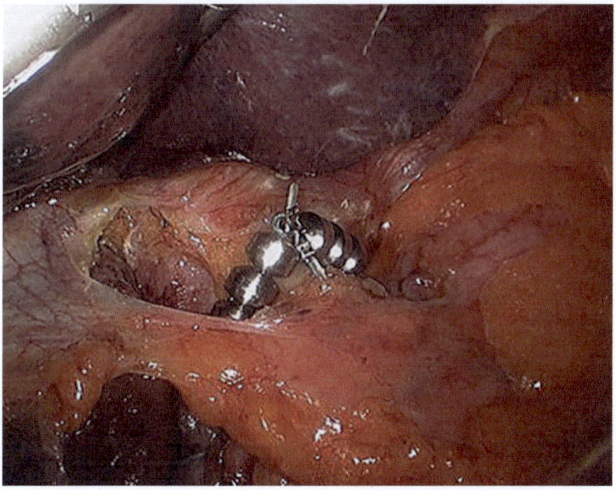

Fig. 34.8 Implanted LINX device at the lower esophageal sphincter (With permission from Palazzo et al. [26])

Implantation of the device is done through a laparoscopic approach. The gastroesophageal junction and distal esophagus is dissected free from surrounding tissue. Care is taken to spare the anterior and posterior vagus nerves. The diaphragmatic edges are dissected free and any hiatal hernia is repaired over a bougie. The esophagus is measured for device placement. The device is implanted around the distal esophagus. Care is taken to exclude the posterior vagus nerve. The device is meant to fit loosely around the esophagus. Patients are started on a regular diet immediately after the surgery. The most common complaint after implantation is dysphagia, which usually resolves after several months (see Fig. 34.8).

Two of the main concerns were its long-term effect on symptomatic reflux, as well as its risk of erosion into the esophagus.

In a safety study published in 2017, over 3000 patients were studied. There were no deaths and no device malfunctions. The device was explanted approximately 3% of the time, most commonly for dysphagia and persistent reflux. Device erosion was a very uncommon event, with only five (0.15%) devices eroding. Device removals can be performed surgically or endoscopically, depending on the amount of scar tissue found. Removals were performed on a nonemergent basis, with most patients returning to baseline in a few weeks [22, 23].

Long-term results show marked improvement at 5 years and beyond. Subjective and objective measurements of patient satisfaction, PPI use, symptomatic reflux score, and acidity within the esophagus all show sustained benefits. Patient satisfaction is as high as 90% after 5 years. Similar improvements with other measures are seen and sustained [24].

Conclusion

Most patients who suffer from gastroesophageal reflux are treated adequately with medication or lifestyle modification. Despite this, there is a population of patients who suffer with symptoms despite maximal medical therapy. In addition, there are patients who remain on proton pump inhibitors long term and wish to be able to weaned off medication. Several recent studies have found many long-term negative consequences of chronic PPI use.

For the correctly selected and worked up patient, antireflux surgery, specifically, laparoscopic Nissen fundoplication can facilitate improvement in symptoms and allow patients to be taken off long-term medications. Laparoscopic Nissen fundoplication has a high patient satisfaction rate with a low complication rate. When compared to other invasive procedures to treat chronic reflux, Laparoscopic Nissen fundoplication still offers the best results. In addition, its long-term efficacy and follow-up makes it a viable option for patients with severe symptomatic gastroesophageal reflux.

Antireflux surgery offers an alternative treatment that is especially useful in situations where long-term reflux and dietary indiscretion have led to obesity and anatomic change of the natural barriers of the gastroesophageal junction. Success rates are initially high regardless of the surgical approach. However, longer term results show an increased failure rate. Recurrent symptoms are most often not from surgical failure but from patient failure to make and maintain long-term dietary and behavioral changes. Surgery should not be used as permission for patients to continue with their standard diet. Postsurgical education, nutritional evaluation, and personal research should be stressed as equally as the risks, benefits, and alternatives of the procedure.

References

1. Costantini M, Zaninotto G, Anselmino M, et al. The role of a defective lower esophageal sphincter in the clinical outcome of treatment for gastroesophageal reflux disease. Arch Surg. 1996;131(6):655–9.
2. Hunter JG, Trus TL, Branum GD, et al. A physiologic approach to laparoscopic fundoplication for gastroesophageal reflux disease. Ann Surg. 1996;223(6):673–87.
3. Worrell SG, DeMeester SR, Greene CL, et al. Pharyngeal pH monitoring predicts a successful outcome for extraesophageal reflux symptoms after antireflux surgery. Surg Endosc. 2006;27(11):4113–8.
4. Campos GM, Peters JH, DeMeester TR, et al. Multivariate analysis of factors predicting outcome after laparoscopic Nissen fundoplication. J Gastrointest Surg. 1999;3(3):292–300.
5. Fein M, Bueter M, Thalheimer A, et al. Ten year outcome of laparoscopic antireflux surgery. J Gastrointest Surg. 2008;12(11):1893–9.
6. Dallemagne B, Weerts J, Markiewicz S, et al. Clinical results of laparoscopic fundoplication at ten years after surgery. Surg Endosc. 2006;20(1):159–65.
7. Morganthal CB, ShaneMD SA, et al. The durability of laparoscopic Nissen fundoplication: 11 year outcomes. J Gastrointest Surg. 2007;11(6):693–700.
8. Csendes A, Orellana O, Cuneo N, et al. Long term (15-year) objective evaluation of 150 patients after laparoscopic Nissen fundoplication. Surgery. 2019;166(5):1–9.
9. Kahrilas PJ, Shaheen NJ, Vaezi MF. American Gastroenterologic Association medical position statement on the management of gastroesophageal reflux disease. Gastroenterology. 2008:593–9.
10. Stefanidis D, Hope WW, Kohn GP, et al. Guidelines for surgical treatment of gastroesophageal reflux disease. Surg Endosc. 2010;24(11):2647–69.
11. Jobe BA, Richter JE, Hoppo T, et al. Preoperative diagnostic workup before antireflux surgery: an evidence and experience-based consensus of the Esophageal Diagnostic Advisory panel. J Am Coll Surg. 2013;217(4):586–97.
12. Tseng D, Rizvi AZ, Fennerty MB, et al. Forty-eight hour pH monitoring increases sensitivity in detecting abnormal esophageal acid exposure. J Gastroint Surg. 2005;9(8):1043–51.
13. Skinner DB, Belsey RH. Surgical management of esophageal reflux and hiatus hernia: long-term results with 1,030 patients. J Thorac Cardiovasc Surg. 1967;53(1):33.
14. Fenton KN, Miller JI, Lee RB, et al. Belsey Mark IV antireflux procedure for complicated gastroesophageal reflux disease. Ann Thor Surg. 1997;64(3):790–4.
15. Richardson WS, Trus TL, Thompson S, et al. Nissen and Toupet fundoplications effectively inhibit gastroesophageal reflux irrespective of natural anatomy and function. Surg Endosc. 1997;11(3):261–3.
16. Heikken TJ, Haukipuro K, Bringman S, et al. Comparison of laparoscopic and open Nissen Fundoplication 2 years after operation. A prospective randomized trial. Surg Endosc. 2000;14(11):1019–23.
17. Thor KB, Silander T. A long-term randomized prospective trial of the Nissen procedure versus a modified Toupet technique. Ann Surg. 1989;210(6):719–24.
18. Guerin E, Betroune K, Closset J, et al. Nissen versus Toupet fundoplication: results of a randomized and multicenter trial. Surg Endosc. 2007;21(11):1985–90.
19. Awais O, Luketich JD, Schchert MJ, et al. Reoperative antireflux surgery for failed fundoplication: an analysis of outcomes in 275 patients. Ann Thor Surg. 2011;92(3):1083–9.
20. Maret-Ouda J, Konings P, Lagergren J, et al. Antireflux Surgery and risk of esophageal adenocarcinoma: a systematic review and meta-analysis. Ann Surg. 2016;263(2):251–7.
21. Bell R, Lipham J, Louie B, et al. Laparoscopic magnetic sphincter augmentation versus double-dose proton pump inhibitors for management of moderate-to-severe regurgitation in GERD: a randomized controlled trial. Gastrointest Endosc. 2019;89(1):14–22.

22. Smith CD, Ganz RA, Lipham JC, et al. Lower esophageal sphincter augmentation for gastroesophageal reflux disease: the safety of a modern implant. J Lap Adv Surg Tech. 2017;27(6):586–92.
23. Alicuben ET, Bell RC, Jobe BA, et al. Worldwide experience with erosion of the magnetic sphincter augmentation device. J Gastro Intest Surg. 2018;22(8):1442–7.
24. Tatum JM, Alicuben E, Bildzukewicz N, et al. Minimal versus obligatory dissection of the diaphragmatic hiatus during magnetic sphincter augmentation surgery. Surg Endosc. 2019;33(3):782–8.
25. Markakis C, Tomos P, Spartalis ED, et al. The Belsey Mark IV: an operation with an enduring role in the management of complicated hiatal hernia. BMC Surgery. 2013;13:24.
26. Palazzo F, Khoraki J, Campos GM. Laparoscopic antireflux surgery. Heidelberg, Switzerland: Springer; 2016. p. 127–52.
27. Gould J. Laparoscopic Nissen fundoplication. London, Great Britain: Springer; 2009.
28. Hinojosa MW, Pellegrini CA. Surgical and endoscopic approaches to GERD. New York, NY: Springer; 2012.
29. Bonavina L, Saino G, Worrell S, et al. Magnetic LES augmentation: the LINX procedure. New York, NY: Springer; 2015.

Chapter 35
State of the Art: Laryngopharyngeal Reflux Treatment

Brian Benson and Corina Din-Lovinescu

Introduction

Compared to gastroesophageal reflux disease (GERD), the concept of LPR is a relatively new idea. Correspondingly, the lack of a robust body of research investigating the various treatments for LPR reflects the nascent stage of research into this relatively common clinical entity. In order to adequately assess response to treatment, standardized methods for diagnosis must exist. Currently, while there are multiple diagnostic tools [Reflux Symptom Index (RSI), Reflux Finding Score (RFS), empiric therapy, combined pH/impedance monitoring, salivary pepsin, and mucosal impedance] to identify LPR, there is no gold-standard testing modality or algorithm, although many have been proposed. Without accurate diagnostic tools, studies assessing the effectiveness of an intervention will invariably include patients whose symptomatology is the result of a different underlying pathophysiology, which in the case of LPR, may include allergic, neurogenic, and other causes of mucosal inflammation. Including these misdiagnosed subjects in the study cohort will decrease the apparent effectiveness of the intervention. Furthermore, the extraesophageal symptoms attributed to reflux include a heterogeneous group of otolaryngologic symptoms including throat clearing, odynophagia, postnasal drip, and ear discomfort as well as abdominal and pulmonary symptoms. Despite these methodological challenges, most investigators accept that patient with symptoms and signs of LPR, with proximal esophageal reflux on multichannel intraluminal impedance-pH monitoring do have LPR. To date, over 1000 publications, including more than

B. Benson (✉)
Department of Otolaryngology-Head & Neck Surgery, Hackensack Meridian School of Medicine at Seton Hall University, Nutley, NJ, USA
e-mail: brian@goldbenson.com

C. Din-Lovinescu
Department of Otolaryngology-Head and Neck Surgery, Rutgers New Jersey Medical School, Newark, NJ, USA

C. H. Zalvan (ed.), *Laryngopharyngeal and Gastroesophageal Reflux*,
https://doi.org/10.1007/978-3-030-48890-1_35

10 placebo randomized-controlled trials (RCTs), have evaluated medical interventions and over 250 studies have assessed surgical fundoplication for LPR [1, 2]. This chapter will review existing evidence in support of the following treatment modalities: lifestyle modification, medical therapy, and surgical intervention.

Lifestyle Modifications

Lifestyle modifications include a wide variety of interventions including decreasing or cessation of known carcinogens and irritants such as alcohol, tobacco, and vaping products, food items including chocolate, caffeine-containing drinks, carbonated beverages, citrus, mint, fried or spicy foods, and medications that are known to be associated with reflux. Nondiet modifications include weight loss, head of bed elevation at night, eating small meals, and avoiding eating several hours prior to bedtime. Although lifestyle modifications are the safest and most beneficial intervention from an overall health perspective, they remain the least-studied intervention for LPR or GERD and have the highest level of noncompliance.

There have been no studies assessing the effects of alcohol and tobacco/vaping cessation on LPR or GERD symptoms; however, the diagnosis of LPR provides an excellent opportunity for the clinician to provide alcohol/tobacco cessation counseling. Similarly, head of bed elevation, consuming small meals, and eating dinner no less than 4 hours prior to bedtime are common-sense interventions in patients who report worsening of LPR, GERD, or regurgitation symptoms when they fail to adhere to these measures, even though these interventions have not been studied. Although there is evidence that weight loss improves GERD symptoms and that weight gain worsens GERD symptoms, there is no high-level evidence showing a relationship between BMI and LPR symptoms [3, 4]. However, a cross-sectional study of patients suspected of having LPR showed a nonlinear relationship between esophageal acid exposure and BMI [5]. In light of the obesity epidemic affecting many communities throughout the world, it is not only appropriate, but encouraged, to use the LPR discussion to encourage patients to achieve and maintain healthy weights, regardless of the paucity of research in this area. Furthermore, those patients with concurrent LPR and GERD symptoms can be reassured that there is evidence that weight loss may improve some of their symptoms.

Some patients with LPR try over-the-counter medications prior to seeking the help of a physician, but few have tried diet modification, because they do not associate classic LPR symptoms with esophageal reflux. However, even in the case of GERD, a systematic review revealed lack of evidence to support diet change to control symptoms [6]. In sharp contrast, Zalvan et al. [7] reported that patients treated with alkaline water and a Mediterranean-style diet exhibited similar improvement in LPR symptoms compared to those taking proton pump inhibitors (PPI). Diet changes have also been shown to potentiate the effects of PPIs [1] and low-acid, low-fat diets were found to be helpful even for patients whose reflux symptoms were refractory to PPIs [8].

The quality of food also might also play a causative role in LPR and GERD. Preservatives used to acidify food to prolong their shelf life and decrease potential contaminants might directly contribute to an acidic environment [9]. Lechien et al. have recently created a "Refluxogenic Diet Score" (REDS) in an attempt to classify various food and beverages according to their ability to cause or propagate LPR symptoms based on a review of the literature. This comprehensive systematic review rates studies assessing food materials according to their ability to cause symptoms, lower the lower esophageal sphincter (LES) and upper esophageal sphincter (UES) pressures, and increase acid and gastrin secretion [10].

Medical Therapy

One of the earliest treatments for dyspepsia was the consumption of coral powders, a practice described by ancient Greek physicians, and later adopted by the Romans. Calcium carbonate has been identified as the key alkali agent in coral powder, which was described by Pilus, The Elder (AD 23–79), a Roman Scientist [11, 12]. Current acid suppression treatment for LPR has, for approximately 30 years, consisted primarily of proton pump inhibitors, although the growing concern about side effects has started to change the prescribing patterns [13]. The first potent acid suppression medication, histamine receptor antagonists (H2RA), was found to aid in esophageal healing in approximately 50% of patients [14], but were never studied in patients with LPR. Several RCTs using H2RA for asthma symptoms produced contradictory results [15].

With the introduction of proton pump inhibitors (PPI) in the late 1980s, the use of H2RA has waned. Early open label studies of PPIs showed promising results [16, 17], but as the number of papers about laryngopharyngeal reflux began to increase rapidly in the early 2000s, less encouraging results were reported. A large, well-designed multicenter randomized double-blinded study in 2006 that treated patients with laryngopharyngeal symptoms and signs using a twice-daily 40 mg dose of esomeprazole showed no benefit of PPI treatment compared to placebo [18]. Subsequent meta-analyses (which included between 8 and 14 studies) in 2006 [19], 2013 [20], and 2016 [21–23] failed to show significant benefit of PPI treatment for patients with laryngopharyngeal reflux. In addition, studies evaluating other extra-esophageal manifestations of GERD, such as asthma [24] and chronic cough [25] also found no improvement compared to placebo. More recently, in 2018, a systematic review and meta-analysis with strict inclusion criteria by the Laryngopharyngeal Reflux Study Group of Young Otolaryngologists of the International Federations of Oto-rhino-laryngological Societies found modest superiority of PPI over placebo, especially in those subjects who combined both PPI and diet modifications [1]. Importantly, the authors noted significant variation in the pH probe inclusion criteria, highlighting the ongoing heterogeneity of studies available for meta-analysis.

Despite the lack of evidence supporting the use of PPIs for LPR, most otolaryngologists continue to prescribe these medications for LPR on an empiric basis for three reasons: (1) diagnostic testing is invasive and expensive, (2) PPIs are well tolerated and are associated with minimal short-term side effects, and (3) most practitioners find them to be helpful to a meaningful proportion of their patient population, especially those with concurrent GERD symptoms.

Prokinetic medications (metoclopramide, domperidone, itopride, and tegaserod) are thought to reduce reflux by improving gastric clearance via multiple mechanisms. Meta-analysis of subjects with GERD on PPIs treated with prokinetic agents [26] found no improvement compared to PPI monotherapy. In contrast, several RCTs studying patients with LPR treated with prokinetics found improvement in LPR symptoms, although meta-analysis of these trials found that the level of evidence was insufficient to make a recommendation [27]. Because prokinetic medications have a significant side-effect profile, including multiple serious adverse reactions, they are not commonly prescribed for LPR. The antispasmodic medication, Baclofen, is a gamma-aminobutyric acid-B (GABA-B) receptor agonist that inhibits LES relaxation. A 2014 meta-analysis of subjects being treated for GERD using baclofen showed efficacy in decreasing number and duration of reflux events as well as transient lower esophageal sphincter relaxation (TLESR) events [28]. There have been no randomized controlled studies in LPR, but a 2019 study of patients with refractory LPR were treated in an open label study with both PPI and baclofen demonstrating improvement in reflux symptom index (RSI) and quality of life (QOL) scores in over 50% [29].

There are also several reports of uncontrolled studies for chronic cough that was treated successfully with baclofen. In light of the side effect profile of baclofen, its use for LPR should be considered only in patients whose LPR symptoms are refractory to more standard interventions.

Alginates are a seaweed-derived food additive that forms a neutral gel within the stomach that functions as a physical barrier to reflux events. pH probe studies of subjects treated with alginate showed significant reduction in both acid and nonacid reflux events [30]. A 2016 multicenter randomized controlled study of patients with GERD refractory to PPI treatment showed improvement of the severity and frequency of heartburn when Gaviscon ® [GSK Company] was administered as an add-on therapy [31]. A 2017 meta-analysis of 15 studies of alginate therapy for GERD reported alginate therapy to be more effective than placebo and antacids, but less effective than H2 blockers or PPIs [32]. A new product, Reflux Gourmet [Reflux Gourmet, Napa, CA, USA] entered the US market in 2019 providing an alternative for alginate therapy.

Several studies have evaluated alginate in the treatment of LPR. A 2009 nonblinded study compared alginate monotherapy to placebo, finding improved symptoms and signs at multiple time points [33], while two studies suggested that alginate was comparable to PPI for both LPR and GERD [34, 35]. A subsequent double-blind placebo-controlled study found that both alginate and placebo significantly reduced RSI as well as pH probe–confirmed reflux events, but alginate was not found to be superior to placebo [36].

Surgical and Endoscopic Antireflux Procedures

In addition to the traditional Nissen fundoplication, multiple other procedures aimed at reducing reflux symptoms, including transoral incisionless fundoplication, radiofrequency ablation, endoluminal anterior fundoplication, and LINX (magnetic sphincter augmentation) currently exist. The absence of high-level evidence for surgical intervention for GERD or LPR can be attributed to a variety of factors [37] and is a reflection of the current state of evidence-based surgery. There are currently no studies comparing surgical treatment to PPI medical therapy for either GERD or LPR. A 2017 meta-analysis of surgical intervention for extra-esophageal manifestations of reflux including cough, laryngopharyngeal reflux, and asthma [38] identified data that were of poor quality, and there was only one randomized study which compared high-dose H2 blockers to surgical intervention for asthma [39] that showed superiority of surgical intervention compared to H2 blockers. A 2019 systematic review of surgical treatment for LPR [2] identified 266 studies, of which 34 met inclusion criteria. Of the 2190 patients with LPR, 83% experienced improvement in their symptoms and 67% reported resolution of symptoms. However, rates of improvement and cure varied between 10% and 98%, owing to inclusion bias, selection bias, and retrospective study design. In most studies, the patients did not undergo laryngoscopy, and only six studies performed multichannel pH impedance testing.

It is generally accepted that patients with LPR respond less favorably to surgical intervention than those with GERD. Furthermore, LPR patients with hiatal hernia are thought to respond favorably to surgical intervention. Conversely, those who are refractory to PPI therapy are unlikely to benefit from surgical intervention. In short, while carefully selected patients are likely to benefit from surgical intervention, the current literature does not support the superiority of surgery over medical management.

Conclusion

While many treatment options exist for patients suffering from LPR symptoms, there is a lack of high-level evidence supporting either lifestyle modification, medical treatment, or surgical intervention for this condition. Even in the absence of robust evidence, lifestyle modifications promoting alcohol, tobacco, and vaping cessation as well as maintenance of a healthy BMI should be promoted. Clinicians should also feel confident in suggesting a mostly plant-based Mediterranean diet with alkaline water as well as alginate medications, since the risk-benefit ratio is extremely favorable [7, 36] and include significant added health benefits. For patients who have failed to improve on the previously mentioned interventions, especially those with concurrent GERD symptoms, a several month trial of PPI medication is likely to result in improvement for some patients. Further workup to rule out hiatal hernia, esophageal dysmotility, and distal esophageal lesions is indicated for patients who fail lifestyle, diet, and medical treatments. In these patients, consideration of neurosensory changes with hypersensitivity should be considered with trigger reduction and potentially neuromodulating medications. Those patients whose symptoms are controlled with PPI and/or have large hiatal hernias may experience benefit from fundoplication; however, there is a paucity of data to support this treatment option in LPR patients. Increased interest among investigators, better understanding of the pathophysiology, and the trend of better-designed research studies bodes well for the future of evidence-based LPR treatment.

References

1. Lechien JR, Saussez S, Schindle A, et al. Clinical outcomes of Laryngopharyngeal reflux treatment: a systematic review and meta-analysis. Laryngoscope. 2018;00:1–14.
2. Lechien JR, Dapri G, Dequanter D, et al. Surgical treatment for Laryngopharyngeal reflux disease: a systematic review. JAMA Otolaryngology – Head & Neck Surgery. 2019;145(7):655–66.
3. Jacobson BC, Somers SC, Fuchs CS, et al. Body-mass index and symptoms of gstroesophageal reflux in women. N Engl J Med. 2006;354:2340–8.
4. Fraser-Moodie CA, Norton B, Gornall C, et al. Weight loss has an independent beneficial effect on symptoms of gastroesophageal reflux in patients who are overweight. Scand J Gastroenterol. 1999;34:337–40.
5. Aslam M, Slaughter JC, Goutte M, et al. Nonlinear relationship between body mass index and esophageal acid exposure in the extraesophageal manifestations of reflux. Clin Gastroenterol Hepatol. 2012;10:874–8.
6. Kaltenbach T, Crockett S, Gerson LB. Are lifestyle measures effective in patients with gastroesophageal reflux disease? An evidence-based approach. Arch Intern Med. 2006;166:965–71.
7. Zalvan CH, Hu S, Greenberg B, Geliebter J. A comparison of alkaline water and Mediterranean diet vs proton pump inhibition for treatment of laryngopharyngeal reflux. JAMA Otolaryngol Head Neck Surg. 2017;143:1023–9.
8. Koufman JA. Low acid diet for recalcitrant laryngopharyngeal reflux: therapeutic benefits and their implications. Ann Otol Rhinol Laryngol. 2011;120:281–7.
9. Koufman JA, Johnston N. Potential benefits of pH 8.8 alkaline drinking water as an adjunct in the treatment of reflux disease. Ann Otol Rhinol Laryngol. 2012;121(7):431–4.
10. Lechien JR, Bobin F, Mouawad F, et al. Development of scores assessing the refluxogenic potential of diet of patients with laryngopharyngeal reflux. Eur Arch Otorhinolaryngol. 2019;276:3389–404.
11. Modlin IM, Kidd M, Lye KD. Historical perspectives on the treatment of gastroesophageal reflux disease. Gastrointest Endosc Clin N Am. 2003;13(1):19–55.. vii–viii
12. Narchi NE, Price LL. Ethnobiology of corals and coral reefs. Springer International Publishing; 2015. https://www.springer.com/gp/book/9783319237626. Accessed 2 Jul 2019.
13. Schubert ML. Proton pump inhibitors: placing putative adverse effects in proper perspective. Curr Opin Gastroenterol. 2019;35(6):509–16.
14. Vaezi MF, Katzka D, Zerbib F. Extraesophageal symptoms and diseases attributed to GERD: where is the pendulum swinging now? Clinical Gastro and Hepatol. 2018;16:1018–29.
15. Sontag SJ, O'Conell S, Khandelwal S, et al. Asthmatics with gastroesophageal reflux: long term results of a randomized trial of medical and surgical antireflux therapies. Am J Gastroenterl. 2003;98:987–99.

16. Park W, Hicks DM, Khandwala F, et al. Laryngopharyngeal reflux: prospective cohort study evaluating optimal dose of proton-pump inhibitor therapy and pretherapy predictors of response. Laryngoscope. 2005;115:1230–8.
17. Williams RB, Szczesniak MM, Maclean JC, et al. Predictors of outcome in an open label, therapeutic trial of high-dose omeprazole in laryngitis. Am J Gastroenterol. 2004;99:777–85.
18. Vaezi MF, Richter JE, Stasney CR, et al. Treatment of chronic posterior laryngitis with esomeprazole. Laryngoscope. 2006;116:254–60.
19. Qadeer MA, Phillips CO, Lopez AR, Steward DL, et al. Proton pump inhibitor therapy for suspected GERD-related chronic laryngitis: a meta-analysis of randomized controlled trials. Am J Gastroenterol. 2006;101(11):2646–54.
20. Megwalu UC. A systematic review of proton-pump inhibitor therapy for laryngopharyngeal reflux. Ear Nose Throat J. 2013;92(8):364–71.
21. Wei C. A meta-analysis for the role of proton pump inhibitor therapy in patients with laryngopharyngeal reflux. Eur Arch Otorhinolaryngol. 2016;273(11):3795–801.
22. Liu C, Wang H, Liu K. Meta-analysis of the efficacy of proton pump inhibitors for the symptoms of laryngopharyngeal reflux. Braz J Med Biol Res. 2016;49(7):e5149.
23. Guo H, Ma H, Wang J. Proton pump inhibitor therapy for the treatment of laryngopharyngeal reflux: a meta-analysis of randomized controlled trials. J Clin Gastroenterol. 2016;50:295–300.
24. American Lung Association Asthma Clinical Research Centers, Mastronarde JG, Anthonisen NR, Castro M, Holbrook JT, Leone FT, Teague WG, Wise RA. Efficacy of esomeprazole for treatment of poorly controlled asthma. N Engl J Med. 2009;360(15):1487–99.
25. Shaheen NJ, Crockett SC, Bright SD, et al. Randomised clinical trial: high-dose acid suppression for chronic cough: a double-blind, placebo-controlled study. Aliment Pharmacol Ther. 2011;33:225–34.
26. Ren LH, Chen WX, Qian LJ, et al. Addition of prokinetics to PPI therapy in gastroesophageal reflux disease: a meta-analysis. World J Gastroenterol. 2014;20:2412–9.
27. Glicksman JT, Mick PT, Fung K, et al. Prokinetic agents and laryngopharyngeal reflux disease: prokinetic agents and laryngopharyngeal reflux disease: a systematic review. Laryngoscope. 2014;124:2375–9.
28. Li S, Shi S, Chen F, Lin J. The effects of baclofen for the treatment of gastroesophageal reflux disease: a meta-analysis of randomized controlled trials. Gastroenterol Res Pract. 2014;2014:307805.
29. Lee YC, Jung AR, Kwon OE, et al. The effect of baclofen combined with a proton pump inhibitor in patients with refractory laryngopharyngeal reflux: a prospective, open-label study in thirty-two patients. Clin Otolaryngol. 2019;44(3):431–4.
30. Zentilin P, Dulbecco P, Savarino E, Parodi A, et al. An evaluation of the antireflux properties of sodium alginate by means of combined multichannel intraluminal impedance and pH-metry. Aliment Pharmacol Ther. 2005;21(1):29–34.
31. Reimer C, Lodrup AB, Smith G, et al. Randomised clinical trial: alginate (Gaviscon Advance) vs. placebo as add-on therapy in reflux patients with inadequate response to a once daily proton pump inhibitor. Aliment Pharmacol Ther. 2016;43:899–909.
32. Leiman DA, Riff BP, Morgan S, Metz DC, et al. Alginate therapy is effective treatment for GERD symptoms: a systematic review and meta-analysis. Dis Esophagus. 2017;30(5):1–9.
33. McGlashan JA, Johnstone LM, Sykes J, et al. The value of a liquid alginate suspension (Gaviscon Advance) in the management of laryngopharyngeal reflux. Eur Arch Otolrhinolaryngol. 2009;266:243–51.
34. Wilkie MD, Fraser HM, Raja H. Gaviscon Advance alone versus co-prescription of Gaviscon Advance and proton pump inhibitors in the treatment of laryngopharyngeal reflux. Eur Arch Otorhinolaryngol. 2018;275:2515–21.
35. Saifullah AM, Ahmed F, Shil BC, et al. Comparative study of alginate and omeprazole in symptomatic treatment of non-erosive gastroesophageal reflux disease. Mymensingh Med J. 2018;27:771–5.

36. Tseng WH, Tseng PH, Wu JF, et al. Double-blind, placebo-controlled study with alginate suspension for laryngopharyngeal reflux disease. Laryngoscope. 2018;128(10):2252–60.
37. Meshikes AWN. Evidence based surgery: the obstacles and solutions. Int J Surgery. 2015;18:159–62.
38. Sidwa F, Moore AL, Alligood E, Fisichella PM. Surgical treatment of extraesophageal manifestations of gastroesophageal reflux disease. World J Surg. 2017;41(10):2566–71.
39. Sontag SJ, O'Connell S, Khandelwal S, et al. Asthmatics with gastroesophageal reflux: long term results of a randomized trial of medical and surgical antireflux therapies. Am J Gastroenterol. 2003;98:987–99.

Chapter 36
Treatment Results for Gastroesophageal Reflux Disease

John O. Clarke

Introduction

Gastroesophageal reflux disease (GERD) is a common condition in the United States that affects approximately 20% of American adults on a weekly basis [1] with similar prevalence in other Western countries [2]. In addition to significant symptoms affecting quality of life, GERD can also lead to numerous complications including esophagitis, esophageal strictures, Barrett's esophagus, and esophageal adenocarcinoma [3]. Data suggest that both reflux disease and esophageal adenocarcinoma have increased over the past decades and are on the rise [4]. Treatment of GERD is thus important as it both reduces symptoms and lessens the risk that reflux may lead to more worrisome downstream consequences. This chapter focuses on treatment results for GERD and how to potentially compare the different options available, as well as reviews what are considered current best practices.

While GERD is a common condition, the pathophysiology and clinical presentation of GERD are not homogeneous, and affected people may develop symptoms due to several potential mechanisms – either in isolation or more often in combination [5]. Proposed etiologies include disruption of the esophagogastric junction (EGJ) via hiatal hernia or a hypotensive lower esophageal sphincter (LES), increased transient lower esophageal sphincter relaxation (TLESR) episodes, impaired esophageal acid clearance, alterations in the postprandial acid pocket, changes in salivary production, impaired gastric emptying, altered esophageal tissue integrity, delayed gastric emptying, microbiome modification, increased intra-abdominal pressure, and esophageal hypersensitivity [6]. This is an important factor when one considers the relative efficacy of different treatment options – as subgroup selection will dictate which therapies are potentially most likely to be effective for specific patients.

J. O. Clarke (✉)
Esophageal Program, Division of Gastroenterology & Hepatology, Stanford University, Redwood City, CA, USA
e-mail: john.clarke@stanford.edu

C. H. Zalvan (ed.), *Laryngopharyngeal and Gastroesophageal Reflux*,
https://doi.org/10.1007/978-3-030-48890-1_36

For example, a patient with a large hiatal hernia and bland nighttime regurgitation may respond well to a hiatal hernia repair with fundoplication but is less likely to respond to medical therapy alone. Conversely, a patient with reflux in the context of scleroderma and absent esophageal contractility may do much better with medical acid suppressive therapy than surgical intervention. These differences in patient selection and subgroup need to be taken into account when discussing GERD treatment results, as often review of the data is not an apple-to-apple comparison.

In addition to differences in GERD phenotype, there are other factors that need to be considered when evaluating treatment response rates for different modalities of treatment. For example, studies sponsored by a large pharmaceutical company may have available resources to pursue a large clinical trial, whereas this would likely be impossible for treatment modalities which are not linked to industry, such as diet, lifestyle, or fundoplication. Likewise, studies that are more accommodative to unselected GERD patients such as many of the proton pump inhibitor (PPI) trials are going to enroll far larger numbers than for example studies evaluating the role of specific endoscopic therapies in very narrowly defined subsets. Definitions of treatment success also vary. For example, acid suppression or resolution of esophagitis is a standard outcome in trials looking at medical antireflux therapy; however, this may not be appropriate for a therapy such as endoscopic radiofrequency which may lead to improvement without necessarily modifying acid parameters [7, 8].

With these caveats, one is left with the questions: how should reflux be treated and how do the various treatment options compare? There are a multitude of options available including diet, lifestyle modification, medical therapy (antacids, histamine-receptor blockers, PPIs, alginates, prokinetics, and baclofen), endoscopic therapies (endoscopic radiofrequency, transoral plication), and surgical therapy (fundoplication, magnetic sphincter augmentation, and gastric bypass). Can they be compared head-to-head and what is best practice at present? This will be the focus of the remainder of this chapter.

Treatment Options for GERD

There are many potential treatment options for reflux, as detailed above, ranging from lifestyle modification to gastric bypass. Each will be addressed in turn, focusing briefly on the published results of each available options.

Diet and Lifestyle Modification

As for most diseases in Western medicine today, there is a clear role for diet and lifestyle modification in the treatment of reflux. Multiple interventions have been described to be of benefit, including elevating the head of the bed, weight loss, restriction of alcohol consumption, elimination of smoking, avoidance of tight-fitting clothing, restriction in late-night eating, and avoidance of certain foods believed to be potential reflux triggers [9–12]. Many of these interventions are difficult to study in large trials for a variety of reasons; however, the available data with regard to outcome for these interventions are encouraging. Of the lifestyle interventions detailed above, weight loss is at present the best studied. Two randomized clinical trials followed esophageal acid exposure time after weight loss and showed reduction (from 5.6% to 3.7% in one study [13] and from 8.0% to 5.5% in the other [14]) and several prospective observational studies have demonstrated reduction in reflux symptoms in parallel with weight loss [9]. Tobacco cessation has been shown to reduce reflux symptoms in a large prospective cohort study. Randomized clinical trials have shown reduction in supine acid exposure with both head-of-the-bed elevation and reduction in late evening meals [15]. A recent study utilizing dietary intervention on GERD patients while monitoring via a 96-hour wireless pH study showed significant improvement in acid exposure with dietary medication alone – in fact, in this study, 32 patients had abnormal esophageal acid exposure on their regular diet and 21 of these patients normalized their acid exposure on reflux-directed dietary intervention [16]. Most of the other suggested lifestyle modifications are based on anecdotal observation and gestalt understanding of underlying mechanisms and are not supported necessarily with data per se.

When one evaluates the outcome data for lifestyle and dietary intervention for GERD, the available data support sensible changes in lifestyle, and in particular weight loss, as an initial approach to treatment. The data with regard to weight loss in particular seem consistent in available reports. Extrapolating from what has been published to date, a 10% reduction in weight seems to be a reasonable target in order to see reduction in GERD symptoms in a patient with GERD and overweight status [17]. Elevating the head of the bed slightly, reducing late night eating, tobacco cessation if appropriate, and eating a healthier diet (smaller portions, higher fiber) also seem supported by the literature – with the caveat that data are limited. However, given the fact that diet and lifestyle interventions carry zero risk and may have other health benefits, this is generally the first step for treatment of GERD in my own personal practice and definitely worth pursuing before engaging in other options that may carry more potential risk.

Medical Reflux Therapy

Medications have been the mainstay of reflux management for years and options include antacids, histamine-receptor antagonists (HRAs), proton pump inhibitors (PPIs), and other less-frequently used options such as alginates, baclofen, and prokinetics. While these therapies will be reviewed in a separate chapter, this discussion will focus briefly on the treatment results that can be expected for these therapies – and the specific subgroups where one may wish to consider these interventions specifically.

Antacids are often the first medication employed and are comprised of a mixture of aluminum, calcium, and/or magnesium with the goal of buffering acid temporarily and reducing immediate symptoms. The main advantage of these medications is quick symptom response and relative safety. However, they do not provide long-term symptom relief, have not been shown to heal esophagitis, and do not prevent long-term consequences from reflux. They are best utilized in patients with rare breakthrough symptoms or as an add-on therapy to other agents [3, 18].

HRAs decrease gastric acid production through antagonism of histamine-2 receptors and were a treatment revolution when initially introduced in the 1970s – as they were by far the best medical therapy available for reflux at that time. This class of medications improves symptoms relatively quickly (within 15–30 minutes) by decreasing acid production and has been shown to improve both symptoms and mucosal healing. Data suggest resolution of esophagitis in approximately 40% of treated patients, as opposed to 20% with placebo [19, 20]. In addition, heartburn can be expected to improve after 4–12 weeks of treatment in approximately half of patients [3]. There is a clear dose response and higher doses can be expected to work better than lower doses or single-day dosing. These agents are not as effective as PPIs and also have tachyphylaxis (as histamine is one of three separate triggers for gastric acid production), which may make them less suitable for long-term maintenance therapy. These medications are best utilized in patients with intermittent reflux symptoms without erosive esophagitis or Barrett's esophagus, as an adjunct to PPI therapy or as an option for step-down therapy after PPI use in patients with uncomplicated GERD.

PPIs have been the mainstay of medical therapy for GERD since their introduction in the late 1980s and provide irreversible blockade of the activated proton pump in gastric parietal cells. PPIs effectively block acid production in the majority of patients; but, of note, they do not affect other potential reflux mechanisms and so do not alter reflux numbers or motility. Their main effect is to change the pH concentration of the refluxate from acid (pH < 4) to either weakly acidic (pH 4–7) or alkaline (pH > 7). Data show that PPIs are the most effective single medical therapy for healing of esophagitis. Short-term PPI therapy heals esophagitis in approximately 75% of patients (as compared to 40% with HRAs and 20% with placebo) [19, 20] and maintains healing of erosive esophagitis in over 90% of patients [21]. However, PPIs are felt to be only effective for acid-mediated symptoms – and as not all reflux is acidic, response rates for symptom resolution for PPI therapy are typically lower than response rates for healing of esophagitis. Even for patients with documented esophagitis, response rates for heartburn resolution ranges from 56% to 77%, and in patients without erosive esophagitis, standard doses of PPI therapy resolves heartburn in only 37–61% of patients [3]. Atypical symptoms such as regurgitation and cough respond less favorably than supposedly acid-mediated symptoms such as heartburn. Putting these data in aggregate, one can surmise that PPIs are quite effective for resolution of esophagitis, although not perfect; however, PPIs are not as effective for symptom control. Their greatest efficacy is with symptoms clearly linked in most cases to abnormal acid exposure or sensitivity, such as heartburn; however, symptom response falls off, as the symptoms become more atypical and less clearly acid mediated. For example, in patients with chronic cough or isolated laryngeal symptoms, response rates to PPIs are believed to be less than 20% [5, 22, 23]. PPIs are best utilized for patients with complicated GERD who need long-term maintenance therapy or for short-term therapy in patients who are not responsive to diet, lifestyle, and HRAs – and despite the limitations detailed above, they remain the mainstay of medical therapy today.

The vast majority of patients with reflux who opt for treatment pursue antacids, HRAs, and PPIs. The use of other agents is far less and not surprisingly data are more limited. Alginates can create a physical barrier against reflux by forming a raft which covers the acid pocket and increasing the viscosity of the gastric contents. As concerns have increased regarding long-term PPI safety, alginates have had a recent renewed interest. A recent randomized controlled trial showed symptom improvement in 47% of patients treated with an alginate formulation as compared to 33% of patients treated with placebo [24]; however, other studies have not demonstrated superiority of alginates over placebo [25, 26]. While data are emerging, the available evidence suggests a modest benefit over placebo and these agents can be considered either for treatment of patients with mild symptoms who do not desire prescription therapy or as add-on therapy for patients with refractory symptoms despite standard therapy.

Sucralfate is a complex of sucrose sulfate and aluminum hydroxide and binds to denuded foregut mucosa. It has been demonstrated to have greater efficacy than placebo in patients with erosive esophagitis; however, it has not been shown to have efficacy in patients with nonerosive reflux disease [27]. Similar to alginates, this may have a role in every selected patient but is certainly not a mainstay of therapy, especially as it requires frequent dosing, can be linked with constipation, and may affect absorption of other medications.

Prokinetics (metoclopramide, domperidone, and prucalopride) are also sometimes utilized for treatment of reflux with the hypothesis that accelerated gastric emptying may lessen reflux burden – and these medications may also increase lower esophageal sphincter pressure and potentially improve esophageal clearance. However, the data do not suggest a clear benefit for these medications in the average GERD patient. A meta-analysis of randomized studies found only modest reductions in symptom scores when these medications were employed, without improvement in esophagitis healing – and with an increased risk of adverse effects [28]. In practice, these medications may have an adjunct role for the treatment of GERD patients with associated dysmotility or impaired gastric emptying but have a far more limited and uncertain future for the average GERD patient.

Finally, baclofen is a gamma-amino butyric acid B receptor agonist, which has been shown to reduce TLESRs and reduce reflux events in healthy volunteers as well as GERD patients. However, side effects are significant, tachyphylaxis may develop, and it also may reduce esophageal clearance. In addition, there are no clinical trials demonstrating efficacy in healing of erosive esophagitis – or in long-term symptom control [29]. Baclofen may have an add-on role for selected patients, but does not play a role at present in management of most GERD patients.

Endoscopic Reflux Therapy

For selected patients who do not tolerate medical therapy or desire nonmedical options, endoscopic therapies have emerged as a potential alternative. While numerous avenues have been explored over the past two decades, only two endoscopic interventions are currently available: radiofrequency ablation (RFA) and transoral incisionless fundoplication (TIF). Patients enrolled in studies evaluating these techniques have been very carefully selected to exclude patients with a significant hiatal hernia, severe esophagitis, or reflux complications (strictures or Barrett's esophagus). The data with regard to these treatment options are significantly limited when compared to the data regarding medical therapies detailed above.

RFA has been approved in the United States for over 15 years. Initial studies suggested improvement with subjective clinical parameters including symptoms; however, there are no available data with regard to esophagitis healing, as these patients were excluded from the clinical trials [3, 30]. Two recent meta-analyses were published with conflicting results. One meta-analysis looking at only randomized clinical trials reported that there was no evidence that RFA improved acid exposure time, lower esophageal sphincter pressure, or quality of life [7]. However, a second meta-analysis evaluating both randomized and nonrandomized studies found improvements in both acid exposure time and quality of life [8]. Given this data, it is impossible to compare RFA with therapies such as PPIs as there are no data with regard to mucosal healing and variable data on symptom improvement. A recent publication highlighted the role of RFA as a potential means to bridge patients off PPI therapy [31]. At present, the role of RFA for GERD patients is still being defined; however, the ideal patient appears to be someone who is either PPI-dependent or unable to take PPI therapy and who has nonerosive reflux disease without a significant hiatal hernia and symptoms severe enough to warrant more aggressive intervention.

TIF operates on the hypothesis that endoscopic therapy can create a more robust structural barrier at the EGJ but use and data remain limited. Similar to RFA, patients enrolled in TIF clinical trials were carefully selected to avoid patients with significant reflux esophagitis, complications of reflux, or a significant hiatal hernia. Hence, the criteria to gauge treatment response are different from those used in assessing medical therapies – and most of the data to date evaluates symptoms, acid exposure time, and PPI use. In a recent systemic review with meta-analysis including 18 studies published over the past decade, the authors concluded that the relative risk of response rate to TIF versus PPIs/sham was 2 [32]; however, the esophageal acid exposure time did not significantly improve, PPI usage increased with time, and most of the patients had resumed PPI therapy (albeit at a reduced dosage) during long-term follow-up. Patient satisfaction with TIF was only 69% at 6 months [33]. While data continue to emerge with regard to TIF, the outcomes seem suboptimal at present (at least in the published data). Similarly to RFA, the ideal patient for TIF appears to be someone who is either PPI-dependent or unable to take PPI therapy and who has nonerosive reflux disease without a significant hiatal hernia and symptoms severe enough to warrant more aggressive intervention.

Surgical Reflux Therapy

Surgery has been a mainstay of therapy for reflux since the introduction of the fundoplication by Dr. Rudolf Nissen in the 1950s. Use of antireflux surgery (ARS) peaked in 2009 and has declined since that point. When one evaluates treatment outcomes with ARS for GERD patients, the main criteria employed are acid exposure time, symptom/quality of life improvement, and absence of esophagitis on postoperative evaluation. Laparoscopic fundoplication [either via a full-thickness (Nissen) wrap or a partial 270-degree (Toupet) wrap] has been the traditional mainstay of ARS therapy. Response rates for ARS are comparable to those of long-term PPI therapy in randomized clinical trials [34–36]. In a seminal European study comparing laparoscopic fundoplication to medical therapy with esomeprazole in 554 GERD patients, remission rates at the end of 5 years were 92% in the PPI group and 85% in the ARS group – not statistically different between the two groups. Similar to the PPI discussion above, ARS is most effective in patients where reflux is unequivocally proven and shown to be the source of symptoms; when symptoms are more atypical and reflux is less well defined, not surprisingly, response rates also are less robust. In a best-case scenario, ARS has been shown to resolve significant symptoms in 90% of patients at 10 years [37]; however, other investigators report less robust results [3]. In a recent nationwide, population-based retrospective cohort study in Sweden, 18% of patients who underwent laparoscopic fundoplication and were followed up for a median of 6.7 years were found to have recurrence. Of those patients with recurrence, 84% were placed on medical therapy and 16% underwent a second antireflux surgery [38]. More recently, a randomized clinical trial of medical versus surgical therapy for refractory heartburn published in *New England Journal of Medicine* suggested that ARS was superior to medical treatment in highly selected patients with symptoms of gastroesophageal reflux disease despite PPI therapy [39]. However, it should be noted that only a minority of patients evaluated for study inclusion qualified for surgery and this study evaluated patients specifically with refractory reflux symptoms despite PPI therapy. When one evaluates this data in aggregate, ARS seems to be a good option for patients who have complicated reflux disease despite medical therapy, patients who have clearly proven GERD with associated symptoms despite medical therapy, patients with a structural abnormality such as a hiatal hernia, and patients who cannot tolerate PPI therapy due to side effects. The role for ARS in a young patient well controlled on PPI therapy remains controversial. However, as ARS is not without risk, side effects can be seen afterward, and recurrence may be a factor, one needs to consider the relative risks/benefits of the intervention on a case-by-case basis.

Magnetic sphincter augmentation (MSA) utilizes a bracelet of titanium-encased magnets which is surgically implanted at the EGJ to augment lower esophageal sphincter pressure and prevent reflux. In a seminal paper evaluating MSA in 100 patients published in *New England Journal of Medicine*, the authors reported normalization or a 50% reduction in acid exposure time in 64% of patients at 1 year [40]. At 5-year follow-up, the authors reported improvement in quality of life (for patients both on and off PPI therapy at baseline), reduction in PPI use from 100% to

15%, reduction in heartburn from 89% to 12%, and reduction in regurgitation from 57% to 1.2% [41]. Patients in these initial studies were carefully selected to include patients with partial PPI response, documented reflux, no significant hiatal hernia, and normal esophageal motility. Short-term dysphagia has been reported as high as 68% but was only 6% at long-term follow-up [40, 41]. Device removal has been required in approximately 3–7% of patients [41, 42]. The outcome data for ARS and MSA appear similar and this was highlighted in a recent systematic review [43]. The main selling point of MSA appears to be the technical ease of implantation and the ability to maintain the patient's ability to belch; however, MSA does not at present have the long-term data available for ARS.

Finally, any discussion of surgical antireflux therapies would not be complete without a brief discussion of bariatric surgery. Roux-en-Y gastric bypass decreases intragastric pressure and decreases reflux burden and symptoms in obese patients. Whether the improvement relates to metabolic factors, reduction in intragastric pressure, weight loss itself, or other mechanisms remains unclear. While long-term outcome data are emerging, a recent white paper from the Society of American Gastrointestinal and Endoscopic Surgeons (SAGES) provided an "expert recommendation" that gastric bypass "should be considered the gold-standard approach to symptoms attributed to reflux in a population with a BMI > 35 kg/m^2" [44]. Magnetic esophageal sphincter augmentation supported by several small studies showed improvement in symptoms, PPI discontinuation, and reduction in esophageal acid exposure in obese GERD patients who underwent gastric bypass [32, 45–47]. However, there remains some question as to the absolute efficacy of gastric bypass, as a recent nationwide cohort study from Sweden of patients undergoing gastric bypass over a 10-year period showed rapid improvement in reflux symptoms following bypass, but recurrence with time with almost half of patients noting recurrence of GERD symptoms requiring intervention within 2 years of surgery [48]. With that caveat, gastric bypass is believed to be the best surgical option for GERD at present in the obese population.

Best Practices

GERD is a heterogenous condition comprised of multiple distinct clinical subsets, with unique associated pathophysiologic and treatment considerations that must be taken into account for each individual patient [49]. While common treatment pathways may exist for individual symptoms, it stands to reason that patients will respond most optimally to therapies tailored specifically for their individual parameters. For example, a patient with reflux symptoms and a large hiatal hernia is unlikely to respond to medical therapy and will likely be most optimally treated with a surgical hiatal hernia repair; however, a patient with reflux in the context of gastroparesis may do dismally with a traditionally antireflux surgery, yet respond well to a combination of acid suppressive therapy and prokinetics.

With this caveat, one can make assumptions about best practices for the majority of GERD patients. If a patient presents with symptoms of GERD and associated alarm findings (for example, weight loss, dysphagia, rapid progression, age >60), then endoscopic evaluation is always warranted as a first step. However, given the high prevalence of reflux and the economic burden which would be invoked if every patient with GERD symptoms underwent diagnostic testing, if a patient presents with GERD symptoms in the absence of alarm findings, then the first step in care before testing is often treatment via either diet and lifestyle modifications or a trial of PPI therapy. If patients do not improve following these initial measures then formal diagnostic testing is often employed to better define whether symptoms truly relate to reflux. This testing may be via a variety of modalities but often consists of endoscopy plus potential formal pH or pH/impedance testing [5, 50]. According to the Lyon Consensus recently published in *Gut*, a diagnosis of GERD can be established by the presence/absence of esophagitis, abnormal parameters on pH testing, or a combination of adjunct tests [5].

For a patient with traditional reflux symptoms or confirmed reflux, best practice would involve a step-up approach. One may begin with diet and lifestyle modification, followed by – or in conjunction with – medical therapy. PPIs are the mainstay of therapy, in particular for complicated GERD (Barrett's esophagus, erosive esophagitis, and peptic strictures); however, they do have potential risks and there has been emerging concern with regard to potential long-term use [51, 52]. If one starts PPI therapy, then the goal is to treat the patient for a finite period of time and then to consider potentially tapering them off if their symptoms are well controlled and they have no evidence of reflux-induced complications. Many patients are able to taper off PPIs entirely through the use of HRA step-down therapy and diet/lifestyle modifications. However, many patients may not be able to taper off PPIs and the goal in those patients is to find the lowest dose that controls symptoms reliably. For patients with reflux-induced complications, data support the use of long-term PPI therapy and recurrence of erosive disease is approximately 80% if PPI therapy is discontinued.

If a patient is not well controlled on PPI therapy, then several steps can be taken. Often, compliance and timing of PPI administration are reviewed, as these can play a clear role in successful treatment. Following that, there may be a benefit in switching to a different PPI or using HRAs, baclofen, alginates or sucralfate as add-on therapy. Diet and lifestyle again become a source of discussion. This is also a point where formal reflux testing can often separate whether symptoms stem from continued acid production, nonacid reflux, or a functional etiology – all of which would change the management algorithm.

If a patient is still symptomatic despite medical therapy or intolerant to medical therapy or unwilling to take medical therapy, then surgical options become very reasonable. This is particularly the case if there is a structural component to their symptoms such as a hiatal hernia. At this point, either traditional ARS via fundoplication or MSA is a very reasonable option based on the outcome data to date. Often, the decision as to which technique to perform is made, based on discussion of the individual risks and benefits with the patient – and via local practice patterns and expertise. Finally, for the obese patient with reflux, gastric bypass surgery remains the ideal option if weight loss cannot be achieved with nonsurgical means, and symptoms, despite medical therapy, are severe enough to require intervention.

Conclusion

GERD is a common condition with multiple potential underlying mechanisms. While outcome data can be used to guide decision-making, the ideal therapy needs to be tailored to the individual patient and their specific mechanisms of symptom pathogenesis and goals of care. The discussion above provides a framework to understand the relative efficacy of treatment outcomes, but it is important to remember that GERD is a heterogeneous collection of different clinically relevant phenotypes and one size will not fit all with regard to treatment. However, by starting with a bottom-up approach and utilizing the armamentarium of treatment approaches detailed in this chapter, the vast majority of GERD patients can be treated successfully.

Conflicts of Interest None.
Funding None.

References

1. Locke GR 3rd, Talley NJ, Fett SL, et al. Prevalence and clinical spectrum of gastroesophageal reflux: a population-based study in Olmsted County, Minnesota. Gastroenterology. 1997;112:1448–56.
2. Hálfdánarson Ó, Pottegård A, Björnsson ES, et al. Proton-pump inhibitors among adults: a nationwide drug-utilization study. Ther Adv Gastroenterol. 2018;11:1756284818777943.
3. Gyawali CP, Fass R. Management of gastroesophageal reflux disease. Gastroenterology. 2018;154:302–18.
4. Boeckxstaens G, El-Serag HB, Smout AJ, et al. Symptomatic reflux disease: the present, the past and the future. Gut. 2014;63:1185–93.
5. Gyawali CP, Kahrilas PJ, Savarino E, et al. Modern diagnosis of GERD: the Lyon Consensus. Gut. 2018;67:1351–62.
6. Tack J, Pandolfino JE. Pathophysiology of gastroesophageal reflux disease. Gastroenterology. 2018;154:277–88.
7. Lipka S, Kumar A, Richter JE. No evidence for efficacy of radiofrequency ablation for treatment of gastroesophageal reflux disease: a systematic review and meta-analysis. Clin Gastroenterol Hepatol. 2015;13:1058–67.e1.
8. Fass R, Cahn F, Scotti DJ, et al. Systematic review and meta-analysis of controlled and prospective cohort efficacy studies of endoscopic radiofrequency for treatment of gastroesophageal reflux disease. Surg Endosc. 2017;31:4865–82.
9. Ness-Jensen E, Hveem K, El-Serag H, et al. Lifestyle intervention in gastroesophageal reflux disease. Clin Gastroenterol Hepatol. 2016;14:175–82.e1–3.
10. Sethi S, Richter JE. Diet and gastroesophageal reflux disease: role in pathogenesis and management. Curr Opin Gastroenterol. 2017;33:107–11.
11. Newberry C, Lynch K. Can we use diet to effectively treat esophageal disease? A review of the current literature. Curr Gastroenterol Rep. 2017;19:38.
12. Ahuja A, Ahuja NK. Popular remedies for esophageal symptoms: a critical appraisal. Curr Gastroenterol Rep. 2019;21:39.
13. Mathus-Vliegen EM, Tygat GN. Gastro-oesophageal reflux in obese subjects: influence of overweight, weight loss and chronic gastric balloon distension. Scand J Gastroenterol. 2002;37:1246–52.

14. Mathus-Vliegen EM, van Weeren M, van Eerten PV. Los function and obesity: the impact of untreated obesity, weight loss, and chronic gastric balloon distension. Digestion. 2003;68:161–8.
15. Navalgund A, Axelrod S, Axelrod L, et al. Colon myoelectric activity measured after open abdominal surgery with a noninvasive wireless patch system predicts time to first flatus. J Gastrointest Surg. 2019;23:982–9.
16. Triadafilopoulos G, Korzilius JW, Zikos T, et al. Ninety-six hour wireless esophageal pH study in patients with GERD shows that restrictive diet reduces esophageal acid exposure. Dig Dis Sci. 2019; https://doi.org/10.1007/s10620-019-05940-9.
17. De Bortoli N, Tolone S, Savarino EV. Weight loss is truly effective in reducing symptoms and proton pump inhibitor use in patients with gastroesophageal reflux disease. Clin Gastroenterol Hepatol. 2015;13:2023.
18. Kroch DA, Madanick RD. Medical treatment of gastroesophageal reflux disease. World J Surg. 2017;41:1678–84.
19. Khan M, Santana J, Donnellan C, et al. Medical treatments in the short term management of reflux oesophagitis. Cochrane Database Syst Rev. 2007:CD003244.
20. Weijenborg PW, Cremonini F, Smout AJ, et al. PPI therapy is equally effective in well-defined non-erosive reflux disease and in reflux esophagitis: a meta-analysis. Neurogastroenterol Motil. 2012;24:747–57.. e350
21. Johnson DA, Benjamin SB, Vakil NB, et al. Esomeprazole once daily for 6 months is effective therapy for maintaining healed erosive esophagitis and for controlling gastroesophageal reflux disease symptoms: a randomized, double-blind, placebo-controlled study of efficacy and safety. Am J Gastroenterol. 2001;96:27–34.
22. Vaezi MF, Richter JE, Stasney CR, et al. Treatment of chronic posterior laryngitis with esomeprazole. Laryngoscope. 2006;116:254–60.
23. Hersh MJ, Sayuk GS, Gyawali CP. Long-term therapeutic outcome of patients undergoing ambulatory pH monitoring for chronic unexplained cough. J Clin Gastroenterol. 2010;44:254–60.
24. Wilkinson J, Wade A, Thomas SJ, et al. Randomized clinical trial: a double-blind, placebo-controlled study to assess the clinical efficacy and safety of alginate-antacid (Gaviscon Double Action) chewable tablets in patients with gastro-oesophageal reflux disease. Eur J Gastroenterol Hepatol. 2019;31:86–93.
25. Tseng WH, Tseng PH, Wu JF, et al. Double-blind, placebo-controlled study with alginate suspension for laryngopharyngeal reflux disease. Laryngoscope. 2018;128:2252–60.
26. Kim JH, Lee YC, Kim EH, et al. The clinical efficacy of a pure alginate formulation (Lamina G) for controlling symptoms in individuals with reflux symptoms: a randomized clinical study. Gut Liver. 2019;13:642–8.
27. Simon B, Ravelli GP, Goffin H. Sucralfate gel versus placebo in patients with non-erosive gastro-oesophageal reflux disease. Aliment Pharmacol Ther. 1996;10:441–6.
28. Ren LH, Chen WX, Qian LJ, et al. Addition of prokinetics to PPI therapy in gastroesophageal reflux disease: a meta-analysis. World J Gastroenterol. 2014;20:2412–9.
29. Clarke JO, Fernandez-Becker NQ, Regalia KA, et al. Baclofen and gastroesophageal reflux disease: seeing the forest through the trees. Clin Transl Gastroenterol. 2018;9:137.
30. Corley DA, Katz P, Wo JM, et al. Improvement of gastroesophageal reflux symptoms after radiofrequency energy: a randomized, sham-controlled trial. Gastroenterology. 2003;125:668–76.
31. Viswanath Y, Maguire N, Obuobi RB, et al. Endoscopic day case antireflux radiofrequency (Stretta) therapy improves quality of life and reduce proton pump inhibitor (PPI) dependency in patients with gastro-oesophageal reflux disease: a prospective study from a UK tertiary centre. Frontline Gastroenterol. 2019;10:113–9.
32. Frezza EE, Ikramuddin S, Gourash W, et al. Symptomatic improvement in gastroesophageal reflux disease (GERD) following laparoscopic Roux-en-Y gastric bypass. Surg Endosc. 2002;16:1027–31.
33. Huang X, Chen S, Zhao H, et al. Efficacy of transoral incisionless fundoplication (TIF) for the treatment of GERD: a systematic review with meta-analysis. Surg Endosc. 2017;31:1032–44.

34. Mehta S, Bennett J, Mahon D, et al. Prospective trial of laparoscopic nissen fundoplication versus proton pump inhibitor therapy for gastroesophageal reflux disease: seven-year follow-up. J Gastrointest Surg. 2006;10:1312–6; discussion 1316–7.
35. Lundell L, Attwood S, Ell C, et al. Comparing laparoscopic antireflux surgery with esomeprazole in the management of patients with chronic gastro-oesophageal reflux disease: a 3-year interim analysis of the LOTUS trial. Gut. 2008;57:1207–13.
36. Galmiche JP, Hatlebakk J, Attwood S, et al. Laparoscopic antireflux surgery vs esomeprazole treatment for chronic GERD: the LOTUS randomized clinical trial. JAMA. 2011;305:1969–77.
37. Dallemagne B, Weerts J, Markiewicz S, et al. Clinical results of laparoscopic fundoplication at ten years after surgery. Surg Endosc. 2006;20:159–65.
38. Maret-Ouda J, Wahlin K, El-Serag HB, et al. Association between laparoscopic antireflux surgery and recurrence of gastroesophageal reflux. JAMA. 2017;318:939–46.
39. Spechler SJ, Hunter JG, Jones KM, et al. Randomized trial of medical versus surgical treatment for refractory heartburn. N Engl J Med. 2019;381:1513–23.
40. Ganz RA, Peters JH, Horgan S. Esophageal sphincter device for gastroesophageal reflux disease. N Engl J Med. 2013;368:2039–40.
41. Ganz RA, Edmundowicz SA, Taiganides PA, et al. Long-term outcomes of patients receiving a magnetic sphincter augmentation device for gastroesophageal reflux. Clin Gastroenterol Hepatol. 2016;14:671–7.
42. Lipham JC, Taiganides PA, Louie BE, et al. Safety analysis of first 1000 patients treated with magnetic sphincter augmentation for gastroesophageal reflux disease. Dis Esophagus. 2015;28:305–11.
43. Skubleny D, Switzer NJ, Dang J, et al. LINX® magnetic esophageal sphincter augmentation versus Nissen fundoplication for gastroesophageal reflux disease: a systematic review and meta-analysis. Surg Endosc. 2017;31:3078–84.
44. Nau P, Jackson HT, Aryaie A, et al. Surgical management of gastroesophageal reflux disease in the obese patient. Surg Endosc. 2020;34(1):450–7.
45. Nelson LG, Gonzalez R, Haines K, et al. Amelioration of gastroesophageal reflux symptoms following Roux-en-Y gastric bypass for clinically significant obesity. Am Surg. 2005;71:950–3; discussion 953–4.
46. Madalosso CA, Gurski RR, Callegari-Jacques SM, et al. The impact of gastric bypass on gastroesophageal reflux disease in morbidly obese patients. Ann Surg. 2016;263:110–6.
47. Mejía-Rivas MA, Herrera-López A, Hernández-Calleros J, et al. Gastroesophageal reflux disease in morbid obesity: the effect of Roux-en-Y gastric bypass. Obes Surg. 2008;18:1217–24.
48. Holmberg D, Santoni G, Xie S, et al. Gastric bypass surgery in the treatment of gastro-oesophageal reflux symptoms. Aliment Pharmacol Ther. 2019;50:159–66.
49. Triadafilopoulos G, Clarke JO, Hawn M. Precision GERD management for the 21st century. Dis Esophagus. 2017;30:1–6.
50. Gyawali CP, de Bortoli N, Clarke J, et al. Indications and interpretation of esophageal function testing. Ann N Y Acad Sci. 2018;1434:239–53.
51. Freedberg DE, Kim LS, Yang YX. The risks and benefits of long-term use of proton pump inhibitors: expert review and best practice advice from the American Gastroenterological Association. Gastroenterology. 2017;152:706–15.
52. Vaezi MF, Yang YX, Howden CW. Complications of proton pump inhibitor therapy. Gastroenterology. 2017;153:35–48.

Part V
Plant Based, Mediterranean Style Diet Based Approach to Reflux Treatment: A Primer

Chapter 37
Overview of the Plant-Based, Mediterranean-Style Diet Approach to Treating Reflux

Craig H. Zalvan

Reflux disease, both gastroesophageal reflux disease (GERD) and laryngopharyngeal reflux (LPR), has been treated for decades with ever-increasing expensive medication, cost-consuming diagnostic testing, endoscopic procedures, and finally a variety of surgical interventions for those that fail conservative treatment. Although diet and behavioral modifications are sometimes, not always, mentioned, time spent is often limited and barely reinforced. The modern patient typically wants, actually demands, a medication as the culture in modern society is pharmacologically based. Eighty-one percent of Americans take at least one prescription drug. Forty percent over age 65 are on more than five prescription with antidepressants, statins, and proton pump inhibitors (PPI) leading the rest by a far margin [1]. With reflux, typically a PPI is tried, often beyond the recommended time frame. Failure leads to a change in brand name, the addition of a second daily dose, a higher dose, and the addition of a different medication, such as an H2 blocker. Ultimately, billions are spent with this pharmacological approach often prolonging patient discomfort and anxiety for months to years.

> "Let your food be medicine and your medicine be food." – Hippocrates

Hippocrates understood then what still applies today. Much of what ails us relates to our environment with our food and beverage intake strongly influencing our health status. The next section of this text will serve to review the overall importance of diet, namely a mostly plant-based, Mediterranean-style diet, in maintaining

C. H. Zalvan (✉)
ENT and Allergy Associates, LLP; Voice and Swallow Division, Tarrytown, NY, USA

The Institute for Voice and Swallowing Disorders, Phelps Hospital, Northwell Health, Sleepy Hollow, NY, USA

Professor of Otolaryngology at the Donald and Barbara Zucker School of Medicine at Hofstra/Northwell, Phelps Hospital Campus, Sleepy Hollow, NY, USA

Communication, Speech Department at Mercy College, Dobbs Ferry, NY, USA
e-mail: czalvan@entandallergy.com

C. H. Zalvan (ed.), *Laryngopharyngeal and Gastroesophageal Reflux*,
https://doi.org/10.1007/978-3-030-48890-1_37

health and reversing disease. Typically, little time is spent in a doctor's visit discussing diet, especially when it comes to reflux. This leads to high levels of noncompliance avoiding the ultimate cure to the disease. This intervention marks the most important step in resolving symptoms, reversing physical changes, and preventing complications of this curable disease.

The last section of this book aims to provide the reader with an understanding of the concept of a plant-based, Mediterranean-style diet as an intervention to control reflux disease. The motivation and hypothetical thinking behind using this dietary approach and the application in a population-based study mark an important step toward diet utilization over prescriptions. In the chapter by Drs. Geliebter, Hu, Tiwari, and Zalvan, the study examining the use of this dietary regimen to control reflux itself is reviewed demonstrating the outcomes of dietary application to patients with LPR. Dr. Aviv then details his approach to acid neutralization based on his concept and book, *The Acid Watcher Diet*. Drs. DeLorgeril, Salen, and Zalvan then review the current concepts of the health benefits of a mostly plant-based, Mediterranean-style diet and its application to overall health and chronic disease. To provide practitioners with important useful concepts on plant-based diets, Dr. Rojido outlines the multiple components of a plant-based diet, nutritional requirements, and other medical conditions that potentially require special attention while eating a plant-based diet. Finally, Linda Arpino, MA, RDN, CDN, outlines a dietary guide meant as a "how to" transition to a plant-based diet. The ultimate goal is to provide the medical professional with a starting resource to delve into the concept of diet, nutrition, and overall health. As a resource, this section of the book will provide the reader with the means to start switching their own diets as they educate themselves on the health benefits. The best way to help patients make these dietary changes is to have made the diet change personally. This section will help the healthcare providers learn to help their patients improve their reflux disease and, in the process, improve their health as well.

Most patients know the concept of reflux precautions. Coffee, tea, chocolate, soda, greasy/fried food, fatty food, mints, and alcohol are the typical foods thought to cause reflux disease. Additionally, wearing tight clothing, lying down after eating, salt, and smoking have also been implicated. However, research into these various "triggers" is lacking in the GERD literature and almost nonexistent in the LPR literature. Most of these "triggers" are just that, triggers of reflux. Avoidance of these triggers is often necessary in the beginning stages of reflux treatment. Often when symptoms subside as patients adopt meaningful dietary and lifestyle changes, many of these can be added back into the diet, within reason.

The concept of utilizing a dietary approach for treatment of LPR was first popularized by Dr. Koufman. Her belief that our modern diet is acidic from a combination of the types of foods we eat and the underlying acidification utilized as preservatives contributes to the reactivation of pepsin resulting in inflammation and thus symptoms. Her concept of a "low-acid" diet was evaluated in a study of 20 patients who demonstrated significant improvement in LPR symptoms as measured by the Reflux Symptom Index (RSI). Patients who had a low acid diet in combination with medication and standard reflux precautions demonstrated over 90% improvement in the RSI compared to 50% in the medication and standard precaution only approach [2]. Additionally, adding alkaline water with pH > 8.0 has been used to counteract acidity within the laryngopharynx and esophagus negating the effect of not only refluxed acid but also acidic food and liquid intake. Dr. Koufman found, in vitro, the ability of alkaline water to irreversibly denature and inactivate pepsin [3]. Following the line of diet-based treatment, Dr. Aviv in *The Acid Watcher Diet: A 28-Day Reflux Prevention and Healing Program* [4] has popularized the concept of acid neutralization in combination with acid avoidance. By adding alkaline foods to acidic foods, the pH can be raised leading to less activation of pepsin and direct stimulation of acid receptors in the laryngopharynx. These concepts with recipes can be found in a recently released follow-up book that provides many dietary options in line with this acid neutralization thought process [5].

The concept of removing acid to prevent pepsin activation undoubtedly makes sense. Much success has been obtained by removing acid through dietary choice and alkalizing acidic foods. However, the endgame intervention is pepsin itself. Pepsin is the digestive enzyme released in the stomach as pepsinogen and activated by acid. The primary role of pepsin is to digest proteins into small-chain amino acids and amino acid constituents. These amino acids collectively trigger gastrin release in the stomach to release more pepsin and more acid in a positive feedback loop. Current pharmacotherapy aims to decrease acid, which can raise gastrin and thus pepsin levels [6]. Pepsin, and its precursor pepsinogen, can remain stable and even active up to pH of 8.0. Thus, acid suppression alone cannot change the course of reflux disease. Intervention with the pepsin pathway does change the course of disease.

Thus, the concept of a low animal protein diet was entertained as a means to change the course of the disease by decreasing the active components, pepsin, and acid, by decreasing the intake of animal-based protein. The hypothesis is being related to the bioavailability of amino acids in animal-based protein vs plant-based protein leading to the positive feedback loop of pepsin and acid secretion. Animal-based proteins are highly bioavailable sources of amino acids that are readily released upon entry into the stomach. Plant-based protein is highly bound to fiber and has lower bioavailability. Most proteolysis of plant-bound protein occurs within the intestines, thus avoiding the gastrin-pepsinogen positive feedback loop. These concepts are reviewed in detail in the chapter by Johnston et al.

In The China Study [7], T. Colin Campbell explores the relationship between animal- vs plant-based diets and the prevalence of chronic Westernized diseases such as diabetes, heart disease, stroke, and cancer. Dr. Campbell has graciously written a foreword in support of using a plant-based diet as a treatment for another chronic disease. Reflux, like heart disease and diabetes, is caused primarily from diet. So, if diet can reverse and prevent many of the chronic diseases that plague our society with morbidity, mortality, and cost, then my thinking is that reflux too is a chronic disease and should respond to the same treatment approach, namely a mostly plant-based, Mediterranean-style diet.

Chronic diseases such as heart disease, diabetes, stroke, and cancer affect millions adding to significant morbidity and mortality. The cost of diagnosing and treating these diseases has also skyrocketed. With obesity rates increasing, alarmingly among the youth, these diseases and costs are expected to rise considerably over the next decade [8].

Data from large population, decades long studies, has provided for multiple and ever-increasing publications demonstrating a significant decline and reversal in chronic disease the more plant based the diet and less animal content. Chicken, popular as a "safe" meat alternative, has been linked to significant increase in rates of colorectal cancer [9]. Data from the Health Professionals and Nurse's Health Studies, with over 100,000 participants, have linked processed and unprocessed red meat, as an independent factor, with significantly increased risk of mortality [10]. The NIH-AARP study population, with over 500,000 participants, concluded that red and processed meat is associated with statistically significant increased risk of dying from cancer, heart disease, and prematurely overall, and "white" meat, in men, is associated with increased cardiovascular mortality [11]. Given the increasing collection of evidence on an international level, the International Agency for Research on Cancer (IARC) of the World Health Organization has declared processed meat as a Group 1 carcinogen – causes cancer in humans, and red meat a Group 2A carcinogen, probably causes cancer in humans (https://www.who.int/features/qa/cancer-red-meat/en/).

Therefore, the thinking behind the plant-based, Mediterranean diet as a treatment to reverse reflux disease by targeting pepsin and acid production represents yet another disease process whose trajectory can be altered by a dietary approach, thus creating the concept for this book. By decreasing the available amino acids in the stomach, less pepsin and acid would be secreted. Complementing that approach by adding alkaline water should neutralize orally consumed acid, as well as refluxed acidity. In addition, utilizing standard reflux precautions would limit triggers of reflux. By combining this approach, the hypothesis for the study by Zalvan et al. was formulated [12].

This section will explore the editor's evolution of thinking in approaching reflux disease. Once one of the highest volume prescribers of proton pump inhibitors (PPI), Dr. Zalvan began to question the daily writing of these drugs to treat a disease. Exploration of the chronic disease literature uncovered compelling evidence that many of the chronic diseases that plague modern society have a cause and propagation rooted in our modern Westernized diets with high-volume animal-based foods predominating at the table. Two cohorts of patients with typical LPR symptoms were evaluated. One group was treated with a standard reflux diet and PPI therapy; the other group was placed on standard reflux diet, alkaline water, and a 90% or more plant-based, Mediterranean-style diet of fruits, vegetables, grains, and nuts. Statistically, both groups improved to the same degree suggesting that LPR could be treated without medication as diet works just as well, if not better. Thus, began a movement toward initiating dietary change to improve reflux disease, just as plant-based diets have begun to surface as perhaps the most logical and successful approaches to many other chronic diseases.

How to Taper PPI Successfully

One of the goals of this textbook is to provide enough data to support a dietary intervention over pharmacological. Many patients are currently taking PPI to help with GERD and LPR symptoms. Transitioning to a dietary approach can allow for successful tapering of these medications. Some patients do experience moderate to severe rebound symptoms if PPI therapy is stopped abruptly. Data are conflicting on this topic [13]; yet, despite conflicting evidence of this rebound phenomenon [14], many patients do report acute worsening of symptoms, especially heartburn, vocal changes, worsening of cough, and other reflux symptoms. The exact mechanism of this rebound symptomatology is unknown. Possible reflexive increased acid and pepsin secretion, or localized hypersensitivity might play a role. Regardless, a tapering process is prudent, especially for patients who have used PPI therapy for long term, at least 3 months.

Once a patient has started on a mostly plant-based, Mediterranean-style diet, most begin to notice symptom improvement within one to 2 weeks. In addition, patients typically notice the loss of two to three pounds of weight during this time frame (ultimately losing 6–8 pounds by the next visit 2 months later). At this point, initiation of PPI tapering should be begun by the patient. Skipping a PPI dose on every third day for 2 weeks begins the slow taper. The patient can then take a PPI every other day for another 2 weeks followed by every third day. If after one to two more weeks, there are no rebound symptoms, no new symptoms, and the patient continues on the plant-based approach, the medication can be stopped. H2 blockers can be used as bridging agents if there are any breakthrough symptoms. In addition, alginate suspensions are excellent agents to allow for this transition. Having two teaspoons after meals, before bedtime, and if awakening during the night can help decrease acid exposure to the affected mucosa, decreasing symptoms. Additionally, alkaline water should be consumed during this transition with most meals, before bed and during sleep when awakening, and when more symptomatic.

However, patients whom have medical conditions such as Barrett's esophagus, esophagitis, gastritis, and other conditions should continue to have long-term follow-up with repeat endoscopies to ensure stabilization or resolution and not progression of any of these diseases during and after cessation of medication. Cessation of any medication should be discussed in detail with all healthcare personal involved in the care and treatment of the disease.

The key to a successful dietary approach, one that affords improved overall health, less medication, better outcome, and less cost starts with the reader of this text. Further self-education of plant-based diets and the overall health benefits will hopefully compel the reader to begin their own journey toward the dietary goals listed. By adopting this plant-based lifestyle and understanding the complexities of transitioning on a personal level, the reader will be better equipped to help their patients understand and adopt these changes. This text is meant as an introduction and includes many references to the plant-based literature that exists.

I started as one of the highest volume prescribers of PPI treatment in my region. My questioning of that practice as not one that made evolutionary sense compelled me to explore the chronic disease literature ultimately concluding that a mostly plant-based, Mediterranean-style diet can and does reverse reflux disease. In the process of dietary change, patients often lose the weight they have desired to shed for many years. They have improved biochemical markers of inflammation and risk. Many decrease or stop their chronic use of medications such as statins, PPI, as well as medication for diabetes. Most report a far more healthy life and lifestyle for which they are repeatedly thankful and finally, live a life without reflux.

The doctor–patient relationship develops through trust, education, and guidance to help a person with a particular medical issue. In modern medicine, most patients now expect some type of medication or test. Diet and behavioral changes are often mentioned, in passing, and rarely with much detail. Perhaps the most important treatment begins with spending more time with these issues. When it comes to changes in diet, there can be a lot of initial resistance to change. People have spent most of their lives eating a certain way and suggesting an acute change can be difficult physically, emotionally, and financially. Perhaps the best way to introduce a dietary change to a more plant-based, Mediterranean-style diet is to adopt this lifestyle change yourself. Self-knowledge and experience of the physician can help a patient overcome some long-held personal beliefs on diet. Here are some guidelines to help the caregiver help their patients, and themselves, start on a pathway of diet transition.

Mediterranean-Style, 90–95% Plant-Based Transition Guidelines

1. Education – Reading, watching, and learning about evidence-based medicine on the health benefits of diet is the most important first step. A well-informed patient who understands the health implications beyond reflux will be more apt to adopt a newer, more plant-based diet. The literature is replete with articles and data, with much of this information synthesized into easy to read books and movies. Please read some of the recommended books, articles, online movies, websites, and other references to understand the importance of diet in overall health. This section of the book will provide such resources.
   (a) Self-understanding and awareness will ensure success.
   (b) Educate your family and friends to join in the transition.
2. Learn about plant-based cooking and eating
   (a) Dining at home – get cookbooks, online videos and recipes, join classes, order online plant-based food delivery.
   (b) Dining out – read guidelines on how and what to order in restaurants and while traveling.
3. Transition SLOWLY – take days, weeks, and even months to transition to a diet that is 90–95% plant based.
   (a) Start with one meal a day that is completely plant based, then two, then three, or start with snacks and work up to meals.
   (b) Chegan attitude – “Cheating Vegan” – the ultimate goal is to have two to three meals per week that have at most 3–4 oz. of any animal product – the rest is plant based.
      (i) “Cheat” when going out, at a friend’s home, or while traveling.
      (ii) “Cheat” with very small amounts of animal products more frequently.

(c) Worth mentioning is the topic of plant-based meat alternatives. Data are lacking on the health benefits of such food sources. Likely "healthier" than animal-based meat, there are potential issues with any foods being processed. These can be included in the "cheat" category, having a few times per month.

References

1. Kantor ED, Rehm CD, Haas JS, Chan AT, Giovannucci EL. Trends in prescription drug use among adults in the United States from 1999–2012. JAMA. 2015;314(17):1818–31. https://doi.org/10.1001/jama.2015.13766.
2. Koufman JA. Low-acid diet for recalcitrant laryngopharyngeal reflux: therapeutic benefits and their implications. Ann Otol Rhinol Laryngol. 2011;120(5):281–7.
3. Koufman JA, Johnston N. Potential benefits of pH 8.8 alkaline drinking water as an adjunct in the treatment of reflux disease. Ann Otol Rhinol Laryngol. 2012;121:431–4.
4. Aviv J. The Acid watcher diet: a 28-day reflux prevention and healing program. New York: Harmony Books; 2017.
5. Aviv J, Kaufmann-Aviv S. The acid watcher cookbook. New York: Harmony Books; 2019.
6. Hirschowitz B. Pepsinogen. Postgrad Med J. 1984;60(709):743–50.
7. Campbell TC, Campbell TM. The China study: startling implications for diet, weight loss and long term health. 1st ed. Texas: BenBella Books, Inc.; 2014.
8. https://stateofobesity.org/wp-content/uploads/2018/09/stateofobesity2018.
9. Singh PN, Fraser GE. Dietary risk factors for colon cancer in a low-risk population. Am J Epidemiol. 1998;148(8):761–74.
10. Pan A, Sun Q, Bernstein AM, Schulze MB, Manson JE, Stampfer MJ, Willett WC, Hu FB. Red meat consumption and mortality: results from 2 prospective cohort studies. Arch Intern Med. 2012;172(7):555–63. https://doi.org/10.1001/archinternmed.2011.2287. Epub 2012 Mar 12.
11. Sinha R, Cross AJ, Graubard BI, Leitzmann MF, Schatzkin A. Meat intake and mortality: a prospective study of over half a million people. Arch Intern Med. 2009;169(6):562–71. https://doi.org/10.1001/archinternmed.2009.6.
12. Zalvan CH, Hu S, Greenberg B, Geliebter J. A comparison of alkaline water and mediterranean diet vs proton pump inhibition for treatment of laryngopharyngeal reflux. JAMA Otolaryngol Head Neck Surg. 2017;143:1023–9.
13. Hunfeld NG, Geus WP, Kuipers EJ. Systematic review: rebound acid hypersecretion after therapy with proton pump inhibitors. Aliment Pharmacol Ther. 2007;25:39–46.
14. Metz DC, Pilmer BL, Han C, Perez MC. Withdrawing PPI therapy after healing esophagitis does not worsen symptoms or cause persistent hypergastrinemia: analysis of dexlansoprazole MR clinical trial data. Am J Gastroenterol. 2011;106(11):1953–60.

Chapter 38
Plant-Based Dietary Approach for the Treatment of LPR

Jan Geliebter, Shirley Hu, Raj K. Tiwari, and Craig H. Zalvan

The gold standard medical treatment for laryngopharyngeal reflux (LPR) has been proton pump inhibitors (PPIs), a multi-billion dollar industry, which exhibits a fair degree of success [1–3]. As the pathology and symptoms of LPR are thought to be mediated by active pepsin in an acidic environment, decreasing the acid environment of the laryngopharynx is an obvious target [4]. Thus, the PPI approach of decreasing acid would result in decreased pepsin activity, hitting the offending enzyme at a very late stage of the underlying causes and processes of LPR. PPI's adverse drug effects include abdominal pain, nausea, diarrhea, and constipation and have been associated with fundic gland polyps secondary to hypergastrinemia, hypomagnesemia, hypocalcemia, bone fractures, decreased absorption of vitamin B12, diarrhea, and pneumonia [5–10]. Importantly, GERD patients treated with PPI have a potentially increased association with myocardial infarction and a twofold increase in association with cardiovascular mortality on survival analysis [11].

A deeper dive into the biology and pathology of LPR reveals that pepsin is derived from the zymogen, pepsinogen, which is activated to pepsin by gastric acid.

J. Geliebter (✉) · R. K. Tiwari
Department of Microbiology and Immunology, Department of Otolaryngology, New York Medical College, Valhalla, NY, USA
e-mail: Jan_geliebter@nymc.edu

S. Hu
Department of Otolaryngolgy, New York Eye and Ear Infirmary of Mt. Sinai, New York, NY, USA

C. H. Zalvan
ENT and Allergy Associates, LLP, Tarrytown, NY, USA

The Institute for Voice and Swallowing Disorders, Phelps Hospital, Northwell Health, Sleepy Hollow, NY, USA

Department of Otolaryngology, New York Medical College, Valhalla, NY, USA

Department of Communications, Mercy College, Dobbs Ferry, NY, USA

C. H. Zalvan (ed.), *Laryngopharyngeal and Gastroesophageal Reflux*,
https://doi.org/10.1007/978-3-030-48890-1_38

The concentration of amino acids in the stomach, gastrin secretion, and vagal stimulation are the main regulators of the secretion of pepsinogen [4, 12]. Targeting these earlier events in the LPR process would serve to decrease ongoing damage to the macroenvironment and microenvironment of the laryngopharynx. Animal-product-based diets contain readily available protein to stimulate the path to activated pepsin and the LPR process [13]. Plant-based diets that are low in animal protein would serve to decrease the concentration of amino acids in the stomach, decrease pepsinogen secretion, decrease pepsin activation by acid, and decrease LPR symptoms and damage [14, 15].

To test the plant-based dietary approach to LPR treatment and prevention, cohorts of patients were compared in a New York Medical College IRB-approved retrospective study [16]. One cohort was treated with a combination of standard reflux precautions (avoidance of coffee, tea, chocolate, soda, greasy and fried food, fatty food, spicy food, other acidic foods, and alcohol) and PPI therapy, designated as "PS." The second cohort was treated with a mostly plant-based, Mediterranean-style diet (90–95% plant-based diet consisting of vegetables, fruits, whole grains, and nuts with 5–10% or less from animal-based products), alkaline water, and standard reflux precautions, designated as "AMS." The study was statistically powered to compare outcomes in these two groups and, in addition, yielded provocative preliminary data for future sub-cohort analyses, as well as combination (PPI and dietary) approaches to LPR.

Six hundred ninety-eight patients were included in the study, out of an initial 1670 patients identified. We exercised rigorous exclusion criteria to provide for well-matched patients with minimal bias and eliminating confounding factors. The instrument used in the study was the Reflux Severity Index (RSI), and only patients with a pretreatment RSI of 10 or greater, who also had a one posttreatment follow-up RSI at 6 weeks, were analyzed. Evidence of compliance with either pharmacological or dietary intervention was provided by documentation submitted by patients. The current first-line treatment of LPR, PPI therapy, guided our null hypothesis – that PPIs would be better than dietary intervention. Rigorous statistical data analysis was performed on a total of 85 patients in the PS cohort and a total of 99 patients in the AMS cohort, which provided statistical power for our hypothesis (Table 38.1). In addition, we had a third cohort of PPI plus Mediterranean-style plant-based diet, alkaline water, and standard reflux precautions, designated as "PAMS." We further subdivide the cohorts into three sub-cohorts based on presenting symptoms – cough (C), dysphonia (DO), and dysphagia (DA). We also collected data at 12 weeks.

Two measures were used to compare cohorts and sub-cohorts-six-point reduction in RSI and percent reduction of RSI. The six-point reduction in RSI has been advanced as a measure of a clinically relevant response [17].

At 6 weeks, a clinically relevant, six-point reduction was observed in 63 percent of the 85 patients in the total dietary, T-AMS6 cohort, compared to 54 percent of the 85 patients receiving PPI therapy (T-PS6) ([16] and Fig. 38.1a). There was no statistical difference in clinical responses (percent of patients with six-point decreases) between the two approaches, indicating that PPI drug intervention is not statistically

Table 38.1 Cohort distribution and mean RSI values before and after treatments

Group	Total (n)	Mean RSI before treatment (SD)	Mean RSI after treatment (SD)
T-PS6	85	20.2 (8.16)	14.3 (8.83)
T-ASM6	99	19.1 (7.44)	12.1 (8.31)
T-PASM6	35	23 (7.55)	16.4 (9.02)
T-PS12	74	18.6 (8.06)	12 (6.53)
T-ASM12	38	21.7 (8.43)	11.9 (8.78)
T-PASM12	20	23 (7.12)	11.4 (7.18)
C-PS6	32	20.5 (8.12)	13.4 (7.8)
C-ASM6	27	19.8 (8.69)	10.9 (9.92)
C-PASM6	10	24.1 (9.07)	16.8 (7.86)
C-PS12	20	18.4 (8.53)	10.6 (6.95)
C-ASM12	9	26.2 (8.36)	15.6 (10.2)
C-PASM12	12	21.4 (7.7)	8.75 (6.3)
DA-PS6	24	23 (9.06)	18.3 (10.5)
DA-ASM6	38	19.2 (7.23)	12.7 (8.42)
DA-PASM6	14	22.9 (7.19)	16.8 (9.43)
DA-PS12	28	20.5 (9.12)	14 (6.22)
DA-ASM12	11	21.1 (8.88)	11.9 (10.5)
DA-PASM12	6	27.3 (6.12)	17.5 (7.23)
DO-PS6	29	17.6 (6.94)	12 (7.53)
DO-ASM6	34	18.4 (6.74)	12.3 (6.8)
DO-PASM6	11	22.3 (7.13)	15.6 (10.2)
DO-PS12	26	16.8 (6.28)	10.9 (6.23)
DO-ASM12	18	19.9 (7.8)	10.1 (6.63)
DO-PASM12	3	21 (3.0)	9.5 (2.78)

Abbreviations: *RSI* reflux symptom index, *T* total, *P* proton pump inhibitor, *A* alkaline water, *S* standard reflux diet and precautions, *M* Mediterranean/plant-based diet, *T* total cohort, *C* cough, *DA* dysphagia, *DO* dysphonia

better than the dietary/AMS intervention. As expected, the combined PPI/alkaline water/standard precautions/diet – PASM) group of 35 patients also had a comparable, 36 percent clinical response rate at 6 weeks (Fig. 38.1a). Sizeable clinical responses were also observed in all three treatment groups when patients were placed in sub-cohorts based on presenting symptoms of cough, dysphonia, or dysphagia (Fig. 38.1a). Robust clinical responses in all cohorts and sub-cohorts were observed when treatment times were extended to 12 weeks (Fig. 38.1b). These data suggest that similar rates of clinical responses may be achieved with a diet-based, non-pharmaceutical approach, as with PPI treatment.

Outcomes were also measured as "percent reduction in RSI," with larger percent reductions representing greater symptom relief. The 99 patients in the combined dietary (T-AMS6) cohort experienced a 39 percent decrease in RSI at 6 weeks, compared to the smaller, 27 percent decrease by patients in the T-PS6 cohort (Fig. 38.2a). This difference in RSI percent reduction between groups was statistically significant in favor of the dietary approach ([16] and Fig. 38.2a). The 35 patients in the

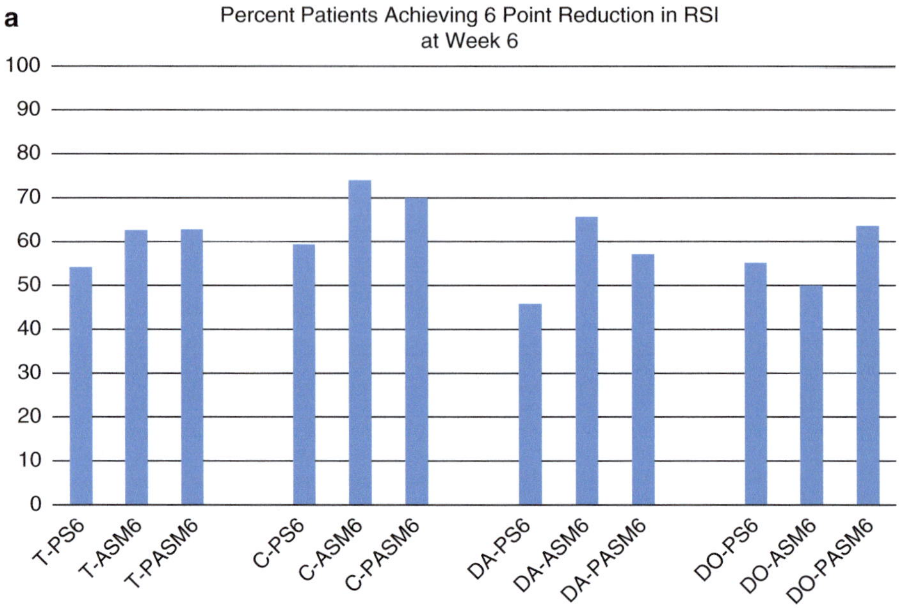

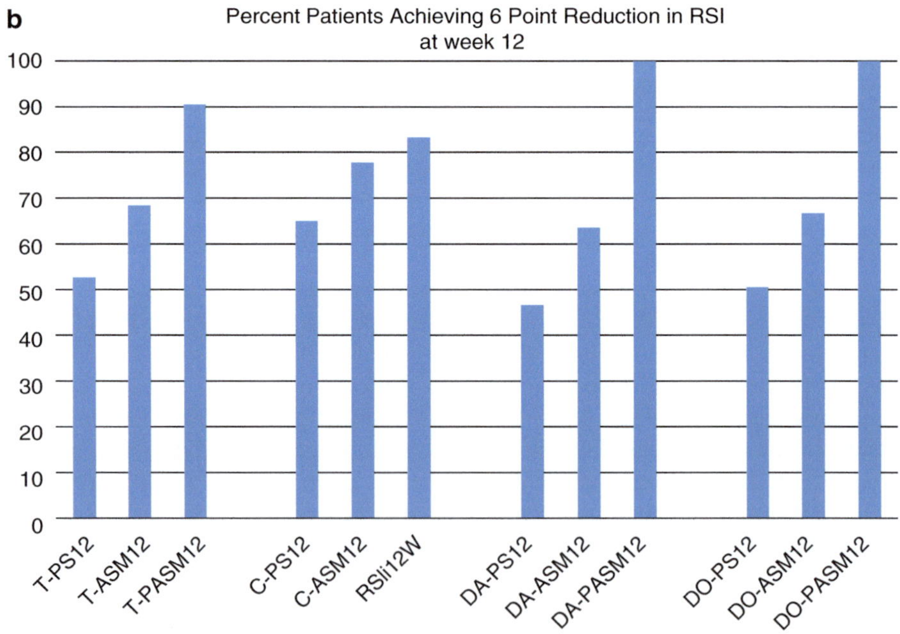

Fig. 38.1 (**a**) Percent Patients Achieving 6 Point Reduction in RSI at Week 6; (**b**) Percent Patients Achieving 6 Point Reduction in RSI at week 12. See Table 1 for number of patients in each group. RSI, reflux symptom index; T, total; P, proton pump inhibitor; A, Alkaline water; S, standard reflux diet and precautions; M, Mediterranean/plant-based diet; T, Total cohort, C, cough; DA, dysphagia; DO, dysphonia

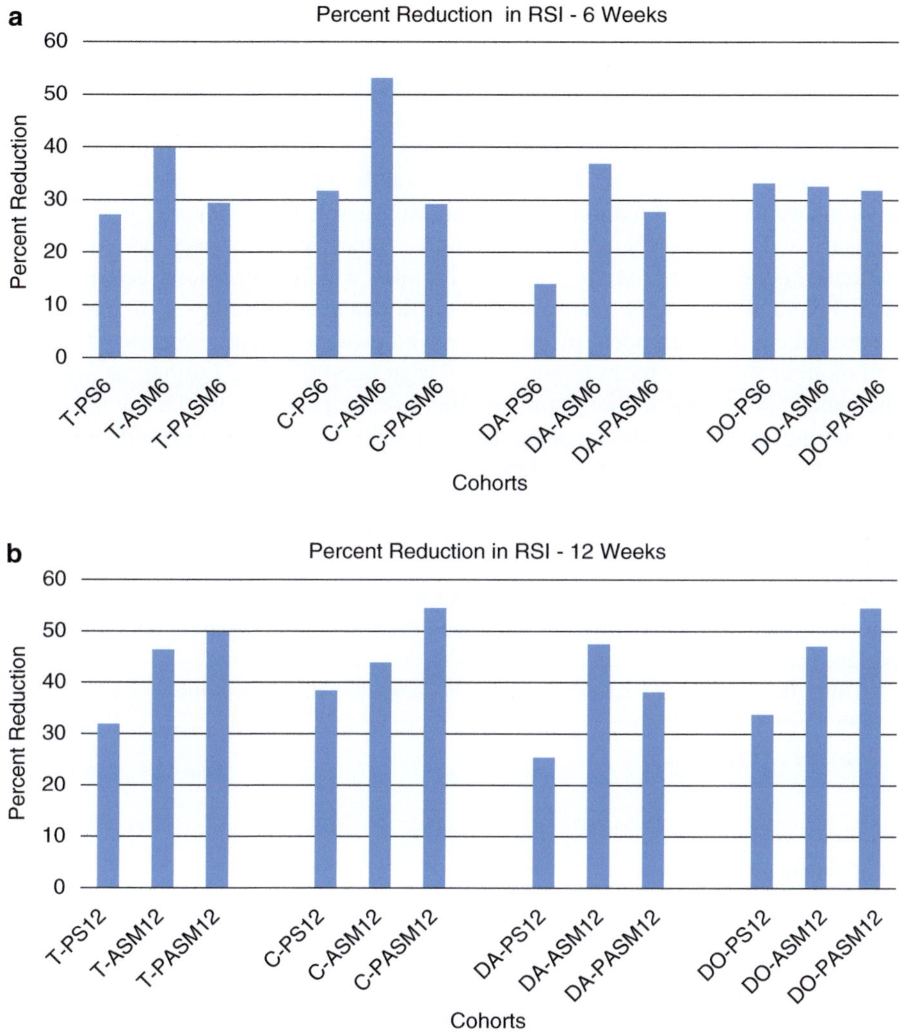

Fig. 38.2 (**a**) Percent Reduction in RSI - 6 Weeks; (**b**) Percent Reduction in RSI - 12 Weeks. See Table 1 for number of patients in each group. RSI, reflux symptom index; T, total; P, proton pump inhibitor; A, Alkaline water; S, standard reflux diet and precautions; M, Mediterranean/plant-based diet; Total cohort, C, cough; DA, dysphagia; DO, dysphonia

combined T-PASM6 group experienced a 29 percent reduction in RSI at 6 weeks. Sizeable percent reductions in RSI were also observed in all three sub-cohorts based on presenting symptoms of cough, dysphonia, or dysphagia. Robust percent reduction in RSI was also observed in cohorts and sub-cohorts at 12 weeks (Fig. 38.2b). Together, the data suggest that a dietary approach to treatment of LPR is as good, if not better, than pharmacological intervention. These data suggest that similar rates of clinical responses may be achieved with a diet-based, non-pharmaceutical approach, as with PPI treatment.

As indicated above, only the two total cohorts (T-PS and T-AMS) at 6 weeks, the main focus of the clinical study, were sufficiently statistically powered to draw firm conclusions. However, our data with combined treatment (T-PASM), the three clinical symptom sub-cohorts (C, DO, and DA), and the 12-week time point do provide preliminary data and direction for a larger, prospective trial. This trial will need to measure and analyze changes in quantitative, objective laboratory parameters in patients, concomitant with changes in the widely accepted, self-reported RSI. Potential laboratory parameters could include measurements of initial and posttreatment oropharyngeal pH, as this would provide crucial, objective data that can monitor the progress in treatment and regression of LPR. Further, as much of the pathology of LPR is thought to be due to active pepsin in the laryngopharynx, measuring pepsin and active pepsin in saliva and mucosal epithelial cells will provide valuable information. Strict dietary controls and food logs can aid in monitoring compliance, but biochemical and physical properties such as body mass index, lipids, and trimethylamine-N-oxide (TMAO) levels can compare diet-based changes to changes in symptoms, objective evidence of reflux, and improvements in overall health. Additional considerations for a future clinical trial include separating the effects of alkaline water from a plant-based diet by having separate and additional patient cohorts.

Thus, the possibility of replacing PPI drugs for the treatment of LPR with a healthy, plant-based dietary regimen appears to be feasible. The proof will be in the plant-based pudding.

References

1. Chiba T, Kudara N, Abiko Y, et al. Effects of proton pump inhibitors in patients with laryngopharyngeal reflux disease. Hepato-Gastroenterol. 2011;58:1580–2.
2. Guo H, Ma H, Wang J. Proton pump inhibitor therapy for the treatment of laryngopharyngeal reflux: a meta-analysis of randomized controlled trials. J Clin Gastroenterol. 2016;50:295–300.
3. Semmanaselvan K, Mukaddam QI, Naik M. An open label, prospective, single centre study to evaluate the efficacy and safety of fixed dose combination of rabeprazole (enteric-coated, EC) 20 mg + domperidone (sustained release, SR) 30 mg capsule in treatment of patients with laryngopharyngeal reflux disease. J Assoc Physicians India. 2015;63:27–32.
4. Johnston N, Dettmar PW, Bishwokarma B, Lively MO, Koufman JA. Activity/stability of human pepsin: implications for reflux attributed laryngeal disease. Laryngoscope. 2007;117:1036–9.
5. Hsu WH, Wu IC, Kuo CH, et al. Influence of proton pump inhibitor use in gastrointestinal polyps. Kaohsiung J Med Sci. 2010;26:76–83.
6. Ngamruengphong S, Leontiadis GI, Radhi S, Dentino A, Nugent K. Proton pump inhibitors and risk of fracture: a systematic review and meta-analysis of observational studies. Am J Gastroenterol. 2011;106:1209–18.. quiz 19
7. Targownik LE, Lix LM, Metge CJ, Prior HJ, Leung S, Leslie WD. Use of proton pump inhibitors and risk of osteoporosis-related fractures. Can Med Assoc J. 2008;179:319–26.

8. Yang YX, Metz DC. Safety of proton pump inhibitor exposure. Gastroenterol. 2010;139:1115–27.
9. Fashner J, Gitu AC. Common gastrointestinal symptoms: risks of long-term proton pump inhibitor therapy. FP Essent. 2013;413:29–39.
10. Lambert AA, Lam JO, Paik JJ, Ugarte-Gil C, Drummond MB, Crowell TA. Risk of community-acquired pneumonia with outpatient proton-pump inhibitor therapy: a systematic review and meta-analysis. PLoS One. 2015;10:e0128004.
11. Shah NH, LePendu P, Bauer-Mehren A, et al. Proton pump inhibitor usage and the risk of myocardial infarction in the general population. PLoS One. 2015;10:e0124653.
12. Hirschowitz BI. The control of pepsinogen secretion. Ann N Y Acad Sci. 1967;140:709–23.
13. Campbell TC. Dietary protein, growth factors, and cancer. Am J Clin Nutr. 2007;85:1667.
14. Guilloteau P, Le Meuth-Metzinger V, Morisset J, Zabielski R. Gastrin, cholecystokinin and gastrointestinal tract functions in mammals. Nutr Res Rev. 2006;19:254–83.
15. Qian JM, Rowley WH, Jensen RT. Gastrin and CCK activate phospholipase C and stimulate pepsinogen release by interacting with two distinct receptors. Am J Phys. 1993;264:G718–27.
16. Zalvan CH, Hu S, Greenberg B, Geliebter J. A comparison of alkaline water and mediterranean diet vs proton pump inhibition for treatment of laryngopharyngeal reflux. JAMA. Otolaryngol Head Neck Surg. 2017;143:1023–9.
17. Lien HC, Wang CC, Lee SW, et al. Responder definition of a patient-reported outcome instrument for laryngopharyngeal reflux based on the US FDA guidance. Value Health. 2015;18:396–403.

Chapter 39
Acid Neutralization Through Diet: Food Is Medicine – It's Not Only What Comes Up; It's What Goes Down

Jonathan E. Aviv

We have a growing nationwide obsession with acid reflux disease [1], especially the type of reflux disease that has extra-esophageal symptoms, that is, the patient has no heartburn complaints, but is complaining of some combination of cough, hoarseness, frequent throat clearing, lump sensation in the throat, and postnasal drip [2]. The typical response from healthcare professionals when encountering a patient with this constellation of symptoms is to recommend a strong acid-reducing agent. However, except for the particular circumstance of eating and then laying down shortly thereafter, many are skeptical that the cause of extra-esophageal symptoms is solely due to refluxed stomach acid, hurtling up from the stomach as if shot out of a canon, to bathe the throat, mouth, and sinuses. A likely culprit of throat-based symptoms in relation to acid reflux disease is the damage caused by the acidity of what one eats and drinks. So the source of the problem may not only be acid that is refluxing upward but also the acidity of what is being ingested, an *acid-ingestion*-related disease.

The reason why acid ingestion is something that should have greater attention paid to it has to do with two relatively recent discoveries, pepsin in the upper aerodigestive tract and the body-wide inflammatory response from acid injury. First, the pepsin story.

Pepsin is an enzyme located in the stomach which breaks down food when it gets activated. Pepsin gets maximally activated below pH 4, and the stomach is generally around pH 2, therefore an environment where pepsin is quite active [3]. However, pepsin can float out of the stomach and lay quietly in the esophagus, chest, vocal folds, pharynx, mouth, paranasal sinuses, and middle ear spaces [4]. When one consumes very acidic foods and beverages, the dormant pepsin gets activated causing an inflammatory response, i.e., what you eat starts eating you.

J. E. Aviv (✉)
Department of Otolaryngology, Icahn School of Medicine, Mount Sinai, New York, NY, USA

Voice and Swallowing Center, ENT and Allergy Associates, LLP, New York, NY, USA
e-mail: javiv@entandallergy.com

C. H. Zalvan (ed.), *Laryngopharyngeal and Gastroesophageal Reflux*,
https://doi.org/10.1007/978-3-030-48890-1_39

Thankfully, very few foods are extremely acidic, defined as having a pH less than four. There are six foods that fall into this category; two are unhealthy and four are healthy, what I call the "dirty half-dozen" [5]. The unhealthies are flavored sodas and bottled ice teas. The soda, diet or sugary, and even flavored sparkling water are almost always below pH 4 and have limited to no discernable health benefits so should be avoided by anyone conscious of their health, let alone people with acid reflux disease [6]. The four healthies are citrus, tomato sauce – not raw tomato, vinegar, and wine. Citrus is lemon, lime, orange, grapefruit, and pineapple. Tomatoes themselves are generally okay to have, as they are typically between pH 4 and pH 5. It is the tomato *sauce* that is the problem since it is generally acidified when it is canned or bottled. Vinegar, including the notorious apple cider vinegar, is extremely acidic. Wine is, by far, the most acidic alcohol beverage. All told, these very acidic half-dozen are to be avoided when preventing or treating those with acid-related injury to the head and neck.

Thus far, the concept is clear; when one eats or drinks foods less than pH 4, tissue-bound pepsin gets activated creating a local inflammatory response. Staying away from these foods will protect these areas.

Second, the body-wide inflammatory response story. In May 2016, Dunbar and colleagues showed that acid reflux or acid ingestion injury initiates a body-wide inflammatory response [7]. As a result, not only will a patient experience what clinicians have seen for years which is swelling of the pharynx, larynx, and esophagus, but also there will be systemic effects. For the past decade, my patients with autoimmune diseases such as irritable bowel syndrome, Crohn's disease, psoriasis, fibromyalgia, and rheumatoid arthritis have commented that their symptoms related to those diseases improved, along with reduced requirements for anti-inflammatory medications such as steroids and other anti-inflammatory drugs while they avoided foods less than pH 4. A diet-based approach to acid-related disease is therefore likely to extend far beyond the elimination of one's reflux symptoms and could ultimately translate to a lower risk for many of the so-called diseases of inflammation that plague so many people today [8].

The facts about pepsin and inflammation led to me spending a lot of time in the kitchen trying to take known very acidic foods and figuring out ways for people to still be able to eat them without suffering the consequences of unwanted acid exposure. It was there that the concept of neutralization of acidic foods with relatively alkaline foods came to fruition.

One of the first mainstays of the acid-neutralization concept was to take fruits less than pH 4 such as red and black berries – strawberries, raspberries, and blackberries – and place them in a blender with dairy-free "milks" such as OSCAR (oat, soy, coconut (or cashew), almond, rice). The same can be done with even an orange and a pineapple. In this way, one can keep the antioxidant properties of these fruits while avoiding their acidic, inflammatory effects. The OSCAR smoothies are not only delicious but also, importantly, quick and easy to prepare.

While the varieties of smoothies one can create are virtually limitless, one does not live on smoothies alone. Patients and followers of the acid-neutralization concept from all over the world – there exist social media-based groups of tens of

Table 39.1 Examples of acid-neutralized popular foods

Apple juice	*Acid-neutralized beet, apple, and ginger juice*
Apple, sugar	Ginger (fresh), beets, Fuji apple
Traditional Caesar dressing	*Acid-neutralized Caesar dressing*
Egg, Parmesan, lemon juice, mustard, raw garlic, black pepper, canola oil, Worcestershire	Cashew, lemon zest, Celtic salt, apple cider vinegar
Traditional tomato soup	*Acid-neutralized tomato basil soup*
Tomatoes (canned), garlic, onion, butter, chicken stock, black pepper, basil leaves	Plum tomatoes (fresh), carrot, Celtic salt, vegetable broth, basil leaves

thousands of people who crave food-based solutions for their reflux disease [9] – were calling for more variety across the entire spectrum of foods.

The next step was then to expand the acid-neutralization principles to include foods and flavors that were previously forbidden, for instance, using tomato, citrus, and even vinegar in highly specific ways by combining (cooking, mixing, blending) them with alkaline foods so that their acidity is neutralized, without losing their flavor. What was created was tasty, healthy, anti-inflammatory recipes that have applications not only for acid reflux sufferers but also for anyone who loves to eat [10], for example, using cucumber or carrot to *neutralize* the acidity of tomato sauce to create a marinara sauce.

Table 39.1 shows three different examples of traditional ingredients for some popular dishes and the acid-neutralization methods implemented to create alternatives either above pH 4 or above pH 5. Fruit juices are often very acidic whether or not they are freshly made or from a can or jar. A great example is traditional apple juice which is a very acidic combination of apple and white sugar. The acid-neutralized version is a beet, apple, and ginger juice where beets and fresh ginger are added to neutralize the acidity of Fuji apples to create a delicious juice that is above pH 5. Another example is Caesar salad dressing. Traditional Caesar dressing with its combination of lemon, mustard, and Worcestershire sauce is very acidic despite the presence of relatively alkaline cheese and egg. The acid-neutralized version uses cashew instead of dairy and lemon zest instead of lemon. The cashew is so concentrated and alkaline that it neutralizes the small amount of apple cider vinegar that is used in the recipe. The zest, or skin, of lemon and lime is above pH 5 so a wonderful replacement for very acidic fruits while still providing the tang, taste, and aroma of fresh citrus. Finally, conventional tomato soup, due to the use of canned tomatoes, is very acidic, while the acid-neutralized version uses carrot to counterbalance the relative acidity of fresh tomatoes.

Food-based solutions utilizing acid-neutralization concepts introduce a myriad of options for those with acid reflux disease. But what can we do as clinicians to better guide our patients, and what can our patients be advised to do?

Step one, and the most basic of all approaches, is to tweak our history taking and to ask our patients what they eat and drink. As a patient myself, it is rare for any of my doctors, no matter the specialty, to ask me what I eat. When patients are initially asked what their beverage is during the day, they are often incredulous, with an answer something along the lines of "Water. I only drink water. All day long. Maybe some coffee." But if one can ask the beverage question in a more detailed fashion such as asking about soda, bottled ice tea, and flavored sparkling water – all very acidic substances generally below pH 4 – a more comprehensive picture of what is actually being consumed and how it may impact upon the patient's throat health and overall health will emerge.

Another example of modifying the food history taking is how to best ask patients if they eat or use vinegar. A direct approach to the question often gives a simple negative response. However, if the question is framed more open ended such as "Do you ever have salad?" this way of asking typically leads to an overall affirmative response, "Of course I have salad, everyday!" which then drills down to what we really want to know, "What's your dressing of choice?"

Clinicians seeing patients should always ask a detailed diet history. The following three to four substances should always be asked about: soda, diet soda, bottled ice tea, or any flavored beverage in a can, bottle, or box. This manner of questioning allows the patient to really think about what they indeed consume on a regular basis and can periodically reveal beverages that one might not typically think of in the initial questioning such as Hawaiian Punch or Diet Red Bull.

The corollary to asking a patient what they eat and drink is to encourage the patient to tell their doctors what they eat and drink. If that fundamental question is asked, a huge step forward to completely treating our patients begins.

Ultimately, people don't want to have to choose between their health and the foods they love and crave. Now we have the ability to advise a wide variety of food-based solutions to satiate these cravings.

#foodismedicine

References

1. Yamasaki T, Hemond C, Eisa M, Ganocy S, Fass R. The changing epidemiology of gastroesophageal reflux disease: are patients getting younger? J Neurogastroenterol Motil. 2018;24(4):559–69. https://doi.org/10.5056/jnm18140.
2. Lechien JR, Akst LM, Hamdan AL, Schindler A, Karkos PD, Barillari MR, Calvo-Henriquez C, Crevier-Buchman L, Finck C, Eun YG, Saussez S, Vaezi MF. Evaluation and management of laryngopharyngeal reflux disease: state of the art review. Otolaryngol Head Neck Surg. 2019;160:762–82. https://doi.org/10.1177/0194599819827488.
3. Bardhan KD, Strugala V, Dettmar PW. Reflux revisited: advancing the role of pepsin. Int J Otolaryngol. 2012;2012:646901. https://doi.org/10.1155/2012/646901.
4. Johnston N, Knight J, Dettmar PW, Lively MO, Koufman J. Pepsin and carbonic anhydrase isoenzyme III as diagnostic markers for laryngopharyngeal reflux disease. Laryngoscope. 2004;114(12):2129–34. https://doi.org/10.1097/01.mlg.0000149445.07146.03.
5. Aviv J. The 28-day blueprint for reducing acid damage, revving up metabolism, and staying healthy for life: the healing phase (days 1 to 28). In: Aviv J, editor. The acid watcher diet: a 28-day reflux prevention and healing program. New York: Harmony Books\Penguin Random House; 2017. p. 119–45.

6. Malik VS, Li Y, Pan A, De Koning L, Schernhammer E, Willett WC, Hu FB. Long-term consumption of sugar-sweetened and artificially sweetened beverages and risk of mortality in US adults. Circulation. 2019;139:2113–25. https://doi.org/10.1161/CIRCULATIONAHA.118.037401.
7. Dunbar KB, Agoston T, Agoston RD, Odze, et al. Association of acute gastroesophageal reflux disease with esophageal histologic changes. JAMA. 2016;315(19):2104–12. https://doi.org/10.1001/jama.2016.5657.
8. Kahrilas PJ. Turning the pathogenesis of acute peptic esophagitis inside out. JAMA. 2016;315(19):2077–8. https://doi.org/10.1001/jama.2016.5827.
9. The Acid Watcher Diet Support Group- Facebook https://www.facebook.com/groups/509489002733660/.
10. Aviv JE, Kaufmann SA. The acid watcher cookbook: 100+ delicious recipes to prevent and heal acid reflux disease. New York: Harmony Books\Penguin Random House; 2019.

Chapter 40
The Mediterranean Diet: A Healthy Diet for the Modern Times

Michel de Lorgeril, Patricia Salen, and Craig H. Zalvan

Introduction

The Mediterranean diet (MD) is the dietary pattern commonly found in South European countries, such as Greece, Spain, Italy, and South France. Populations of Northern Africa and Middle East also influence the MD model.

This diet is widely embraced by medical doctors and nutritionists, as numerous studies have shown that adhering to the MD can reduce the risk of many diseases, such as cardiovascular disease (CVD), cancers, cognitive decline, and dementia. Adherence to the MD model is however challenged in the present times due to the Western diet model spreading across the world.

We now are aiming at providing an overview of the fundamentals of the MD model. We will summarize some important findings regarding its definition and health effects. The biological mechanisms explaining the health effects of the MD and the totality of epidemiological evidence supporting the benefits of the MD are not fully discussed in this text. Preedy and Watson have contributed an authoritarian text on this subject that encompasses the finer details of epidemiology, mechanism, and specific health advantages [1].

M. de Lorgeril (✉) · P. Salen
Laboratoire Coeur et Nutrition, School of Medicine, Grenoble Alps University, Grenoble, France

C. H. Zalvan
The Institute for Voice and Swallowing Disorders, Northwell Health/Phelps Hospital, Sleepy Hollow, NY, USA

Professor of Otolaryngology at the Donald and Barbara Zucker School of Medicine at Hofstra/Northwell, Phelps Hospital Campus, Sleepy Hollow, NY, USA

ENT and Allergy Associates, LLP; Voice and Swallowing Division, Tarrytown, NY, USA
e-mail: czalvan1@northwell.edu

C. H. Zalvan (ed.), *Laryngopharyngeal and Gastroesophageal Reflux*,
https://doi.org/10.1007/978-3-030-48890-1_40

What the Mediterranean Diet Is?

Historical Overview

The traditional MD diet is an eating pattern typical of the people living in the Mediterranean Sea areas. It likely originated before the modern eating habits emerged with energy-dense, highly processed, and mass-produced foods.

The MD was first defined by the controversial American biochemist Ancel Keys, who launched the Seven Countries Study in the 1950s [2]. The MD was the eating pattern of Italians and Greeks at that time with a very low risk of CVD and coronary heart disease (CHD) mortality especially among middle-aged men living in Crete and Corfu. The Seven Countries Study was in fact the first epidemiological study that examined whether CVD could be influenced by factors such as diet and lifestyle.

The main finding was that the farmers of Crete and Corfu, despite high intake of fat, had very low CHD mortality and the highest life expectancy in comparison to the other cohorts, in particular American and Northern European people. Only the Japanese cohort was comparable to the Greek, but because of the recent world war, the Japanese example did not attract the attention of Keys.

This quite surprising finding was first attributed by Ancel Keys to the low blood cholesterol levels of the people in Crete and Corfu. Ancel Keys was thinking that the reason of low cholesterol was the low intake of saturated fat and high intake of unsaturated fat. The MD being characterized by high consumption of olive oil (rich in unsaturated fat), along with low consumption of fatty meat and cow milk products (rich in saturated fat), the main advantage of the MD as seen by Ancel Keys was its effect on blood cholesterol. Thus, for Ancel Keys, the main finding of the Seven Countries Study was the role of blood cholesterol in CHD, a theory he had been defending for many years and before launching the Seven Countries Study. All the other aspects of the MD, including polyphenols of olive oil and wine (for instance), had no importance for Ancel Keys who was focusing almost exclusively on the cholesterol-lowering effect of the MD [2].

However, since that introduction, a great amount of work has been carried out highlighting the protective role of several components of the MD against chronic diseases, such as CHD and cancer.

This plethora of evidence on the positive health benefits of the MD, which is not present for other dietary patterns, led to the MD being recognized by the United Nations Educational, Scientific, and Cultural Organization (UNESCO) in 2010 as an "intangible cultural heritage of humanity" [3].

The Traditional Mediterranean Diet

The traditional MD is characterized by abundant plant foods, such as fruits, vegetables, legumes, potatoes, nuts, seeds, and unrefined cereals (e.g., whole grain bread and pasta, brown rice). Olive oil is the principal source of fat, and intake of animal and plant saturated fat is low. Dairy products (mostly in the form of cheese and yogurt), fish, and poultry are consumed in low to moderate amounts, and several eggs are consumed weekly. Red meat is consumed in low amounts, and wine is consumed in low to moderate amounts, normally with meals. Between-meal snacks are frequent with nuts, cheese, bread, and some alcoholic beverage. Fresh and dried fruit is often and seasonally consumed. The energy from fats of the MD can range according to the area; it could be high, around 40%, as in Greece, or moderate, around 30%, as in Southern Italy, but in any case, the intake of the monounsaturated fats, primarily originating from olive oil, is higher than the saturated fats [4–6].

What Is the Evidence on Health Benefits of the MD?

Cardiovascular Diseases

According to WHO, CHD and stroke remain the major causes of death around the globe. It is estimated that 15.2 million deaths occurred from CHD and stroke in 2016, out of which 9.4 million were due to CHD and 5.8 due to stroke [7].

Many epidemiological and ecological studies have examined the association between the MD and cardiovascular diseases (CVD). For instance, a meta-analysis of cohort studies up to 2010 assessed the relationship between the degree of adherence to the MD – using an MD score – and CVD mortality and morbidity. It was shown that a two-point increase in the MD score was associated with an 8% reduction in mortality and a 10% reduction in morbidity [8].

In 2011, a Spanish cohort of 13,000 participants concluded that participants with the highest MD score (>6 out of 9) had a lower CVD risk compared to those with the lowest adherence score (<3 out of 9). It was found that a 20% risk reduction for total CVD and a 26% risk reduction for CHD were associated with a two-point increase in the MD score [9].

Interestingly, the benefits of adhering to the MD are not confined to the Mediterranean populations. For instance, in the Dutch European Prospective Investigation into Cancer and Nutrition (EPIC)-NL cohort study, analyzing data from 40,000 participants, a two-point increase in the MD score (on a nine-point scale) was inversely associated with fatal CVD, total CVD, myocardial infarction, stroke, and pulmonary embolism [10].

Similarly, in the US cohort Northern Manhattan Study (NOMAS), investigators found that the MD score was inversely associated with the risk of ischemic stroke, myocardial infarction, and CVD death [11].

More importantly, data from randomized clinical trials (RCT) supported the epidemiological evidence. The Lyon Diet Heart Study was a single-blinded RCT aimed at testing secondary prevention with the MD on recurrence rates of myocardial infarction in comparison to the diet recommended in the Western world after myocardial infarction or other heart attacks. The study showed that the protective effect of the MD was considerable (70% reduction of the risk) and maintained up to 4 years after the first infarction [12, 13].

The Prevención con Dieta Mediterránea (PREDIMED) RCT investigated the effect of the MD on CVD risk in primary prevention. The researchers randomized 7.447 participants into an MD diet group supplemented with extra-virgin olive oil, an MD diet group supplemented with mixed nuts, or a control diet group. Results showed that the MD extra-virgin olive oil group had a 30% lower CVD risk and the MD nuts group a 28% lower risk compared with the control group. The results of multivariate analyses showed a similar protective effect of the two Mediterranean diet versions versus the control diet [14].

Taken together, a plethora of epidemiological, clinical, and meta-analytic evidence highlights the cardioprotective effect of the MD.

Cancer

Cancer is the second cause of death worldwide and in developed countries. According to WHO, about one-third of deaths due to cancer are attributed to deleterious lifestyle, i.e., low fruit and vegetable intake, lack of physical activity, and tobacco and alcohol use [15]. Therefore, a healthy dietary pattern can play an important role in cancer prevention.

The first randomized trial showing an anticancer effect of the MD was again the Lyon Diet Heart Study [16]. Revisiting the updated review and meta-analysis of Sofi et al. [8], data of the Lyon Diet Heart Study were confirmed, as it was found that adherence to the MD (assessed by an MD score) was associated with a lower cancer risk. Later, the Multicase-Control Study on Common Tumors in Spain (MCC-Spain), a study performed in seven Spanish provinces between 2008 and 2013, investigated the influence of environmental factors in certain tumors. They recently came up with data showing that high adherence to the MD is associated with a lower risk of aggressive prostate cancer [17]. Sub-analysis of the Adventist study found an association of eating red meat one or more times per week with nearly twice the risk of colon cancer. In the same population, an association of eating "white meat," both chicken and fish, one or more times per week was found to confer a risk with colon cancer over three times than that of nonmeat eaters. Eating legumes two or more times per week predicted half the risk [18].

Data on breast cancer are also supportive of the protective role of MD. Breast cancer is the leading type of cancer in European women, followed by colorectal and lung cancers [19]. The Greek EPIC cohort study followed up 14,807 women and found that adherence to the MD (assessed by an MD score) was associated with a lower breast cancer risk [20]. The same was found in an American case-control study, showing that a high MD score is associated with a decreased risk of breast cancer [21]. In the Nurses' Health Study cohort, investigators also found that high MD scores were associated with a lower risk of breast cancer [22]. The PREDIMED study showed a 62% lower risk of malignant breast cancer in the group of women receiving supplements of extra-virgin olive oil compared to the control group [23]).

In contrast, some other studies have not found an association between breast cancer and the MD. For instance, a British study with 33,731 women found no significant associations between the MD and breast cancer [24]. A similar result was reported in Sweden [25]. An important issue is the control of many confounding factors including genetic predisposition and lifestyle characteristics other than diet.

Taken together, the above scientific evidence, especially data from randomized trials (Lyon Diet Heart Study and PREDIMED), points toward a protective effect of the MD against several cancer types. Additionally, the association of excess body weight, often mitigated in a plant-based, MD-style diet, has been linked independently to a number of cancers including breast, colon, esophageal, liver, ovarian, and thyroid [26].

Cognitive Function

Cognitive aging has become an important concern of the modern times. It decreases the quality of life and is predictive of cognitive decline and dementia.

Dietary patterns, including the MD, have been investigated for their influence on cognitive function. Higher adherence to the MD appears to be associated with a lower risk of cognitive impairment. In subjects with mild cognitive impairment, adhering to the MD seems to reduce the risk of progressing to Alzheimer disease [27]. The MD has also been associated with a risk reduction of Alzheimer disease [28, 29]. A cohort study examined the relations between the MD score and cognitive performance [30]. It was found that higher MD scores are associated with slower cognitive decline. Another prospective study concluded that adherence to the MD is associated with lower subjective cognitive function [31]. Meta-analyses have also shown a protective effect of the MD against cognitive decline [32, 33]. Another meta-analysis provided evidence that adherence to the MD results in benefits on cognition in healthy adults [34]. Finally, the PREDIMED trial showed that in the MD group supplemented with extra-virgin olive oil, cognition scores were higher than the control group [35].

Thus, overall evidence indicates that the MD protects cognitive health. This is a critical finding in the context of aging population.

Nonalcoholic Fatty Liver Disease

Nonalcoholic fatty liver disease (NAFLD) is a common cause of chronic liver disease in the developed world, and the patients who suffer from it have increased mortality and morbidity [36]. It will probably emerge as the leading cause of end-stage liver disease in the coming decades, with the disease affecting both adults and children [37]. NAFLD is characterized by the accumulation of fat in the liver, not related to alcohol drinking. The prognosis can vary in severity, from simple steatosis to hepatocellular carcinoma. Mechanisms of NAFLD are not well defined.

A diet high in refined sugars and saturated fats has been associated with NAFLD [38]. General advice however simply refers to weight loss. Interestingly, low adherence to the MD was associated with the severity of both NAFLD and insulin resistance [39].

A randomized 6-week dietary trial showed that the MD reduces liver steatosis and improves insulin sensitivity without weight loss [40]. Another study found that a low adherence to the MD and a high body mass index predict fatty liver disease in obese children [41]. More recently, in children 10–17 years of age, poor adherence to the MD was shown to be higher in patients with NAFLD [42].

Thus, the MD might be associated with a reduction in NAFLD risk and severity, but more studies, in particular randomized trials, are needed to confirm the point.

Rheumatoid Arthritis

Rheumatoid arthritis (RA) is an autoimmune disorder that affects joints and causes pain, swelling, and stiffness. The main treatment is medications, which can provoke side effects. Dietary interventions can improve the symptoms of RA [43].

A diet rich in vegetables can improve the symptoms of RA. The MD, being primarily based on plant products and low in red meat, dairy foods, and alcohol, can decrease inflammatory activity in RA. It could also increase physical function and improve vitality [44]. The precise components of the MD that are responsible for the amelioration are not clearly defined.

A recent cohort study reported that the intake of MUFA, pulses, total vegetables, meat, milk, and other dairy products was significantly lower in RA patients than in controls [45]. In contrast, grain intake was higher in the RA group. Finally, it was found that monounsaturated fat was the main factor that decreases risk. The study has highlighted the importance of MUFA, which the MD is rich in [45].

Recent studies suggest a link to RA from *Proteus mirabilis*, a pathogenic bacterium potentially found in the urinary tract. Through molecular mimicry, the immune system reacting to an antigen of the *P. mirabilis*, an autoimmune reaction results in RA deposits and symptoms [46]. Potentially, switching to an MD-style plant-based diet can alter the microbiome of the urine and colon resulting in a decline in *P. mirabilis* leading to less onset and a decline in symptoms. This has been clinically supported by a study demonstrating a vegan then lactovegetarian diet resulting in significant decline in pain, morning stiffness, and improved function in patients with RA [47].

Chronic Respiratory Diseases

Among chronic respiratory diseases, one of the most common is asthma. In particular, it is the most common chronic disease in children. However, most asthma deaths occur in the elderly, and with the increasing aging population, deaths from asthma will considerably increase in the next 20 years.

Lifestyle characteristics, such as tobacco, air pollutants, and nutrition, are thought to play a role in asthma. Antioxidants, such as vitamins A, C, and E, carotenoids, and polyphenols, may be protective against asthma during childhood, because it is the time when airways are most vulnerable to oxidative stress [48].

Since the MD is high in antioxidants (fruit, vegetables, and extra-virgin olive oil), studies have investigated the relations of MD with asthma.

A study among 7–18-year-old children in Crete was performed to assess whether adherence to the MD is protective effect against allergic rhinitis, asthma, and atopy [49]. Another study showed that high adherence to the MD reduces by about 80% the risk of asthma in adults, in particular because of high intake of fresh fruit [50]. Three studies reported a protective effect of the MD for wheezing in children [51]; reduced asthma, wheezing, and rhinitis in Mexican children [52]; and a protective effect in girls aged 6–7 years with current severe asthma [53]. A cohort study showed that high adherence to the MD had a protective effect against persistent wheeze, atopic wheeze, and atopy [54]. In 2011, a Greek study found that high adherence to the MD was inversely associated with wheeze, in particular exercise wheeze. One-unit increase in the MD adherence score was associated with 14% lower risk of asthma [55].

Finally, a randomized trial, where asthmatic adults were allocated to an MD or a control diet, found improvements in the quality of life of patients in the MD group [56].

There appears to be a significant rate of misdiagnosis of asthmatics with over 30% demonstrating no objective evidence of asthma resulting in cessation of medication in 90% of the group [57]. Exercise-induced asthma is a misnomer as most cases are not asthmatic at all and are instead related to "exercise-induced laryngeal obstruction" or EILO. EILO occurs during physical activity and presents as inspiratory stridor, on inhalation, and not a "wheeze" as it is commonly described. This occurs from a hypersensitive larynx reflexively causing closure of the vocal folds and thus stridor, when stimulated. Treatment consists of trigger reduction of postnasal drip, laryngopharyngeal reflux, and exercise-induced laryngeal obstruction therapy and not asthma medication [58]. A diet-based approach using alkaline water and a plant-based MD with EILO therapy can improve symptoms significantly and avoid the long-term unnecessary use of medications, steroids, and other asthmatic treatments [59].

Given the scope of this book, only a few of the many benefits of an MD have been discussed. A plant-based, MD-style diet can result in significant improvement in glycemic control in diabetes, both type 1 and type 2. Decreased rates of cerebrovascular disease as well as neuropsychiatric diseases with better outcomes are seen in an MD. A mostly plant-based MD lifestyle leads to far less obesity. In fact, a mostly plant-based MD results in overall decline in morbidity and mortality. The authoritarian text by Preedy and Watson [1] encompasses the wide range of health benefits and disease improvements afforded by a mostly plant-based MD.

What Are the Main Foods of the Mediterranean Diet?

A synergistic effect of the different food components in the MD is suggested to play the main role in the protective effect of the MD. Studies have examined the effects of individual components of the MD. There is evidence that some components of the MD are important. Most nutritional studies are observational and epidemiological in nature and thus exposed to multiple confounding factors and variables. Studies focusing on a specific nutrient or compound often miss the forest through the trees. The focus on the compound often does not take into account the complex interactions of the multitude of components within the whole food and the complex biochemical and biophysical reactions within the body during digestion and metabolism. The emphasis on a mostly plant-based, whole food MD should be the focus rather than the individual components of the particular foods in order to see the marked potential improvement in overall health.

Fish and Marine Omega-3 Polyunsaturated Fats

Marine long-chain omega-3 fatty acids (LCO3) are found in fatty fish and have been studied for their health effects. Fatty fish is a component of the MD. It is unknown so far whether the health effects of fatty fish are independent from full adherence to the MD. Conceivably, evidence from these studies may be skewed to represent a trend toward a healthier lifestyle that has incorporated far more fruits, vegetables, grains, and nuts into the diet.

Eicosapentaenoic acid (EPA) and docosahexaenoic acid (DHA) are the main LCO3 in fish and are thought to be partly responsible for the cardioprotective effect of marine foods. A systematic review of RCT showed that LCO3 reduce the risk of CVD by 23% [60]. A meta-analysis of RCT found a significant CHD risk reduction with LCO3 among high-risk populations, and from the analysis of cohorts, it found a statistically significant 18% reduced risk of CHD [61]. On the other hand, studies showed that supplementation with LCO3 had no significant effect on fatal and non-fatal cardiovascular complications [62].

However, it is important to distinguish between the consumption of fish and that of LCO3 supplements. The health benefits related to consuming fish/seafood are not limited to the consumption of LCO3. Sea and most freshwater fish contain in various amounts high-quality proteins, iodine, selenium, and vitamin D, all this in addition to LCO3, cholesterol, and other lipids. In other words, testing the benefits of fish is not equivalent to testing the effects of fish oil and/or LCO3 supplements [63].

However, there is not yet a published randomized trial testing the effect of fish, so one has to rely on epidemiological studies. Studies, such as the Zutphen [64] and Western Electric studies [65], showed an inverse association between fish and CHD mortality. The US Physicians Health Study also showed that one fish meal per week reduced the risk of sudden cardiac death by 52%, compared to a fish meal once a month [66]. The Nurses' Health Study reported that frequent fish consumption was associated with a lower risk of CHD [67]. A meta-analysis showed that an increased consumption of fish was associated with a 19% reduced risk of coronary heart disease [60].

In contradiction, other studies, such as the Health Professionals Follow-Up Study [68], the EPIC-Spain [69], and the EPIC-Germany cohort [70], found no association between fish consumption and the risk of myocardial infarction and/or stroke. A meta-analysis found a nonsignificant trend toward decreased risk with fish consumption [71]. The reason for the nonsignificant results could be that the amount of fish was less than suggested by previous studies, for example, about 30 g/d in the study of Grosso versus more than 100 g/d from previous positive studies.

Importantly, fish consumption also results in lower risk of other diseases such as cancers. Studies have shown an inverse association between fish intake and various types of cancers [72–74]. However, as mentioned earlier, an increase rate of colon cancer was found among a population of Seventh-Day Adventists eating one or more serving of fish weekly [18].

Finally, in a randomized trial, high consumption of DHA was shown inversely associated with cerebral amyloidosis, a preclinical stage of Alzheimer [75].

The human body can process LCO3 into EPA and DHA bringing into question the amount required to be consumed on a daily basis. Chia seeds and walnuts are simple sources of LCO3, and as little as a tablespoon a day is sufficient to provide the sources required.

It is always important to balance the potential benefits and risks of any particular type of food material. The benefit of fish, though suggested in some studies, is not completely clear as other studies have shown potential risks. In addition, the majority of fish stocks are contaminated with heavy metals such as lead, mercury, and cadmium, organic pollutants such as dioxins and other polychlorinated, and polybrominated diphenyls, not to mention antibiotics, other pharmaceuticals, and most recently microplastics.

Keeping the consumption of fish to no more than one to two servings per week in the setting of a mostly plant-based diet can be a guide for those who choose to keep fish and marine animals in their diet.

Plant Omega-3 Fatty Acids

The traditional MD is rich in plant n-3 fatty acids, the main one being alpha-linolenic acid (ALA). This n-3 fatty acid is *essential* to humans, meaning that they cannot synthesize it independently. The major sources of ALA in the Western diet are vegetable oils (for instance, rapeseed oil and soybean oil), seeds (for instance, flaxseed), and nuts (mainly walnuts). In the traditional MD and besides walnuts, ALA is found in wild plants consumed by goats, sheep, chickens, and rabbits, products of which (eggs, fermented milk, meat) are then consumed by the Mediterraneans [76]. The intake of ALA is definitely associated with health benefits [77–79].

ALA is in fact a precursor molecule that can be converted into LCO3 such as EPA and DHA, discussed in the previous section [80, 81]. The enzymatic system acts through a series of elongation and desaturation steps. The conversion of ALA to EPA and DHA is influenced by genetic variations, hormonal status, and nutrient substrate competition [82–85]. This conversion efficiency is thought to be low in non-Mediterranean populations, leading to the necessity of consuming certain amounts of LCO3.

Another interesting aspect lies in consumption of polyphenols, which seems to increase the conversion of ALA to DHA and EPA, as shown in epidemiological and animal studies [86–88]. These data were however not confirmed in human trials [89]. This might have been due to the fact that in these studies, the polyphenol ingestion was increased through supplementations and/or pure substances and not through the consumption of a healthy diet as in the positive studies [86–88]. This is a critical issue as the active forms of polyphenols – the substances that actually increase the synthesis of LCO3 from ALA – need a specific microbiota to be activated and acquisition of that specific microbiota needs specific nutrients (specific fibers in particular) absent from the supplements [90]. In other words, to get benefits from ALA intake and obtain more blood and tissue LCO3, the Mediterranean polyphenols and microbiota are both required.

Olive Oil

Olive oil is a traditional component of the MD. For a long time, olive oil has been the main source of fat for the Mediterranean population. Extra-virgin olive oil is obtained from the fruit of the olive tree, and more than 95% of if consists of fatty acids. Its fatty acids are mainly monounsaturated, such as oleic acid, whereas polyunsaturated fatty acids, such as linoleic acid, and saturated fatty acids, such as stearic or palmitic acid, are in very low amounts. Olive oil also contains major phenolic compounds, oleuropein being the most abundant one. Other minor components of olive oil may have a potential cardioprotective effect. The amounts of these compounds in the final olive oil depend on the cultivar, climate, and ripeness of the olives at harvesting.

Studies have found an inverse association between olive oil consumption and risk of cardiovascular diseases and also risk of various cancers, diabetes, and neurodegenerative disorders [91–95]. The most recent finding comes from the PREDIMED study reporting a 39% risk reduction of stroke in the group consuming extra-virgin olive oil. For each 10 g/day increase in olive oil consumption, mortality decreased by 7% [96].

The proposed mechanisms of the protective effect of olive oil are the improvement of insulin resistance, reduction of blood pressure, improvement of endothelial function, decrease of inflammatory markers, and reduction of coagulation factors and platelet aggregation [97]. Just as with fish, there are also studies suggesting the consumption of oils, including olive oils, can lead to increased endothelial stiffness lasting for hours potentially suggesting that overconsumption can lead to cardiovascular disease [98]. Evaluation of the Spanish cohort of the EPIC study, with over 40,000 people evaluated, demonstrated that although extra-virgin olive oil seemed to confer a slight advantage over regular olive oil with regard to cardiac events, neither significantly differed when controlled for other healthy diets including more vegetables and fruits [99]. In fact, the benefits of olive oil consumption are related to the anti-inflammatory phytonutrients which are in far higher concentration in the olive itself, again suggesting the whole food is more important than an isolated component.

Fruit and Vegetables

Most healthy diet required high fruit and vegetable intake. Fruit and vegetable are major components of the MD. The Healthy Eating Plate created by the Harvard School of Public Health advices that ½ of our plate should consist of fruit and vegetables [100]. The American Heart Association also recommends five or more servings per day for adults [101]. This advice is based on epidemiological studies. In 2003, WHO concluded that the evidence on the preventive effect of fruit and vegetables against CHD is powerful enough and advised on an intake of about 500 g/day (5–6 portions of 80 g each) [102].

In the European Prospective Investigation into Cancer and Nutrition (EPIC)-Heart, investigators found that fruit and vegetable consumption was associated with a 22% lower risk of fatal CHD for subjects consuming at least eight portions (80 g each) of fruits and vegetables a day, in comparison to those consuming fewer than three portions a day [103]. In the Health Survey of England data, there was inverse association between fruit and vegetable intake and all-cause, cancer, and cardiovascular mortality [104]. The cardioprotective effects of fruit and vegetables could be linked to their high content of antioxidant vitamins and phytochemicals [105–107].

Several meta-analyses have been conducted to examine the issue. Wang analyzed 16 studies and found a significant association between consumption of fruit and vegetables and all-cause and cardiovascular mortality [108]. The study found a threshold around five servings of fruit and vegetable per day, after which the effect of all-cause mortality does not persist. In the systematic review and meta-analysis, a reduced risk of CHD, stroke, cancer, and all-cause mortality was observed with increased intake of fruit and vegetables [109].

As expected, the results from RCTs regarding the health effects of fruit and vegetables are less evident. In a small trial, individuals consuming a standardized meal of 500 g of fruit and vegetables per day, as well as 200 ml of fruit juice per day, were compared to a group who consumed only 100 g of fruit and vegetables per day [110]. It was found that over a 4-week follow-up, the serum lipids, blood pressure, and hemostatic parameters were not modified. Conversely, in a 6-month RCT including 690 healthy individuals, those allocated in the intervention group (increased fruit and vegetable consumption) had higher plasma concentrations of carotenoids and ascorbic acid and a significant decrease of blood pressure, compared to the control group [111].

Studies examined the effects of specific fruits or vegetables. In a study where subjects had low intake of fruit and vegetables, consumption of blackcurrant juice (high in vitamin C and polyphenols) resulted in decreased oxidative stress and improvement of vascular health, within a 6-week time frame [112]. Fruits and vegetables are the primary source of abundant antioxidants, phytochemicals, and other nutrients that can protect against oxidative stress and against a chronic inflammatory state.

Another study reported that high-sulforaphane broccoli sprouts reduced production of noxious nitric oxide metabolites in *H. pylori*-infected patients [113]. Obviously, we need RCT testing the intake of specific Mediterranean fruit and vegetables in the context of full adherence to the MD.

Nuts and Seeds

Nuts and seeds are nutrient-dense foods, high in vitamins and minerals, and they have been part of the MD diet since early times. These products contain, among other components, beneficial fatty acids and proteins. Main nuts of the MD are almonds, hazelnuts, walnuts, and pistachios [114]. Saturated fatty acids in these nuts are low, whereas mono- and polyunsaturated fatty acids are high. For instance, walnuts provide the omega-6 linoleic acid and the omega-3 ALA; both have been linked to health benefits. Nuts are also sources of fiber, protein, and micronutrients, such as potassium, calcium, magnesium, folate, antioxidant vitamins, and polyphenols [115].

Several studies have studied the association between nuts consumption and health outcomes. A summary of the data from the Adventist Health Study, Iowa Women's Health Study, Nurses' Health Study, and Physician's Health Study found a dose-response relationship, estimating an 8% reduction of CHD death for each weekly serving of nuts [116]. The cross-sectional Multi-Ethnic Study of Atherosclerosis found that frequent nut and seed consumption was associated with lower levels of inflammatory markers. This could explain the inverse association of nut consumption with cardiovascular disease and diabetes risk [117].

Clinical trials confirmed epidemiological studies. For example, in the PREDIMED trial, participants allocated to the intervention group with 30 g/day mixed nuts had a lower prevalence of high blood pressure, compared to the control group [118].

Nuts and seeds are integral components of the MD, and even though the specific mechanisms of their protective effects are still unclear, nut consumption is highly recommended, especially in individuals with a high risk of CHD.

Dietary Fiber

Dietary fiber traditionally refers to the indigestible part of plants. It is found in fruits, vegetables, legumes, nuts, seeds, and whole grain and cereals. Examples are lignin and polysaccharides. Oligosaccharides, such as inulin and resistant starches, have been recently added to the definition of dietary fiber [119]. The recommended intake of fibers is 25–30 g/day.

Most available data are from epidemiological studies. A large body of evidence exists on the inverse association between dietary fiber intake and CHD, diabetes, and gastrointestinal disease. Knowledge on the effects of fiber on weight management and gastrointestinal health is more widespread than the benefits against CHD and diabetes.

High intake of dietary fiber has been associated with a decreased CHD and stroke risk. Early evidence came from the Iowa Women's Health Study where postmenopausal women with high intake of whole grains had a lower risk of CHD [120]. In the Nurses' Health Study, women in the highest quintile of whole grain consumption had a 30% lower risk of CHD than women in the lowest quintile [121]. Similar results were reported in subsequent studies [122]. An inverse association between fiber intake and risk of stroke was found in epidemiological studies and meta-analyses [123, 124].

Increased dietary fiber intake is useful in diabetes prevention [125, 126]. In addition, total grain and whole grain were inversely associated with the risk of type 2 diabetes [127]. In a randomized crossover study of participants following a diet with moderate amounts of fiber (24 g) or a high-fiber diet (50 g), improvement of glycemic control and decreased blood insulin were observed [128]. Finally, a meta-analysis found a dose-response relationship, where the risk of type 2 diabetes decreased by 6% for each 2 g/day increment in cereal fiber intake [129].

Wine

Wine is the preferred alcoholic drink of the Mediterranean population, except in Muslims. Wine consumption has been shown to reduce risk of CVD throughout the world. The first report of the possible protective effect of wine was in 1979 [130]. The term "French paradox" was used to describe the fact that French people, despite their high saturated fat intake and lifestyle characteristics often similar to other Western populations, have a low incidence of CHD [131–133]. Wine and ethanol drinking has been associated with several protective effects including antiplatelet [134, 135] and vasodilating action but also myocardial preconditioning [136, 137] and increasing plasma LCO3 (as discussed above in the fish section), all these factors being critical in the prognosis of heart attack and ischemic stroke.

Many studies have shown a cardioprotective effect of wine, including systematic reviews and meta-analyses. For instance, Di Castelnuovo analyzed 26 studies and found a J-shaped association between wine intake and CHD risk [138]. A subsequent meta-analysis included 84 prospective cohort studies and found that light to moderate alcohol consumption is linked to a reduced CHD risk [139].

One of the main principles of the MD is moderation. This implies that when wine is consumed in the setting of an MD, it is critical to respect the Mediterranean "way of drinking." That means in moderate quantities and most of the time during the meals and not Saturday night binge drinking. Is there a safe amount of alcohol to consume? This question was addressed in a large multi-institutional study published in Lancet suggesting that the current limits for alcohol consumption should be lower than what is currently recommended. In over 600,000 studied, the risk of all causes of mortality, especially cancer, rises with increasing alcohol intake. Recommendations from this study suggest that "no level of alcohol consumption" should be considered safe [140]. Again, the epidemiological nature of this research is prone to confounding factors. Does alcohol use in a vegan or mostly plant-based MD population have less of a negative effect than in a more meat-heavy, standard American diet?

Is the MD Adapted to the Present Times?

Level of Adherence to the MD

To determine whether a population is adhering to the MD, we need a specific methodology. So far, the usual methodology to evaluate adherence to the MD has been the scoring of the dietary habits of sample populations. In most cases, higher score stands for higher adherence [141]. In the Greek EPIC cohort study, investigators used a Mediterranean Diet Score (MDS) and observe that a two-unit increase of the MDS was associated with a 25% reduction in mortality [142]. This MDS was based on nine major components of the MD: vegetables, legumes, fruits and nuts, cereals, fish and seafood, meat and meat products, dairy products, moderate alcohol intake, and MUFA/SFA ratio. A value of 0 or 1 was assigned to subjects whose consumption was below the median (value: 0) or at or above the median (value: 1). The MDS ranges from 0 to 9.

The Mediterranean Adequacy Index (MAI) is another MD score [143]. The reference MD was that from Nicotera (Southern Italy) in 1960, and the data for the calculation of the MAI were derived from the Seven Countries Study.

The MD 55 Score is based on the Greek ATTICA study and aimed at detecting clinical characteristics associated with cardiovascular disease [144]. Eleven main components of the MD (non-refined cereals, fruits, vegetables, potatoes, legumes, olive oil, fish, red meat, poultry, full-fat dairy products, and alcohol) are used. Scores from 0 to 5 are assigned depending on the frequency of consumption of each of these foods (from 0: no consumption to 5: daily). A score (from 0 to 55) is calculated. The study reported, for instance, that the score was 23.5 in hypertensive subjects versus 26.8 in normotensive subjects, 22.2 in diabetic subjects versus 26.2 in nondiabetic subjects, and 22.2 in obese subjects versus 26.5 in normal/overweight subjects.

The 14-point MD Adherence Screener (MEDAS) is another index created to provide a rapid control of compliance with the dietary intervention of the Spanish PREDIMED study (135). It consists of 14 food consumption frequency questions.

Each question is scored as 0 (no fulfillment) or 1 (fulfillment criterion). The study reported that for men, MEDAS was 8.7 ± 2.0 and 8.5 ± 2.0 for women [145].

Recently, a Spanish study developed a self-efficacy scale for adherence to the MD (SESAMeD) [146].

Challenges of Adhering to the MD

Despite the plethora of health benefits resulting from adherence to the MD, adherence can be challenging. Globalization and economic, urban, and technology-driven developments have led to a significant shift toward the Western diet high in refined sugars and saturated and industrial *trans* fats and low in fruits, vegetables, legumes, nuts, and seeds.

At present in many developed countries, the low-income groups show the highest prevalence in CVD, and it is thought that it is, at least partly, a result of the shift toward the Western diet. The higher prices of healthy, high-quality, and fresh foods, compared to the low prices of unhealthier snacks and fast food, also reduce adherence to the MD, as it has been found in the MOLI-SANI study, in which adherence to the MD was highly related to material resources [147].

The greater the income is, the higher the adherence to the MD. During the economic crisis in Italy (between 2008 and 2010), adherence to the MD decreased dramatically (18.3%) especially in the elderly, the less affluent, and the urban inhabitants [148].

Two additional factors that might be important for adhering to the MD are nutrition knowledge and exposure to media [149, 150]. Thus, it is likely that material resources are one of the most important factors influencing adherences to the MD. Other factors, such as mass media exposure and information, might play a role as well.

The Updated Mediterranean Diet Recommendations

Despite a general consensus in the scientific community on the characteristics of the MD, issues have been raised that the traditional MD should be updated to cover the changing lifestyle, as well as the environmental and health challenges of the modern society.

Main recommendations for a new (modernized) MD are food related. It is recommended to consume plant-based foods on a daily basis, such as fruit and vegetables, whole grain bread/pasta/rice, grains, cereals, and nuts. The overall goal is to obtain the vast amount of nutritional intake from a 90–95% whole food, plant-based, Mediterranean-style diet with only 10% of the dietary intake from any animal-based product. This translates to a diet of two to three meals out of twenty-one meals with snacks containing three to four ounces of any type of animal product, meat, or dairy.

These recommendations are in line with the most recent online dietary recommendations for the population of Canada [151].

To cover the intake of monounsaturated fatty acids, foods like extra-virgin olive oil (sparingly) and avocado can be consumed. Extra-virgin olive oil might be considered expensive compared to other oils, but due to its high caloric content, it does not need to be consumed in large amounts. Rapeseed canola oil can be used alternatively with olive oil, again sparingly. Selecting organic oils could be a major issue despite their costs. Nuts are recommended, as they are a rich source of important amino acids, unsaturated fats, fiber, and micronutrients. Mediterranean nuts include almonds, hazelnuts, pine nuts, pistachios, and walnuts. Walnuts especially are a rich source of ALA and have the highest level of phenolic compounds in comparison to other nuts [152].

Another important component of the MD is water. Hydration is important, and a daily intake of 1.5–2 L of water is strongly advised. This intake can be complemented with non-sugar herbal infusions, such as tea. Dairy products are recommended in moderate amounts, primarily in the form of yogurt, cheese, and other fermented dairy products though limited to the overall meal of less than five percent. For those who desire alcohol, a minimal consumption of wine during meals is recommended, but religious and social beliefs should be taken into account. On a weekly basis, it is suggested to consume fatty fish and seafood no more than two to three times per week, in line with a 95% whole food, plant-based MD-style diet. Fish can provide *essential* protein and lipids and other major nutrients such as iodine and selenium. Fish is a nonvegetarian source of LCO3, but until recently, vegetarians and vegans had only a few options, like flaxseeds and nuts to get ALA, but these options do not provide the LCO3 such as EPA and DHA. As the conversion of plant omega-3 to LCO3 is limited in humans in the absence of adequate microbiota and polyphenols, a solution could be algae, which is an emerging food rich in LCO3. By eating a mostly plant-based diet, adequate levels through endogenous conversion can be achieved.

White meat, such as poultry, rabbit, and eggs, can be consumed on a weekly basis, as they are sources of high-quality proteins, a major nutrient in the aging population but again limited to part of the two to three meals per week with three to four ounces per meal. Red and certainly processed meats should be consumed rarely, if at all, and in low amounts. Instead, legumes (lentils and chickpeas, for instance) and soy are alternatives.

Potatoes and other starches should be consumed weekly, as they often form a part of many traditional MD recipes. They should be consumed with moderation because of their high glycemic index, and the fried version should be consumed on an occasional basis. The seasonality of fruit and vegetables is a factor that should be taken into account. Fresh, seasonal, non-processed organic foods are the basis of the new and traditional MD. It is important to remember that it is not only about choosing a fruit but also considering its journey to the table and the way (organic or not) it has been produced, harvested, and stored.

Sweets and beverages high in sugars should be avoided, except for special occasions.

Socializing during meals is important, and sharing foods with family is recommended as a supportive factor of healthy eating and learning.

Sustainability

Adhering to sustainable diets is now a critical issue in modern societies. It is definitely recognized that the MD is not only a healthy dietary model but also a sustainable diet. In the first World Conference on the MD held in Milan in 2016, the International Mediterranean Diet Foundation illustrated the MD as a sustainable, human-centered dietary pattern.

The four sustainable benefits of the MD have been very well highlighted in a review article on the Med Diet 4.0 framework (142). These are as follows:

1. Major health benefits
2. Low environmental impact
3. High sociocultural values
4. Positive local economic returns

Regarding the lower environmental impact of the MD, many studies have documented it. As the MD is a plant-based diet with low animal product consumption, it has a small water footprint, low greenhouse gas emissions, and low energy consumption [153, 154].

The MD is a biodiverse diet, as it uses a large range of cereals, fruits, and vegetables that not only are cultivated but also can be wild; in the latter case, they come with specific local and traditional knowledge on their use.

The seasonality of the plant-based products of the MD is another important factor that contributes to its biodiversity.

Regarding the sociocultural value, the MD populations have had so many traditions and religious and cultural differences throughout their history, with values such as family and common meals all contribute to the MD being considered as an Intangible Cultural Heritage of Humanity.

Finally, about the positive local economic returns, it is clear that the MD encourages the sustainable development of rural areas producing local and traditional food products, with low dependence on external food imports. Local producers should be empowered, supported, and protected, and typical Mediterranean food products should be properly labelled, identified, and promoted [155].

Conclusions

The MD has definitely earned its title as a healthy-eating dietary pattern and a sustainable model. A plethora of medical studies, meta-analyses, and clinical trials supports the notion that the MD is a protective diet against several noncommunicable diseases. Finally, the MD is not static but rather a dynamic model that brings together food, nutrition, sociocultural elements, and sustainability to create one of the world's most valuable lifestyles. Further exploration into the health benefits of a mostly plant-based, whole food, Mediterranean-style diet is encouraged with resources such as "The Mediterranean Diet" by Preedy and Watson [1], "How not to Die" by Michael Greger [156], and online resources such as "Forks over Knives" [157] that can be the basis for educated decisions on diet for the treatment and prevention of most chronic disease.

References

1. Preedy V, Watson R. The Mediterranean diet 1st edition: an evidence-based approach. Waltham, MA, USA: Academic Press; 2015.
2. Keys A. Seven countries. A multivariate analysis of death and coronary heart disease, 1st ed. Cambridge, MA, USA: Harvard University Press; 1980.
3. Mediterranean diet – Intangible cultural heritage – UNESCO. 2013. https://www.ich.unesco.org/en/RL/mediterranean-diet-00884. Accessed April 2019.
4. Simopoulos AP. The Mediterranean diets: what is so special about the diet of Greece? The scientific evidence. J Nutr. 2001;131:3065S–73S.
5. de Lorgeril M, Salen P, Rabaeus M. New and traditional foods in a modernized mediterranean diet model. Eur J Clin Nutr. 2018; https://doi.org/10.1038/s41430-018-0308-6.
6. Trichopoulou A, Martínez-González MA, Prabhakaran D, Mozaffarian D, de Lorgeril M. Definitions and potential health benefits of the mediterranean diet: views from experts around the world. BMC Med. 2014;12:112.
7. The top ten causes of death – World Health Organization. 2018. https://www.who.int/news-room/fact-sheets/detail/the-top-10-causes-of-death. Accessed April 2019.
8. Sofi F, Abbate R, Gensini GF, Casini A. Accruing evidence on benefits of adherence to the mediterranean diet on health: an updated systematic review and meta-analysis. Am J Clin Nutr. 2010;92:1189–96.
9. Martínez-González MA, García-López M, Bes-Rastrollo M, Toledo E, Martínez-Lapiscina EH, Delgado-Rodriguez M, et al. Mediterranean diet and the incidence of cardiovascular disease: a Spanish cohort. Nutr Metab Cardiovasc Dis. 2011;21:237–44.
10. Hoevenaar-Blom MP, Nooyens AC, Kromhout D, Spijkerman AM, Beulens JW, Van Der Schouw YT, et al. Mediterranean style diet and 12-year incidence of cardiovascular diseases: the EPIC-NL cohort study. PLoS One. 2012;7:e45458.
11. Gardener H, Wright CB, Gu Y, Demmer RT, Boden-Albala B, Elkind MS, et al. Mediterranean-style diet and risk of ischemic stroke, myocardial infarction, and vascular death: the Northern Manhattan Study. Am J Clin Nutr. 2012;94:1458–64.
12. de Lorgeril M, Renaud S, Mamelle N, Salen P, Martin JL, Monjaud I, et al. Mediterranean alpha-linolenic acid-rich diet in secondary prevention of coronary heart disease. Lancet. 1994;343:1454–9. Erratum in: Lancet 1995;345:738
13. de Lorgeril M, Salen P, Martin JL, Monjaud I, Delaye J, Mamelle N. Mediterranean diet, traditional risk factors, and the rate of cardiovascular complications after myocardial infarction: final report of the Lyon Diet Heart Study. Circulation. 1999;99:779–85.
14. Estruch R, Ros E, Salas-Salvadó J, Covas M, Corella D, Arós F, et al. Primary prevention of cardiovascular disease with a Mediterranean diet supplemented with extra-virgin olive oil or nuts. N Engl J Med. 2018;378:e34.
15. WHO fact sheet on cancer providing key facts – World Health Organization. 2018. https://www.who.int/news-room/fact-sheets/detail/cancer. Accessed April 2019.

16. de Lorgeril M, Salen P, Martin JL, Monjaud I, Boucher P, Mamelle N. Mediterranean dietary pattern in a randomized trial: prolonged survival and possible reduced cancer rate. Arch Intern Med. 1998;158:1181–7.
17. Castelló A, Boldo E, Amiano P, Castaño-Vinyals G, Aragonés N, Gómez-Acebo I, et al. Mediterranean dietary pattern is associated with low risk of aggressive prostate cancer: MCC-Spain study. J Urol. 2018;199:430–7.
18. Singh PN, Fraser GE. Dietary risk factors for Colon Cancer in a low-risk population. Am J Epidemiol. 1998;148:761–74.
19. Ferlay J, Steliarova-Foucher E, Lortet-Tieulent J, Rosso S, Coebergh JWW, Comber H, et al. Cancer incidence and mortality patterns in Europe: estimates for 40 countries in 2012. Eur J Cancer. 2013;49:1374–403.
20. Trichopoulou A, Bamia C, Lagiou P, Trichopoulos D. Conformity to traditional Mediterranean diet and breast cancer risk in the Greek EPIC (European Prospective Investigation into Cancer and Nutrition) cohort. Am J Clin Nutr. 2010;92:620–5.
21. Wu AH, Yu MC, Tseng CC, Stanczyk FZ, Pike MC. Dietary patterns and breast cancer risk in Asian American women. Am J Clin Nutr. 2009;89:1145–54.
22. Fung TT, Hu FB, McCullough ML, Newby PK, Willett WC, Holmes. Diet quality is associated with the risk of estrogen receptor–negative breast cancer in postmenopausal women. J Nutr. 2006;136:466–72.
23. Toledo E, Salas-Salvadó J, Donat-Vargas C, Buil-Cosiales P, Estruch R, Ros E, et al. Mediterranean diet and invasive breast cancer risk among women at high cardiovascular risk in the PREDIMED trial: a randomized clinical trial. JAMA Intern Med. 2015;175:1752–60.
24. Cade JE, Taylor EF, Burley VJ, Greenwood DC. Does the Mediterranean dietary pattern or the healthy diet index influence the risk of breast cancer in a large British cohort of women? Eur J Clin Nutr. 2011;65:920–8.
25. Couto E, Sandin S, Löf M, Ursin G, Adami HO, Weiderpass E. Mediterranean dietary pattern and risk of breast cancer. PLoS One. 2013;82:e55374.
26. Sing H, Siegel RL, Torre LA, et al. Global patterns in excess body weight and the associated cancer burden. CA Cancer J Clin. 2018;69:1–25.
27. Scarmeas N, Stern Y, Mayeux R, Manly JJ, Schupf N, Luchsinger JA. Mediterranean diet and mild cognitive impairment. Arch Neurol. 2009;66:216–25.
28. Gardener S, Gu Y, Rainey-Smith SR, Keogh JB, Clifton PM, Mathieson SL, et al. Adherence to a Mediterranean diet and Alzheimer's disease risk in an Australian population. Transl Psychiatry. 2012;2:e164.
29. Scarmeas N, Stern Y, Tang MX, Mayeux R, Luchsinger JA. Mediterranean diet and risk for Alzheimers disease. Ann Neurol. 2006;59:912–21.
30. Feart C, Samieri C, Rondeau V, Amieva H, Portet F, Dartigues JF, et al. Adherence to a Mediterranean diet, cognitive decline, and risk of dementia. JAMA. 2009;302:638–48.
31. Bhushan A, Fondell E, Ascherio A, Yuan C, Grodstein F, Willett W. Adherence to Mediterranean diet and subjective cognitive function in men. Eur J Epidemiol. 2018;33:223–34.
32. Psaltopoulou T, Sergentanis TN, Panagiotakos DB, Sergentanis IN, Kost R, Scarmeas N. Mediterranean diet, stroke, cognitive impairment, and depression: a meta-analysis. Ann Neurol. 2013;74:580–91.
33. Singh B, Parsaik AK, Mielke MM, Erwin PJ, Knopman DS, Petersen RC, et al. Association of Mediterranean diet with mild cognitive impairment and Alzheimer's disease: a systematic review and meta-analysis. J Alzheimer Dis. 2014;39:271–82.
34. Loughrey DG, Lavecchia S, Brennan S, Lawlor BA, Kelly ME. The impact of the Mediterranean diet on the cognitive functioning of healthy older adults: a systematic review and meta-analysis. Adv Nutr. 2017;8:57186.
35. Martínez-Lapiscina EH, Clavero P, Toledo E, Estruch R, Salas-Salvad J, San Julián B, et al. Mediterranean diet improves cognition: the PREDIMED-NAVARRA randomised trial. J Neurol Neurosurg Psychiatry. 2013;84:1318–25.

36. Adams LA, Lymp JF, Sauver JS, Sanderson SO, Lindor KD, Feldstein A, et al. The natural history of nonalcoholic fatty liver disease: a population-based cohort study. Gastroenterology. 2015;129:113–21.
37. Younossi Z, Anstee QM, Marietti M, Hardy T, Henry L, et al. Global burden of NAFLD and NASH: trends, predictions, risk factors and prevention. Nat Rev Gastroenterol Hepatol. 2018;15:11–20.
38. Bray GA, Popkin BM. Calorie-sweetened beverages and fructose: what have we learned 10 years later. Pediatr Obes. 2013;8:242–8.
39. Kontogianni MD, Tileli N, Margariti A, Georgoulis M, Deutsch M, Tiniakos D, et al. Adherence to the Mediterranean diet is associated with the severity of non-alcoholic fatty liver disease. Clin Nutr. 2014;33:678–83.
40. Ryan MC, Itsiopoulos C, Thodis T, Ward G, Trost N, Hofferberth S, et al. The Mediterranean diet improves hepatic steatosis and insulin sensitivity in individuals with non-alcoholic fatty liver disease. J Hepatol. 2013;59:138–43.
41. Cakir M, Akbulut UE, Okten A. Association between adherence to the Mediterranean diet and presence of nonalcoholic fatty liver disease in children. Child Obes. 2016;12:279–85.
42. Della Corte C, Mosca A, Vania A, Alterio A, Iasevoli S, Nobili V. Good adherence to the Mediterranean diet reduces the risk for NASH and diabetes in pediatric patients with obesity: the results of an Italian study. Nutrition. 2017;39:8–14.
43. Rennie K, Hughes J, Lang R, Jebb SA. Nutritional management of rheumatoid arthritis: a review of the evidence. J Hum Nutr Diet. 2003;16:97–109.
44. Sköldstam L, Hagfors L, Johansson G. An experimental study of a Mediterranean diet intervention for patients with rheumatoid arthritis. Ann Rheum Dis. 2003;62:208–14.
45. Matsumoto Y, Sugioka Y, Tada M, Okano T, Mamoto K, et al. Monounsaturated fatty acids might be key factors in the Mediterranean diet that suppress rheumatoid arthritis disease activity: the TOMORROW study. Clin Nutr. 2018;37:675–80.
46. Ebringer A, Rashid T. Rheumatoid arthritis is caused by a Proteus urinary tract infection. APMIS. 2014;122(5):363–8.
47. Kjeldsen-Kragh J. Rheumatoid arthritis treated with vegetarian diets. Am J Clin Nutr. 1999;70(3):594S–600S.
48. Devereux G, Seaton A. Diet as a risk factor for atopy and asthma. J Allergy Clin Immunol. 2005;115:1109–17.
49. Chatzi L, Apostolaki G, Bibakis I, Skypala I, Bibaki-Liakou V, Tzanakis N, et al. Protective effect of fruits, vegetables and the Mediterranean diet on asthma and allergies among children in Crete. Thorax. 2007;62:677–83.
50. Barros R, Moreira A, Fonseca J, Ferraz de Olivei J, Delgado L, Castel-Branco MG, et al. Adherence to the Mediterranean diet and fresh fruit intake are associated with improved asthma control. Allergy. 2008;63:917–23.
51. Castro-Rodriguez JA, Garcia-Marcos L, Rojas JDA, Valverde-Molina J, Sanchez-Solis M. Mediterranean diet as a protective factor for wheezing in preschool children. J Pediatr. 2008;152:823–8.
52. De Batlle J, Garcia-Aymerich J, Barraza-Villarreal A, Antó JM, Romieu I. Mediterranean diet is associated with reduced asthma and rhinitis in Mexican children. Allergy. 2008;63:1310–6.
53. Garcia-Marcos L, Canflanca IM, Garrido JB, Varela ALS, Garcia-Hernandez G, Grima FG, et al. Relationship of asthma and rhinoconjunctivitis with obesity, exercise and Mediterranean diet in Spanish schoolchildren. Thorax. 2007;62:503–8.
54. Chatzi L, Torrent M, Romieu I, Garcia-Esteban R, Ferrer C, Vioque J, et al. Mediterranean diet in pregnancy is protective for wheeze and atopy in childhood. Thorax. 2008;63:507–13.
55. Arvaniti F, Priftis KN, Papadimitriou A, Papadopoulos M, Roma E, Kapsokefalou M, et al. Adherence to the Mediterranean type of diet is associated with lower prevalence of asthma symptoms, among 10–12 years old children: the PANACEA study. Pediatr All Immunol. 2011;22:283–9.

56. Sexton P, Black P, Metcalf P, Wall CR, Ley S, Wu L, et al. Influence of Mediterranean diet on asthma symptoms, lung function, and systemic inflammation: a randomized controlled trial. J Asthma. 2013;50:75–81.
57. Aaron SD, Vandemheen KL, FitzGerald JM, Ainslie M, Gupta S, Lemière C, Field SK, McIvor RA, Hernandez P, Mayers I, Mulpuru S, Alvarez GG, Pakhale S, Mallick R, Boulet LP. Reevaluation of diagnosis in adults with physician-diagnosed asthma. JAMA. 2017;317(3):269–79. https://doi.org/10.1001/jama.2016.19627.
58. Liyanagedera S, McLeod R, Elhassan HA. Exercise induced laryngeal obstruction: a review of diagnosis and management. Eur Arch Otorhinolaryngol. 2017;274(4):1781–9. https://doi.org/10.1007/s00405-016-4338-1. Epub 2016 Oct 11
59. Zalvan CH, Yuen E, Geliebter J, Tiwari R. A trigger reduction approach to treatment of paradoxical vocal fold motion disorder in the pediatric population. J Voice. 2019. https://doi.org/10.1016/j.jvoice.2019.08.013.
60. Mente A, de Koning L, Shannon HS, Anand SS. A systematic review of the evidence supporting a causal link between dietary factors and coronary heart disease. Arch Intern Med. 2009;169:659–69.
61. Alexander DD, Miller PE, Van Elswyk ME, Kuratko CN, Bylsma LC. A meta-analysis of randomized controlled trials and prospective cohort studies of eicosapentaenoic and docosahexaenoic long-chain omega-3 fatty acids and coronary heart disease risk. Mayo Clin Proc. 2017;92:15–29.
62. Aung T, Halsey J, Kromhout D, Gerstein HC, Marchioli R, Tavazzi L, et al. Associations of Omega-3 fatty acid supplement use with cardiovascular disease risks: meta-analysis of 10 trials involving 77 917 individuals. JAMA Cardiol. 2018;3:225–34.
63. Siscovick DS, Barringer TA, Fretts AM, Wu JH, Lichtenstein AH, Costello RB, et al. Omega-3 polyunsaturated fatty acid (fish oil) supplementation and the prevention of clinical cardiovascular disease: a science advisory from the American Heart Association. Circulation. 2017;135:e867–84.
64. Kromhout D, Bosschieter EB, Coulander CDL. The inverse relation between fish consumption and 20-year mortality from coronary heart disease. N Engl J Med. 1985;312:1205–9.
65. Daviglus ML, Stamler J, Orencia AJ, Dyer AR, Liu K, Greenland P, et al. Fish consumption and the 30-year risk of fatal myocardial infarction. N Engl J Med. 1997;336:1046–53.
66. Albert CM, Hennekens CH, O'donnell CJ, Ajani UA, Carey VJ, Willett WC, et al. Fish consumption and risk of sudden cardiac death. JAMA. 1998;279:23–2.
67. Hu F, Bronner L, Willett WC, Stampfer MJ, Rexrode KM, Albert CM, et al. Fish and omega-3 fatty acid intake and risk of coronary heart disease in women. JAMA. 2002;287:1815–21.
68. Ascherio A, Rimm EB, Stampfer MJ, Giovannucci EL, Willett WC. Dietary intake of marine n-3 fatty acids, fish intake, and the risk of coronary disease among men. N Engl J Med. 1995;332:977–83.
69. Amiano P, Chamosa S, Etxezarreta N, Arriola L, Moreno-Iribas C, Huerta JM, et al. No association between fish consumption and risk of stroke in the Spanish cohort of the European Prospective Investigation into Cancer and Nutrition (EPIC-Spain): a 13· 8-year follow-up study. Public Health Nutr. 2016;19:674–81.
70. Kühn T, Teucher B, Kaaks R, Boeing H, Weikert C. Buijsse. Fish consumption and the risk of myocardial infarction and stroke in the German arm of the European Prospective Investigation into Cancer and Nutrition (EPIC-Germany). Br J Nutr. 2013;110:1118–25.
71. Grosso G, Marventano S, Yang J, Micek A, Pajak A, Scalfi L, et al. A comprehensive meta-analysis on evidence of Mediterranean diet and cardiovascular disease: are individual components equal? Crit Rev Food Sci Nutr. 2017;57:3218–32.
72. Yu XF, Zou J, Dong J. Fish consumption and risk of gastrointestinal cancers: a meta-analysis of cohort studies. World J Gastroenterol. 2014;20:15398–412.
73. Huang RX, Duan YY, Hu JA. Fish intake and risk of liver cancer: a meta-analysis. PLoS One. 2015;10:e0096102.

74. Lian W, Wang R, Xing B, Yao Y. Fish intake and the risk of brain tumor: a meta-analysis with systematic review. Nutr J. 2017;16:1.
75. Yassine HN, Feng Q, Azizkhanian I, Rawat V, Castor K, Fonteh AN, et al. Association of serum docosahexaenoic acid with cerebral amyloidosis. JAMA Neurol. 2016;73:1208–16.
76. de Lorgeril M, Salen P. Alpha-linolenic acid and coronary heart disease. Nutr Metab Cardiovasc Dis. 2004;14:162–9.
77. Hu FB, Stampfer MJ, Manson JE, Rimm EB, Wolk A, Colditz GA, et al. Dietary intake of α-linolenic acid and risk of fatal ischemic heart disease among women. Am J Clin Nutr. 1999;69:890–7.
78. Fleming JA, Kris-Etherton PM. The evidence for α-linolenic acid and cardiovascular disease benefits: comparisons with eicosapentaenoic acid and docosahexaenoic acid. Adv Nutr. 2014;5:863S–76S.
79. Yamagishi K, Ikeda A, Chei CL, Noda H, Umesawa M, Cui R, et al. Serum α-linolenic and other ω-3 fatty acids, and risk of disabling dementia: community-based nested case–control study. Clin Nutr. 2017;36:793–7.
80. Voss A, Reinhart M, Sankarappa S, Sprecher H. The metabolism of 7, 10, 13, 16, 19-docosapentaenoic acid to 4, 7, 10, 13, 16, 19-docosahexaenoic acid in rat liver is independent of a 4-desaturase. J Biol Chem. 1991;266:19995–20000.
81. Sprecher H. Metabolism of highly unsaturated n-3 and n-6 fatty acids. BBA Mol Cell Biol Lipids. 2000;1486:219–31.
82. Glaser C, Heinrich J, Koletzko B. Role of FADS1 and FADS2 polymorphisms in polyunsaturated fatty acid metabolism. Metab Clin Exp. 2010;59:993–9.
83. Horrobin DF. Fatty acid metabolism in health and disease: the role of delta-6-desaturase. Am J Clin Nutr. 1993;57:732S–6S.
84. Burdge GC, Wootton SA. Conversion of α-linolenic acid to eicosapentaenoic, docosapentaenoic and docosahexaenoic acids in young women. Br J Nutr. 2002;88:411–20.
85. de Lorgeril M, Salen P, Martin JL, Boucher F, De Leiris J. Interactions of wine drinking with omega-3 fatty acids in patients with coronary heart disease: a fish-like effect of moderate wine drinking. Am Heart J. 2008;155:175–81.
86. di Giuseppe R, de Lorgeril M, Salen P, Laporte F, Di Castelnuovo A, Krogh V, et al. European Collaborative Group of the IMMIDIET Project. Alcohol consumption and n-3 polyunsaturated fatty acids in healthy men and women from 3 European populations. Am J Clin Nutr. 2009;89:354–362.
87. Toufektsian MC, Salen P, Laporte F, Tonelli C, de Lorgeril M. Dietary flavonoids increase plasma very long-chain (n-3) fatty acids in rats. J Nutr. 2010;141:37–41.
88. Vauzour D, Tejera N, O'Neill C, Booz V, Jude B, Wolf IM, et al. Anthocyanins do not influence long-chain n-3 fatty acid status: studies in cells, rodents and humans. J Nutr Biochem. 2015;26:211–8.
89. Burak C, Wolffram S, Zur B, Langguth P, Fimmers R, Alteheld B, et al. Effects of the flavonol quercetin and α-linolenic acid on n-3 PUFA status in metabolically healthy men and women: a randomised, double-blinded, placebo-controlled, crossover trial. Br J Nutr. 2017;117:698–711.
90. Ounnas F, Privé F, Salen P, Gaci N, Tottey W, Calani L, et al. Whole Rye consumption improves blood and liver n-3 fatty acid profile and gut microbiota composition in rats. PLoS One. 2016;11:e0148118.
91. Schwingshackl L, Hoffmann G. Monounsaturated fatty acids, olive oil and health status: a systematic review and meta-analysis of cohort studies. Lipids Health Dis. 2014;13:154.
92. Alonso A, Ruiz-Gutierrez V, Martínez-González MÁ. Monounsaturated fatty acids, olive oil and blood pressure: epidemiological, clinical and experimental evidence. Public Health Nutr. 2006;9:251–7.
93. Psaltopoulou T, Kosti RI, Haidopoulos D, Dimopoulos M, Panagiotakos DB. Olive oil intake is inversely related to cancer prevalence: a systematic review and a meta-analysis of 13800 patients and 23340 controls in 19 observational studies. Lipids Health Dis. 2011;10:127–35.

94. Schwingshackl L, Lampousi AM, Portillo MP, Romaguera D, Hoffmann G, Boeing H. Olive oil in the prevention and management of type 2 diabetes mellitus: a systematic review and meta-analysis of cohort studies and intervention trials. Nutr Diabetes. 2017;7:e262.
95. Rodríguez-Morató J, Xicota L, Fitó M, Farré M, Dierssen M, de la Torre R. Potential role of olive oil phenolic compounds in the prevention of neurodegenerative diseases. Molecules. 2015;20:4655–80.
96. Guasch-Ferré M, Hu FB, Martínez-González MA, Fitó M, Bulló M, Estruch R, et al. Olive oil intake and risk of cardiovascular disease and mortality in the PREDIMED study. BMC Med. 2015;12:78.
97. Villegas AS, Sanchez-Taínta A. The prevention of cardiovascular disease through the Mediterranean diet. 1st ed. San Diego, CA, USA: Academic Press; 2017.
98. Rueda-Clausen CF, Silva FA, Lindarte MA, Villa-Roel C, Gomez E, Gutierrez R, Cure-Cure C, López-Jaramillo P. Olive, soybean and palm oils intake have a similar acute detrimental effect over the endothelial function in healthy young subjects. Nutr Metab Cardiovasc Dis. 2007;17(1):50–7. Epub 2006 Mar 20
99. Buckland G, Travier N, Barricarte A, Ardanaz E, Moreno-Iribas C, Sánchez MJ, Molina-Montes E, Chirlaque MD, Huerta JM, Navarro C, Redondo ML, Amiano P, Dorronsoro M, Larrañaga N, Gonzalez CA. Olive oil intake and CHD in the European prospective investigation into cancer and nutrition Spanish cohort. Br J Nutr. 2012;108(11):2075–82. https://doi.org/10.1017/S000711451200298X. Epub 2012 Sep 25.
100. Harvard School of Public Health, Healthy Eating Plate & Healthy Eating Pyramid. https://www.hsph.harvard.edu/nutritionsource/healthy-eating-plate/. Accessed April 2019.
101. Krauss RM, Eckel RH, Howard B, Appel LJ, Daniels SR, Deckelbaum RJ, et al. AHA dietary guidelines: revision 2000: a statement for healthcare professionals from the nutrition Committee of the American Heart Association. Circulation. 2000;102:2284–99.
102. World Health Organization. Nutrition and the prevention of chronic diseases. WHO. Technical Report Series 916. Geneva: World Health Organization; 2003.
103. Crowe FL, Roddam AW, Key TJ, Appleby PN, Overvad K, Jakobsen MU, et al. Fruit and vegetable intake and mortality from ischaemic heart disease: results from the European Prospective Investigation into Cancer and Nutrition (EPIC)-Heart study. Eur Heart J. 2011;32:1235–43.
104. Oyebode O, Gordon-Dseagu V, Walker A, Mindell JS. Fruit and vegetable consumption and all-cause, cancer and CVD mortality: analysis of health survey for England data. J Epidemiol Community Health. 2014;68:856–62.
105. Pounis G, Costanzo S, Di Giuseppe R, De Lucia F, Santimone I, Sciarretta A, et al. Consumption of healthy foods at different content of antioxidant vitamins and phytochemicals and metabolic risk factors for cardiovascular disease in men and women of the Moli–sani study. Eur J Clin Nutr. 2013;67:207–14.
106. Pounis G, Bonaccio M, Di Castelnuovo A, Costanzo S, De Curtis A, Persichillo M, et al. Polyphenol intake is associated with low-grade inflammation, using a novel data analysis from the Moli-sani study. Thromb Haemost. 2016;115:344–52.
107. Bonaccio M, Pounis G, Cerletti C, Donati MB, Iacoviello L, Gaetano G. Mediterranean diet, dietary polyphenols and low grade inflammation: results from the MOLI-SANI study. Br J Clin Pharmacol. 2017;83:107–13.
108. Wang X, Ouyang Y, Liu J, Zhu M, Zhao G, Bao W, Hu FB. Fruit and vegetable consumption and mortality from all causes, cardiovascular disease, and cancer: systematic review and dose-response meta-analysis of prospective cohort studies. BMJ. 2014;349:4490.
109. Aune D, Giovannucci E, Boffetta P, Fadnes LT, Keum N, Norat T, et al. Fruit and vegetable intake and the risk of cardiovascular disease, total cancer and all-cause mortality—a systematic review and dose-response meta-analysis of prospective studies. Intern J Epidemiol. 2017;46:1029–56.
110. Broekmans WM, Klöpping-Ketelaars WAA, Kluft C, Van den Berg H, Kok FJ, Van Poppel G. Fruit and vegetables and cardiovascular risk profile: a diet controlled intervention study. Eur J Clin Nutr. 2001;55:636–44.

111. John JH, Ziebland S, Yudkin P, Roe LS, Neil HAW. Effects of fruit and vegetable consumption on plasma antioxidant concentrations and blood pressure: a randomised controlled trial. Lancet. 2002;359:1969–74.
112. Khan F, Ray S, Craigie AM, Kennedy G, Hill A, Barton KL, et al. Lowering of oxidative stress improves endothelial function in healthy subjects with habitually low intake of fruit and vegetables: a randomized controlled trial of antioxidant-and polyphenol-rich blackcurrant juice. Free Rad Biol Med. 2014;72:232–7.
113. Mirmiran P, Bahadoran Z, Ghasemi A, Jeddi S, Azizi F. High-sulforaphane broccoli sprout powder reduces serum nitric oxide metabolites in helicobacter pylori infected patients. J Funct Foods. 2017;34:356–68.
114. de Lorgeril M, Salen P, Laporte F, Boucher F, de Leiris J. Potential use of nuts for the prevention and treatment of coronary heart disease: from natural to functional foods. Nutr Metab Cardiovasc Dis. 2001;11:362–71.
115. Manach C, Scalbert A, Morand C, Rémésy C, Jiménez L. Polyphenols: food sources and bioavailability. Am J Clin Nutr. 2004;79:727–47.
116. Kelly JH, Sabaté J. Nuts and coronary heart disease: an epidemiological perspective. Br J Nutr. 2006;96:S61–7.
117. Jiang R, Jacobs DR Jr, Mayer-Davis E, Szklo M, Herrington D, Jenny NS, et al. Nut and seed consumption and inflammatory markers in the multi-ethnic study of atherosclerosis. Am J Epidemiol. 2005;163:222–31.
118. Salas-Salvadó J, Fernández-Ballart J, Ros E, Martínez-González MA, Fitó M, Estruch R, et al. Effect of a Mediterranean diet supplemented with nuts on metabolic syndrome status: one-year results of the PREDIMED randomized trial. Arch Intern Med. 2008;168:2449–58.
119. Jones JR, Lineback DM, Levine MJ. Dietary reference intakes: implications for fiber labeling and consumption: a summary of the international life sciences institute North America fiber workshop, June 1–2, 2004, Washington, DC. Nutr Rev. 2006;64:31–8.
120. Jacobs DR Jr, Meyer KA, Kushi LH, Folsom AR. Whole-grain intake may reduce the risk of ischemic heart disease death in postmenopausal women: the Iowa Women's Health Study. Am J Clin Nutr. 1998;68:248–57.
121. Liu S, Stampfer MJ, Hu FB, Giovannucci E, Rimm E, Manson JE, et al. Whole-grain consumption and risk of coronary heart disease: results from the Nurses' Health Study. Am J Clin Nutr. 1999;70:412–9.
122. Jensen MK, Koh-Banerjee P, Hu FB, Franz M, Sampson L, Grønbæk M, et al. Intakes of whole grains, bran, and germ and the risk of coronary heart disease in men. Am J Clin Nutr. 2004;80:1492–9.
123. Ascherio A, Rimm EB, Hernan MA, Giovannucci EL, Kawachi I, Stampfer MJ, et al. Intake of potassium, magnesium, calcium, and fiber and risk of stroke among US men. Circulation. 1998;98:1198–204.
124. Threapleton DE, Greenwood DC, Evans CE, Cleghorn CL, Nykjaer C, Woodhead C, et al. Dietary fiber intake and risk of first stroke: a systematic review and meta-analysis. Stroke. 2013;44:1360–8.
125. Salmeron J, Manson JE, Stampfer MJ, Colditz GA, Wing AL, Willett WC. Dietary fiber, glycemic load, and risk of noninsulin-dependent diabetes mellitus in women. JAMA. 1997;277:472–7.
126. Schulze MB, Liu S, Rimm EB, Manson JE, Willett WC, Hu FB. Glycemic index, glycemic load, and dietary fiber intake and incidence of type 2 diabetes in younger and middle-aged women. Am J Clin Nutr. 2004;80:348–56.
127. Meyer KA, Kushi LH, Jacobs DR Jr, Slavin J, Sellers TA, Folsom AR. Carbohydrates, dietary fiber, and incident type-2 diabetes in older women. Am J Clin Nutr. 2000;71:921–30.
128. Chandalia M, Garg A, Lutjohann D, von Bergmann K, Grundy SM, Brinkley LJ. Beneficial effects of high dietary fiber intake in patients with type 2 diabetes mellitus. N Engl J Med. 2000;342:1392–8.

129. Yao B, Fang H, Xu W, Yan Y, Xu H, Liu Y, et al. Dietary fiber intake and risk of type 2 diabetes: a dose–response analysis of prospective studies. Eur J Epidemiol. 2014;29:79–88.
130. St Leger AS, Cochrane AL, Moore F. Factors associated with cardiac mortality in developed countries with particular reference to the consumption of wine. Lancet. 1979;313:1017–20.
131. Renaud SD, de Lorgeril M. 1992. Wine, alcohol, platelets, and the French paradox for coronary heart disease. Lancet. 1992;339:1523–6.
132. de Lorgeril M, Salen P, Paillard F, Laporte F, Boucher F, de Leiris J. Mediterranean diet and the French paradox: two distinct biogeographic concepts for one consolidated scientific theory on the role of nutrition in coronary heart disease. Cardiovasc Res. 2002;54:503–15.
133. de Lorgeril M, Salen P, Martin JL, Boucher F, Paillard F, de Leiris J. Wine drinking and risks of cardiovascular complications after recent acute myocardial infarction. Circulation. 2002;106:1465–9.
134. de Lorgeril M, Salen P. Wine ethanol, platelets, and Mediterranean diet. Lancet. 1999;353:1067.
135. Grønbaek M, Di Castelnuovo A, Iacoviello L, Furman K, Donati MB, de Gaetano G, Trichopoulou A, La Vecchia C, Corrao G, De Lorgeril M, Salen P. Wine, alcohol and cardiovascular risk: open issue. J Thromb Haemost. 2004;2:2041–8.
136. de Lorgeril M, Salen P, Guiraud A, Boucher F, de Leiris J. Resveratrol and non-ethanolic components of wine in experimental cardiology. Nutr Metab Cardiovasc Dis. 2003;13:100–3.
137. Guiraud A, de Lorgeril M, Boucher F, Berthonneche C, Rakotovao A, de Leiris J. Cardioprotective effect of chronic low dose ethanol drinking: insights into the concept of ethanol preconditioning. J Mol Cell Cardiol. 2004;36:561–6.
138. Di Castelnuovo A, Rotondo S, Iacoviello L, Donati MB, de Gaetano G. Meta-analysis of wine and beer consumption in relation to vascular risk. Circulation. 2002;105:2836–44.
139. Ronksley PE, Brien SE, Turner BJ, Mukamal KJ, Ghali WA. Association of alcohol consumption with selected cardiovascular disease outcomes: a systematic review and meta-analysis. BMJ. 2011;342:d671.
140. GBD 2016 Alcohol Collaborators. Alcohol use and burden for 195 countries and territories, 1990-2016: a systematic analysis for the global burden of disease study 2016. Lancet. 2018;392(10152):1015–35. https://doi.org/10.1016/S0140-6736(18)31310-2. Epub 2018 Aug 23
141. Bach A, Serra-Majem L, Carrasco JL, Roman B, Ngo J, Bertomeu I, et al. The use of indexes evaluating the adherence to the Mediterranean diet in epidemiological studies: a review. Public Health Nutr. 2006;9:132–46.
142. Trichopoulou A, Costacou T, Bamia C, Trichopoulos D. Adherence to a Mediterranean diet and survival in a Greek population. N Engl J Med. 2003;348:2599–608.
143. Alberti-Fidanza A, Fidanza F. Mediterranean adequacy index of Italian diets. Public Health Nutr. 2004;7:937–41.
144. Panagiotakos DB, Pitsavos C, Arvaniti F, Stefanadis C. Adherence to the Mediterranean food pattern predicts the prevalence of hypertension, hypercholesterolemia, diabetes and obesity, among healthy adults; the accuracy of the MedDietScore. Prev Med. 2007;44:335–40.
145. Martínez-González MA, García-Arellano A, Toledo E, Salas-Salvado J, Buil-Cosiales P, Corella D, et al. A 14-item Mediterranean diet assessment tool and obesity indexes among high-risk subjects: the PREDIMED trial. PLoS One. 2012;7:e43134.
146. Cuadrado E, Gutiérrez-Domingo T, Castillo-Mayen R, Luque B, Arenas A, Taberneroa C. The self-efficacy scale for adherence to the Mediterranean diet (SESAMeD): a scale construction and validation. Appetite. 2018;120:6–15.
147. Bonaccio M, Donati M, Iacoviello L, de Gaetano G. Socioeconomic determinants of the adherence to the Mediterranean diet at a time of economic crisis: the experience of the MOLI-SANI Study1. Agr Agricult Science Proc. 2016;8:741–7.

148. Bonaccio M, Di Castelnuovo A, Bonanni A, Costanzo S, De Lucia F, Persichillo M, et al. Decline of the Mediterranean diet at a time of economic crisis. Results from the Moli-sani study. Nutr Metab Cardiovasc Dis. 2014;24:853–60.
149. Bonaccio M, Di Castelnuovo A, Costanzo S, De Lucia F, Olivieri M, Donati MB, et al. Mass media information and adherence to Mediterranean diet: results from the Moli-sani study. Intern J Public Health. 2012;57:589–97.
150. Bonaccio M, Di Castelnuovo A, Costanzo S, De Lucia F, Olivieri M, Donati MB, et al. Nutrition knowledge is associated with higher adherence to Mediterranean diet and lower prevalence of obesity. Results from the Moli-sani study. Appetite. 2013;68:139–46.
151. Canada's Food Guide. Canadian Government. Accessed August 2019. https://food-guide.canada.ca/en/.
152. Souza RG, Gomes AC, Naves MM, Mota JF. Nuts and legume seeds for cardiovascular risk reduction: scientific evidence and mechanisms of action. Nutr Rev. 2015;73:335–47.
153. Dernini S, Berry EM, Serra-Majem L, La Vecchia C, Capone R, Medina FX, et al. Med diet 4.0: the Mediterranean diet with four sustainable benefits. Public Health Nutr. 2017;20:1322–30.
154. Pimentel D, Pimentel M. Sustainability of meat-based and plant-based diets and the environment. Am J Clin Nutr. 2003;78:660S–3S.
155. Sáez-Almendros S, Obrador B, Bach-Faig A, Serra-Majem L. Environmental footprints of Mediterranean versus Western dietary patterns: beyond the health benefits of the Mediterranean diet. Environ Health. 2013;12:118–22.
156. Greger M, Stone M. How not to die: discover the foods scientifically proven to prevent and reverse disease. New York: Flatiron Books; 2015.
157. Forks over Knives. Online resource for plant-based nutrition. https://www.forksoverknives.com/. Accessed August 2019.

Chapter 41
Mediterranean-Style Whole-Food, Plant-Based Diet: Dealing with Common Myths and Transitioning with Complex Medical and Surgical History

Maria Carolina Rojido

When people transition to a plant-based diet, they may be confronted with many myths and doubts. This chapter answers many of those questions, starting with some essential concepts.

First of all, let us clarify what is a whole foods, plant-based diet (WFPB): it is a way of eating that emphasizes the consumption of minimally processed and nutrient-dense vegetables, fruits, whole grains, legumes, nuts, and seeds. WFPB minimizes or eliminates meat, poultry, fish, eggs, dairy products, and processed foods of animal (sausages and cured meats) or plant origin (refined grains, added refined sugars and oils, and artificial ingredients). Veganism avoids completely any foods or products of animal origin but can include highly processed foods that are detrimental to health. Therefore, the emphasis on whole foods in WFPB is essential [1, 2]. A 90–95% Mediterranean-style whole-food, plant-based diet differs in that it encompasses a spectrum of eating patterns that are predominantly plant-based but that (like vegetarianism, pescatarianism, and the Mediterranean diet) may include some animal products. The WFPB diet may include up to 5% of whole foods of animal origin (red meat and processed meat is completely excluded) and still retain the overall health benefits. However, the therapeutic effects of this diet appear to be more significant the closer a person is to being 100% plant based [3–6].

To those new to nutrition, the importance of "whole foods" may sound like a new concept. But it is central to healthful nutrition, because as any creature that belongs to the natural world, humans are not intended to consume processed foods and drinks, much less the "ultra-processed" ones dominant in the modern Western society.

Homo sapiens appeared about 315,000 years ago [7]. Since then, we survived and progressed consuming whatever we could find in our environment. Food was minimally processed, if at all, and we tended to eat mostly plants partly because they are easier to collect than animals are to hunt. But in the last 10,000 years, our lifestyle

M. C. Rojido (✉)
Plant-based Nutrition Certificate, Freelance Medical Writer, Ségoufielle, France

C. H. Zalvan (ed.), *Laryngopharyngeal and Gastroesophageal Reflux*,
https://doi.org/10.1007/978-3-030-48890-1_41

habits have changed considerably, especially our diet. The advent of dairy products, refined plant derivatives (cereals, sugars, and vegetable oils), fatty meats, and salt changed the glycemic load, macronutrient content, fatty acid composition, micronutrient density, acid-base balance, sodium–potassium ratio, and fiber content of our diet [8]. Over the last century, these changes have become much more pronounced and our health and weight have changed accordingly.

Although whole foods may seem simple, they are actually quite complex. Containing hundreds of nutrients that are intended to act synergistically, they interact with each other in ways that we are only starting to understand. For example, 100 g of apple contains just 5.7 mg of vitamin C, but its antioxidant activity is equivalent to that of 1500 mg of the vitamin because that amount of vitamin C in the fruit is only one of the multiple antioxidants in a fresh apple that work together and potentiate each other [9]. The problem with food processing is that it divides whole foods and separates nutrients. When whole wheat is refined into white flour, we lose its fiber, vitamins, minerals, and phytochemicals; decrease its protein content, and are left with only its carbohydrate part. This refined product may later be fortified with a couple of elements like iron and folic acid, but not the rest that were lost during processing.

There is a practical tool that helps to categorize foods in terms of processing: NOVA. It is a useful classification that categorizes foods according to the extent and purpose of their processing, rather than in terms of nutrients. It includes four categories: unprocessed or minimally processed, processed culinary ingredients, processed, and ultra-processed foods and drinks. This last category includes snacks, drinks, and ready meals made of refined ingredients and additives that make them highly convenient, palatable, and profitable [10]. However, they are directly linked with degenerative chronic diseases and should not be consumed at all.

Last but not least, "Wholism" is also a very important concept in nutrition and in general medicine. The opposite, "reductionism" is what medical science has relied upon to progress over the last century. This "divide and conquer" approach, where processes are reduced into simpler units for better understanding, has allowed for amazing advances in diagnosing, treating, and preventing diseases. As a consequence, chronic diseases are treated with modern miracles like medicines or surgeries that alleviate and slow down disease progression but do not target the reason why people get sick in the first place: their lifestyle and particularly their diets. Nowadays, it is possible to explore biological processes underlying a disease at the molecular level, but sometimes, the complex interactions between these processes result in effects different from those that might be expected. The same thing happens in nutrition science where we reduce foods to macronutrients, micronutrients, etc. to understand them, but in the process, we lose sight of the fact that nutrients interact with each other in incredibly complex ways. In other words, the whole is greater than the sum of its parts [11]. This essential concept needs to be kept in mind when we look at our diets because if someone chooses to eat a lot of vegetables, this may lead to healthy outcomes. However, if they also consume processed meats, high-fat dairy, and ultra-processed foods, the diet would no longer be considered health promoting. Consuming vegetables in the presence of a higher portion of animal-based products does not ameliorate the negative effect of the non-plant-based component of the diet.

Addressing Common Myths

People considering a whole-food, plant-based diet may have many doubts rising from long-standing popular beliefs. This is perfectly normal and the following section aims at providing well-founded answers.

Myth #1: The Quantity of Protein in Plant-Based Diets Is Poor

Whole foods contain all macronutrients, meaning protein is readily available within them. It is abundant throughout the plant kingdom, including in all vegetables. Foods that are particularly rich in protein include legumes, nuts and nut butters, seeds and seed butters, soy foods, and intact whole grains. Adequate intake of protein is based on weight and is estimated at:

- 1.5 g/kg/d for infants
- 1.1 g/kg/d for 1- to –3-year-olds
- 0.95 g/kg/d for 4- to 13-year-olds
- 0.85 g/kg/d for 14- to 18-year-olds
- 0.8 g/kg/d for adults
- 1.1 g/kg/d for pregnant (using prepregnancy weight) and lactating women [12]

This adds up to 46 and 56 g per day for women and men of average size and activity, about 10% of daily caloric needs, which is very easily met on plant-based diets.

Myth #2: The More Protein the Better

People consume an average of 80 g/day globally, while in North America, we are at 109 g/day [13]. That amounts to 1.9 and 1.5 g/kg/d for average women and men. Considering the numbers provided in the previous paragraph, this is a clear excess.

Excess protein is linked with:

- *Early puberty* in girls and boys
- Increased *cancer development and growth*
- Formation of *cholesterol plaques* in our blood vessels
- Poor *bone health* (higher dairy and animal protein consumption is linked with a higher incidence of bone fractures)
- More *allergic, autoimmune, and inflammatory* disorders
- And *metabolic disorders* like gout and kidney stones [11]

When considering protein, as with all nutrients, it is important to consider the "*package*" it comes in:

- Protein from animal sources comes with saturated fat, dietary cholesterol (present in animal cell walls, so all animal products contain it), trans fats, hormones, antibiotics, insulin-like growth factor 1 (IGF-1), and lipophilic environmental

contaminants which concentrate in animal tissues (persistent organic pollutants) [14]. And all these are linked through research to most chronic degenerative diseases.
- On the other hand, protein from plant sources comes with soluble and insoluble fiber, vitamins, minerals, phytochemicals, and other antioxidants [11, 15], all of which are paramount to good health and linked through research as being protective.

Myth #3: Plant-Based Protein Is Incomplete

The protein we obtain from food is considered to be of different quality depending on how efficiently it provides the amino acids we need to replace the protein in our bodies. Because animals and humans are similarly built, their flesh, milk, and eggs contain the amino acids we need, that is what is called complete protein. However, as mentioned above, the "package" this protein comes with is not necessarily healthful to us, much less at the disproportionate large quantities we consume.

Plant-based protein sometimes may miss one essential amino acid, for example: beans and vegetables do not contain enough methionine; grains, nuts, and seeds are deficient in lysine. That is where the idea of combining these foods or "protein complementation" comes from. However, it is known now that as long as people consume mostly whole or minimally processed plant foods, their bodies are perfectly able to derive all the essential amino acids they need from different plant sources. It is not necessary to meticulously plan each meal, just eat a varied plant-based diet [11, 16].

Myth #4: You Need Lots of Protein to Build Muscle

Muscle hypertrophy occurs as a result of mechanical tension, microtrauma, and metabolic stress that occur during exercise. It does not occur due to excess protein consumption.

As stated above, because most people, including those on plant-based diets, tend to consume excess protein, any additional need they may have due to exercising is covered with normal consumption.

Of course, those in constant and strenuous exercise routines may have increased needs: the International Society of Sports Nutrition recommends 1.0–1.6 g/kg/day for endurance athletes (depending on intensity and duration of exercise) and 1.6–2.0 g/kg/day for strength athletes [17].

Please note, again, that this is about the same amount that average people consume in America. Which brings us to another thing that happens when we consume excess protein: instead of being used for structural and functional purposes, ANY excess protein is treated as ANY excess calories: it is used as energy and deposited as fat.

Myth #5: Plant-Based Eating Is High in Carbohydrates and Carbs Are Bad for Us

Yes, plant-based diets are high in carbohydrates, ideally somewhere around 70–75% of daily caloric needs. That is not necessarily a bad thing considering they provide the fuel for our bodies and our brains and exercising muscles prefer them above anything else.

And they are not bad for us, but just as with protein, there is a "package" concept around them. In this case, refined carbohydrates (flours, sugars, syrups, juices, etc.) have been stripped of their packages, while whole carbohydrates still have them. It has been clearly established that refined carbohydrates are deleterious to our health precisely because they do not have any more the fiber, vitamins, minerals, and phytochemicals they should be consumed with.

Myth #6: You Will Get Weak

As long as we consume whole, plant-based foods, we actually become healthier and stronger. In fact, athletes, including elite professionals, are increasingly turning to plant-based diets because they experience faster recovery, better performance, less injuries, and better general health when they eat this way [18].

Myth #7: It Is Time Consuming

Shopping and cooking the whole foods plant-based way may take a bit more time, especially in the beginning, while you are learning to read ingredients lists in packages and trying out new recipes.

Some helpful strategies include the following:

- Planning (look a week in advance at what you would like to make and shop accordingly)
- Batch cooking (cook, for example, 1 kg of beans to make salads, veggie burgers, stews/soups, even brownies)
- Involving family members in this new endeavor
- Following some of the free kickstart programs listed at the end of this chapter to learn more quickly and rest assured you are getting what you need

On the other hand, thanks to improved overall health and higher energy levels, you will be performing better mentally and physically. Plus, if you are using little added oils and parchment paper for baking, it is easier to clean.

Myth #8: It Is Expensive

On the contrary, it is considerably cheaper as long as you focus on minimally processed or unprocessed plant-based foods, namely beans, pulses, whole grains, vegetables, fruits, nuts, and seeds. Avoid buying trendy foods or those that come from far away, as they are unnecessarily expensive. Regular, local foods' nutrients are usually just as good as those from fancy foods.

Regarding conventional versus organically grown items, organic foods have less environmental contaminants on them, but they are usually pricey and their nutritional benefits are not necessarily higher. If you can afford them, be wise about which ones to buy. The Environmental Working Group's website (https://www.ewg.org/foodnews/) updates every year its "Dirty Dozen" and "Clean 15" lists of fruits and vegetables that are better when organic or safe when conventional.

Local and seasonal foods are usually fresher and cheaper plus their large amounts of anticarcinogenic and anti-inflammatory phytochemicals counteract the effect of environmental contaminants in food [19].

Myth #9: You Will Be Exposed to More Environmental Contaminants

As mentioned above, a plant-based diet provides very high levels of phytochemicals and antioxidants that have powerful protective effects against the potential harm from pesticides, herbicides, heavy metals, and other substances in foods.

Animal-based foods are actually higher in these substances because they are lipophilic, that is, they concentrate in fat, cell walls, milk, and eggs. Additionally, the saturated fats, dietary cholesterol, IGF-1, and hormones they contain have additional carcinogenic and inflammatory properties that potentiate the harm environmental contaminants may cause [19]. As you may notice, the "package" concept works here too.

How to avoid environmental contaminants then?

- Avoid animal-based foods.
- If consuming fish, avoid fish that are higher in the food chain (tuna, salmon, and swordfish) because due to their carnivorous nature, environmental contaminants concentrate in their tissues.
- Simply washing and peeling produce help reduce environmental contaminant exposure.
- If able to afford them, buy organic "Dirty Dozen" produce.

Myth #10: We Must Consume Dairy to Have Strong Bones

Countries where dairy is consumed the most are the ones with the highest hip fracture incidences, including the United States, New Zealand, and European countries. High animal protein consumption, with its greater amount of sulfur-containing amino acids, increases the acid load in our body. However, our preferred pH is approximately 7.4: to maintain this pH, our bodies neutralize the acidosis with a very effective base: calcium from our bones. In short, the more dairy we consume, the more calcium we need [11].

Have you considered that the animals we use to obtain milk, like cows and sheep, only get their calcium from plants? Plants contain adequate calcium, especially green vegetables (bok choy, broccoli, cabbage, collard greens, dandelion greens, kale, turnip greens, and watercress), beans, lentils, nuts (especially almonds), seeds (such as sesame seeds and tahini), dried figs, calcium-set tofu, tempeh, sweet potatoes, and fortified drinks [12].

To have strong bones then, consume calcium-rich plant foods, practice weight-bearing exercise regularly, and get adequate amounts of vitamin D, through the sun, or a supplement if you live far from the equator, and especially if you have dark skin.

Myth #11: Soy Is Bad for Health

Soybeans and minimally processed soy foods are good sources of protein, fiber, vitamins, minerals, mono- and poly-unsaturated fats, and isoflavones, which have beneficial antioxidant and phytoestrogenic activity. But, as with any other food or drink, soy is problematic when it is ultra-processed. It is very frequently broken down and used as soy protein isolate or soybean oil which lack all of the other nutrients listed earlier in this paragraph. Ultra-processed soy products should be avoided as much as possible, just as any other food in the ultra-processed category.

The belief that soy can be harmful comes from studies using very high levels of soy products rarely consumed on a daily basis. On the contrary, many studies and epidemiologic data show that soy consumption has many beneficial effects when not consumed in ultra-processed form. So, eat whole soybeans (edamame or dry soybeans), fermented soybeans (tempeh, miso, natto), soy milk (only soybeans and water), tofu, or soy flour (made from whole soybeans).

Myth #12: We Need Meat to Get Enough Iron

Women of childbearing age, pregnant women, infants, children, and teenage girls need more iron than other people. However, iron-deficiency anemia is no more common in vegetarians than in omnivores.

The iron in plant foods is nonheme iron, and its absorption can be increased or decreased depending on what we consume with it. To offset this, vegans and vegetarians need to consume more iron-containing foods which is fairly easy on a plant-based diet: leafy greens, beans and legumes, soy products, dark chocolate, blackstrap molasses, sesame seeds, tahini, pumpkin seeds, sunflower seeds, raisins, prunes, and cashews are all great sources of iron.

To improve iron absorption, it is recommended to eat iron-rich foods in combination with foods high in vitamin C, which happens almost naturally on a plant-based diet because we tend to mix them together (beans with tomatoes and nut butters on apple, for example) [12].

Moreover, plant-based females tend to have lighter periods and, therefore, need less iron [11].

Myth #13: Anemia

As stated above, iron is not a problem when consuming a whole-food, plant-based diet.

However, lack of vitamin B12 can cause anemia and other severe health problems (neurologic and gastrointestinal) for people not consuming animal products. Vitamin B12 is the only nutrient the vegetable kingdom cannot provide, because it is synthesized only by microorganisms like bacteria and fungi. Animals consume these microorganisms along with their food, either in nature or through supplements added to their feed, which is why this vitamin can be found in their meat, organs, eggs, and milk.

Our body has stores of this vitamin that can last 3–5 years, but because deficiency could be asymptomatic and eventual consequences are very serious, it is much safer to take it in supplements. Nutritional yeast and fortified plant milks may have it, but still, taking this vitamin as a supplement is highly recommended [12].

Myth #14: In My Family, Despite Our Animal-Based Diets, We Live into Our Nineties

There are always outliers who live longer despite illness or exposure. However, the quality of life from chronic disease must also be taken into account. Animal-based diets promote chronic diseases. Thus, one may live long but often with the burden of illness. In fact, there is a significant gap between life expectancy and healthy life expectancy (the number of years that a person is expected to live without an activity limitation or disability) [20], with men spending a fifth of their life in poor health and women nearly a quarter [21].

Myth #15: We Should Consume Everything in Moderation, and Going 100% Plant-Based Is Too Extreme

Numerous studies, including WHO recommendations, have shown that many foods (like processed and red meat being cancerogenic, ultra-processed foods of any type causing earlier death) are very unhealthy and that they should not be consumed. As

Dr. Esselstyn has said "Having our chest open in half and arteries in our heart replaced is a bit extreme too, not to mention all the other blood vessels in our body will remain partially clogged."

A full whole-food, plant-based diet is the only one so far that has been proven to reverse cardiovascular disease and diabetes and prevent and help fight cancer [11].

Myth #16: Not Enough Essential Fatty Acids

These polyunsaturated fatty acids include both omega-3 and omega-6 fatty acids. They can be found in flaxseeds, hemp seeds, chia seeds, leafy green vegetables (terrestrial and marine), soybeans and soy products, walnuts, and wheat germ, and in their respective oils.

Cold-water fish are rich in omega 3 fatty acids because these do not become solid at freezing temperatures. They get them from microalgae, and we can do the same and limit fish since they are generally contaminated with heavy metals and industrial pollutants, and are depleted or overfished [12].

Also, what really matters is the ratio between omega 6 and 3 fatty acids, as high amounts of omega 6s inhibit omega 3 activity. Our ideal omega 6 to 3 ratio is about 1, whereas in the typical Western diet, it is at least 15 to 1. When consuming a whole-food, plant-based diet, the amount of omega 6s consumed decreases since omega 6 oils are more common in ultra-processed foods and added oils. So, the ratio improves. The addition of the omega 3-rich plant foods cited above usually is enough to satisfy our needs for these nutrients.

Medical and Surgical Conditions to Keep in Mind and Important Considerations or Precautions for These Cases

Antihypertensives, Diabetes Medications, and Insulin Therapy

Patients taking these drugs need to be closely monitored for dose adjustments if they decide to follow a whole-food, plant-based diet because blood pressure and diabetes (especially type 2) can respond rapidly as the patient loses weight and metabolism normalizes with this diet.

Proton Pump Inhibitors

These drugs can be tapered off as the patient transitioning to a plant-based diet starts losing weight and acid reflux symptoms start improving. H2 blockers can be taken before bed to help with nighttime symptoms. Alginate-containing liquids can coat the throat and esophagus providing a safe alternative to oral pharmaceuticals during a transition to a mostly plant-based diet.

Laxatives

It is very likely that these will need to be stopped as fiber intake on a whole-food, plant-based diet is naturally high.

Steroids

Patients on long-term steroid treatments for chronic inflammatory and autoimmune diseases need to be warned that they must not stop their treatment abruptly. As they transition to a more plant-based diet, levels of inflammation, symptoms, and flare ups can decrease. Steroids should only then, and only with medical supervision, be weaned slowly.

Warfarin

Dietary supplements, high-protein diets, foods high in vitamin K (green leafy vegetables including broccoli, brussels sprouts, kale, parsley, and spinach), and cranberry juice can alter warfarin levels. As a rule of thumb, patients taking this drug should be watchful of making any sudden diet changes because they can alter warfarin levels in blood and risk life-threatening consequences [22]. However, these plant-based foods need not be avoided as they have many other benefits to healthful living. With medical guidance, transitioning to a plant-based diet can include these foods as long as close attention is paid to changes in laboratory parameters and warfarin levels adjusted accordingly.

Other Food–Drug Interactions

- Grapefruit juice: can alter the way many drugs are metabolized (psychotropics, anticonvulsants, felodipine, midazolam, cyclosporine, and many other drugs).
- High-fiber diets: may reduce the efficacy of some statins and other cholesterol lowering medications. However, they have their own cholesterol lowering effects.
- Tyramine-containing foods (matured cheese, red wine, ripe bananas, yogurt, shrimp paste, and salami) can produce hypertensive crises in patients taking monoamine oxidase inhibitors.
- Celiprolol's (a beta-blocker) intestinal absorption is inhibited when taken with orange juice. It seems that the hesperidin in orange juice is responsible [22].

Bloating, Digestive Discomfort

For some people going from very little to lots of fiber quickly could cause some benign bloating and digestive discomfort. The websites provided in the resources section of this chapter include dietician-designed diet plans to help manage these problems.

Short Gut

When part of the intestines is removed, the remaining sections adapt by absorbing the nutrients and liquids that would have normally been absorbed by the removed part. But this adaptation can take time and some nutrient deficiencies may occur.

During this time, it is recommended to:

- Consume 6–8 small meals a day accompanied by little water. Most liquid should be consumed between meals.
- Consume foods rich in protein, refined or low-fiber complex carbohydrates (white bread, rice, pasta, flour, skinned potatoes, low sugar-added breakfast cereals with less than 1 g of fiber per serving), or foods rich in soluble fiber (oatmeal, soy, nut butters, fruit, fruit pectin, psyllium, legumes, barley).
- Avoid foods rich in insoluble fiber (whole grains, dried fruit, fruit and vegetable peels, whole nuts and seeds, and coconut).
- Consume moderate amounts of fats, and limit simple sugars [23].

Sleeve Gastrectomy, Gastric Bypass, Postbariatric Surgery

Patients having had these procedures could be at risk of nutrient deficiencies due to reduced stomach capacity or because a part of the intestine where many vitamins and other nutrients are absorbed are being bypassed. Experts have not expressed concern about this for patients who decide to follow a whole-food, plant-based diet because this way of eating is very nutrient dense and may help to offset the possible problems those surgeries may cause [24].

Conclusion

Although it is important to keep in mind interactions between foods, drugs, and some surgeries, the benefit of switching to a whole-food, plant-based diet is so great that it outweighs the risks. Many diseases get better including GERD, cardiovascular disease, diabetes, cancer, autoimmune disease, gout, kidney, and liver diseases among others [11].

Patients should be advised to consult with their doctor or dietician if they have any doubts about particular conditions, prescription medications, and any dietary changes they are considering.

Resources

The resources listed below provide information that can be useful in clearing doubts and covering any topics not touched upon in this chapter.

Network of plant-based doctors	https://www.plantbaseddoctors.org/find
Organizations offering articles, recipes, diet plans, etc.	Physicians' Committee for Responsible Medicine, https://www.pcrm.org/ Center for Nutrition Studies at Cornell University, https://nutritionstudies.org/ Dr. Esselstyn's website, http://www.dresselstyn.com/site/ Ornish Lifestyle Medicine, https://www.ornish.com/ Nutrition Facts Dr. Greger, https://nutritionfacts.org/ Forks over Knives, https://www.forksoverknives.com/ Bluezones, https://www.bluezones.com/ Physicians Association for Nutrition, https://pan-int.org/ Plantrician Project, https://www.plantricianproject.org/ American College of Lifestyle Medicine, https://www.lifestylemedicine.org/ Lifestyle Medicine Global Alliance, https://lifestylemedicineglobal.org/
For recipes, many of the above provide free recipes, diet plants, etc. plus:	Engine2 diet, https://engine2diet.com/ https://plantbasedonabudget.com/
Books	Dr. T. Colin Campbell: *The China Study*, *Whole* Dr. Neal Barnard: *Power Foods*, *The Cheese Trap*, *Reversing Diabetes* Dr. John McDougall and Mary McDougall: *The Starch Solution* Dr. Caldwell B. Esselstyn Jr.: *Prevent and Reverse Heart Disease* Dean Ornish: *Dr. Dean Ornish's Program for Reversing Heart Disease*, *Undo-It!*, *The Spectrum* Dr. Michael Greger: *How Not to Die* Dr. Garth Davis: *Proteinaholic* Dr. David Katz: *The Truth About Food*
Movies	Forks over Knives The Game Changers Plant Pure Nation What the Health Eating You Alive Hungry for Change Fat, Sick, and Nearly Dead Before the Flood

References

1. Fiolet T, Srour B, Sellem L, Kesse-Guyot E, Alles B, Mejean C, et al. Consumption of ultra-processed foods and cancer risk: results from NutriNet-Sante prospective cohort. BMJ (Clin Res ed). 2018;360:k322.
2. Hall KD, Ayuketah A, Brychta R, Cai H, Cassimatis T, Chen KY, et al. Ultra-processed diets cause excess calorie intake and weight gain: an inpatient randomized controlled trial of Ad libitum food intake. Cell Metab. 2019;30:67.
3. Ornish D, Scherwitz LW, Billings JH, Brown SE, Gould KL, Merritt TA, et al. Intensive lifestyle changes for reversal of coronary heart disease. JAMA. 1998;280(23):2001–7.
4. Ornish D, Weidner G, Fair WR, Marlin R, Pettengill EB, Raisin CJ, et al. Intensive lifestyle changes may affect the progression of prostate cancer. J Urol. 2005;174(3):1065–9; discussion 9–70
5. Allen KE, Gumber D, Ostfeld RJ. Heart failure and a plant-based diet. A case-report and literature review. Front Nutr. 2019;6(82):82.
6. Barnard ND, Cohen J, Jenkins DJ, Turner-McGrievy G, Gloede L, Green A, et al. A low-fat vegan diet and a conventional diabetes diet in the treatment of type 2 diabetes: a randomized, controlled, 74-wk clinical trial. Am J Clin Nutr. 2009;89(5):1588s–96s.
7. Tuttle RH. Human evolution: Encyclopædia Britannica; 2019 [updated May 24, 2019]. Available from: https://www.britannica.com/science/human-evolution.
8. Cordain L, Eaton SB, Sebastian A, Mann N, Lindeberg S, Watkins BA, et al. Origins and evolution of the Western diet: health implications for the 21st century. Am J Clin Nutr. 2005;81(2):341–54.
9. Boyer J, Liu RH. Apple phytochemicals and their health benefits. Nutr J. 2004;3:5.
10. Monteiro CA, Cannon G, Moubarac JC, Levy RB, Louzada MLC, Jaime PC. The UN Decade of Nutrition, the NOVA food classification and the trouble with ultra-processing. Public Health Nutr. 2018;21(1):5–17.
11. Campbell TC. The China study: the most comprehensive study of nutrition ever conducted and the startling implications for diet, weight loss and long-term health/T. Colin Campbell and Thomas M. Campbell II. Campbell TM, editor. Kent Town, S. Aust: Wakefield Press; 2007.
12. Hever J. Plant-based diets: a Physician's guide. Perm J. 2016;20(3):15–082.
13. Data OWi. Protein supply by region: University of Oxford, Global Change Data Lab. Available from: https://ourworldindata.org/grapher/protein-supply-by-region?time=1961..2013.
14. Ruzzin J. Public health concern behind the exposure to persistent organic pollutants and the risk of metabolic diseases. BMC Public Health. 2012;12:298.
15. The Nutrition Source: Protein: Harvard T. Chan School of Public Health. Available from: https://www.hsph.harvard.edu/nutritionsource/what-should-you-eat/protein/.
16. Protein Complementation: American Society for Nutrition. Available from: https://nutrition.org/protein-complementation/.
17. Fuhrman J, Ferreri DM. Fueling the vegetarian (vegan) athlete. Curr Sports Med Rep. 2010;9(4):233–41.
18. Esposito L. Athletes can thrive on plant-based diets: U.S. News and World Report; 2019. Available from: https://health.usnews.com/wellness/fitness/articles/2019-01-11/athletes-can-thrive-on-plant-based-diets.
19. Greger M. How not to die. London: Pan Books; 2018.
20. Eurostat. Number of healthy years of life: countries compared [updated 04/02/2019. Available from: https://ec.europa.eu/eurostat/web/products-eurostat-news/-/DDN-20190204-1.
21. EPHA E, NCDA. Joint paper: towards an EU strategic framework for the prevention of Non-communicable Diseases (NCDs). 2019 May 2019.
22. Bushra R, Aslam N, Khan AY. Food-drug interactions. Oman Med J. 2011;26(2):77–83.
23. Center MSKC. Nutrition guidelines for people with short bowel syndrome. NY, USA: Memorial Sloan Kettering Cancer Center; 2017. Available from: https://www.mskcc.org/cancer-care/patient-education/nutrition-guidelines-patients-short-bowel-syndrome.
24. Medicine PCfR. Vegan after weight loss surgery. Available from: https://www.pcrm.org/news/exam-room-podcast/vegan-after-weight-loss-surgery.

Chapter 42
Reflux Cure - Transitioning to a Plant-Based Diet from the Standard American Diet (SAD)

Linda Arpino

Symptoms of gastroesophageal reflux disease (GERD) and laryngopharyngeal reflux (LPR) improve without the use of medication following a plant-based diet based on numerous studies [1–4]. Current standards of care focus on the use of proton pump inhibitors (PPI) with significant cost and potential side effects [7]. Often, certain trigger foods and behaviors are discussed briefly. Rarely are diet and lifestyle changes "prescribed" as the primary modality to treat the disease. Scientific evidence [6] has produced objective data on the role of certain trigger foods such as fatty foods or chocolate and lifestyle choices, including moderate regular exercise are critical in management [13, 14].

The National Institutes of Health and the American College of Gastroenterology endorses nutrition intervention as the first line of treatment for GERD and LPR [3].

According to the Nutrition Care Manual of the Academy of Nutrition and Dietetics [8], "it is recommended that a trial of limiting or eliminating the following foods may reduce the symptoms of reflux."

- Citrus
- Alcohol
- Chocolate
- Spearmint and peppermint
- Tomato products
- Coffee and tea
- Spicy foods
- Total fat intake: especially fried foods (French fries, fried meats, bacon, sausage, pepperoni, salami, bologna, frankfurters/hot dogs), gravy, whole milk dairy, and cream
- Large meals

L. Arpino (✉)
Life Focus Nutrition, LLC, Stamford, CT, USA
e-mail: la@lifefocusnutrition.com

C. H. Zalvan (ed.), *Laryngopharyngeal and Gastroesophageal Reflux*,
https://doi.org/10.1007/978-3-030-48890-1_42

Lifestyle habits that trigger symptoms include the following: overeating, smoking, and eating prior to lying down, lack of daily physical activity, and sleep. Other triggers are reviewed elsewhere in this text [14, 33].

Tips in Healthy Eating Include the Following:

- Eat approximately every 4 hours.
- Smaller portions at all meals.
- Meals should include at least three food groups that offer fiber and protein from grains, legumes, fruits, and vegetables to create low glycemic load.
- Eat several small snacks throughout the day if mealtimes are over 4 hours apart.
- Eat in a calm, relaxed place. Sit down while you eat.
- Wait at least 3 hours after eating before lying down.
- Preparing home-cooked meals rather than relying on take-out food or eating out.

Why Plant Based?

There are over 25,000 phyto (plant) nutrients in plant-based foods that combat inflammation [10], inhibit cancer cell proliferation, remove cholesterol and arterial plaque formation, and protects against neurological decline [11]. Animal proteins including chicken, fish, turkey, beef, pork, cheese, eggs, milk, yogurt, and bison do not offer any of the more than 25,000 phytonutrients. Lack of these important nutrients in the diet, and foods rich in animal protein drive chronic disease such as diabetes, heart disease, cancer, and reflux [11]. Research has found that whole plant-based fruits, vegetables, grains, and legumes act in a synergistic way to lower inflammation unlike nutrition supplements [12]. Symptoms of GERD and LPR can also be controlled by removing these animal-based trigger foods. According to the Position of the Academy of Nutrition and Dietetics on Vegetarian Diets, "Vegetarians and vegans are at reduced risk of certain health conditions, including ischemic heart disease, type 2 diabetes, hypertension, certain types of cancer, and obesity. Low intake of saturated fat and high intakes of vegetables, fruits, whole grains, legumes, soy products, nuts, and seeds (all rich in fiber and phytochemicals) are characteristics of vegetarian and vegan diets that produce lower total and low-density lipoprotein cholesterol levels, and better serum glucose control. These factors contribute to reduction of chronic disease. Vegans need reliable sources of vitamin B-12, such as fortified foods or supplements" [9]. Foods fortified with vitamin B12 include many brands of soy milk and cereals. Encouraging a 95 percent plant-based diet not only helps with GERD and LPR [7] but many other medical conditions. Weight management is also critical, and increasing whole, not processed plant-based foods allows for greater satiety with less calories, sodium or fat (coconut fat is added to most plant-based cheese). Refer to the Nutrition Rainbow, at the end of this text, for the many functions' phytonutrients have in promoting health to share with your patients.

Active phytonutrients in plants have health benefits [23, 24]. They have in the past been categorized as nonessential nutrients, but as evidence emerges, there is reason these micronutrients may be added as essential in chronic disease prevention. Hippocrates coined the term "Food is Thy Medicine." It is only now that we are finding the true meaning of this.

Select Phytonutrients in Common Foods [23, 24]

Anthocyanins Plant colors are red and purple. Food plants rich in anthocyanins include blue berries, red onions, kidney beans, pomegranates, grapes (including wine), tomatoes, acai, and tart cherries.

Carotenoids These include α-carotene, β-carotene, β-cryptoxanthin, lutein, zeaxanthin, and lycopene**:** Plant colors are orange, red, and yellow**,** such as carrots, sweet potatoes, carrot juice, pumpkin, and winter squash.

Isoflavones The popular foods include soy, alfalfa sprouts, chickpeas, red clover, peanuts, and other legumes.

Organosulfides/Organosulfur The allium and allicin compounds are found in garlic, onions, leeks, chives, shallots and wasabi or horseradish.

Phytoestrogens Foods include seeds such as soy beans, flax, sesame, sunflower and pumpkin; whole grains, fruit, and vegetable**s.**

Suggested Foods

A healthy diet should include a DAILY intake of fruits, vegetables, legumes, or other plant protein such as tofu and high fiber, unprocessed whole grains. Many people follow the Standard American Diet (SAD), which is quite different: 10% fruit and vegetables, 30% or more animal protein, and 60% processed grains. The Center for Disease Control, 2018 State Indicator Report on Fruits and Vegetables [35] cites that overall Americans remain low in both food groups. The number of servings of each food group depends on age, weight, gender, and other nutritional needs.

Low glycemic load meals [8] rich in carbohydrate foods high in fiber and low in sugar have been demonstrated to lower the risk of esophageal adenocarcinoma [5]. Adherence to a predominantly Mediterranean diet decreases the risk of gastroesophageal reflux disease [6].

The United States Dietary Guidelines (USDG) states, "the goal of the *Dietary Guidelines* is for individuals throughout all stages of the lifespan to have eating patterns that promote overall health and help prevent chronic disease" [16]. "Dietary Guidelines for Americans is a set of evidence-based recommendations intended to help people choose an overall healthy diet." USDG purpose is to be used by healthcare professionals and legislators for reference and setting policy in federal nutrition programs [16]. Healthcare professionals can obtain the most updated recommendations for calories per age and the number of servings per food group for each calorie level. Refer to these links: (https://health.gov/dietaryguidelines/2015/guidelines/appendix-2/) (https://health.gov/dietaryguidelines/2015/guidelines/appendix-3/). Obesity ranks high as a health risk especially for women not only for GERD and LPR but for the top health related causes of death, hence recommendations have been scrutinized [15].

Currently, food groups are being challenged by many healthcare providers because many cultures worldwide consume limited dairy products and evidence links full fat dairy to many medical conditions, especially saturated fat in whole milk products. This group was used to meet calcium needs, but with a guided meal plan, this can be achieved without dairy or in limited fat-free or 1% fat choices. The United States Dietary Guidelines are updated every 5 years. The next update is in 2020. This is important to follow because a lot of nutrition education materials used both on the Internet and in schools reference these guidelines for education on a healthy diet. Often the expert panel can represent a wide variety of stakeholders in food industry such as dairy or meat and not always what evidence-based science suggests.

Many experts, such as Neal Bernard, MD from the Physicians Committee for Responsible Medicine, Walter C. Willett, M.D., Dr. P.H., Professor of Epidemiology and Nutrition at Harvard T.H. Chan School of Public Health and Professor of Medicine at Harvard Medical School, Healthy Eating Plate [37], and Michael Gregor, MD in his book, "How Not to Die" [38] have suggested the dairy group be removed from the My Plate concept. The dairy industry is a billion-dollar industry and despite efforts toward more sustainable food systems, there is great influence from the funding they provide to professional speakers at organizations, such as Academy of Pediatrics, American Heart Association and the Academy of Nutrition and Dietetics as well as universities research projects. The influence from big business is an obstacle. Good sources of plant-based calcium foods for GERD and LPR include organic fortified soymilk and other fortified plant-based food such as, tempeh, tofu using calcium in processing, almond butter, and figs [38].

The primary source of protein in the SAD diet is from animals (lean meat, fish, poultry, and dairy products). Concerns continue that a plant-based diet will not provide adequate protein. The information in this chapter provides numerous sources of plant-based protein to help healthcare professionals encourage patients to eat a wide variety of grains, legumes, nuts, seeds, and soy products to achieve adequate protein. Symptoms of protein deficiency are fatigue, inability to maintain sufficient muscle mass, and high blood sugar or triglycerides [17]. Monitoring for these symptoms is important. Eating disorders, liver disease, kidney disease, and malnutrition due to poor food choices are heightened reasons for protein deficiency. Low blood levels of protein are called hypoproteinemia. Diagnostic tests include measuring total protein, albumin, and albumin/globulin (A/G) ratio [18]. The Academy of Nutrition and Dietetics position paper on vegetarian diets confirms that vegetarian diets can provide adequate nutrients at all stages of life when properly planned [9].

By making simple diet and lifestyle changes, one can reduce the risk for most chronic diseases, including GERD and LPR [1, 14, 15]. A Mediterranean-style, plant-based diet emphasizes vegetables, fruits, legumes, nuts, seeds, and whole grains. These foods are complete sources of protein, carbohydrates, fat, vitamins, minerals, and over 25,000 phytonutrients. Plant-based diets are becoming more mainstream and can include foods that are unfamiliar to many. Americans are obsessed with the need for protein, especially animal protein. Most adults only require 0.8 g/kg of body weight. As we age and with encouraged increased daily activity, these requirements may increase slightly. Adequate protein intake can be achieved with a whole food, plant-based diet. There are nine essential amino acids out of the 20 that exist. These are histidine, isoleucine, leucine, lysine, methionine, phenylalanine, threonine, tryptophan, and valine. They are essential because they cannot be made by the body. There are other conditional essential amino acids, meaning they are essential only in certain conditions such as illness or cancer. Essential amino acids are needed in the body for diverse functions such as building tissue, wound healing, blood cells, hormone production, cellular functions, and nervous system including mental clarity [17]. Amino acids are composed of nitrogen, carbon, hydrogen, and oxygen, along with a side chain group. While animal protein sources have all essential amino acids, plants do not. According to the Position of the Academy of Nutrition and Dietetics on Vegetarian Diets, "Protein from a variety of plant foods, eaten during the course of a day, supplies enough of all indispensable (essential) amino acids when caloric requirements are met. Regular use of legumes and soy products will ensure adequate protein intake for the vegetarian. This is especially important for older adults" [9].

The information below is to help you become more familiar with the common foods of a plant-based diet. A simple suggestion for achieving all amino acids from plant protein is by consuming grains and legumes.

Glossary of Plant-Based Terms

The grains below are sold dry and are cooked similar to rice.

Amaranth This gluten-free ancient grain was eaten by the Aztecs and called huauhtli [19]. It cooks quickly and can be used as a breakfast porridge or in soups or stews.

Bulgur This grain is a whole-wheat grain used in soups, side dishes, and vegetable salads. This nutty taste grain is a great source of fiber, folic acid, and iron. Tabbouleh is a common recipe.

Barley Barley was one of the first cultivated grains, particularly in Eurasia as early as 10,000 years ago [19]. It is a major cereal grain, commonly found in bread, beverages, soups, and in various cuisines of every culture.

Buck Wheat This gluten-free grain belongs to a group of foods classified as pseudo cereals, it is not a grass or contains wheat. It contains heart-healthy compounds such as rutin, an antioxidant, magnesium, copper, *fiber,* and certain proteins [19].

Faro Faro is a wheat species, sold dried, and prepared by cooking (70–90 minutes) in water until soft, but has a firmer texture than other grains. Soaking overnight lowers cooking time. Faro is rich in protein and fiber.

Just Egg Just Egg is a product made from mung bean and is a cholesterol-free egg alternative for scrambles, omelets, fried rice, French toast, and waffles providing 5 g of protein per serving.

Legumes The vegetable family that includes beans, lentils, peas, and peanuts, all of which are excellent sources of vegetable protein.

Nutritional Yeast This health supplement is grown on molasses, sugar beets, or wood pulp, and in some products, a rich source of vitamin B12 and protein.

Quinoa Quinoa is a gluten-free grain grown primarily for its edible seeds which contain essential amino acids and acceptable quantities of fiber, calcium, phosphorus, and iron.

Spelt This ancient wheat light red grain is widely cultivated in southwest Asia, the Near East, and Europe during the Bronze Age and is now grown chiefly in Europe [19].

Wheat Berries or Whole-Grain Wheat The wheat berry is a *wheat* kernel, composed of bran, germ, and endosperm, *high in fiber and* protein. Soaking overnight shortens the cooking time.

Seitan (Also Called Wheat Gluten) Seitan is made of protein (gluten) extracted from flour and is a replacement for meat.

Soybean Soybean is a legume, which is an excellent, inexpensive source of protein and iron.

Soybeans are used to make a number of substitutions for meat, dairy, and eggs.

Soy Cheese A cheese-like product made from soybeans. Soy cheeses come in most of the same varieties as dairy cheeses, such as parmesan, mozzarella, and cheddar.

Soy Yogurt Soy yogurt is made from soy milk and yogurt cultures.

Soy Milk Soy milk is a product made from soybeans, with a similar amount of protein and less fat than cow's milk. It is known to have benefits over other plant-based milk because of its anticancer properties and high protein content [20].

Tempeh Tempeh is a replacement for meat, a traditional Indonesian soy product, made from fermented soybeans.

Textured Vegetable Protein Derived from soy flour, TVP is commonly used as a substitute for ground beef.

Tofu Tofu is a replacement for meat, eggs, and cheese, made from condensed soy milk and pressed into blocks and originated in China. Tofu can be eaten fresh or cooked in many different ways and is an excellent source of protein.

Types and Uses of Tofu:

- Extra-firm tofu: frying, roasting, grilling or marinating.
- Firm tofu: stir-frying, boiling or to use as filling.
- Soft tofu: pureeing.
- Silken tofu: pureeing, simmering, egg substitution, used in desserts and smoothies.
- Sprouted tofu: soybeans are sprouted before being made into tofu to lower the phytate level over 50% and trypsin inhibitors by up to 81% while also increasing the protein content by up to 13%, allowing for better utilization of nutrients [38].

The chart below shows you how quickly protein can add up on a plant-based, Mediterranean diet [21].

Plant-based protein in foods

Food	Amount	Grams of protein
Black bean spaghetti, cooked	¼ cup	25
Tempeh	½ cup	21
Seitan	3 ounces	20
Soybeans, cooked	1 cup	29
Faro, cooked	½ cup	6
Buck wheat, cooked	½ cup	13
Spelt, cooked	½ cup	13
Bulgur, cooked	1 cup	6
Lentils, cooked	1 cup	18
Black beans, cooked	1 cup	13
Kidney beans, cooked	½ cup	13
Veggie burger	1 patty	13
Chickpeas, cooked	1 cup	12
Veggie baked beans	1 cup	12
Pinto beans, cooked	1 cup	12
Black-eyed peas, cooked	1 cup	11
Tofu, firm	4 ounces	11
Lima beans, cooked	1 cup	10
Quinoa, cooked	1 cup	9
Tofu, regular	4 ounces	9
Peas, cooked	1 cup	9
Textured vegetable protein (TVP), cooked	½ cup	8
Peanut butter	2 Tbsp	8
Sprouted tofu	3 ounces	10
Sunflower seed butter	**2** Tbsp	**7**
Spaghetti, cooked	1 cup	8
Almonds	¼ cup	8
Quinoa	1 cup	8
Soy milk, commercial, plain	1 cup	7–8
Soba noodles (buckwheat)	1 cup	6
Soy yogurt, plain	6 ounces	6
Bulgur, cooked	1 cup	6

(continued)

Food	Amount	Grams of protein
Sunflower seeds	1/4 cup	6
Cashews	1/4 cup	5
Almond butter	2 tbsp	5
Brown rice, cooked	1 cup	5
Spinach, cooked	1 cup	5
Broccoli, cooked	1 cup	4
Grits, cooked	½ cup	4
Potato (medium size), baked	6 oz	4
Coconut, shredded	¼ cup	3
Whole wheat tortilla	6 inch	4–7
Whole wheat Pita bread	5 inch	4
Oat Non-Dairy Beverage	1 cup	4
Whole wheat bread	1 slice	3–2
Hemp nondairy beverage	1 cup	3
Almond nondairy beverage	1 cup	1
Cashew nondairy beverage	1 cup	1
Coconut nondairy beverage	1 cup	0
Oat nondairy beverage	1 cup	4

Meatless Plant Protein Products

There are many reasons the plant-based food industry is exploding with new products. Besides benefit in chronic disease prevention, sustainable food systems are necessary to preserve our planet and feeding our growing population estimated to be 9.7 billion by 2050. Plant-based meat alternatives, such as Beyond Meat, are an example. According to the Beyond Meat website, the ingredients are water, pea protein isolate*, expeller-pressed canola oil, refined coconut oil, rice protein, natural flavors, cocoa butter, mung bean protein, methylcellulose, potato starch, apple extract, salt, potassium chloride, vinegar, lemon juice concentrate, sunflower lecithin, pomegranate fruit powder, beet juice extract (for color). One four-ounce patty contains 20 g of protein, 0 cholesterol, 18 g of fat, and 390 g of sodium. An 85 percent lean beef burger offers 27 g protein, 100 mg of cholesterol, 18 g of fat, and 81 mg of sodium. Even if sodium is slightly higher, using these types of products a few times a week fits and balanced with other meals including vegetables, fruits, nuts, seeds, whole grains, and legumes. The American Heart Association recommendations a daily intake of sodium of 2300 mg, but 1500 mg per day is more desirable for most adults [40].

Another popular product is the Impossible Burger. The ingredients are water, soy protein concentrate, coconut oil, sunflower oil, natural flavors, 2% or less of potato protein, methylcellulose, yeast extract, cultured dextrose, food starch modified, soy leghemoglobin, salt, soy protein isolate, mixed tocopherols (vitamin E), zinc

*The ingredients are important to know when making recommendations in plant based alternatives since this is a growing industry and not all plant based foods maybe of benefit. These and the ones mentioned below are choices that fit into a plant based diet a few times a week.

gluconate, thiamine hydrochloride (vitamin B1), sodium ascorbate (vitamin C), niacin, pyridoxine hydrochloride (vitamin B6), riboflavin (vitamin B2), vitamin B12.

Consumers are going to be confronted with a lot of new products like those mentioned above and the main point is that using these products as a meat alternative one or two times a week is fine but more processed foods such as these should not replace the whole unprocessed plant-based foods.

Other products include fishless fish filets, chickenless chicken filets, beefless ground and tofurkey. Popular brands are Morning Star, Gardien, Upton's, Tofurkey, and Beyond Meat.

These types of products are found in the frozen food and refrigerator sections of the supermarket and are in most large chain food stores such as Target, Walmart, Stop and Shop, Whole Foods, and Trader Joes.

Tips to Add Phytonutrients:

- Add different colored berries and fruit to breakfast. As a general guide, the darker the fruit, the more anti-oxidants and phytonutrients.
- Keep ready to eat fruit and vegetables handy. Dried fruit is more concentrated in sugar so smaller portions are suggested.
- In sandwiches, add far more vegetables than meat or poultry: Spinach, mushrooms and other grilled vegetables. Better to substitute hummus instead of animal protein.
- Cook oatmeal with soy milk instead of water and add cinnamon, walnuts, almonds, and fruit.
- In Salads: Use dark greens such as spinach or kale, carrots, chickpeas, beets, fresh herbs.
- Try tempeh for a firmer texture in a stir fry with ginger, baby corn, bok choy and soy beans.

Meal Suggestions

Breakfast

- High-fiber cereal with skimmed milk or ORGANIC SOY milk with banana
- Whole-wheat toast with peanut butter or margarine or jelly and slices of fresh ORGANIC apple
- Oatmeal with cinnamon, walnuts, raisins, and organic soy or fat-free cow's milk
- Whole grain toast, ½ sliced avocado, sliced tomato, soy milk or yogurt
- Fat-free or 1% cottage cheese OR ricotta cheese with cinnamon, organic berries, slivered almonds in a whole-wheat tortilla (warm in microwave for a taste like a warm cheese Danish)
- Just Egg or Egg white omelet or tofu scramble with spinach and mushrooms sliced or diced potatoes sautéed in olive oil

Lunch

- Grilled vegetable sandwich (zucchini, eggplant, peppers, onions, and avocado) with or without whole-grain bread, hummus or Chickenless filet (Beyond Meat), fresh fruit
- Vegetable soup with a piece of whole-grain toast with hummus or nut butter, apple
- Pasta and bean soup with Ryvita crackers or whole-wheat pita bread, grapes
- Vegetable burger or falafel with (soy) cheese, mushrooms, and tomato on whole-grain bread
- Pita bread filled with vegetables, wild salmon, and orange
- Meatless Chili with beans and rice or organic corn or sweet potato, corn bread, grapes
- Asian stir fry with tofu and vegetables, brown rice
- Rice and beans, salad or raw vegetables, fresh fruit

Dinner

- Thai Soup with tofu or edamame, vegetables, light coconut milk, Asian noodles
- Vegetable Sushi with cucumber, carrots and avocado, vegetable spring roll with tofu and peanut sauce
- Whole-grain pasta with tomato sauce plus vegetables (mushrooms, tomatoes, eggplant, peppers, and onions)
- Tacos or burritos filled with vegetables, beans, quinoa, tofu, and/ or tempeh Pizza with or without cheese and topped with vegetables, tofu or a meat substitute
- Black rice and beans and salad with olive oil and vinegar
- Pasta and beans with escarole
- Indian curry vegetables & chickpeas over rice
- Tempeh sautéed with mushrooms and bok choy, miso soup
- Stuffed peppers with rice and beans
- Wheat berries with pasta and broccoli
- Broccoli Rabe with pasta and a sprinkle of nutritional yeast
- Impossible burger or other vegetable burgers with sweet potato fries and a pickle
- Black bean soup with crusty bread, salad with dried cranberries and walnuts

Snacks

- Fresh fruits or vegetables
- Vegetable spring roll in rice wrap not fried
- Trail mix with dried fruits and nuts and bran chex

- Popcorn (air popped or microwave type), no butter or salt
- Rice cakes or high fiber, low fat cracker, nut or seed butter
- Fat-free plain soy or cow's yogurt with pineapple, strawberries, or blueberries
- Smoothies made with nut butter, calcium fortified soy milk, fresh vegetables, or fruit
- Hummus with unsalted pretzels or high-fiber cracker or raw vegetables
- Raw vegetables with hummus
- Broth with veggies or miso soup
- Fat-free bean or yogurt dip with herbs and celery, cherry tomatoes, and carrots

Key Nutrients to Monitor for Nutritional Adequacy

The values required of all nutrients are found in the Dietary Intake References (DRI) of the National Academy of Sciences, Engineering and Medicine [22]. In the 1990s, the DRI replaced the Recommended Dietary Allowances (RDA), but both are referred to in literature. The National Institute of Health (NIH) Fact Sheet for Healthcare Professionals cites Dietary Reference Intakes (DRIs) developed by the Food and Nutrition Board (FNB) of the Institute of Medicine (IOM) [2]. DRIs is the general term for a set of reference values used for planning and assessing nutrient intakes of healthy people. These values, which vary by age and sex, include the following:

- Recommended Dietary Allowance (RDA): Average daily level of intake sufficient to meet the nutrient requirements of nearly all (97–98%) healthy individuals; often used to plan nutritionally adequate diets for individuals.
- Adequate Intake (AI): Intake at this level is assumed to ensure nutritional adequacy; established when evidence is insufficient to develop an RDA.
- Estimated Average Requirement (EAR): Average daily level of intake estimated to meet the requirements of 50% of healthy individuals; usually used to assess the nutrient intakes of groups of people and to plan nutritionally adequate diets for them; can also be used to assess the nutrient intakes of individuals.
- Tolerable Upper Intake Level (UL): Maximum daily intake unlikely to cause adverse health effects.'

Below are key nutrients on a predominantly plant-based diet to monitor.

Vitamin B12 This vitamin is required daily because it is not made by the body. Animal foods and fortified plant foods are the only source in the diet. When lowering animal protein, encourage patients to use vitamin B12-fortified foods such as tofu with calcium additive and vitamin B12 fortified cereals, meat alternatives, and soy milk.

The National Institute for Health (NIH) has an excellent Vitamin B12 Fact Sheet for professionals [21]. The table they list is as follows:

Recommended Dietary Allowances (RDAs) for vit**amin B12**

Age	Male (μg)	Female pregnancy lactation
0–6 months[a]	0.4	0.4
7–12 months[a]	0.5	0.5
1–3 years	0.9	0.9
4–8 years	1.2	1.2
9–13 years	1.8	1.8
14+ years	2.4	2.4 2.6 2.8

[a]Adequate Intake

According to the National Academy of Sciences, Engineering and Medicine, Health and Medicine Division, The Dietary Reference Intakes (DRIs) are nutrient reference values developed by the Institute of Medicine of The National Academies. They are intended to serve as a guide for good nutrition and to provide the scientific basis for the development of food guidelines in both the United States and Canada. These nutrient reference values are specified on the basis of age, gender, and life stage and cover more than 40 nutrient substances [21].

Calcium Calcium is found in dark green leafy vegetables, tofu made with calcium sulfate, calcium-fortified soy milk, and orange juice. Daily recommended intake of calcium is 1000 milligrams (mg) a day for women and men of ages 19–50 and 1200 mg for women over 50. For men of ages 51–70, 1000 mg, men over age 71, 1200 mg. Food is always recommended over supplements because it is better absorbed and utilized. While fat-free and low-fat cow's milk and yogurt have been emphasized as good sources of calcium, a well-planned, plant-based meal provides sufficient calcium. One serving of tofu or soy milk provides about one-third of the daily needs for an adult. A 3.5 oz serving of almonds provides about 295 mg, almost one-third compared to 85 mg in one cup of collard greens.

Choline The liver produces choline but it is not enough. Adding foods rich in choline such as tofu, quinoa, broccoli, brussels sprouts, beans, peas, edamame, soymilk, peanut butter, and pistachio nuts will allow for adequate intake. Animal food sources such as eggs, meat, fish, and poultry are rich in choline as well. The National Institute for Health (NIH) offers a Fact Sheet and summarizes the recommendations and food sources below. This fact sheet is available for healthcare professionals at https://ods.od.nih.gov/factsheets/Choline-HealthProfessional/#h2. It also cites 'Choline deficiency can cause muscle damage, liver damage, and nonalcoholic fatty liver disease (NAFLD or hepatosteatosis) [29] (Table 42.1).

Although many people consume less than the recommendations, deficiency is rare since the body produces some endogenously [29]. Choline intake in pregnancy and for children in the first years of life is important for cognitive brain development [30, 31].

Iron Iron is an essential nutrient for red blood cells, DNA synthesis, and our immune system.

There are two types of iron: heme and nonheme iron. Much of the iron in meat is heme iron, which is more easily absorbed from food and used by your body. Plant foods contain only nonheme iron.

Table 42.1 Adequate intakes (AIs) for choline

Age	Male (mg/day)	Female (mg/day)	Pregnancy (mg/day)	Lactation (mg/day)
Birth to 6 months	125	125		
7–12 months	150	150		
1–3 years	200	200		
4–8 years	250	250		
9–13 years	375	375		
14–18 years	550	400	450	550
19+ years	550	425	450	550

Several food sources of choline are listed in Table 42.2

Table 42.2 Selected food sources of choline [11, 39]

Food	Milligrams (mg) per serving	Percent DV*
Calves liver, pan fried, 3 oz	356	65
Egg, hard boiled, 1 large egg	147	27
Beef top round, separable lean only, braised, 3 oz	117	21
Soybeans, roasted, ½ cup	107	19
Chicken breast, roasted, 3 oz	72	13
Beef, ground, 93% lean meat, broiled, 3 oz	72	13
Fish, cod, Atlantic, cooked, dry heat, 3 oz	71	13
Mushrooms, shiitake, cooked, ½ cup pieces	58	11
Potatoes, red, baked, flesh and skin, 1 large potato	57	10
Wheat germ, toasted, 1 ounce	51	9
Beans, kidney, canned, ½ cup	45	8
Quinoa, cooked, 1 cup	43	8
Milk, 1% fat, 1 cup	43	8
Yogurt, vanilla, nonfat, 1 cup	38	7
Brussels sprouts, boiled, ½ cup	32	6
Broccoli, chopped, boiled, drained, ½ cup	31	6

*Daily Value

Some plant-based foods are good sources of iron, such as beans and chickpeas and black-eyed peas. A compound called phytate can reduce iron absorption and is present in whole grains and dried beans. Compounds in coffee and tea also reduce iron absorption. Other plant-based foods that are rich in iron are enriched cereals, spinach, molasses, and nuts. Recommend vitamin C-rich foods with these foods and avoid calcium supplements at meals which could interfere with absorption. The recommended daily intake of iron is 18 mg for menstruating women, 8 mg for postmenopausal women and men and 27 mg for pregnant women. Considering one cup of raw soybeans contains 29 mg, it is not hard to achieve a well-planned diet without animal protein. In athletes, special consideration is needed to assure additional needs which can be 30–70 percent higher than the recommended intake.

For further summary on nutrition considerations recommending plant-based diets, refer to the Academy of Nutrition and Dietetics Position on Vegetarian Diets [9].

Dining Out, Travel, and Holiday Menu Suggestions

Whether a patient is preparing a family holiday meal, going out to eat or traveling, there are basic suggestions to remember.

- Choose foods that are prepared without frying.
- Be sure to emphasize no butter, oil, or gravy!
- Keeping in mind that BAKED, BROILED, GRILLED, AND STEAMED cooking method to LOWER FAT.
- Choosing recipes that fit and using seasonings recommended for GERD and LPR.

Emphasize Boosting Flavor with Spices and Herbs Using spices and herbs are recommended with the exception of onions, pepper, and mint which may cause GERD and LPR symptoms. Little research has been done on the health effects of herbs and spices specifically as it relates to GERD and LPR but the phytonutrients in herbs and spices have medicinal benefits as mentioned earlier. A spice comes from a part other than the leaf, usually the seed, root, and bark. Herbs come from the leafy green part of the plant. Allium is found in garlic, chive, onion, and leeks; some people with GERD may be sensitive to the allium flavors if used in higher amounts. The health benefits of specific phytonutrients in herbs are well known [25]. Christine M. Kaefer and John A. Milner cite, "Spices may be a key to determining the balance between pro- and anticancer factors that regulate risk and tumor behavior" [25]. Future investigation needs to identify the processes in consuming herbs and spices affect DNA repair, carcinogen metabolism, hormonal regulation, cell cycle, inflammatory responses, and apoptosis in health.

Multiple cancer-related processes may account for the ability of spices to inhibit experimentally induced cancers. While these processes are likely critical for determining the risk of cancer and tumor behavior in humans, only limited clinical evidence exists that spices in physiological relevant exposures can alter one or more of these processes. The type of microbiome in the gut driven by the foods consumed and specific pathways on how it impacts chronic diseases is emerging.

Research continues to reveal more and more benefits of phytochemicals in herbs and spices. Encourage multicultural restaurants that offer plant-based eating options and cuisines that utilize a wide variety of spices and herbs. Greater flavor is achieved on a plant-based diet when cooking techniques utilize these phytonutrient-rich additives – soups with lentils or beans, salads without cheese, and small plate servings or sharing. Many restaurant's serving sizes are double of what is needed, and ordering for the meal with two or three side dishes such as rice, beans, and salad is often enough.

Holidays Every culture has selective food traditions that need to be considered. There are many cookbooks and online sites that offer plant-based options to traditional recipes or at least lowering the sugar salt and fat in the recipes or total animal protein. An example is switching a traditional chopped liver recipe to a vegan recipe made from mushrooms. Each culture has recipes that may be high in sugar, fat, and sodium but there are many ways to alter recipes to make them healthier alternatives.

Choosing Restaurants There are a growing number of plant-based alternatives being offered in fast food chains and for take-out. When eating in a restaurant, seek places that offer healthier plant-based alternatives. An international resource is called Happy Cow. Visit the website, https://www.happycow.net/, when seeking a restaurant that offers greater selection of vegan or vegetarian menus options. When preparing meals with animal protein, choose half the amount usually used and add more side dishes using whole grains, legumes, and fresh vegetables.

Examples:

- An Italian *restaurant* maybe choosing an animal protein as an appetizer such as tomatoes and mozzarella cheese, and pasta with beans or vegetables and the main course.
- **Japanese Restaurant**: Miso soup with ramen noodles with shiitake mushrooms, edamame.
- **Mexican Restaurant:** Vegetable Fajitas with a side dish of rice and beans limit the nachos and salsa.

In summary, the meal planning goals should be as follows:

1. Increase plant-based food to 90–95%
2. Limit animal to 2–3 meals per week
3. Limit the serving size of the animal protein to 3–4 oz and use the 3–4 finger rule
4. Drink Alkaline Water as the beverage of choice [32]

Helping patients transition to eating a 95% Mediterranean plant-based diet is a process that needs guidance for long-term adherence. A suggestion is to first select none animal protein for one meal a day such as breakfasts, after doing that for a week or two, reduce the animal protein to one meal a day for a week, then add a meatless Monday and gradually by the fourth week consume all meatless meals except two to three meals a week. Refer to the My Plate in the appendix and encourage a fist portion of a grain or starchy vegetable along with two thirds of the plate with vegetables. When selecting animal protein, remind patients to choose lean animal protein such as chicken or turkey breast, London broil, fish from less contaminated waters. It is recommended to check local fish consumption advisory for guidance on environmental protection agency websites for the region the fish comes from. Our waters are becoming more contaminated and fish from many regions have high levels of mercury and other contaminants [26–28]. The highest in mercury is Swordfish, Shark, Gulf of Mexico Tile fish, and big eye tuna [28]. A simple formula in guiding patients in meal planning is to suggest a meal that includes grain + beans or other legumes = complete protein and color from a variety of vegetables and fruits. Below is a list of menu suggestions:

- Black beans and rice
- Whole wheat pita with hummus and veggies
- Soy milk and oatmeal and walnuts and raisins
- Whole grain pasta with cannellini beans and escarole
- Minestrone soup with salad and stuffed mushrooms
- Tofu with bok choy, water chestnuts, carrots, broccoli and brown rice

- Quinoa, chickpea and vegetable salad with fresh parsley
- Lentil soup with thyme and carrots. Crusty brown bread with avocado
- Stuffed baked potato with cilantro, beans and mild salsa
- Moroccan chili: sweet potato with cinnamon, apples, quinoa and black bean
- Wild salmon with dill, quinoa and asparagus
- Mushroom barley soup with three bean salad and vegetable wrap with fresh parsley
- Poke bowl: greens, rice, pineapple, fish or edamame (soy beans) with fresh ginger

At Home Easy Meals Could Be

- Corn and lima beans succotash and an impossible burger or beyond meat, sliced tomato and basil
- Tempeh or beefless ground bolognese over pasta with chopped tomato and pesto
- Black bean pasta and mixed vegetables with asian peanut sauce
- Pasta with basil beans, spinach, and a few diced tomatoes
- Turmeric flavored tofu scramble, oven home fries, melon, kale chips
- Veggie burger on a whole grain bun, corn, watermelon
- Just egg scramble with mushrooms and spinach and avocado on whole grain toast
- Thai soup: made with lemon grass, light coconut milk, tofu and asian vegetables

Consumer handouts and resources listed in the Academy of Nutrition and Dietetics Vegetarian Nutrition Position Paper [19] include the Following:

- www.vegetariannutrition.net VNDPG's consumer website provides a blog with evidence-based vegetarian nutrition plus RDN resources for consumers.
- www.vrg.org The Vegetarian Resource Group provides nutrition information, recipes, meal plans, and recommended readings for vegetarian nutrition.
- www.PCRM.org The Physicians Committee for Responsible Medicine promotes preventive medicine through innovative programs and offers free patient educational materials.
- www.veganhealth.org This website offers evidence-based recommendations covering the nutritional features of plant-based diets.
- www.nutritionfacts.org This website provides brief, referenced video clips and articles on numerous aspects of vegetarian nutrition.
- www.vegweb.com VegWeb offers vegetarian recipes, community, and a blog.
- The websites above offer a wide array of patient resources and are continually updated with current information.

In conclusion, a well-balanced meal should include foods rich in plant protein, grains rich in fiber and fruits and vegetables rich in colors to gain the phytonutrient benefits. Seasoning plant-based foods with herbs and spices will add diversity not only in cultural cuisine but also in nutrients.

The Plant Based Plate can be used as a guide to help patients make new choices Omit from this section.

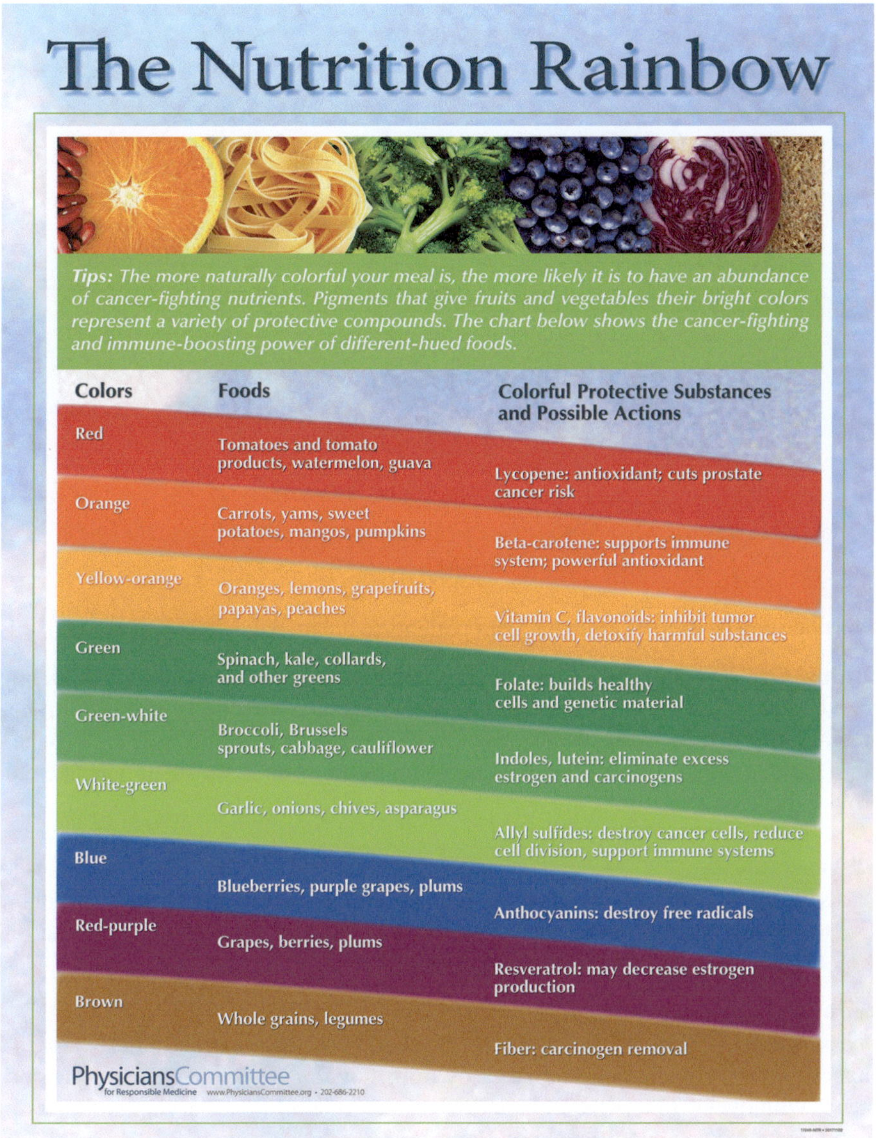

Permission obtained from Physicians Committee for Responsible Medicine

Healthy Plant-Based Plate

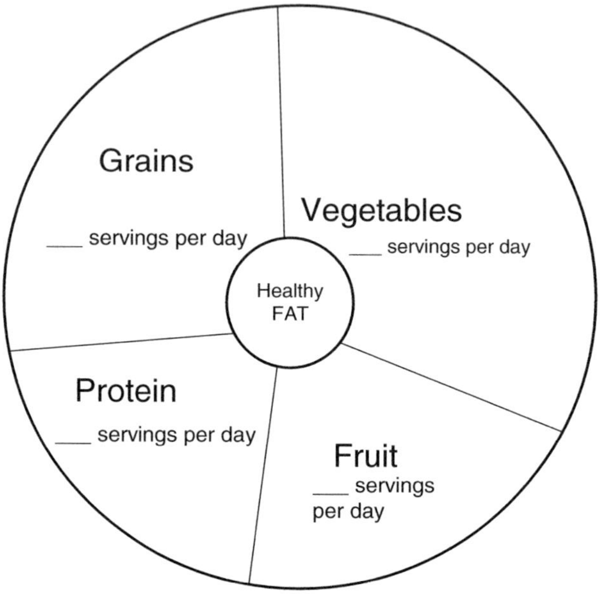

This plate can be used as guide by your patients to create balanced plant based meals.

Grains One serving = 3+ g fiber1 c. cold cereal such as organic Nature's Path, bran cereal, shredded wheat, ½ c. hot unsweetened cereal-steel cup or old fashion oatmeal, ½ cup beans, lentils, rice; millet, bulgur, organic corn or corn meal, whole grain pasta, 1 ounce whole grain breads, 3 inch home cooked waffle or pancake (add ground flaxseed)

All Vegetables
One serving = 1 cup raw vegetable such as lettuce, radish, cucumber, sprouts or tomato, ½ cup cooked green beans, cauliflower, broccoli, mushroom, carrots, bok choy, onion, peas, beets, squash or cabbage

Eat more plant protein:
One serving= 1/3 cup bean lentils, black eyed peas, green peas; wheat berries 2 ounces tofu or tempeh 1 cup organic soy milk, soy yogurt, avoid plant yogurts and cheese with over 4 grams fat and under 7 grams protein in one serving and/or using coconut cream such as Follow Your Heart brand

All Fruits
One serving= banana: 3 in; tennis ball size: pear, apple, peach, plum orange; ½ cup pineapple, 1 cup melon, or mixed fruit; 15 grapes or cherries, 2 figs, ¼ cup dried fruit, ½ grapefruit

Choose less than 5% or no animal protein
Better bets: Fat free or 1% cow's milk or yogurt or cheese, white meat chicken or turkey, fish, 90 % lean cuts of lamb, beef, or pork.

Eliminate high sodium and or high nitrate cold cut, hot dogs, and bacon.

Skip the high fat cheese, chicken wings, ribs, and fried foods.

Fat: One serving = 75–100 calories 1/4 avocado, or 2 tablespoons seeds, 10–15 nuts, 1 tablespoon olive oil or canola oil, nut butters (peanut, almond, sunflower seed, soy) without hydrogenated oil, sugar, or palm oil and 1/4 c. shredded coconut.

Less heart beneficial fat sources: Cream, ghee, butter, lard, chicken fat, palm oil, hydrogenated fats

Beverages: Water, especially Alkaline water [32] is best, unsweetened tea, vegetable juice, soy milk, fat free milk

Cooking Methods: Limit frying any food. Best bets: *Steaming, baking, poaching, broiling, stir-frying, or sautéing* (in water or non-fat, low sodium broth). Grilling foods from animals causes known carcinogens to form; grilled chicken is one of the highest according to the Cancer Project. http://www.pcrm.org/health/reports/the-five-worst-foods-to-grill.

The typical American diet: Is high in saturated fats. Sources of these unhealthy and heart-hurtful fats come from animal products such as cheese, whole milk, meats, and ice cream. By swapping out, these choices are more healthful ones you will strengthen your heart and cut down on calories.

How to create great habits:

1. Incorporate plant-based proteins into your diet. These foods will help eliminate much of your saturated from your diet, as they are lower in calories and higher in nutrients.
2. Choose low fat or non-fat options when you can, which will be lower in calories and lower in fat.
3. Downsize your portions, when eating out most entrees that are served to you are 1000+ calories and contain multiple portions. Set some aside at the start of the meal to not overindulge or order some sides of vegetables and grains as your meal such as rice and beans.
4. Don't drink your calories, choose lower calorie options like water. Stay away from drinks with added sugar.
5. Eat mindfully, set time aside to be able to enjoy food's quality over quantity and avoid eating on the run or multi-tasking.

Try something new: We often get stuck in ruts and form habits that can be unhealthy. Take a step back to analyze why you do something a certain way. Can you make a change or improvement? Don't be afraid to start you journey on the road to a healthier life. If you even try one new food and recipe a week, it helps you on your journey.

Choose restaurants that help you eat healthy. Visit the restaurant's website and look at the menu. Below are some tips:

Appetizers: Choose raw vegetables such as salad *without* rich toppings such as bacon bits, cheese, and croutons. *Skip the tomatoes, hot peppers, and salsa*

Choose clear broth soups such as vegetable, bean, lentil, or minestrone, **not** cream soups rich in fat.

Entrees:

Breakfast: Choose old fashion oatmeal, fresh fruit, unsweetened cereal (organic corn, rice bran, millet or quinoa as alternative to always eating wheat types), pancakes with fruit (blueberry pancake) or waffles with fruit **NOT** cream or chocolate. Skip the fried eggs, bacon and cheese sandwiches, or bagels with high fat cream cheese! Fruit should be eaten whole not in a smoothie.

Lunches and Dinners: *Choose baked, broiled, grilled or steamed foods*. Avoid fried food with sauces in cream, butter or gravy. Hold the CHEESE!

- *Choose salads* with vegetable toppings such as cucumber, beans, nuts, or avocado with vinaigrette dressing **NOT** cheese, bacon, salami or ham, tuna or egg salads, potato salad or creamy dressings.
- *Choose sandwiches* with peanut butter or grilled vegetables in a wrap, humus and veggie burgers or Impossible burger. Use whole grain breads, **NOT** the rolls and heroes or wedges. *Skip the fried foods! Foods such as lean roast turkey or chicken breast in deli's or restaurants are much higher in portions than recommended.*

Asian

Choose sushi rolls with cooked fish or vegetables NOT fried fish or tempura. Try a vegan option with vegetables and avocado and brown rice.

Choose steamed *vegetable and tofu or chicken stir fry with brown rice* – ask for sauce on side. Vegetables in a rice spring roll or miso soup is good. Skip the fat-rich appetizers such as fried egg rolls, entrees drowning in oil or with fried foods or noodles, ice cream for dessert.

Italian

Limit pasta or pizza. Choose thin crust type, add vegetables, not loads of cheese and high-fat meats such as pepperoni, fried chicken, or sausage. Broiled fish or pasta with beans is nice with broccoli rabe or escarole. Try escarole, minestrone, bean, or lentil soups.

Mexican

Bean burrito or rice and beans (no cheese or meat) with vegetables, tacos with beans and vegetables.

Vegetable Fajitas with a side dish of guacamole and beans.

Indian

Dishes with *lentils, mung beans, or chickpeas* are great! Limit the creamy curries, dishes rich in coconut cream or ghee. Skip the fried options including the bread. Plain naan is fine.

In all restaurants, a good habit is saying no to the breadbasket with butter and caffeinated and alcoholic beverages! Drink water as your beverage!

Fruits and Vegetables: Organic, GMO Free Suggested

- All fresh, frozen or jarred (skip the canned if it does not say BPA FREE) Citrus, garlic, onion and tomato use in small amounts if tolerated. Omit if sensitive.
- Dried fruit in small amounts.
- Vegetable juices (100% juice varieties): Carrot, juice containing tomato may not be tolerated.
- Choose a variety of fruits and vegetables to maximize your vitamin and mineral intake.
- Limit fruit and vegetable or juices that have added sugar or salt, choose "100%," not "drinks."

- Limit 100% fruit juice to 6 oz and day and use whole fresh fruit most often.

Herbs and Spices

- *All herbs and spices are recommended except limit spicy Cajun seasonings or pepper. Try Mrs. Dash or Trader Joes*
- Example of using herbs: Kale, Cashew, and Basil Pesto
- Mediterranean herbs: Bay leaves, Basil, Oregano, Thyme, Parsley

Grain Products: Organic, GMO Free, 3+ Grams Fiber, Less Than 4 Grams Sugar

- Hot and cold cereals (Look for 3+ g fiber, less than 4 g sugar, whole-grain, and cereals)
- Cereals and snacks made from beans. Keep sugar under 5 g and salt under 200 mg if possible
- Whole wheat, whole grain breads, tortillas, pita, crackers, and other bread products (Choose less processed types with at least 3 g of fiber and unbleached flour)
- Rice (red, brown or wild are good choices)
- Pasta (whole grain, bean, lentil, pea, and yolk-free varieties)
- Flour (whole grain, soy, corn, spelt)
- Great grains: Amaranth, barley: black or pearl, bran, bulgur, faro, millet, quinoa: red or white; spelt, wheat berries, and whole-grain wheat germ
- Polenta
- Newer cereals made with beans and lentils

Protein Selections

- Peas, beans, lentils, and other legumes (fresh, dried, boxed, canned if BPA free or frozen).
- All nuts and seeds (*limit if sensitive or trying to lose weight*).
- All nut or seed butters: almond, peanut, soy, sunflower, and sesame (tahini) (limit if sensitive *or trying to lose weight*).
- Roasted seeds (sesame, pumpkin, or sunflower), ground flax seed, chia seed, hemp *(limit if sensitive or trying to lose weight).*
- Organic soy products: tofu: extra firm, firm, silken; tempeh; soy milk.
- Just Egg Scramble (made from mung beans), eggs, egg whites, and egg substitutes.
- Beyond Meat, Impossible Burger, Gardien Beefless ground, Morning Star Veggie Burger. Trader Joes Veggie burgers, Soy Chorizo.
- Limit more processed meat analogues over 350 mg of sodium such as some soy burgers, soy chickenless or fishless patties, soy hot dogs, soy sausage, and soy cold cuts.
- Limit lean meats, poultry and eggs to 2–3 meals a week.

Plant-Based Combination/Main Entrée Foods

- Boxed or canned prepared vegetarian bean, lentil, or vegetable soups
- Pasta salad or Primavera
- Vegetable Wontons
- Tofu/ Vegetable Spring Roll
- Frozen vegetarian burritos, burgers, and spring rolls
- Boxed vegetarian entrees such as a bente box with mushrooms and brown rice

- Frozen Indian Paneer
- Salads with vegetables, grains such as rice, quinoa, or lentils

Dairy and Plant Alternates
- Organic milk (check the food label use zero or 1% fat).
- Organic almond, soy or rice milk (check the label; use only types that have *8 g of protein,* fortified with 20%+ calcium and vitamin D).
- Cheese (dairy or alternative, reduced fat- part skim or 1%). Limit animal cheeses and choose low fat types: one serving under 8 g of fat. Most vegan cheese is made with coconut cream and is high in saturated fat but still better than full fat whole milk cheese.
- 1% fat or fat-free yogurt (dairy) or soy or unsweetened coconut yogurt is high in fat, so limit intake if it is made with coconut cream.
- Frozen desserts: Limit flavors with nuts. Good options are vanilla, lemon, and berry. Read label for reduced fat ice cream or frozen yogurt or tofutti or Trader Joe's Soy Frozen Dessert or fruit ice or sorbet. One serving should be under 130 calories.
- Bencol, Smart Balance or Earth Balance Margarine Spreads.

Oil
- Olive, canola, sesame seed, flaxseed, walnut, avocado oils.

Sandwich Spreads
- Hellmann's Vegan Dressing and Sandwich Spread (48 calories/ tablespoon)
- Veganaise (80 calories/ tablespoon)

Vegan Jams and Spreads
- MacCay's Preserves
- Smucker's Jelly and Jams
- Crofters Organic Just Fruit Spread

Beverages
- Alkaline water [32]
- Caffeine-free herbal tea
- Water

Conclusions

Choosing a 95 percent plant-based Mediterranean diet to aid in the treatment of GERD and LPR using alkaline water will reduce the need for proton pump inhibitors. The following summarizes management:

- Eliminate trigger foods.
- Encourage plant protein instead of animal protein.
- Maintain a healthy body mass index and weight.
- Eat small meals and snacks every 3–4 hours.
- When eating, sit upright and remain upright 40–60 minutes after eating [34].

- Avoid eating at least 3 hours before bed time [34].
- Eliminate high fat foods such as cheese, fried foods, and excess oil or butter.

Maintaining a healthy lifestyle and the above recommendations has proven successful outcomes.

References

1. Sethi S, Richter JE. Diet and gastroesophageal reflux disease: role in pathogenesis and management. Curr Opin Gastroenterol. 2017;33(2):107–11. https://doi.org/10.1097/MOG.0000000000000337.
2. Kim JS, Kim BW. Are diet and micronutrients effective in treating gastroesophageal reflux disease especially in women? J Neurogastroenterol Motil. 2019;25(1):1–2. https://doi.org/10.5056/jnm18198.
3. Kubo A, Block G, Quesenberry CP Jr, Buffler P, Corley DA. Dietary guideline adherence for gastroesophageal reflux disease. BMC Gastroenterol. 2014;14:144. https://doi.org/10.1186/1471-230X-14-144.
4. Newberry C, Lynch K. Can we use diet to effectively treat esophageal disease? A review of the current literature. Curr Gastroenterol Rep. 2017;19(8):38. https://doi.org/10.1007/s11894-017-0578-5.
5. Mulholland HG, Cantwell MM, Anderson LA, Johnston BT, Watson RG, Murphy SJ, Ferguson HR, McGuigan J, Reynolds JV, Comber H, Murray LJ. Glycemic index, carbohydrate and fiber intakes and risk of reflux esophagitis, Barrett's esophagus, and esophageal adenocarcinoma. Cancer Causes Control. 2009;20(3):279–88. https://doi.org/10.1007/s10552-008-9242-6. Epub 2008 Oct 7.
6. Mone B, Kraja A, Bregu V, Duraj E, Sadiku J, Hyska G, Burazeri. Adherence to a predominantly Mediterranean diet decreases the risk of gastroesophageal reflux disease: a cross-sectional study in a South Eastern European population. Dis Esophagus. 2016;29(7):794–800. https://doi.org/10.1111/dote.12384.
7. Olson NR. Laryngopharyngeal manifestations of gastroesophageal reflux disease. Otolaryngol Clin N Am. 1991;24(5):1201–13.
8. Biesemeier, C. Editor in chief. Academy of nutrition and dietetics nutrition care manual. Copyright 2018, Academy of Nutrition and Dietetics.
9. Melina V, Craig W, Levin S. Position of the academy of nutrition and dietetics on vegetarian diets. J Nutr Diet. 2016;116(12):1970–80.
10. Zhu F, Du B, Xu B. Anti-inflammatory effects of phytochemicals from fruits, vegetables, and food legumes: a review. Crit Rev Food Sci Nutr. 2018;58(8):1260–127. Accessed 10 Oct 2019.
11. Liu RH. Dietary bioactive compounds and their health implications. J Food Sci. 2013;78(Suppl 1):A18–25. Accessed 10 Oct 2019.
12. Liu RH. Health-promoting components of fruits and vegetables in the diet. Adv Nutr. 2013;4(3):384S–92S. Accessed 10 Oct 2019.
13. Bodai BI, Nakata TE, Wong WT, Clark DR, Lawenda S, Tsou C, Liu R, Shiue L, Cooper N, Rehbein M, Ha BP, Mckeirnan A, Misquitta R, Vij P, Klonecke A, Mejia CS, Dionysian E, Hashmi S, Greger M, Stoll S, Campbell TM. Perm J. Lifestyle medicine: a brief review of its dramatic impact on health and survival. 2018;22:17–025 Accessed 10 Oct 2019.
14. Dağlı Ü, Kalkan İH. The role of lifestyle changes in gastroesophageal reflux diseases treatment. Turk J Gastroenterol. 2017;28(Suppl 1):S33–7. Accessed 1 Oct 2019.
15. Dore MP, Maragkoudakis E, Fraley K, Pedroni A, Tadeu V, Realdi G, Graham DY, Delitala G, Malaty HM. Diet, lifestyle and gender in gastro-esophageal reflux disease. Dig Dis Sci. 2008;53(8):2027–32. Accessed 1 Oct 2019.
16. 2015–2020 Dietary Guidelines. https://health.gov/dietaryguidelines/2015/. Accessed 14 Oct 2019.
17. Amino Acids Guide. https://aminoacidsguide.com/. 2007–2019. Accessed 14 Oct 2019.

18. Medical News Today. https://www.medicalnewstoday.com/articles/320050.php. Accessed 14 Oct 2019.
19. Wikopedia. https://en.wikipedia.org/wiki/. Accessed 16 Oct 2019.
20. American Cancer Society. Soy and cancer risk: our expert's advice. April 29, 2019. https://www.cancer.org/latest-news/soy-and-cancer-risk-our-experts-advice.html. Accessed 16 Oct 2019.
21. US Department of Agriculture, Agricultural Research Service, Nutrient Data Laboratory. USDA national nutrient database for standard reference, legacy. Version current: April 2018. Internet: https://www.ars.usda.gov/northeast-area/beltsville-md-bhnrc/beltsville-human-nutrition-research-center/nutrient-data-laboratory/docs/usda-national-nutrient-database-for-standard-reference/. Accessed 19 Oct 2019.
22. Institute of Medicine. Food and Nutrition Board. Dietary reference intakes: thiamin, riboflavin, niacin, vitamin B6, folate, vitamin B12, pantothenic acid, biotin, and choline. Washington, D.C.: National Academy Press, 1998. https://www.ncbi.nlm.nih.gov/books/NBK114310/. Accessed 17 Oct 2019.
23. Institute for Functional Medicine. Phytonutrient spectrum comprehensive guide. 2014 The Institute for Functional Medicine. Accessed 17 Oct 2019.
24. http://www.thehealthedgepodcast.com/wp-content/uploads/2015/07/Phytonutrient-Spectrum-Comprehensive-Guide.pdf
25. Tapsell LC, Hemphill I, et al. Health benefits of herbs and spices: the past, the present, the future. Med J Aust. 2006;185(4 Suppl):S4–24. https://doi.org/10.5694/j.1326-5377.2006.tb00548.x.
26. Benzie IF, Wachtel-Galor S, editors. Herbal medicine: biomolecular and clinical aspects. 2nd ed. Boca Raton: CRC Press/Taylor & Francis; 2011.
27. Ahmed FE. Seafood Safety. In: Institute of Medicine (US), editor. Committee on evaluation of the safety of fishery products. Washington, D.C.: National Academies Press (US); 1991.
28. US Food and Drug Administration. Advice about eating fish. Updated 2 of July 2019. https://www.fda.gov/food/consumers/advice-about-eating-fish. Accessed 17 Oct 2019.
29. Zeisel SH, Corbin KD. Choline. In: Erdman JW, Macdonald IA, Zeisel SH, editors. Present knowledge in nutrition. 10th ed. Washington, D.C.: Wiley-Blackwell; 2012. p. 405–18. Accessed 17 Oct 2019.
30. Sanders LM, Zeisel SH. Choline: dietary requirements and role in brain development. Nutr Today. 2007;42:181–6, [PubMed abstract] Accessed 17 October 2019.
31. Mills JL, Fan R, Brody LC, Liu A, Ueland PM, Wang Y, et al. Maternal choline concentrations during pregnancy and choline-related genetic variants as risk factors for neural tube defects. Am J Clin Nutr. 2014;100:1069–74. [PubMed abstract] Accessed 17 of October 2019.
32. Zalvan CH, Hu C, Greenberg B, Geliebter J. A comparison of alkaline water and mediterranean diet vs proton pump inhibition for treatment of laryngopharyngeal reflux. JAMA Otolaryngol Head Neck Surg. 2017;143(10):1023–9. https://doi.org/10.1001/jamaoto.2017.1454. Published online September 7, 2017.
33. International Foundation for Functional Gastrointestinal Disorders. Diet & lifestyle changes. https://www.iffgd.org/. Accessed 18 Oct 2019.
34. Cleaveland Clinic. https://my.clevelandclinic.org/health/diseases/17019-gerd-or-acid-reflux-or-heartburn-overview/prevention. Accessed 6/8/2020.
35. Center for Disease Control. 2018 state indicator report on fruits and vegetables. https://www.cdc.gov/nutrition/downloads/fruits-vegetables/2018/2018-fruit-vegetable-report-508.pdf. Accessed 19 Nov 2019.
36. Harvard School of Public Health. Healthy Eating Plate Vs USDA Plate. https://www.hsph.harvard.edu/nutritionsource/healthy-eating-plate-vs-usda-myplate/. Accessed 4 Nov 2019.
37. Michael Greger, Gene Stone. How not to die: discover the foods scientifically proven to prevent and reverse disease. New York: Flatiron Books; 2015.
38. Murugkar DA. Effect of sprouting of soybean on the chemical composition and quality of soymilk and tofu. J Food Sci Technol. 2014;51(5):915–21. https://doi.org/10.1007/s13197-011-0576-9. Epub 2011 Nov 3.
39. U.S. Department of Agriculture, Agricultural Research Service. Food Data Central, 2019. fdc.nal.usda.gov. Accessed 11 Nov 2019.
40. American Heart Association. Healthy Living. https://www.heart.org/en/healthy-living/healthy-eating/eat-smart/sodium/how-much-sodium-should-i-eat-per-day. Accessed 12 Nov 2019.

Index

C. H. Zalvan (ed.), *Laryngopharyngeal and Gastroesophageal Reflux*,
https://doi.org/10.1007/978-3-030-48890-1

T

Z

MIX
Papier aus verantwortungsvollen Quellen
Paper from responsible sources
FSC® C105338

If you have any concerns about our products,
you can contact us on
ProductSafety@springernature.com

In case Publisher is established outside the EU,
the EU authorized representative is:
Springer Nature Customer Service Center GmbH
Europaplatz 3, 69115 Heidelberg, Germany

Printed by Libri Plureos GmbH
in Hamburg, Germany